INTEGRATIVE
NUTRITION THERAPY

INTEGRATIVE
NUTRITION THERAPY

EDITED BY

MARY J. MARIAN, DCN, RDN, CSO, FAND
UNIVERSITY OF ARIZONA
TUCSON, USA

GERARD E. MULLIN, MD
DIVISION OF GASTROENTEROLOGY AND HEPATOLOGY
ASSOCIATE PROFESSOR OF MEDICINE
THE JOHNS HOPKINS UNIVERSITY SCHOOL OF MEDICINE
BALTIMORE, MARYLAND, USA

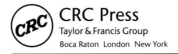

CRC Press
Taylor & Francis Group
Boca Raton London New York

CRC Press is an imprint of the
Taylor & Francis Group, an **informa** business

CRC Press
Taylor & Francis Group
6000 Broken Sound Parkway NW, Suite 300
Boca Raton, FL 33487-2742

© 2016 by Taylor & Francis Group, LLC
CRC Press is an imprint of Taylor & Francis Group, an Informa business

No claim to original U.S. Government works

Printed on acid-free paper
Version Date: 20150223

International Standard Book Number-13: 978-1-4665-9613-9 (Hardback)

Library of Congress Cataloging-in-Publication Data

Integrative nutrition therapy / edited by Mary J. Marian and Gerard Mullin.
    p. ; cm.
    Includes bibliographical references and index.
    ISBN 978-1-4665-9613-9 (hardcover : alk. paper)
    I. Marian, Mary, 1956- , editor. II. Mullin, Gerard E., editor.
    [DNLM: 1. Nutrition Therapy--methods. 2. Digestive System Diseases--diet therapy.
3. Integrative Medicine. 4. Neoplasms--diet therapy. WB 400]

    RM217.2
    615.8'54--dc23   2015007177

Visit the Taylor & Francis Web site at
http://www.taylorandfrancis.com

and the CRC Press Web site at
http://www.crcpress.com

To our families and loved ones for their unwavering support, to the pioneers of integrative medicine, to the clinicians who practice "The New Medicine," to the researchers who provide us evidence and confirmation, to the organizations and philanthropists who promote integrative medicine awareness and support research, and to our mentors, colleagues, administrators, and staff who support our careers.

Contents

Preface

Integrative medicine is a whole systems approach to wellness that embodies all healing modalities and emphasizes natural and traditional approaches and favors noninvasive low-risk interventions. The movement of integrative medicine dates back several decades to a more evolutionary process whose growth was organic and a number of pioneers who collectively increased public awareness and ultimately popularity. Due to consumer demand of integrative medicine, congressional legislation established the Office of Alternative Medicine in October 1991 and appropriated $2M for its inception under the auspices of the National Institutes of Health (NIH).* The goal was to fund research studies to confirm the validity of integrative medicine healing modalities. Despite economic fluxes, there has been a steady growth in funding for this office whose name was changed in 2000 as the National Center for Complementary and Alternative Medicine (NCCAM), which was refined as the federal government's lead agency for scientific research on the diverse medical and health-care systems, practices, and products that are not generally considered part of conventional medicine. Ultimately, the goal of the 65 FTE-staffed agency is to advance the science and practice of complementary and alternative medicine and promote evidence-based personalized strategies while enabling practitioner's data to incorporate evidence-based strategies to promote wellness and health care.† NCCAM and philanthropic funding of research encouraged research and rapid growth of integrative medicine with ample evidence supporting its benefits. In 1994, Dr. Andrew Weil, philanthropists, and colleagues formed the nation's first university-based training program in integrative medicine at the University of Arizona. In 2001, a conversation began the formation of The Bravewell Collaborative, a community of philanthropists that are devoted to the growth of integrative medicine and partnered with leading academic physicians to transform health care into a more humanistic integrative model.‡ The Bravewell Collaborative then brought together over 50 major academic centers in the United States to form the Consortium of Academic Health Centers for Integrative Medicine. In 2014, The American Board of Integrative Medicine came together under the American Board of Physician Specialties to provide the public a means to recognize physicians who are qualified in the practice of integrative medicine.

There have been many studies regarding the use of integrative medicine in health care. The most transformative study was published by Dr. David Eisenberg of the Harvard School of Public Health, which showed that complementary and alternative modalities are used by approximately one-third of the U.S. population (Eisenberg et al. 1993). According to the most recent National Health Survey data, complementary and alternative medicine (CAM) is being used by

---

* http://nccam.nih.gov/about/budget/appropriations.htm.
† http://nccam.nih.gov/about/ataglance.
‡ http://www.bravewell.org/bravewell_collaborative/.

almost 40% of adults and 12% of children in the United States (Barnes et al. 2008). Interestingly, those with chronic diseases utilize CAM the most and often report greater satisfaction than with conventional therapies alone (Jonas et al. 2013). Among the CAM modalities, nutrition-based therapies (i.e., special diets and dietary supplements) are consistently among the highest utilized across the board by consumers and patients with a wide variety of illnesses. This area of integrative medicine is among the most controversial as dietary supplements are largely unrelated under the Dietary Supplement Health and Education Act (DSHEA)* and dietary therapeutic trails are tedious to execute; however, there are abundant data with a message that is oftentimes difficult to unify into cohesive recommendations. In 2006, *Integrating Therapeutic and Complementary Nutrition (Modern Nutrition)* was published to offer the CAM provider an evidence-based foundation in delivering nutrition recommendations to the educated consumer (Marian et al. 2006). This first-of-a-kind textbook served a broad audience and across life spectrums to provide an extensive resource for complementary nutrition. Since the publication of *Integrating Therapeutic and Complementary Nutrition (Modern Nutrition)*, the research in the area of specialized therapeutic diets and dietary supplements for disease prevention and remediation has literally exploded, requiring a new approach to message this exhaustive database. In *Integrative Nutrition Therapy*, we have reorganized the subject matter in a systematic manner that emphasizes an evidence-based translational how-to approach of the scientific data. An overview of integrative medicine is written by Dr. Roberta Lee, a leading authority in the field. The need for practical knowledge for the integrative practitioner is covered in depth by award-winning academic-based nutrition experts; the topics covered include "Nutrition Assessment," "Popular Diets" as a search for the holy grail of the optimum diet, "Functional Foods," "Sports Nutrition and Physical Activity," and "Nutrition through the Life Cycle." Finally, the evidence regarding the use of complementary nutrition is presented for cardiovascular, gastrointestinal, and liver disorders; diabetes; obesity; and neurological disorders.

We are pleased to provide you with this cutting-edge desk reference and hope this will transform the lives of many.

Mary J. Marian, DCN, CSO, FAND
Assistant Professor of Practice
Arizona Center for Integrative Medicine
University of Arizona
Tucson, Arizona

Gerard E. Mullin, MD
Associate Professor of Medicine
The Johns Hopkins University School of Medicine
Baltimore, Maryland

---

* http://www.anh-usa.org/dshea/.

REFERENCES

Barnes PM, Bloom B, and Nahin RL. (2008). Complementary and alternative medicine use among adults and children: United States, 2007. *National Health Statistics Reports*, 12, 1–23.

Eisenberg DM, Kessler RC, Foster C, Norlock FE, Calkins DR, and Delbanco TL. (1993). Unconventional medicine in the United States. Prevalence, costs, and patterns of use. *The New England Journal of Medicine*, 328(4), 246–252.

Jonas WB, Eisenberg D, Hufford D, and Crawford C. (2013). The evolution of complementary and alternative medicine (CAM) in the USA over the last 20 years. *Forsch Komplementmed*, 20(1), 65–72.

Marian MJ, Wiliams-Mullen P, and Muir-Bowers J. (2006). *Integrating Therapeutic and Complementary Nutrition (Modern Nutrition)*, 1st edn. Taylor & Francis/CRC Press, Boca Raton, FL.

Acknowledgments

My sincere thanks to my coeditor Dr. Mary Marian for her fortitude, support, and outstanding editorial management. A big thank-you to Randy Brehm and Kari Budyk from Taylor & Francis Group/CRC Press, for all of their efforts in producing this book. I express my gratitude to the many experts whose exceptional contributions made this book possible. There are many individuals I would like to recognize who have guided my career and sparked my interest in nutrition and integrative medicine—to my mentors who have guided my career over the years, in particular, Drs. Anthony Kalloo, Andrew Weil, Victoria Maizes, Tieraona Low Dog, and Ben Caballero and to the nutritionists whose collaborations have fostered career development and friendships over the years: Drs. Laura E. Matarese, Carol Irenton-Jones, Mark DeLegge, Steve McClave, Kelly Tappenden, Jeanette Hasse, and Amy Brown. A special thank-you to those who have supported my clinical practice at Johns Hopkins: my medical office assistants Julie McKenna-Thorpe and Roseann Wagner; administrators Erin O'Keefe, Lisa Bach-Burdsall, and Nathan Smith; administrative director of the Division of Gastroenterology and Hepatology Tiffany Boldin; Dr. Myron L. Weisfeldt, chairman of medicine; and Dr. Linda A. Lee, clinical director of the Division of Gastroenterology and Hepatology.

Gerard E. Mullin, MD
Baltimore, Maryland

Editors

Dr. Mary J. Marian is an assistant professor of practice and director of the Didactic Program in Dietetics in the Department of Nutritional Sciences at The University of Arizona, Tucson, Arizona. Dr. Marian is also the nutritionist and dietitian for Arizona Oncology Associates, Tucson, Arizona. She is a faculty member with the Integrative Medicine Program at the University of Arizona. She is widely published and has given numerous presentations both nationally and internationally. She has also served on numerous committees for the Academy of Nutrition and Dietetics as well as the American Society for Parenteral and Enteral Nutrition (ASPEN). She has been the chair for Dietitians in Nutrition Support and served on the board of directors for ASPEN.

Dr. Marian is the recipient of numerous honors and awards, including the Excellence in Clinical Practice from the American Dietetics Association. In 2014, she received the Academy of Nutrition and Dietetics' Medallion Award. She is also associate editor for the journal *Nutrition in Clinical Practice* published by the ASPEN and has served as lead editor for several books, including *Integrating Therapeutic and Complementary Nutrition*.

Dr. Gerard E. Mullin is an associate professor in the Department of Medicine at The Johns Hopkins Hospital, Baltimore, Maryland, where he chairs the hospital's Nutrition Advisory Committee. He is an internist, gastroenterologist, and nutritionist. Dr. Mullin is nationally and internationally renowned for his work in integrative gastroenterology and nutrition. He has accumulated more than 20 years of clinical experience in the field of integrative gastroenterology and earned his master's degree in nutrition while in practice.

In 2009, he was named by the American Dietetic Association as an honorary member. He is chair of the CNSC exam committee for the NBNSC and is chair-elect of the Medical Practice section of American Society for Parenteral and Enteral Nutrition (ASPEN). Dr. Mullin is on the editorial boards of several nutrition and integrative medicine journals and serves on several certification exam committees and boards. He has authored and edited several books in nutrition and integrative medicine. He has been interviewed on radio and television and has contributed to many stories in print media. Dr. Mullin's biography has been included in Marquis and Covington's *Who's Who* numerous times and continues to be selected as one of America's top physicians since 2004. Learn more about Dr. Mullin by visiting his website http://thefoodmd.com.

Contributors

Ryan Bradley, ND, MPH
Helfgott Research Institute
and
School of Research and Graduate
    Studies
National College of Natural
    Medicine
Portland, Oregon

Michelle Bratton, RDN, CSO
Nutrition Services
University of Arizona Cancer Center
Tucson, Arizona

Britta Brown, MS, RD, LD, CNSC
Medical Nutrition Therapy
Hennepin County Medical Center
Minneapolis, Minnesota

Danielle Flug Capalino, MSPH, RD
New York Gastroenterology
    Associates
New York, New York

Kristi Crowe-White, PhD, RD
College of Human Environmental
    Sciences
University of Alabama
Tuscaloosa, Alabama

Alia S. Dadabhai, MD
Division of Gastroenterology and
    Hepatology
School of Medicine
Johns Hopkins University
Baltimore, Maryland

**Dwight L. Davidson, PhD, MA,
LHMC**
Department of Health
College of Health Sciences
West Chester University of Pennsylvania
West Chester, Pennsylvania

**Patricia G. Davidson, DCN, RDN,
CDE, LDN**
Department of Nutrition
College of Health Sciences
West Chester University of
    Pennsylvania
West Chester, Pennsylvania

**Jennifer Doley MBA, RD, CNSC,
FAND**
Food and Nutrition Services
Carondelet St. Mary's Hospital
Tucson, Arizona

**Lindsay Dowhan, MS, RD, CSO, LD,
CNSC**
Center for Gut Rehabilitation and
    Transplant
Digestive Disease Institute
Cleveland Clinic
Cleveland, Ohio

Sherif El Behiry, MD
Division of Gastroenterology,
    Hepatology and Nutrition
Department of Internal Medicine
Suez Canal University
East Carolina University
Greenville, North Carolina

Coni Francis, PhD, RD
School of Human Sciences
University of Northern Colorado
Greeley, Colorado

Nora Galil, MD, MPH, FAACAP
School of Medicine and Health Sciences
George Washington University
Washington, DC

Karen M. Gibson, RDN, CD, CSSD
Nutrition and Dietetics
Viterbo University
La Crosse, Wisconsin

Mimi Guarneri, MD, FACC
Integrative Medicine Atlantic Health
    System
Morristown, New Jersey
and
Scripps Integrative Medicine
San Diego, California

Monica Habib, MS, RD, LD, CNSC
Holy Cross Nutrition Center
Holy Cross Hospital
Fort Lauderdale, Florida

Robert Hedaya, MD, DLFAPA
School of Medicine
Georgetown University
Washington, DC

Neha Jakhete, MD
Department of Medicine
Johns Hopkins Hospital
Baltimore, Maryland

Hossam M. Kandil, MD, PhD
Division of Gastroenterology,
    Hepatology and Nutrition
Department of Internal Medicine
Brody School of Medicine
East Carolina University
Greenville, North Carolina

Roberta Lee, MD, CaC
Department of Internal Medicine
Banner-University Medical Center
Tucson, Arizona

Laura E. Matarese, PhD, RND, LDN, FADA, CNSC, FASPEN, FAND
Division of Gastroenterology,
    Hepatology and Nutrition
Department of Internal Medicine
Brody School of Medicine
and
Department of Nutrition Science
East Carolina University
Greenville, North Carolina

Hilary H. McClafferty, MD, FAAP
Departments of Pediatrics and
    Medicine
University of Arizona College of
    Medicine
Tucson, Arizona

Gerard E. Mullin, MD
Division of Gastroenterology and
    Hepatology
The Johns Hopkins University School
    of Medicine
Baltimore, Maryland

Francis Okeke, MD, MPH
Department of Medicine
Johns Hopkins University
Baltimore, Maryland

Alyssa Parian, MD
Department of Gastroenterology
The Johns Hopkins University School
    of Medicine
Baltimore, Maryland

Bani Chander Roland, MD
New York-Presbyterian
Columbia University Medical Center
New York, New York

Maya Shetreat-Klein, MD
New York Medical College
Bronx, New York

Vikesh K. Singh, MD, MSc
Division of Gastroenterology
School of Medicine
Johns Hopkins University
Baltimore, Maryland

Deborah Straub, MS, RDN
Canyon Ranch Resort
Tucson, Arizona

Laurie Tansman, MS, RD, CDN
Department of Clinical Nutrition
The Mount Sinai Hospital
and
Department of Preventive Medicine
Icahn School of Medicine at Mount Sinai
New York, New York

Cynthia A. Thomson, PhD, RD
College of Public Health
The University of Arizona
Tucson, Arizona

List of Reviewers

Audrey Caspar-Clark, MA, RD, CSO, LDN
Department of Radiation Oncology
Hospital of the University of Pennsylvania
Philadelphia, Pennsylvania

Jennifer Doley, MBA, RD
Carondelet
Tucson, Arizona

David O. Garcia, PhD
Mel & Enid Zuckerman College of Public Health
The University of Arizona
Tucson, Arizona

Mindy Hermann, MBA, RDN
Hermann Communications
Mt. Kisco, New York

John Mark, MD
Stanford Hospital and Clinics
Stanford University
Palo Alto, California

Mary Russell, MS, RDN, LDN, FAND
Medical Affairs
Baxter Healthcare Corporation
Deerfield, Illinois

Ashley Vargas, PhD, MPH, RDN
Cancer Prevention Fellowship Program
National Cancer Institute
Bethesda, Maryland

Valaree Williams, MS, RDN, CSO, LDN
Department of Radiation Oncology
Hospital of the University of Pennsylvania
Philadelphia, Pennsylvania

1 Nutrition Assessment

Britta Brown, MS, RD, LD, CNSC

CONTENTS

INTRODUCTION

Nutrition screening and assessment are important steps in identifying individuals who may have nutrition-related health problem(s) and/or malnutrition. According to the American Society for Parenteral and Enteral Nutrition (ASPEN), nutrition screening is defined as "a process to identify an individual who is malnourished or who is at risk for malnutrition to determine if a detailed nutrition assessment is indicated" [1]. Nutrition screening is mandated by the Joint Commission, and it must be completed within 24 h of admission in the acute care setting [2]. In most facilities, nursing staff complete the nutrition screen. A variety of nutrition screening tools have been developed and validated, including the Malnutrition Screening Tool (MST) and the Malnutrition Universal Screening Tool (MUST) [3]. In general, nutrition screening tools should be quick and easy to complete and validated for the population they will be used with. However, each healthcare system may establish institution-specific nutrition screening criteria that may not be exclusive to malnutrition. For example, some healthcare facilities may choose to include screening criteria to identify individuals who may benefit from nutrition education or who have food allergies. Individuals with a positive nutrition screen (i.e., presence of nutritional risk factors identified following completion of the screening) are selected to receive a nutrition assessment. ASPEN defines nutrition assessment as "a comprehensive approach to diagnosing nutrition problems that uses a combination of the following: medical, nutrition, and medication histories; physical examination; anthropometric measurements, and laboratory data" [1]. The Academy of Nutrition and Dietetics has created the Nutrition Care Process and Model (NCPM), with the first step being assessment. The Academy's definition of assessment is more broad compared to the ASPEN criteria and is characterized as "a systemic approach to collect, record, and interpret relevant data from patients, clients, family members, caregivers, and other individuals and groups. Nutrition assessment is an ongoing, dynamic process that

1

Screening and referral system

• Identify risk factors
• Use appropriate tools and methods
• Involve interdisciplinary collaboration

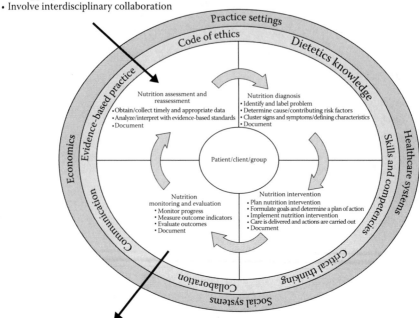

Outcomes management system

• Monitor the success of the Nutrition Care Process Implementation
• Evaluate the impact with aggregate data
• Identify and analyze causes of less than optimal performance and outcomes
• Refine the use of the Nutrition Care Process

FIGURE 1.1 Nutrition care process and model (NCPM). (From Lacey, K. and Pritchett, E., *J. Am. Diet. Assoc.*, 103, 1061, 2003.)

involves initial data collection as well as continual reassessment and analysis of the patient's/client's status compared to specific criteria" [4,5]. The four steps of the NCPM are described in Figure 1.1 [4].

COMPONENTS OF A NUTRITION ASSESSMENT

Several validated nutrition assessment tools are widely referenced in the literature [6–11]. The Mini Nutritional Assessment (MNA®) has been validated among adults over age 65 who are malnourished or who are at risk for malnutrition [6–8]. The original MNA, now referred to the as the "full MNA," consists of 18 questions and includes questions regarding dietary habits, living situation, use of prescription medications, self-view of nutritional status, mid-arm circumference (MAC), and calf circumference (CC) [8]. In addition to the "full MNA," there is also the MNA-short form that has also been validated and only includes six questions. Due to increased ease of use, the MNA-short form is typically used in clinical practice and includes questions on food intake over the past 3 months, weight loss during the last 3 months, mobility, psychological stress over the past 3 months, neuropsychological problems (i.e., dementia or depression), and body mass index (BMI) [8]. Although the MNA has been validated among the elderly population, there is still debate about the sensitivity of this tool since its use has been associated with the "over-diagnosis" of malnutrition [7]. Although the ASPEN Clinical Guidelines for nutrition screening, assessment, and intervention in adults classify the MNA as a nutrition assessment tool [3], it is important to note, the MNA was originally developed as a screening tool to be used by non-RD practitioners. This is one reason debate exists whether the MNA is an appropriate assessment tool for "diagnosing" malnutrition.

A second nutrition assessment tool that has been validated and demonstrated to have excellent reliability is the Subjective Global Assessment (SGA) tool, described by Detsky and colleagues in 1987 [9]. This tool was designed to be easily used at the bedside without the need for specialized equipment to assess nutritional status [10–11]. This tool includes questions on weight and diet history, gastrointestinal symptoms, functional capacity, and physical assessment (subcutaneous fat or muscle loss, edema, and ascites [Figure 1.2]) [9]. Patients are classified as (1) well nourished, (2) moderately malnourished, or (3) severely malnourished [9]. This tool has been successfully used and validated in the surgical, oncology, HIV, acute kidney injury, chronic kidney disease, kidney and liver transplant, and elderly populations [10–11]. SGA has been positively regarded since it is simple and quick to administer, low-cost, requires no special equipment, and it assesses functional capacity [10,11]. It also has the advantage of excellent interobserver reproducibility [11]. Historically, some clinicians have been reluctant to use SGA due to unfamiliarity with conducting a nutrition-focused physical exam (NFPE), but this skill can be readily taught [10] and more training and standardized resources are available since NFPE is recognized as an important component of diagnosing malnutrition [12].

Jensen and colleagues have combined aspects of the MNA and SGA in their approach to nutrition assessment based on the joint ASPEN and Academy consensus guidelines on adult malnutrition [13,14] and our current understanding of inflammation in the pathogenesis of malnutrition [15]. The ASPEN and Academy consensus guidelines on adult malnutrition were developed to standardize the process for diagnosing malnutrition and to reduce confusion and possible misdiagnosis [14]. In addition, this approach is etiology based and criteria may change over time as validity evidence accrues. The identification of two or more of the following six criteria is needed for the diagnosis of malnutrition: insufficient energy intake, weight loss, loss of muscle mass, loss of subcutaneous fat, localized or generalized fluid accumulation that may mask weight loss, and diminished functional status measured by handgrip strength [14]. Clinical characteristics for diagnosing malnutrition are defined in Table 1.1 [14].

Jensen advocates a systematic approach to nutrition assessment based on six criteria, including history and clinical diagnosis, clinical signs and physical examination,

SUBJECTIVE GLOBAL ASSESSMENT OF NUTRITIONAL STATUS
select appropriate category with a checkmark, or enter numerical value

A. HISTORY
1. Weight change: Normal weight = #_____ kg IBW = #_____ kg
Overall change in past 6 months = #_____ kg loss/gain Current weight =
#_____ kg
% change in past 6 months = _____ % loss/gain %IBW = _____ %
Change in past 2 weeks: no change ↑ ↓ Amt = #_____ kg
2. Dietary intake change (relative to normal)
_____ No change _____ ↑'d intake _____ ↓'d intake
Duration of change = # _____ weeks
If intake ↓'d: Type of change _____ Suboptimal solid diet _____ Full liquid
diet
_____ Hypocaloric liquids _____ Starvation
3. Gastrointestinal symptoms persisting for >2 weeks
_____ None _____ Nausea _____ Vomiting _____ Diarrhea _____ Anorexia
4. Functional Capacity
_____ No dysfunction (full capacity) _____ Dysfunction: duration = # _____ weeks
Dysfunction: _____ Working suboptimally _____ Ambulatory _____ Bedridden
        Specific handicap(s):

5. Disease and its relation to nutritional requirements
Primary diagnosis:

Metabolic demand (stress) _____ None _____ Low _____ Moderate _____ High

B. PHYSICAL FINDINGS: 0 = normal 1+ = mild 2+ = moderate 3+ = severe
_____ loss of subcutaneous fat (triceps, chest) _____ ankle edema _____ ascites
_____ muscle wasting (quadriceps, deltoids) _____ sacral edema

C. SUBJECTIVE GLOBAL ASSESSMENT RATING (select one)

A Nourished
B Moderately malnourished
C Severely malnourished

FIGURE 1.2 Subjective global assessment (SGA). (From Detsky, A.S. et al., *J. Parenter. Enteral. Nutr.*, 11, 8, 1987.)

anthropometric data, laboratory indicators of inflammatory response, dietary data, and functional outcomes (Table 1.2) [15]. The first step of the etiology-based approach to the diagnosis of malnutrition is identification of nutrition risk (compromised intake or loss of body mass), followed by the presence of inflammation (no/yes) [16]. Individuals identified at nutritional risk who are not experiencing inflammation are categorized as having starvation-related malnutrition (pure chronic starvation and anorexia nervosa) [16]. Individuals identified at nutritional risk who are experiencing inflammation are categorized into two groups based on the severity of the inflammatory response. Those identified with a mild-to-moderate degree of malnutrition are classified with chronic disease-related malnutrition (i.e., cancer, rheumatoid arthritis, and sarcopenic obesity), whereas those identified with a marked inflammatory response are classified with acute disease or injury-related malnutrition (i.e., major

TABLE 1.1

A.S.P.E.N./Academy Clinical Characteristics Supporting the Diagnosis of Malnutrition

	Malnutrition in the Context of Acute Illness or Injury		Malnutrition in the Context of Chronic Illness		Malnutrition in the Context of Social or Environmental Circumstances	
	Moderate Malnutrition	Severe Malnutrition	Moderate Malnutrition	Severe Malnutrition	Moderate Malnutrition	Severe Malnutrition
Clinical characteristic						
Energy intake	<75% of estimated energy requirement for >7 days	≤50% of estimated energy requirement for ≥5 days	<75% of estimated energy requirement for ≥1 month	≤75% of estimated energy requirement for ≥1 month	<75% of estimated energy requirement for ≥3 months	≤50% of estimated energy requirement for ≥1 month
Interpretation of weight loss	1%–2% loss in 1 week 5% loss in 1 month 7.5% loss in 3 months	>2% loss in 1 week >5% loss in 1 month >7.5% loss in 3 months	5% loss in 1 month 7.5% loss in 3 months 10% loss in 6 months 20% loss in 1 year	>5% loss in 1 month >7.5% loss in 3 months >10% loss in 6 months >20% loss in 1 year	5% loss in 1 month 7.5% loss in 3 months 10% loss in 6 months 20% loss in 1 year	>5% loss in 1 month >7.5% loss in 3 months >10% loss in 6 months >20% loss in 1 year
Physical findings						
Body fat Loss of subcutaneous fat	Mild	Moderate	Mild	Severe	Mild	Severe
Muscle mass Muscle loss	Mild	Moderate	Mild	Severe	Mild	Severe
Fluid accumulation: Localized fluid accumulation evidence (e.g., extremities; vulvar/scrotal edema)	Mild	Moderate to severe	Mild	Severe	Mild	Severe
Reduced hand-grip strength	N/A	Measurably reduced	N/A	Measurably reduced	N/A	Measurably reduced

Source: Malone, A. and Hamilton, C., *Nutr. Clin. Pract.*, 28, 639, 2013.

TABLE 1.2

Systematic Approach to Nutrition Assessment

Clinical Domain	Possible Indicators and Considerations
History and clinical diagnosis	May identify possible medical conditions associated with malnutrition or inflammation
	May identify social/environmental factors associated with malnutrition
Clinical signs and physical examination	Nonspecific indicators of inflammation—fever, hypothermia, and tachycardia
	Identify signs of edema, weight gain/loss, and nutrient deficiencies
Anthropometric data	Height, weight, body mass index, skin folds, and circumferences
Laboratory indicators	Avoid use of albumin or prealbumin
	Markers of inflammation C-reactive protein, white blood cell count, and blood glucose
	Others—negative nitrogen balance and elevated resting energy expenditure
Dietary data	Modified diet history or 24 h dietrecall
	REAP tool [20]
Functional outcomes	Hand-grip strength measured by dynamometer
	Others—wound healing; performance batteries (timed gait, chair stands, and stair steps)

Source: Jensen, G.L. et al., *J. Parenter. Enteral Nutr.*, 36, 267, 2012.

infection, burns, and trauma) [16]. A listing of acute and chronic conditions associated with the inflammatory response has been previously published [12]. Based on currently available data, the prevalence of malnutrition in the hospital setting is estimated to range from 15% to 60% [3].

Many practitioners can proficiently review medical and dietary histories, anthropometric measurements, and laboratory indicators to determine the likelihood of nutritional problems. However, performing a nutrition-focused physical examination (NFPE) may be a new skill for some clinicians. Conducting a NFPE occurs after the other assessment criteria have been reviewed. This tool can be especially useful when other nutrition assessment parameters are inconclusive, but a nutrient deficiency or toxicity is suspected. A NFPE is a head-to-toe inspection of body systems using the techniques of inspection, palpation, percussion, and auscultation [17]. To complete a thorough NFPE, a clinician will conduct a general visual inspection of the patient or client, followed by an assessment of vital signs, skin, hair, nails, head and neck, oral cavity, teeth, the respiratory system, the cardiovascular system, abdomen, and the neurologic system [17]. The abdominal exam included in an NFPE is particularly important since findings from this exam can provide insight into the functional status of the GI tract and whether a patient or client will be able to adequately consume, digest, and absorb nutrients [18]. Resources on performing an abdominal exam, and a complete review of body systems with corresponding physical signs, possible nutrient deficiencies, and nonnutritional causes of similar findings has been previously published [17,18]. There are now published standards to guide the clinician in assessing subcutaneous fat and muscle loss and the corresponding characteristics observed with severe malnutrition, mild to moderate malnutrition, and well-nourished states [12].

Anthropometric nutrition assessment data typically consists of height, weight, weight history, body mass index (BMI), and possibly skin fold and circumference measurements, and/or body composition measurements (i.e., bioelectrical impedance, ultrasound, and CT imaging). Height, weight, weight history, and body mass index can easily be documented in the electronic health record (EHR) and clinicians can follow trends over time. Given the obesity epidemic and the role of obesity in chronic illness, BMI should be closely followed as nutrition interventions may need to be adjusted to promote weight loss or weight maintenance (Table 1.3) [19].

Historically, laboratory indices such as serum albumin, prealbumin, and transferrin have been used to assess nutritional status. However, we now know these negative acute-phase proteins lack both sensitivity and specificity as markers of nutritional status. These proteins can be affected by injury, disease, and inflammation [15]. In addition, it is possible to have severely depleted albumin and prealbumin levels and not be malnourished based on a comprehensive nutrition assessment [15]. Urinary nitrogen balance is still a useful marker of protein catabolism, particularly in critical illness, but performing a 24 h urine collection and capturing a patient/client's 24 h protein intake is not practical in most settings.

Dietary data obtained through a 24 h diet recall, modified diet history, or a food frequency tool can be one of the most useful nutrition assessment components. Patients/clients, family members, and caregivers can all contribute valuable information on dietary intake. It is useful for clinicians to get a picture of both general intake patterns and overall quality of macro- and micronutrient consumption. It is important to recognize exacerbations of acute or chronic illnesses that compromise nutritional intake and to clarify the duration of decreased intake [15]. In addition to food intake, clinicians must also evaluate intake of vitamin, mineral, or herbal

---

TABLE 1.3

International Classification of Adult Underweight, Overweight, and Obesity According to BMI

BMI (kg/m²)	Classification
<18.5	Underweight
18.5–24.9	Normal weight
25.0–29.9	Overweight
30.0–34.9	Class I obesity
35.0–39.9	Class II obesity
≥40.0	Class III obesity

Source: Global Database on Body Mass Index, BMI classification, The Word Health Organization, http://apps.who.int/bmi/index.jsp?introPage=intro_3.html, published November 2013, accessed November 26, 2013.

Note: BMI = weight (kg)/height (m)².

supplements; oral nutrition supplements; and nutrition support (i.e., parenteral or enteral nutrition) intake (if applicable).

In the ambulatory care setting, clinicians may use a tool such as the Rapid Eating Assessment for Patients (REAP) developed by the Institute for Community Health Promotion, Brown University [20,21]. This tool was designed to assess diet related to the 2000 U.S. Dietary Guidelines [20]. It includes questions to assess intake of whole grains, calcium-rich foods, fruits, vegetables, fat, saturated fat, cholesterol, sugary beverages and foods, alcohol, and physical activity [20]. It also captures information on whether the patient/client prepares his/her own food, encounters difficulty shopping or preparing food, follows a special diet, eats or limits certain foods, and has an interest in changing eating habits [20,22]. The developers of REAP suggest having patients/clients complete this tool prior to their clinic visit or while they are in the waiting room. The physician can then review this tool and provide a targeted nutrition counseling message during the office visit. A REAP Physician Key for Diet Assessment and Counseling has been developed and guidelines exist for implementing nutrition counseling in as little as 1–2 min [22]. Patients/clients should be referred to the registered dietitian (RD) if they are interested in more thorough nutrition education, counseling, and behavior modification strategies for improving their overall diet.

Functional outcomes are a newer aspect of nutrition assessment, and our understanding of functional status is evolving as more research becomes available. At this time, measurements of hand-grip strength using a dynamometer are advocated to assess the presence of malnutrition [13–15]. However, this tool is limited to patients or clients who are neurologically intact and who can participate in this exercise, and to those who do not have conditions that impair hand strength (i.e., arthritis). Researchers are evaluating other markers of functional status such as wound healing and physical tests such as timed gait, chair stands, and stair steps [15]. In the future, there will likely be more collaboration between nutrition professionals and other therapies (i.e., physical, occupational, and speech language pathology) in assessing functional outcomes as they relate to nutritional status.

NUTRITION DIAGNOSIS

After a nutrition assessment has been generated following the analysis and synthesis of pertinent data, the practitioner develops a nutrition diagnosis. According the NCPM, a nutrition diagnosis can be described as "identification and labeling that describes an actual occurrence, risk of, or potential for developing a nutritional problem that dietetics professionals are responsible for treating independently" [4]. RDs document the nutrition diagnosis using the International Dietetics and Nutrition Terminology (IDNT) [23]. These standardized nutrition diagnoses are categorized into three domains: intake, clinical, and behavioral and environmental [23]. These diagnoses are simply labels for nutrition problems such as "Inadequate oral intake" (NI-2.1), "malnutrition" (NI-5.2), "underweight" (NC-2.1), "food and nutrition knowledge-related deficit" (NB-1.1), or "limited access to food or water" (NB-3.2) [23]. Nutrition diagnoses are not medical diagnoses. Rather, a nutrition diagnosis can change over time as a patient or client's response changes. Making an accurate nutrition diagnosis aids in setting realistic, measurable goals; developing interventions; as well as monitoring progress toward the desired outcomes [4].

Nutrition diagnoses included in the IDNT are terms used by RDs to identify, describe, and communicate aspects of a nutrition problem. Healthcare facilities utilize information provided by RD assessments, including nutrition diagnoses, to guide medical coding for reimbursement. Current International Classification of Disease (ICD) codes for malnutrition do not match the etiology-based definitions of malnutrition adopted by ASPEN and the Academy. Various ICD-9 codes for nutrition deficiencies can be applied to adult malnutrition. At this time, it is recommended that the term "other, severe protein-calorie malnutrition" (code 262) be used for the diagnosis of severe malnutrition and "moderate malnutrition" (code 263.0) be used for the diagnosis of nonsevere (moderate) malnutrition [12]. The definitions of these ICD codes best match the definitions of malnutrition criteria established in the ASPEN/Academy consensus guidelines [12]. New ICD-10 codes will be implemented by October 2015, but they are not expected to differ significantly from the current ICD-9 malnutrition codes.

NUTRITION INTERVENTION

Developing nutrition intervention(s) is the next step in the NCPM. It entails selecting, planning, and implementing appropriate actions to meet a patient or client's nutritional needs [4]. When developing nutrition interventions, it is important to prioritize the nutrition diagnoses to be addressed. For example, nutrition diagnoses and corresponding interventions may be prioritized based on severity of the condition, safety, urgency, patient/client's perceived importance of the issue, and/or the likelihood that addressing the issue will result in the resolution of the problem. In this step of the NCPM, it is important to first plan the intervention and then to implement the intervention [4]. During the planning stage, providers may utilize evidenced-based practice guidelines, determine patient/client-centered outcomes, assess how progress toward reaching goals will be measured, define the care plan (i.e., nutrition prescription, nutrition education, behavior modification counseling, etc.), define the frequency and intensity of nutrition interventions, and provide additional resources/referrals as indicated (i.e., education materials and community programs) [4]. The implementation stage involves providing nutrition care, gathering appropriate data to assess the effectiveness of the plan, collaborating with the patient/client and other healthcare team members, and modifying the plan as needed. Effective interventions must be realistic and include clear timelines and methods for measuring progress toward meeting established goals.

A key component of the intervention step is developing a nutrition prescription that is appropriate for the patient/client's overall health condition and nutrition diagnosis [5]. Nutrition prescriptions can contain specific information on goal requirements for macronutrients (energy, protein, and fat), micronutrients (vitamins and minerals), water, and dietary fiber or for selected whole foods. For healthy individuals, nutrition prescriptions may be based on reference standards such as the Dietary Guidelines for Americans, 2010 [24] and the Dietary Reference Intakes (DRI) [25]. The nutrition prescription will vary based on the presence of underweight or overweight/obesity, activity level, and medical conditions. Guidelines for developing nutrition prescriptions for various medical conditions (i.e., diabetes, critical illness, weight management, heart failure, etc.) can be accessed through the Academy's Evidence Analysis Library [26]. These guidelines are rigorously developed and continually updated to reflect current research findings.

Nutrition interventions can have a profound positive effect on clinical outcomes. For example, one systematic review that included hospitalized patients with chronic disease-related malnutrition, the intervention of providing a high-protein oral nutrition supplement (ONS), was associated with fewer complications (p < 0.001), reduced likelihood of hospital readmission (0.004), improved hand-grip strength (p < 0.014), increased protein and energy intake (p < 0.001), and improved weight (p < 0.001) [27]. Other nutrition interventions, such as Medical Nutrition Therapy (MNT), provided by an RD can have a profound impact on clinical outcomes for individuals with diabetes mellitus (DM). In this population, when a variety of nutrition therapy interventions, such as a reduced energy and fat intake, carbohydrate counting, simplified meal plans, healthy food choices, individualized meal planning strategies, exchange lists, insulin-to-carbohydrate ratios, and behavioral strategies, were implemented, reductions in A1C have ranged from 0.25%–2.9% at 3–6 months following initiation of MNT [28].

NUTRITION MONITORING AND EVALUATION

Simply stated, the monitoring and evaluation step "identifies the amount of progress made and whether goals/expected outcomes are being met" [4,5]. With enhanced technology, patients/clients can self-monitor data through various smart phone, tablet, or computer applications. Electronic communication from healthcare providers to patients or clients can be valuable in monitoring progress toward established health goals. Using the EHR, it is also easy for clinicians to monitor trends in anthropometric measurements, laboratory data, medical tests/procedures, and other healthcare issues [5]. In the monitoring and evaluation stage, it is important for the clinician to determine if the nutrition diagnosis has resolved or whether a new approach is necessary to meet the specified outcomes/goals and to improve overall care.

IMPLEMENTATION OF A NUTRITION ASSESSMENT PROGRAM

Implementing a nutrition assessment program in a primary care setting is challenging due to many factors, including lack of resources and time constraints. As previously mentioned, REAP is a validated nutrition assessment tool designed to be used by physicians and other healthcare providers to evaluate nutrition intake and physical activity patterns [20,21] (Table 1.4). The same group who developed REAP have also created WAVE, an acronym that stands for weight, activity, variety, and excess [22]. The goals of WAVE include (1) provide a quick tool for primary care providers to discuss weight, physical activity, and eating habits; (2) use a simple acronym that is easy to remember; (3) identify weight, nutrition, and/or physical activity issues that need to be addressed during the visit or through referral to a dietitian; and (4) reinforce the role of nutrition and physical activity in wellness and disease prevention [22]. Simple pocket cards have been developed to guide physicians in assessing these four categories as well as making corresponding recommendations [22] (Table 1.5). This same information could easily be built into an EHR for real-time use during the office visit.

TABLE 1.4
Rapid Eating Assessment for Patients (REAP)

Rapid Eating Assessment for Patients (REAP)

Please check the box that best describes your habits.

TOPIC	In an average week, how often do you:	Usually/ Often	Sometimes	Rarely/ Never	Does not apply to me
MEALS	1. Skip breakfast?	O	O	O	
	2. Eat <u>4 or more</u> meals from sit-down or take out restaurants?	O	O	O	
GRAINS	3. Eat <u>less than 3 servings</u> of whole grain products a day? **Serving** = 1 slice of 100% whole grain bread; 1 cup whole grain cereal, high fiber cereal, oatmeal; 3-4 whole grain crackers; 1/2 cup brown rice or whole wheat pasta	O	O	O	
FRUITS AND VEGETABLES	4. Eat <u>less than 2-3 servings</u> of fruit a day? **Serving** = 1/2 cup or 1 med. fruit or 4 oz. 100% fruit juice	O	O	O	
	5. Eat <u>less than 3-4 servings</u> of vegetables/potatoes a day? **Serving** = 1/2 cup vegetables/potatoes, or 1 cup leafy raw vegetables	O	O	O	
DAIRY	6. Eat or drink <u>less than 2-3 servings</u> of milk, yogurt, or cheese a day? **Serving** = 1 cup milk or yogurt; 1.5 - 2 ounces cheese	O	O	O	
	7. Use <u>2% (reduced fat)</u> or <u>whole milk</u> instead of skim (non-fat) or 1% (low-fat) milk?	O	O	O	Rarely use milk O
	8. Use <u>regular cheese</u> (like American, cheddar, Swiss, Monterey Jack) instead of low fat or part skim cheeses as a snack, on sandwiches, pizza, etc?	O	O	O	Rarely eat cheese O
MEATS/CHICKEN/TURKEY	9. Eat beef, pork, or dark meat chicken <u>more than 2 times a week</u>?	O	O	O	
	10. Eat <u>more than</u> 6 ounces (see sizes below) of meat, chicken, turkey or fish <u>per day</u>? ***Note***: *3 ounces of meat or chicken is the size of a deck of cards or ONE of the following:* *1 regular hamburger, 1 chicken breast or leg (thigh & drumstick), or 1 pork chop.*	O	O	O	Rarely eat meat, chicken, turkey or fish O
	11. Choose <u>higher fat red meats</u> like prime rib, T-bone steak, hamburger, ribs, etc. instead of lean red meats?	O	O	O	Rarely eat meat O
	12. Eat the <u>skin</u> on chicken and turkey and the <u>fat</u> on meat.	O	O	O	Rarely eat meat, chicken, turkey or fish O
	13. Use <u>regular processed meats</u> (like bologna, salami, corned beef, hot dogs, sausage or bacon) instead of low fat processed meats (like roast beef, turkey, lean ham; low-fat cold cuts/hotdogs)?	O	O	O	Rarely eat processed meats O
FRIED FOODS	14. Eat <u>fried foods</u> such as fried chicken, fried fish or French fries?	O	O	O	

OVER

(Continued)

TABLE 1.4 (*Continued*)
Rapid Eating Assessment for Patients (REAP)

TOPIC	In an average week, how often do you:	Usually/ Often	Sometimes	Rarely/ Never	Does not apply to me
SNACKS	15. Eat <u>regular potato chips, nacho chips, corn chips, crackers, regular popcorn, nuts</u> instead of pretzels, low-fat chips or low-fat crackers, air-popped popcorn?	O	O	O	Rarely eat these snack foods O
FATS AND OILS	16. Use <u>regular salad dressing & mayonnaise</u> instead of low-fat or fat-free salad dressing and mayonnaise?	O	O	O	Rarely use dressing/mayo O
	17. <u>Add butter, margarine or oil</u> to bread, potatoes, rice or vegetables at the table?	O	O	O	
	18. <u>Cook with oil, butter or margarine</u> instead of using non-stick sprays like Pam or cooking without fat?	O	O	O	Rarely cook O
SWEETS	19. Eat <u>regular sweets</u> like cake, cookies, pastries, donuts, muffins, and chocolate instead of <u>low fat or fat-free</u> sweets?	O	O	O	Rarely eat sweets O
	20. Eat <u>regular ice cream</u> instead of sherbet, sorbet, low fat or fat-free ice cream, frozen yogurt, etc.?	O	O	O	Rarely eat frozen desserts O
	21. Eat <u>sweets</u> like cake, cookies, pastries, donuts, muffins, chocolate and candies more than 2 times per day?	O	O	O	Rarely eat sweets O
SOFT DRINKS	22. <u>Drink 16 ounces or more</u> of non-diet soda, fruit drink/punch a day? **Note:** *1 can of soda = 12 ounces*	O	O	O	
SODIUM	23. Eat high sodium <u>processed foods</u> like canned soup or pasta, frozen/packaged meals (TV dinners, etc.), chips?	O	O	O	
	24. <u>Add salt</u> to foods during cooking or at the table?	O	O	O	
ALCOHOL	25. Drink <u>more than</u> 1-2 alcoholic drinks a day? (One drink = 12 oz. beer, 5 oz. Wine, one shot of hard liquor or mixed drink with 1 shot)	O	O	O	
ACTIVITY	26. Do <u>less than</u> 30 total minutes of physical activity 3 days a week or more? (Examples: walking briskly, gardening, golf, jogging, swimming, biking, dancing, etc.)	O	O	O	
	27. Watch <u>more than</u> 2 hours of television or videos a day?	O	O	O	

Do you....	Yes	No
28. Usually shop and prepare your own food?	O	O
29. Ever have trouble being able to shop or cook?	O	O
30. Follow a special diet, eat or limit certain foods for health or other reasons?	O	O

31. How willing are you to make changes in what, how or how much you eat in order to eat healthier?
(Circle the number that best describes how you feel)

Very willing				Not at all willing
5	**4**	**3**	**2**	**1**

Source: Research Tools and Resources, Brown University, Institute for Community Health Promotion. http://www.brown.edu/academics/public-health/centers/community-health-promotion/research-tools-and-resources, published 2005, accessed January 13, 2014.

TABLE 1.5

Weight, Activity, Variety, Excess (WAVE) Assessment and Recommendations

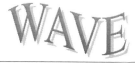 Assessment

Weight	Activity
Assess patient's Body Mass Index.* Patient is overweight if BMI>25.	Ask patient about any physical activity in the past week: walking briskly, jogging, gardening, swimming, biking, dancing, golf, etc.

Height	Body Weight lbs.	Height	Body Weight lbs.
4'10"	≥119	5'8"	≥164
4'11"	≥124	5'9"	≥169
5'0"	≥128	5'10"	≥174
5'1"	≥132	5'11"	≥179
5'2"	≥136	6'0"	≥184
5'3"	≥141	6'1"	≥189
5'4"	≥145	6'2"	≥194
5'5"	≥150	6'3"	≥200
5'6"	≥ 155	6'4"	≥205
5'7"	≥159		

1. Does patient do **30 minutes** of moderate activity on **most days/wk.?**

2. Does pt do "lifestyle" activity like taking the **stairs** instead of elevators, etc.?

3. Does patient usually watch less than **2 hours of TV or videos/day?**

* Certain pts may require assessment for underweight and/or unintentional weight loss

If pt answers **NO** to above questions, assess whether pt is willing to increase physical activity.

Variety	Excess
Is patient eating a variety of foods from important sections of the food pyramid?	Is patient eating too much of certain foods and nutrients?

Grains (6-11 servings)
Fruits (2-4 servings)
Vegetables (3-5 servings)
Protein (2-3 servings)
Dairy (2-3 servings)

Determine **Variety** and **Excess** using one of the following methods:

• Do a quick one-day recall.

• Ask patient to complete a self-administered eating pattern questionnaire.

Too much fat, saturated fat, calories
• > 6 oz/day of meat
• Ice cream, high fat milk, cheese, etc.
• Fried foods or foods cooked with fat
• High fat snacks and desserts
• Eating out > 4 meals/wk

Too much sugar, calories
• High sugar beverages
• Sugary snacks/desserts

Too much salt
• Processed meats, canned/frozen meals, salty snacks, added salt

• *What does pt think are pros/cons of his/her eating pattern?*
• *If pt needs to improve eating habits, assess willingness to make changes.*

 Brown University School of Medicine Nutrition Academic Award

(Continued)

TABLE 1.5 (*Continued*)
Weight, Activity, Variety, Excess (WAVE) Assessment and Recommendations

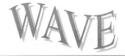 **Recommendations**

Weight	Activity

If pt is overweight:
 1. **State concern** for the pt, e.g., "I am concerned that your weight is affecting your health."
 2. Give the pt **specific advice**, i.e.,
   a) Make 1 or 2 changes in eating habits to reduce calorie intake as identified by diet assessment.
   b) Gradually increase activity/decrease inactivity.
   c) Enroll in a weight management program and/or consult a dietitian.
 3. If patient is ready to make behavior changes, jointly **set goals** for a plan of action and arrange for follow-up.
 4. **Give pt education materials/ resources.**
	Examples of moderate amounts of physical activity:
	 • Walking 2 miles in 30 minutes
	 • Stair walking for 15 minutes
	 • Washing and waxing a car for 45-60 minutes
	 • Washing windows or floors for 45-60 minutes
	 • Gardening for 30-45 minutes
	 • Pushing a stroller 1 ½ miles in 30 minutes
	 • Raking leaves for 30 minutes
	 • Shoveling snow for 15 minutes
	
	 1. If patient is ready to increase physical activity, jointly **set specific activity goals** and arrange for a follow-up
	 2. **Give pt education materials/ resources.**

Variety	**Excess**
What is a serving? **Grains** (6-11 servings) 1 slice bread or tortilla, ½ bagel, ½ roll, 1 oz. ready-to-eat cereal, ½ cup rice, pasta, or cooked cereal, 3-4 plain crackers *Is patient eating whole grains?* **Fruits** (2-4 servings) 1 medium fresh fruit, ½ cup chopped or canned fruit, ¾ cup fruit juice **Vegetables** (3-5 servings) 1 cup raw leafy vegetables, ½ cup cooked or chopped raw vegetables, ¾ cup vegetable juice **Protein** (2-3 servings) 2-3 oz. poultry, fish, or lean meat, 1-1 ½ cup cooked dry beans, 1 egg equals 1 oz. meat, 4 oz. or ½ cup tofu **Dairy** (2-3 servings) 1 cup milk or yogurt, 1½ oz. cheese **See instructions 1-4 under Excess.**	1. **Discuss pros and cons** of pt's eating pattern keeping in mind Variety & Excess. 2. If patient is ready, jointly **set specific dietary goals** and arrange for follow-up. 3. **Give pt education materials/resources.** 4. **Consider referral** to a dietitian for more extensive counseling and support. **Suggestions for decreasing excess**: • Eat chicken and fish (not fried)or meatless meals instead of red meat • Choose leaner cuts of red meat • Choose skim or 1% milk • Eat less cheese/choose lower fat cheeses • Bake, broil, grill foods rather than fry • Choose low fat salad dressings, mayo, spreads, etc. • Eat more whole grains, fruits & vegetables • Drink water instead of sugary drinks • Use herbs instead of salt

Source: Research Tools and Resources, Brown University, Institute for Community Health Promotion. http://www.brown.edu/academics/public-health/centers/community-health-promotion/ research-tools-and-resources, published 2005, accessed January 13, 2014.

Going forward, it is imperative that the whole healthcare team collaborates and partners with patients and clients to promote health and wellness and to minimize the effects of chronic disease. Many simple nutrition interventions can be initiated by medical assistants, nurses, physicians, and other providers with referrals made to dietitians for those who would benefit from more comprehensive nutrition assessment and intervention.

ADDITIONAL RESOURCES

Additional information on nutrition guidelines, assessment tools, or implementing a nutrition assessment program can be found in Table 1.6 [24–26,29–32].

TABLE 1.6
Nutrition Assessment and Guideline Resources

Organization	Website
Academy of Nutrition and Dietetics	http://www.eatright.org
Academy of Nutrition and Dietetics Evidence Analysis Library	http://andevidencelibrary.com/default.cfm
American Society for Parenteral and Enteral Nutrition (A.S.P.E.N.)	http://www.nutritioncare.org
Alliance to Advance Patient Nutrition	http://malnutrition.com/
Dietary Guidelines for Americans, 2010	http://www.health.gov/dietaryguidelines/2010.asp
Rapid Eating Assessment for Patients (REAP)	http://www.brown.edu/academics/public-health/
Weight, activity, variety, excess (WAVE)	centers/community-health-promotion/
	research-tools-and-resources
United States Department of Agriculture dietary reference intakes	http://fnic.nal.usda.gov/dietary-guidance/ dietary-reference-intakes

Sources: Dietary Guidelines for Americas, 2010, http://www.health.gov/dietaryguidelines/dga2010/ DietaryGuidelines2010.pdf, The U.S. Department of Agriculture, the U.S. Department of Health and Human Services, 2010 Dietary Guidelines Committee, published January 2011, accessed November 12, 2013; Dietary Reference Intakes Tables, The U.S. Department of Agriculture, National Agriculture Library, Food and Nutrition Information Center, published 2010, accessed November 12, 2013; Academy of Nutrition and Dietetics Evidence Analysis Library, Evidenced-based nutrition practice guidelines, http://andevidencelibrary.com/category. cfm?cid=14&cat=0, published 2013, accessed November 12, 2013; Academy of Nutrition and Dietetics, http://www.eatright.org, published 2013, accessed December 1, 2013; American Society for Parenteral and Enteral Nutrition, http://www.nutritioncare.org., published 2013, accessed December 1, 2013; Research Tools and Resources, Brown University, Institute for Community Health Promotion, http://www.brown.edu/academics/public-health/centers/ community-health-promotion/research-tools-and-resources, published 2005, accessed January 13, 2014; Alliance to Advance Patient Nutrition, http://malnutrition.com., published 2013, accessed January 13, 2014.

REFERENCES

1. American Society for Parenteral and Enteral Nutrition (A.S.P.E.N.) Board of Directors and Clinical Practice Committee. Definition of terms, style, and conventions used in A.S.P.E.N. Board of Directors-approved documents. American Society for Parenteral and Enteral Nutrition. http://www.nutritioncare.org/Professional_Resources/Guidelines_and_Standards/Guidelines/2012_Definitions_of_Terms,_Style,_and_Conventions_Used_in_A_S_P_E_N__Board_of_Directors-Approved_Documents/. Published July 2010, accessed November 12, 2013.
2. The Joint Commission. Provision of care, treatment, and services. PC.01.02.03 EP7. http://www.e-dition.jcrinc.com/Maincontent.aspx. Published July 1, 2013, accessed November 22, 2013.
3. Mueller CM, Compher C, Druyan ME. American Society for Parenteral and Enteral Nutrition (A.S.P.E.N.) Board of Directors. A.S.P.E.N. Clinical guidelines: nutrition screening, assessment, and intervention in adults. *J Parenter Enteral Nutr* 2011;35:16–24.
4. Lacey K, Pritchett E. Nutrition care process and model: ADA adopts road map to quality care and outcomes management. *J Am Diet Assoc* 2003;103:1061–1072.
5. Nutrition Care Process/Standardized Language Committee. American Dietetic Association. Nutrition care process and model part I: The 2008 update. *J Am Diet Assoc* 2008;108:1113–1117.
6. Guigoz Y. The mini-nutrition assessment (MNA®) review of the literature—What does it tell us? *J Nutr Health Aging* 2006;10:466–487.
7. Cereda E. Mini nutritional assessment. *Curr Opin Clin Nutr Metab Care* 2012;15:29–41.
8. MNA® Mini-Nutritional Assessment. Nestlé Nutrition Institute. http://www.mna-elderly.com/. Published 2013, accessed November 13, 2013.
9. Detsky AS, McLaughlin JR, Baker JP et al. What is subjective global assessment of nutritional status? *J Parenter Enteral Nutr* 1987;11:8–13.
10. Day LN. Subjective global assessment: Fundamentals of a powerful technique. *Support Line* 2004;26:3–7.
11. Makhija S, Baker J. The subjective global assessment: A review of its use in clinical practice. *Nutr Clin Pract* 2008;23:405–409.
12. Malone A, Hamilton C. The Academy of Nutrition and Dietetics/The American Society for Parenteral and Enteral Nutrition Consensus Malnutrition Characteristics: Application in practice. *Nutr Clin Pract* 2013;28:639–650.
13. Jensen GL et al. Adult starvation and disease-related malnutrition: A proposal for etiology-based diagnosis in the clinical practice setting from the International Consensus Guideline Committee. *JPEN J Parenter Enteral Nutr* 2010;34:156–159.
14. White J et al. The Academy Malnutrition Workgroup; the A.S.P.E.N. Malnutrition Task Force; and the A.S.P.E.N. Board of Directors. Consensus Statement of the Academy of Nutrition and Dietetics/American Society for Parenteral and Enteral Nutrition: Characteristics recommended for the identification and documentation of adult malnutrition (undernutrition). *J Acad Nutr Diet* 2012;112:730–738.
15. Jensen GL, Hsiao PY, Wheeler D. Adult nutrition assessment tutorial. *JPEN J Parenter Enteral Nutr* 2012;36:267–274.
16. Jensen GL, Bistrian B, Roubenoff R, Heimburger DC. Malnutrition syndromes: A conundrum vs. continuum. *JPEN J Parenter Enteral Nutr* 2009;33:710–716.
17. Pogatshnik C, Hamilton C. Nutrition-focused physical examination (NFPE): Skin, nails, hair, eyes, and oral cavity. *Support Line* 2011;33:7–13.
18. Moccia L, DeChicco R. Abdominal examinations: A guide for dietitians. *Support Line.* 2011;33:16–21.

19. Global Database on Body Mass Index. BMI classification. The Word Health Organization. http://apps.who.int/bmi/index.jsp?introPage=intro_3.html. Published November 2013, accessed November 26, 2013.

20. Eaton CB, McBride PE, Gans KA, Underbakke GL. Teaching nutrition skills to primary care practitioners. *J Nutr* 2003;133:563S–566S.

21. Gans KM, Risica PM, Wylie-Rosett J, Ross EM, Strolla LO, McMurray J, Eaton CB. Development and evaluation of the nutrition component of the rapid eating and activity assessment for patients (REAP): A new tool for primary care providers. *J Nutr Educ Behav* 2006;38:286–292.

22. Gans KM, Ross E, Barner CW, Wylie-Rosett J, McMurray J, Eaton C. REAP and WAVE: New tools to rapidly assess/discuss nutrition with patients. *J Nutr* 2003;133:556S–562S.

23. *International Dietetics and Nutrition Terminology (IDNT) Reference Manual: Standardized Language for the Nutrition Care Process*, 4th Ed. Academy of Nutrition and Dietetics, Chicago, IL, 2012.

24. Dietary Guidelines for Americans, 2010. http://www.health.gov/dietaryguidelines/dga2010/DietaryGuidelines2010.pdf. The U.S. Department of Agriculture; the U.S. Department of Health and Human Services; 2010 Dietary Guidelines Committee. Published January2011, accessed November 12, 2013.

25. Dietary Reference Intakes Tables. The U.S. Department of Agriculture. National Agriculture Library. Food and Nutrition Information Center. Published 2010, accessed November 12, 2013.

26. Academy of Nutrition and Dietetics Evidence Analysis Library. Evidenced-based nutrition practice guidelines. http://andevidencelibrary.com/category.cfm?cid=14&cat=0. Published 2013, accessed November 12, 2013.

27. Cawood A et al. Systematic review and meta-analysis of the effects of high protein oral nutritional supplements. *Ageing Res Rev* 2012;11:278–296.

28. Academy of Nutrition and Dietetics Evidence Analysis Library. How effective is MNT provided by Registered Dietitians in the management of type 1 and type 2 diabetes? http://andevidencelibrary.com/conclusion.cfm?conclusion_statement_id=250595. Published 2013, accessed January 9, 2014.

29. Academy of Nutrition and Dietetics. http://www.eatright.org. Published 2013, accessed December 1, 2013.

30. American Society for Parenteral and Enteral Nutrition. http://www.nutritioncare.org. Published 2013, accessed December 1, 2013.

31. Research Tools and Resources. Brown University, Institute for Community Health Promotion. http://www.brown.edu/academics/public-health/centers/community-health-promotion/research-tools-and-resources. Published 2005, accessed January 13, 2014.

32. Alliance to Advance Patient Nutrition. http://malnutrition.com. Published 2013, accessed January 13, 2014.

2 Integrative Medicine

Roberta Lee, MD, CaC

CONTENTS

FOOD, NUTRITION, AND HEALTH IN MEDICINE

The role of food and its relationship to health is as old as the healing arts. Examine any ancient traditional medical system such as Ayurveda or Chinese medicine and you will find a likely list of specific foods and herbs as part of the therapy plan. Nutrition is central to health. Even in western medicine, Hippocrates, considered the father of medicine, reflects his high esteem for food in the role of health in his quotes "let food be thy medicine and let medicine be thy food" and "Leave your drugs in the chemist's pot if you can heal the patient with food." Despite these deep philosophical roots on the role of nutrition in health as science became more reductionistic nutrition was marginalized. In 1962 [1], the Council on Foods and Nutrition devoted a conference to grapple with the problems of nutritional teaching in medical training. At that time, clinical literature was beginning to link the role of diet in disease prevention and the formation of chronic diseases with poor dietary choices. Yet, medical training focused on rarely seen nutritional deficiencies. Fifty years later, in 2010, a study analyzing nutritional training in U.S. medical schools documented that little had changed with respect to nutritional education medical training. The share of schools requiring a dedicated course in nutrition was down from 27% in 1985 [2] to 25% with the average amount of nutritional course work reduced from 21 to 19.6 h [3]. In June 2014, the debate over the paucity of nutritional education continues as Nathaniel Morris, a medical student at Harvard Medical School, in a *Journal of the American Medical Association* (*JAMA*) commentary, worries that the limited training that he is receiving will not be enough to address the dietary challenges his patients will present when he finally becomes a practicing clinician [4]. In answer to Morris's commentary, Nestle and Brown in the *JAMA* invited commentary to broaden the context of the problem surrounding the needs of medical education and nutrition:

> Learning the basic biochemical, metabolic and clinical facts about nutrition is necessary but not sufficient. Medical students and residents must also develop competence in the interpersonal and communication skills needed to counsel patient about behavior change and to perform motivational interviewing ... They must learn to work in inter-professional teams with dieticians and other skilled health professionals. Just as medical students and residents must be taught to become antismoking advocates, they need to be taught to how to advocate for a healthier food environment as part of their role as future physician-citizens. [5]

Similarly, in the September 2014 issue of *The American Journal of Medicine*, leading academic educators of integrative medicine comment on the schism between the public's view of its physicians [6] as sources of "very credible sources" of nutritional information (61%) [7] and the percentage of medical residents feeling adequately trained in nutrition (14%) [8].

PUBLIC INTEREST IN COMPLEMENTARY AND ALTERNATIVE MEDICINE AND CHANGE IN MEDICAL EDUCATION

The 1960s were a pivotal time in American culture. Environmental awareness and novel healing systems different from mainstream medicine captured the public's interest and created a powerful consumer-driven economic movement focused on a more natural approach to health and medicine. The public turned to many new or alternative medical techniques and systems for self-care. By the early 1990s public demand for a better patient–provider relationship, and more humanistic and natural approach to treating health and chronic disease, was finally evident to the medical community. A groundbreaking study published in the *New England Journal of Medicine* in 1993 revealed that $13 billion a year was being spent out of pocket by the public on complementary and alternative medical care [9]. Subsequent studies demonstrated that the public trend was continuing. This made the medical community realize it was ill prepared to advise patients on the risks or benefits in any meaningful evidence-based way.

Government health agencies began to address the gap by creating the Office of Alternative Medicine in 1993. It was started with a paltry budget of $2 million (of $80 billion annual budget). By 2010, the office was upgraded to become the National Center for Complementary and Alternative Medicine (NCCAM) and its budget grew to $127 million. At the same time as academic awareness grew, it became evident that a new evidence-based approach was needed to train physicians more about complementary and alternative (CAM) practices that were not part of the American medical training.

INTEGRATIVE MEDICINE EMERGES AS A NEW MEDICAL EDUCATION MODEL

To answer the medical education gap in CAM, Andrew Weil, a Harvard-trained physician and educator, founded a new medical education to introduce education in CAM at the University of Arizona in 1997. The curriculum was designed to incorporate conventional medical practices with CAM and he defined this model as integrative medicine (IM). Similarly, within a 2-year period a national organization known as the Consortium for Academic Health Centers for Integrative Medicine (CAHCIM) was founded in 1999. CAHCIM's mission was and continues to be to bring medical institutions together who are committed to including integrative medicine teachings into its medical school curriculum. CAHCIM started out with 11 members and is now comprised of 57 members, including some Canadian and Latin American participants. Through this collaboration a universal definition of integrative medicine has been developed:

> Integrative Medicine is the practice of medicine that reaffirms the importance of the relationship between practitioner and patient, focuses on the whole person, is informed by evidence, and makes use of all appropriate therapeutic approaches, healthcare professionals and disciplines to achieve optimal health and healing. [10]

To date, despite 20 years of evolution in forging a new IM training model, a seamless integration of the core principles of IM in medical school has not been achieved. Rather IM exists in small modules much as nutritional education exists in the medical school curriculum. However, core competencies in IM for medical school have been proposed [11]. Nevertheless, comprehensive integrative training at the postdoctoral level has flourished. In addition to the University of Arizona's Center for Integrative Medicine IM fellowship, many members of CAHCIM have postdoctoral fellowships in IM. The types of fellowships are varied from those focused on research to those designed for IM primary care.

PRINCIPLES OF INTEGRATIVE MEDICINE

The principles of IM encompass a whole person approach that has been defined by its founder Andrew Weil [12] as including the following:

1. Patient and practitioner are partners in the healing process.
2. All factors that influence health, wellness, and disease are taken into consideration, including mind, spirit, and community, as well as the body.
3. Appropriate use of both conventional and alternative methods facilitates the body's innate healing response.
4. Effective interventions that are natural and less invasive should be used whenever possible.
5. Integrative medicine neither rejects conventional medicine nor accepts alternative therapies uncritically.
6. Good medicine is based in good science. It is inquiry-driven and open to new paradigms.
7. Alongside the concept of treatment, the broader concepts of health promotion and the prevention of illness are paramount.
8. Practitioners of integrative medicine should exemplify its principles and commit themselves to self-exploration and self-development.

The overarching goal of IM has not been a new one—to provide effective high quality of care to its patients. At the very core of IM principles lies the philosophy that the most pivotal cornerstones of focus between patient and healthcare practitioner is a collaboration that addresses healthy lifestyle practices including diet, nutrition, exercise, stress reduction, and so forth. The IM model has extended the tools of healthcare providers not only in knowledge of CAM and training in evaluation of evidence for its use but also in increasing new skills. IM education includes the evaluation of and techniques in more effective methods of communication (motivational interviewing and teaching), as well as familiarity with and the ability to educate patients on the use of techniques in stress reduction, other mind/body practices, and CAM modalities.

Terms describing a whole person approach have changed as the movement to accommodate CAM into the mainstream medical model evolved. Initially the IM approach was commonly referred to as alternative, complementary, and alternative or holistic with little awareness of any distinction between these terms. However, though these terms share the objective to implement practices into healthcare that are not commonly taught in U.S. medical schools and are whole person oriented, they do not necessarily require an evidence-based analysis to evaluate whether these other practices are scientifically sound enough to be implemented in an IM approach. The IM philosophy is a synthesis of both worlds neither rejecting conventional medicine nor accepting alternative therapies uncritically.

Embedded in the IM approach is the belief that IM practitioners should strive to act as advocates for patients and the health needs of society. There is also an expectation within the IM community that practitioners themselves will aspire to live and model the philosophy they teach to their patients. With respect to nutrition this means the IM practitioner is encouraged to educate, motivate, and empower his or her patients to make sound and healthy food choices while doing the same themselves! Additionally, in this whole person approach, it should be noted that while it is important to select high-quality nutritious foods, the context of how foods are prepared, whether the foods are savored, and the presence or lack of important cultural social rituals are of equal importance.

Over the 20 years that the IM approach has come into being as a whole person model for medical training, new areas of science have emerged. Areas of neuroscience, psychoneuroimmunology, epigenetics, and genetics have helped to flesh out the connections in health that previously seemed plausible to address but whose mechanisms were not well understood—especially in the area of mind and body medicine and the impact of environment on health. Much of this new-found knowledge has underscored the complex nature in human health and disease. For example, one recent study by Kiecolt-Glaser, a long-time researcher in the field of psychoneuroimmunology and stress, has shown how a Mediterranean diet could possibly be protective in preventing depression [13]. Kiecolt-Glaser suggests that the pro-inflammatory influences of chronic psychosocial stress and depression in combination with poor diets (also pro-inflammatory) have more than additive negative inflammatory effects. The physiologic state of chronic stress creates maladaptive cellular responses to the metabolism that amplifies poor food processing (e.g., delayed gastric emptying, abnormal intestinal absorption, exaggerated post-prandial hyperlipidemia) resulting in excessive oxidative stress. She illustrates how much of this negative synergism is facilitated by the inhibition of the vagal activation that would naturally rebalance and downregulate inflammatory responses in a timely fashion [14]. The end result of this perfect unfortunate inflammatory storm is increased and prolonged inflammation that is the common link among all leading causes of death. However, we know that many modalities known in mind/body medicine facilitate noninvasive vagal stimulation that can reduce the physiologic damage of chronic stress [15]. Thus mind/body practices if strategically implemented in an integrated care plan—in this case for a nutritional issue—could be a plausible antidote. Given this information, Kiecolt-Glaser's comprehensive perspective increases the necessity for practitioners and policy makers to create a more conducive environment to change behavior for better nutritional outcomes. This plan would need to include resilience, coping, and stress reduction training.

Since people are known to make poor dietary choices while stressed and stressed states amplify untoward physiological outcomes in health, it makes sense that an integrative medicine practitioner (or other whole person–oriented practitioner) skilled in motivational interviewing, stress reduction while having a deeper base of nutritional knowledge would be the appropriate healthcare practitioner to effectively coach patients out of this unfortunate conundrum.

GASTROINTESTINAL INFLUENCES ON HEALTH, NEW AREAS OF SCIENCE, AND FUNCTIONAL MEDICINE

The role of digestion with respect to an integrative approach to health represents an area of IM that integrates known areas of basic science research that have been slow to enter into clinical practice. It is estimated that more than two million Americans are affected in some way by digestive system–related illnesses. Digestive diseases are the second leading cause of disability due to illness in the United States with an economic impact on the U.S. economy that is more than $141 billion [16]. From an IM framework, beyond the analysis of food quality and its psychosocial impact, further concerns focused at the microscopic and intracellular level have become increasingly important in ways that we could not have imagined. We have understood for several decades how much the quality and type of gastrointestinal organisms within our digestive system impacts on our ability to metabolize foods. But until recently we had not anticipated that the gut brain axis also could be modified to reduce anxiety, depression, and attention deficit disorder [17]. Stool analysis is one of the many ways in which this problem is analyzed. There are other areas of health that represent other new areas of science to uncover root causes of disease and health. The initial source of these aspects of care identified as a functional medicine approach are derived from applied clinical biochemistry initially developed by Jeffery Bland, PhD, a biochemist himself who worked with Dr. Linus Pauling for many years [18]. Around the same time Weil developed integrative medicine, Bland realized much of what he was teaching medical students in the basic science years was being lost in their clinical training. Worst still doctors were focused on disease identification leaving behind analyzing primary causes of these events unique to each patient. Functional medicine is also inclusive of modalities and practices not initially taught in U.S. medical schools. It is science based and is integrative but has a special focus on incorporating the latest in genetic science, systems biology, and environmental factors. It represents another "face" of analysis of whole person care that seeks to transform disease and maintain health. It is beyond the purview of this chapter to cover this area in more depth but more information can be accessed on the Institute of Functional Medicine's website (www.functionalmedicine.org) [18].

CONCLUSION

Now more than ever, new ways to educate and manage nutrition-related illnesses such as obesity, diabetes, and heart disease are needed especially as these diseases reach epidemic proportions. The Centers for Disease Control and Prevention now estimates that one in three U.S. adults are obese with a cost of $147 billion annually to manage the problem [19]. These trends and their effects on healthcare and healthcare expenditures are compelling arguments for accelerating the role of nutritional education in medical education as well as in the clinical arena. Furthermore, with new evidence on the complexity of how nutrition and disease affect the body, most notably in the areas of the mind/body axis, gastrointestinal microbiome, and environment, it makes sense that a twenty-first-century approach will require a whole person approach open to multidisciplinary collaboration, rooted in science, and open to all therapeutic interventions that promote healing. Integrative medicine, functional medicine, and other modalities and medical systems willing to apply these principles represent the next iteration of future healthcare approaches that will most effectively transform healthcare, protect health, and promote true healing.

REFERENCES

1. Council on Foods and Nutrition. Nutrition teaching in medical schools. *JAMA.* 1963;183(11):955–957.
2. National Academy of Science. *Nutrition Education in US Medical Schools.* Washington, DC: National Academy Press, 1985.
3. Adams KM, Kohlmeier M, Zeisel S. Nutrition education in U.S. medical schools: Latest update of a national survey. *Acad Med.* 2010;85(9):1537–1542.
4. Morris NP. The neglect of nutrition in medical education: A firsthand look. *JAMA Intern Med.* 2014;174(6):841–842.
5. Nestle M, Baron R. Nutrition in medical education: From counting hours to measuring competence. *JAMA Intern Med.* 2014;174(6):843–844.
6. Devries S, Dalen J, Eisenberg D, Maizes V, Ornish D et al. A deficiency of nutrition education in medical training. *Am J Med.* 2014;127(9):804–806.
7. American Dietetic Association. Nutrition and you: Trends 2008. Available at http://www.eatright.org/WorkArea/Downtown Asset.aspx?id=644245139. Accessed September 27, 2014.
8. Vetter ML, Herring SJ, Sood M, Shah NR, Kalet AL. What do residents physicians know about nutrition? An evaluation of attitudes, self-perceived proficiency and knowledge. *J Am Coll Nutr.* 2008;27(2):287–298.
9. Eisenberg DM, Kessler RC, Foster C, Norlock FE, Calkins DR et al. Unconventional medicine in the United States—Prevalence, costs, and patterns of use. *N Engl J Med.* 1993;328(4):246–252.

10. Consortium for Academic Health Centers for Integrative Medicine. Definition of integrative medicine, 2014. Available at http://www.imconsortium.org/about/home.html. Accessed September 14, 2014.

11. Kligler BL, Maizes V, Schachter S, Park CM, Gaudet T, Benn R, Lee R, Remen RN. Education Working Group, Consortium of Academic Health Centers for Integrative Medicine. *Acad Med.* 2004;79(6):521–531.

12. Center for Integrative Medicine. The University of Arizona, Tucson, AZ. http://integrativemedicine.arizona.edu/about/definition.html. Accessed October 4, 2014.

13. Sanchez-Villegas A, Delgado-Rodríguez M, Alonso A, Schlatter J, Lahortiga F, Majem LS, Martínez-González MA. Association of the Mediterranean Dietary Pattern With the Incidence of Depression: The Seguimiento Universidad de Navarra/University of Navarra Follow-up (SUN) Cohort. *Arch Gen Psychiatry.* 2009;66(10):1090–1098.

14. Kiecolt-Glaser J. Stress, food and inflammation: Psychoneuroimmunology and nutrition at the cutting edge. *Psychosom Med.* 2010;72(4):365–369.

15. Clancy J, Mary D, Witte K, Greenwood J, Deuchars J. Non-invasive vagus nerve stimulation in healthy humans reduces sympathetic nerve activity. *Brain Stimul.* 2014;7(6):871–877.

16. Mullin G. Why integrative gastroenterology? In: Mullin G. ed. *Integrative Gastroenterology.* New York: Oxford Press, 2011 pp. 3–12.

17. Foster JA, McVey Neufeld KA. Gut-brain axis: How the microbiome influences anxiety and depression. *Trends Neurosci.* 2013;36:305–312.

18. Institute of Functional Medicine. Digital Millennium Copyright Act ("DMCA") notice, Federal Way, WA. Available at: www.functionalmedicine.org. Accessed October 4, 2014.

19. Centers for Disease Control and Prevention. Obesity facts. Available at http://www.cdc.gov/obesity/data/adult.html. Accessed October 4, 2014.

3 Searching for the Optimal Diet
Which Is Best?

*Danielle Flug Capalino, MSPH, RD
and Gerard E. Mullin, MD*

CONTENTS

INTRODUCTION

In this chapter, we present diets that have made headlines, and the latest science that looks at the important questions—Do these diets work? What are the outcomes? We are your guides on the search for the dietary "holy grail"—a diet that is sustainable to eat for a lifetime, promotes long life, keeps us lean, and tastes good too. We will review the rationale and evidence for the diets that you might have tried, and that your patients ask about, to provide you with the most up-to-date answer to the question we all want to know: *What should we be eating?*

Our Paleolithic ancestors did not have the option of opening up a refrigerator, or even a pantry, to decide what to eat for dinner. We emerged from a lineage of hunter-gatherers (HGs), who ate what was available, when it was available, out of necessity for survival. With the explosion of the field of food science, our grocery stores now have literally hundreds of thousands of products available 24 h a day, and we are left with big questions—*What should we eat to optimize our health and well-being? How can we choose a diet to stay slim and look and feel our very best?*

Every year, there are hundreds of new diet books on the market that make a wide range of promises about what we should be eating, and because consumers are always looking for the newest, latest, and greatest diet, these books continue to top the bestsellers lists. You cannot walk past a bookstore or magazine stand without seeing a claim for the *best* new diet—and it gets confusing for consumers and even health professionals to make sense of all of the claims, especially when they seem to contradict each other, seemingly diametrically opposed at times.

Because many of these meal plans are not sustainable, or even questionable in their approaches, the consumer is ultimately left to continue their search guided by publicists rather than scientists. Thus, the search for the optimal diet continues to be the "holy grail" for many of us today, presenting a challenge for nutritionists and practitioners to provide sound advice to consumers.

STANDARD AMERICAN DIET

Let us start by looking at what most Americans are currently eating. We are well aware that the typical American diet has rapidly digressed from its reliance on foods we could catch and kill, or grow, to foods that are highly processed and last for long periods of time on store shelves. Our Western-based Standard American Diet (aptly abbreviated SAD) has rapidly devolved into a processed, refined, and less nutritious selection of foods. The rising of epidemic chronic-degenerative diseases since the 1950s parallels the increase in our consumption of daily caloric intake via refined grains, sugars, trans-fats, fast foods, and high-energy dense snacks. As a society our Western-based SAD with its inherent low intake of foods that have been associated with preventing and fighting degenerative diseases (i.e., fruits, vegetables, whole-grains)[1,2] runs countercurrent with science-based recommended dietary guidelines.[3–5] Overall, clever marketing, taste appeal, availability, and affordability of fast foods drive the aforementioned consumption of the SAD.

PALEOLITHIC DIET

There has been much media attention in the past several years given to this diet, which mimics that of our Paleolithic or "hunter-gatherer" ancestors. To use the definition from Loren Cordain's widely popular book *The Paleo Diet*, the diet is comprised of lean meats, fruits and vegetables, nuts, and seeds—it excludes grains, dairy, and legumes entirely.[6] Early work on this subject came from Konner and Eaton's landmark review of a "Paleolithic" diet that they associated with optimal health, and a 2010 follow-up to the study reaffirming the validity of the model initially presented based on more current research.[7,8] Their original observations are that societies that adopt a "caveman" or "hunter-gatherer" diet has sparse obesity, type 2 diabetes mellitus (T2DM), and cardiovascular disease. It is important to note how the Paleolithic diet was defined in this research because of the original 50 tribes that were studied, diets varied considerably based on location—but in general are "very low in refined carbohydrates and sodium, much higher levels of fiber and protein, and comparable levels of fat (primarily unsaturated fat) and cholesterol" to our modern-day SAD.

A major critique of this diet has been its *perceived* recommendation of high red meat consumption that appears to contradict the known harmful effects of ingesting animal flesh on cardiovascular health. However, the sources of animal protein for HGs are game animals (i.e., deer, bison, horses, and mammoths), which have more mono- and polyunsaturated fatty acids (MUFA and PUFA) than the domesticated meat we find in supermarkets—even if it is grass fed.[9] One claim to address the weight disparity between our ancestors and us is that despite the higher consumption of macronutrients by HGs, the heavy exercise that was required in order to procure enough food for family and tribe made obesity rare in primitive times.[10] However, there are a plethora of claims aside from lifting boulders that can attribute for the disparity in weight between us and our HG predecessors.

Studies have looked both retrospectively at what happens to communities that change from HG to a modern diet as well as intervention studies looking at outcomes from introducing an HG diet. In one epidemiological study, tribes such as the Australian Aborigines who have abandoned their HG diets have been shown to have decreased cardiovascular diseases and diabetes when they return to the HG diet and lifestyle.[11]

The therapeutic effect of the Paleolithic diet has been tested in a scientific model as well. A randomized controlled trial of 29 patients with ischemic heart disease and either glucose intolerance or T2DM were randomized to 12 weeks of a "Paleolithic" (i.e., lean meat, fish, fruit, vegetables, root vegetables, eggs, and nuts) or a Mediterranean-like "consensus" diet based on whole grains, low-fat dairy products, vegetables, fruits, fish, oils, and margarines. The Paleolithic group showed an improved glucose control and a greater decrease in waist circumference when compared to the consensus group.[12]

Fifteen patients with T2DM were randomized to either a Paleolithic diet or a diabetes diet then crossed over after 3 months.[13] Subjects were on each diet for 3 months. Compared to the diabetes diet, the Paleolithic diet produced lower mean levels of hemoglobin A1C, triacylglycerol, diastolic BP, weight, body mass index (BMI), and waist circumference and higher mean high-density lipoprotein (HDL).

Whether the Paleolithic diet will become a suitable "prescriptive" alternative remains to be determined by more extensive studies on a larger number of subjects.

VEGETARIAN DIET

One of the most popular "healthy" diets in today's Western culture and arguably worldwide is a vegetarian diet. Vegetarianism is a plant-based diet that may vary from being exclusive of all animal products (i.e., vegan), include dairy (i.e., lacto-vegetarianism), or dairy and eggs as a protein source (i.e., lacto-ovo-vegetarianism).

A number of studies have demonstrated that a plant-based diet (fruits, vegetables, whole-grains, legumes, nuts, and various soy products) promotes improved cardiovascular health and blood glucose regulation. Vegetarians typically have a lower body mass index, lower total and low-density lipoprotein cholesterol levels, lower rates of death from ischemic heart disease, lower blood pressure, lower rates of hypertension and stroke, a lower incidence of obesity and T2DM, and certain cancers than do nonvegetarians.[14] On a macronutrient level, these health-promoting benefits have been ascribed to a diet with a relatively low intake of saturated fat, high dietary fiber, and many health-promoting phytochemicals.

VEGAN DIET

As mentioned earlier, a vegan diet is the strictest form of vegetarianism where all animal products are excluded entirely. A recent meta-analysis of over 1500 participants on a low-fat (≤10% of calories), high-carbohydrate (~80% of calories), moderate-sodium, purely plant-based diet ad libitum for 7 days indicated that predicted risk markers of cardiovascular disease and metabolic disease were significantly reduced by only 1 week on this diet. The results indicated that the participants lost weight (median 3 lb) and improved blood pressure, blood lipids, and blood sugar levels.[15]

In one randomized controlled trial of dietary intervention with a vegan diet, 93 early-stage prostate cancer patients were assigned to a very-low-fat (10% fat) vegan diet and lifestyle changes or to usual care. Diets were monitored for changes at baseline and at 1 year after the intervention. The results showed that diets in the intervention group had significantly increased many protective dietary factors (including fiber increase from a mean of 31 to 59 g/day) and significantly decreased intake of most pathogenic dietary factors (e.g., saturated fatty acids decreased from 20 to 5 g/day and cholesterol decreased from 200 to 10 mg/day) in the intervention compared to controls. These changes are thought to improve diet to reduce the risk of disease and show that it is manageable and sustainable to make long-term changes toward a vegan diet.[16]

Like any health practice that is restrictive, there are potential pitfalls and concerns. Due to the exclusion of animal and fish protein sources, vegetarians may require supplementation with vitamin B12 and D, omega-3 fatty acids, iron, zinc, and calcium or else run the risk of deficiency. Those vegetarians who restrict dairy should supplement with calcium and vitamin D to maintain bone health among other benefits.[17]

LOW-CARBOHYDRATE DIET

A low-carbohydrate diet can take many shapes and sizes. Though the term conjures up thoughts of Dr. Atkins' diet and the cheeseburger with no bun, a low-carbohydrate diet might also be a diet without refined grains that does include lots of highly soluble fiber vegetables. Intuition and clinical experience suggest that in the realm of low carbohydrate, there are healthy and unhealthy ways to go about it. However, much of the literature does not consider components of the diet outside of the percentage of macronutrients assigned.

A recent randomized controlled trial of 148 healthy adults sought to test a low-carbohydrate diet (less than 40 g/day net minus fiber) versus a low-fat diet (less than 30% of total daily calories from fat, less than 7% saturated fat) and look at weight and cardiovascular risk factors as outcomes. After 1 year, the low-carbohydrate diet compared with the low-fat diet correlated with better body composition, HDL cholesterol level, ratio of total-HDL cholesterol, triglyceride level, CRP level, and estimated 10-year risk of coronary artery disease.[18] It is interesting to note that fiber intake slightly *decreased* throughout the study in both groups, begging the question about dietary composition of the low-carbohydrate diet.

LOW-FAT DIET

There is much overlap between a low-fat diet and the vegetarian/vegan diets, should the diets be conducted in a responsible way. While one can certainly eat potato chips on a vegan diet, if it is done healthfully, then it will likely also be a low-fat diet.

In the preceding section, we reviewed an important recent randomized study on low-carbohydrate and low-fat diets. Interestingly, the threshold that the investigators used to identify a "low fat" diet, was not particularly different from the participants baseline. In fact if you look at the baseline characteristics of the people put on a low-fat diet (less than 30% caloric intake), they started out on average with 34.7% caloric intake from fat—in other words, this was not a significant dietary intervention when looking at the fat content. For that reason, the study does give a representation of effects from a low-carbohydrate diet, but not from a low-fat diet.

Dean Ornish has been a pioneer in the field of low-fat diets in the treatment of heart disease. With a landmark paper in the Lancet, "Can Lifestyle Changes Reverse Coronary Heart Disease," the team showed a resounding "yes" to that question with a vegetarian diet (less than 10% of calories from fat) plus other lifestyle measures (smoking cessation, stress management, exercise). The results showed that patients were motivated to continue the lifestyle changes throughout the yearlong study. The participants' lipid levels were lowered as would be expected with lipid lowering medications. Improvements were also demonstrated measurably with arteriography.[19] It is not possible to isolate the low-fat component of the intervention from other lifestyle interventions, but the efficacy and adherence are robust.

GLUTEN-FREE DIET

It seems remiss not to include a mention of a gluten-free diet in a chapter about searching for the "holy grail" in diet and health. In recent years, gluten free has become the biggest diet craze in history. Though individuals with celiac disease have a medical necessity to follow a 100% gluten-free diet, there is increasing evidence that individuals with non-celiac gluten sensitivity (NCGS) benefit as well. Though these people may have found their "holy grail" by eliminating gluten (and in many cases also dairy), this is not necessarily an optimal diet for the population at large. There have been no controlled trials to date (that we are aware of) looking at the safety or efficacy of long-term gluten-free diets for health or weight control in individuals without celiac disease.

MACROBIOTIC DIET

Though the macronutrient foundation of this diet is mainly whole grains with plant-based carbohydrates and protein, its principal tenet is person-centered, whereby the focus is on lifestyle adherence and spirituality. Another distinguishing feature is the built-in flexibility that allows variation based upon health status, gender, age, etc. The present-day culture of eating local, organic, and seasonal stems from this Eastern (Japanese)-based way of life.[20] Foods that are encouraged include beans, lentils, brown rice, sea vegetables (i.e., seaweed), and miso soup. Though used by many alternative practitioners as an adjunct to cancer therapy, no studies to date have successfully demonstrated an impact of this diet upon its outcome in a controlled clinical trial.[21] The most well-publicized study using the macrobiotic diet was the China Study. Individuals from rural China following a macrobiotic diet, compared to subjects living in the United States, were reported to consume one-third less daily fat, 10 times less animal protein, and 3 times more fiber with profoundly less cardiovascular disease (5.6- to 16.7-fold).[22] Factors aside from diet (i.e., spirituality, stress reduction, etc.) may play a key role as was previously noted in the Paleolithic diet (i.e., exercise).

NUTRITIONAL GENOMICS

A newly emerging concept in the search for the "holy grail" is nutritional genomics, the study of how foods affect our genes.[23] Scientific investigation into the influence of nutrients upon gene expression commenced over 70 years ago. Food can influence genetic expression without altering the sequence of DNA by chromatin remodeling, DNA methylation, genomic imprinting, or RNA interference (RNAi).[24] The human genome has changed little over the past 40–50,000 years but diet and morphology barely resemble our ancestors. In terms of the scientific advances in understanding the effects of nutritional genomics with the goal of creating personalized medicine— a diet that is designed to allow your genetics to be best expressed—there is still a tremendous amount of research needed.

ANTI-INFLAMMATORY DIET

The availability of serum markers of inflammation (notably highly sensitive-C-reactive protein, or HS-CRP) has permitted scientific investigation into the mechanism of action of specific food-derived nutrients upon inflammation.[25] The anti-inflammatory or Mediterranean diet is composed largely of fruits and vegetables but includes nuts and fish (rich in omega-3 fatty acids), berries and red wine (antioxidants), and limits red meat (saturated fat). When compared to the SAD, the anti-inflammatory diet is low in the glycemic index and glycemic impact and has a higher fiber content that was shown in the Women's Health study to lower inflammatory markers.[26] Furthermore, the higher omega-3 fatty acids have been demonstrated to lower multiple serum markers (i.e., HS-CRP), prevent cardiovascular disease, and improve T2DM.[27,28] Numerous studies have evaluated the impact of anti-inflammatory foods upon inflammatory markers, the prevention of degenerative diseases (i.e., cardiovascular disease, cancer, Alzheimer's disease), and the variation in response by specific cultures (i.e., Mediterranean vs. non-Mediterranean). Diets that are high in fruits and vegetables have been shown across cultures (i.e., Western vs. non-Western) and ages (i.e., adults vs. children) to reduce inflammatory markers.[29] Micronutrients in the anti-inflammatory diet that may play an important role in controlling inflammation include omega-3 fatty acids, polyphenols (i.e., resveratrol), magnesium, calcium, monounsaturated fatty acids (i.e., oleic acid, olive oil, avocado), fiber, flavonoids, and carotenoids.

CONCLUSIONS

There is a vast array of diets in the lay and scientific literature for practitioners and consumers to consider in formulating a food-based wellness plan. Though many of the diets that receive hype seem like they are complete opposites, when you get down to the details they are quite similar. None of the diets that we analyzed promote processed or sugar-laden foods. Responsible forms of each diet—from Vegan to Paleolithic—should contain healthy fats, lean proteins, and lots of plants. The foundation of all diets should be whole foods with ingredient names that you can pronounce. Animal protein sources, if included, should be rich in omega-3 fatty acids while low in saturated fat. Given what we know today, the best diet we can prescribe is intuitive, as said by Michael Pollan and summed up in a recent review: "Eat food. Not too much. Mostly plants."[30]

However, nutritional genomics is an emerging field that accounts in part for the diversity of responses to food among individuals. It is likely that diets are like shoes; one size does not fit all. Our microbiomes—the bacteria that make up the bulk of our cells—are in part responsible for digesting and metabolizing our food, and with unique microbial compositions, we are just beginning to understand the individual implications for how this factors into the emerging science of personalized nutrition. Further investigation of these diets in the prevention and treatment of illness according to disease and genetic background of the individual will help practitioners apply the science to their client's health and well-being. It may in fact be the "holy grail" that we are searching for.

Type of Diet	What It Entails	Research Evidence
Standard American Diet	Processed and refined carbohydrates, high in saturated fats.	The SAD has paralleled the obesity epidemic in the United States.
Paleolithic diet	Lean meats, fruits and vegetables, nuts and seeds. Excludes grains, dairy, and legumes.	Epidemiological evidence that the diet correlates with reduced cardiovascular disease (CVD) and T2DM. Intervention studies show weight, lipid, and glucose control.
Vegetarian diet	Plant-based diet exclusive of animals.	Numerous studies show beneficial health effects ranging from better glucose control to lower incidence of T2DM.
Vegan diet	Plant-based diet exclusive of all animal products including eggs and dairy.	Improved glucose, lipids, and weight control.
Low-carbohydrate diet	Limited proportion of carbohydrate; in one clinical trial defined as less than 40 g.	Improved weight control, lipid levels, CVD risk, and inflammatory markers.
Low-fat diet	Ranging in definition from less than 30% of calories to less than 10% of calories from fat.	Improved CVD factors and improved arteriography.
Gluten-free diet	Diet exclusive of the protein gluten, which is found in wheat, barley, rye, and derivatives.	Only known treatment for Celiac disease is 100% gluten-free diet. No research on benefits for general population.

(Continued)

Type of Diet	What It Entails	Research Evidence
Macrobiotic diet	Whole grains with plant-based carbohydrates and protein; lifestyle and spiritual components.	No benefits demonstrated in clinical trials.
Nutritional genomics	Personalized diet based on individual genome.	Research ongoing.
Anti-inflammatory diet	Limited saturated fat, low glycemic index, high fiber.	Reduction in inflammatory markers, prevention of CVD.

REFERENCES

1. Gross LS, Li L, Ford ES, Liu S. Increased consumption of refined carbohydrates and the epidemic of type 2 diabetes in the United States: An ecologic assessment. *Am J Clin Nutr.* May 2004; 79(5): 774–779.
2. Streppel MT, Ocké MC, Boshuizen HC, Kok FJ, Kromhout D. Dietary fiber intake in relation to coronary heart disease and all-cause mortality over 40 years: The Zutphen Study. *Am J Clin Nutr.* October 2008; 88(4): 1119–1125.
3. U.S. Department of Agriculture and U.S. Department of Health and Human Services. Dietary Guidelines for Americans, 2010. 7th Edn., Washington, DC: U.S. Government Printing Office, December 2010.
4. U.S. Department of Agriculture. ChooseMyPlate.gov Website. Washington, DC. http://www.choosemyplate.gov/. Accessed May 19, 2015.
5. Institute of Medicine. *Dietary Reference Intakes: Energy, Carbohydrate, Fiber, Fat, Fatty Acids, Cholesterol, Protein, and Amino Acids (Macronutrients).* Washington, DC: National Academies Press, 2005.
6. Cordain L. *The Paleo Diet.* New York: Houghton Mifflin, 2011.
7. Eaton SB, Konner M. Paleolithic nutrition: A consideration of its nature and current implications. *New Engl J Med.* 1985; 312: 283–289.
8. Eaton SB, Konner M. Paleolithic nutrition: Twenty-five years later. *Nutr Clin Pract.* December 2010; 25: 594–602.
9. Cordain L, Eaton SB, Miller JB, Mann N, Hill K. The paradoxical nature of hunter-gatherer diets: Meat-based, yet non-atherogenic. *Eur J Clin Nutr.* 2002; 56(Suppl. 1): S42–S52.
10. Cordain L, Miller JB, Eaton SB, Mann N. Macronutrient estimations in hunter-gatherer diets. *Am J Clin Nutr.* 2000; 72(6): 1589–1592.
11. Rowley KG, O'Dea K. Diabetes in Australian aboriginal and Torres Strait Islander peoples. *PNG Med J.* 2001; 44(3–4): 164–170.
12. Jönsson T et al. Beneficial effects of a Paleolithic diet on cardiovascular risk factors in type 2 diabetes: A randomized cross-over pilot study. *Cardiovas Diabetol.* 2009; 8: 35.
13. Jenike MR. Nutritional ecology: Diet, physical activity and body size. In: Panter-Brick C, Layton RH, Rowley-Conway P, eds. *Hunter-Gatherers: An Interdisciplinary Perspective.* Cambridge, U.K.: Cambridge University Press, 2001, pp. 205–238.
14. Craig WJ, Mangels AR. Position of the American Dietetic Association: Vegetarian diets. American Dietetic Association. *J Am Diet Assoc.* July 2009; 109(7): 1266–1282.
15. McDougall J et al. Effects of 7 days on an ad libitum low-fat vegan diet: The McDougall Program cohort. *Nutr J.* 2014; 13(1): 99.
16. Dewell A, Weidner G, Sumner MD, Chi CS, Ornish D. A very-low-fat vegan diet increases intake of protective dietary factors and decreases intake of pathogenic dietary factors. *J Am Diet Assoc.* 2008; 108(2): 347–356.
17. Craig WJ. Health effects of vegan diets. *Am J Clin Nutr.* 2009; 89(5): 1627S–1633S.

18. Bazzano LA et al. Effects of low-carbohydrate and low-fat diets: A randomized trial. *Ann Intern Med.* 2014; 161(5): 309–318.
19. Ornish D et al. Can lifestyle changes reverse coronary heart disease? The lifestyle heart trial. *Lancet.* 1990; 336(8708): 129–133.
20. Kotzsch R. *Macrobiotics Yesterday and Today.* New York: Japan Publications, 1985.
21. Kushi LH, Cunningham JE, Hebert JR, Lerman RH, Bandera EV, Teas J. The macrobiotic diet in cancer. *J Nutr.* November 2001; 131(11 Suppl.): 3056S–3064S.
22. Campbell TC, Parpia B, Chen J. Diet, lifestyle, and the etiology of coronary artery disease: The Cornell China study. *Am J Cardiol.* November 26 1998; 82(10B): 18T–21T.
23. DeBusk R. The role of nutritional genomics in developing an optimal diet for humans. *Nutr Clin Pract.* 2010; 25(6): 627–633.
24. Kauwell GP. Epigenetics: What it is and how it can affect dietetics practice. *J Am Diet Assoc.* 2008; 108(6): 1056–1059.
25. Galland L. Diet and inflammation. *Nutr Clin Pract.* 2010; 25(6): 634–640.
26. Ma Y et al. Association between dietary fiber and markers of systemic inflammation in the Women's Health Initiative Observational Study. *Nutrition.* October 2008; 24(10): 941–949.
27. Farzaneh-Far R, Harris WS, Garg S, Na B, Whooley MA. Inverse association of erythrocyte n-3 fatty acid levels with inflammatory biomarkers in patients with stable coronary artery disease: The Heart and Soul Study. *Atherosclerosis.* August 2009; 205(2): 538–543.
28. Murakami K et al. Total n-3 polyunsaturated fatty acid intake is inversely associated with serum C-reactive protein in young Japanese women. *Nutr Res.* May 2008; 28(5): 309–314.
29. Holt EM, Steffen LM, Moran A, Basu S, Steinberger J, Ross JA, Hong CP, Sinaiko AR. Fruit and vegetable consumption and its relation to markers of inflammation and oxidative stress in adolescents. *J Am Diet Assoc.* March 2009; 109(3): 414–421.
30. Katz DL, Meller S. Can we say what diet is best for health? *Annu Rev Public Health.* 2014; 35: 83–103.

4 Functional Foods

Kristi Crowe-White, PhD, RD and
Coni Francis, PhD, RD

CONTENTS

DEFINITION OF FUNCTIONAL FOODS

No single definition for the term "functional foods" is recognized globally by regulatory bodies.[1] The term "functional foods" is considered more of a marketing term.[2,3] All food is essentially functional as it provides energy and nutrients needed to sustain life.[4] A number of working definitions, however, are used to define functional foods, as summarized by organization in Table 4.1.

The terms "nutraceuticals" and "functional foods" are often used interchangeably. However, the two terms are not interchangeable, as the term nutraceutical refers to nearly any bioactive component that delivers a health benefit. Nutraceuticals are commonly found in supplement form, while functional foods are always in food form.[11] Medical foods and dietary supplements are also not considered functional foods. Medical foods are foods formulated to be administered by a physician for the management of a condition, disease, or life stage, such as phenylalanine-free formula for patients with phenylketonuria, or infant formula for babies. In contrast, dietary supplements are products in non-food form intended to supplement the diet.[12]

FUNCTIONAL FOODS AS A VEHICLE FOR DELIVERY OF BIOACTIVE COMPOUNDS

Eating for health and wellness can be an elusive goal for many consumers, especially given the complex marketplace and the influx of mixed messages in the media. Nevertheless, consumer desire for health has led to market penetration by foods and supplements containing increased amounts of bioactive food compounds (BFCs)

TABLE 4.1

Functional Foods "Working" Definitions

Organization	Definition
Academy of Nutrition and Dietetics	"Foods defined as whole foods along with fortified, enriched, or enhanced foods that have a potentially beneficial effect on health when consumed as part of a varied diet on a regular basis at effective levels."[5]
International Food Information Council	"Foods or dietary components that may provide a health benefit beyond basic nutrition and may play a role in reducing or minimizing the risk of certain diseases and other health conditions."[6]
Institute of Food Technologists	"Foods and food components that provide a health benefit beyond basic nutrition (for the intended population)."[4]
International Life Sciences Institute	"Foods that by virtue of the presence of physiologically active food components provide health benefits beyond basic nutrition."[7]
European Commission	A food that "beneficially affects one or more target functions in the body, beyond adequate nutritional effects, in a way that is relevant to either an improved state of health and well-being and/or reduction of risk of disease. Functional foods must remain foods and they must demonstrate their effects in amounts that can normally be expected to be consumed in the diet: they are not pills or capsules, but part of a normal food pattern."[8]
Health Canada	"A *functional food* is similar in appearance to, or may be a conventional food, is consumed as part of a usual diet, and is demonstrated to have physiological benefits and/or reduce the risk of chronic disease beyond basic nutritional functions."[9]
Japanese Ministry of Health, Labor, and Welfare	"FOSHU refers to foods containing ingredients with functions for health and officially approved to claim its physiological effects on the human body. FOSHU is intended to be consumed for the maintenance/promotion of health or special health uses by people who wish to control health conditions, including blood pressure or blood cholesterol."[10]

or physiologically active nutrients and non-nutrients that impart health benefits. Antioxidant vitamins and omega-3 fatty acids are examples of nutrient-based BFCs garnering strong market share whereas flavonoids, catechins, and other lesser known phytochemicals are non-nutrient BFCs that are being incorporated into various products marketed as functional foods. A listing of some common foods containing BFCs and their proposed health benefits is provided in Table 4.2.

With the increase in awareness of potential benefits derived from BFC intake, consumers often subscribe to the age-old adage that "if a little is good, then a lot must be better." This can lead to BFC intake outside of normal dietary patterns and/or supplemental intake of BFCs. Unfortunately, the supplemental approach may not be the most efficacious means of BFC acquisition. For example, according to results of the Iowa Women's Health Study published by Mursu et al.,[26] several commonly consumed vitamin and mineral supplements were associated with increased total mortality risk among older women. Likewise, a systematic review on antioxidant supplement intake and health risks by Bjelakovic et al.[27] reported that supplementation with beta-carotene, vitamin A, and vitamin E does not impart beneficial effects

TABLE 4.2

Example Functional Foods and Their Principal Bioactive Compounds

Functional Food	Principal Bioactive Compound	Proposed Health Benefit
Berries	Polyphenols	Antioxidant activity[13,14]
		Anti-inflammatory properties[13,14]
		Improved heart health[13,14]
		Improved cognitive function[15]
Allium vegetables	Organosulfur compounds	Cancer preventative effects[16]
		Antimicrobial activity[16]
Green tea	Catechins	Improved metabolic health[17]
		Antioxidant activity[17]
Coffee	Caffeine,	Cancer preventative effects[18]
	Chlorogenic acid	Improved metabolic health[18]
		Stimulant[18]
Cocoa	Polyphenols	Antioxidant activity[19]
		Anti-inflammatory properties[19]
Cruciferous vegetables	Sulfur containing glucosinolates and *S*-methylcysteine sulfoxide	Antioxidant activity[20]
		Improved heart health[20]
	Flavonoids	Cancer preventative effects[20]
	Anthocyanins	
	Coumarins	
	Carotenoids	
	Antioxidant enzymes	
	Terpenes	
Omega-3 fatty acids	Docosahexaenoic acid (DHA)	Anti-inflammatory properties[21]
	Eicosapentaenoic acid (EPA)	Improved heart health[21]
	Alpha-linolenic acid (ALA)	Improved central nervous function[21]
Prebiotics	Undigestible oligosaccharides	Improved digestive health[22]
		Improved immune health[22]
Probiotics	Beneficial bacteria	Reduction of inflammatory bowel disease[23]
		Improved lactose tolerance[23]
Soy	Soy protein	Improved heart health[24]
	Isoflavones	Improved metabolic health[24]
	Genistein	Prevent postmenopausal osteoporosis[25]
	Daidzein	Improved bone strength[25]
	Glycitein	

with regard to overall mortality and development of cardiovascular disease, but rather supplementation with these vitamins can increase the risk of death. In contrast to these results, epidemiological studies report inverse correlations between consumption of foods containing naturally high levels of nutrient and non-nutrient BFCs, primarily fruits and vegetables, and risk and/or prevalence of various chronic diseases.[28–31] Additionally, studies have demonstrated a strong inverse relationship between dietary intake of antioxidant-rich foods and markers of inflammation or oxidative stress.[32,33] At first glance, the research on BFC intake appears to be conflicting, yet these highlighted studies differ in the vehicle of delivery—supplement versus food. Such results underscore the complexity of food, especially foods considered functional due to their inclusion of compounds providing health benefits beyond basic nutrition. Nevertheless, it should be acknowledged that while there are clinical justifications for recommending targeted supplementation to specific subgroups of the population, food-focused intake guided by the *Dietary Guidelines for Americans 2010* remains the most scientifically substantiated approach to fostering health and wellness among the general population.[34]

ROLE OF FUNCTIONAL FOODS IN THE HEALTH CARE CONTINUUM

Rising health care costs, the growing trend to self-medicate to keep costs lower,[35] the increasing age of the population, the obesity epidemic, and the high prevalence of lifestyle-related diseases such as cancer, cardiovascular disease, and diabetes have led consumers to look for ways to prevent illness.[36] Functional foods are an option offered by the food industry in response to consumer health concerns.[37,38] Fortunately, functional foods have been shown to minimize health care costs while improving health and wellness, giving consumers greater control over their health by providing a convenient food form of health-enhancing ingredients.[4] Figure 4.1 shows the role of functional foods in the health care continuum.

Health is no longer considered just the absence of disease, but rather is the optimization of mental and physical well-being[12]; thus, the continued interest of consumers in the prevention of disease and optimal health will likely increase the consumption of functional foods.[39] Nutrition science is more focused on optimal nutrition than just on the role essential nutrients play in the prevention of disease.[8,40] For many years, the primary focus of the food industry was on subtracting ingredients

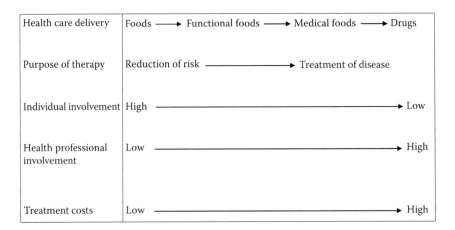

FIGURE 4.1   The role of functional foods in the health care continuum. (From Institute of Food Technologists, Functional foods: Opportunities and challenges, Expert Report, March 2005, http://www.ift.org/knowledge-center/read-ift-publications/science-reports/scientific-status-summaries/~/media/Knowledge%20Center/Science%20Reports/Expert%20Reports/Functional%20Foods/Functionalfoods_expertreport_full.pdf, accessed January 29, 2014.)

considered less healthy from processed foods in an effort to make foods healthier. Functional foods shift the focus from eliminating less healthy ingredients to adding beneficial ingredients for similar effects.[37] Evidence is growing that some food components not considered nutrients in the traditional sense can provide positive health benefits beyond basic nutrition. The use of food to provide health benefits beyond the prevention of deficiencies is a reasonable progression of traditional nutrition intervention.[4]

EVALUATING FUNCTIONAL FOODS: SHIFTING THE PARADIGM AWAY FROM REDUCTIONISM

For decades, nutrition research has been guided by a reductionist approach that advocates an additive character of linear cause-and-effect constructs such that the whole can be explained by the sum of its parts.[41] While it is imperative to reduce confounding factors in order to ascertain the bioactivity of compounds of interest, the breadth of functionality of BFCs may not be completely understood by isolating and supplementing single compounds or combinations of compounds from foods. For example, providing isolated BFCs or even cocktails of BFCs has been found not to have the same effects as whole foods, and, in the case of several studies, previously unrecognized risks resulting from nutrient toxicities and interactions have been identified.[42] Furthermore, under conditions of excessive intake, bioactive compounds with antioxidant properties can shift the antioxidant-oxidant balance within the body such that antioxidants can behave as pro-oxidants and contribute to oxidative stress.[43–45]

The need to broaden the nutrition perspective was highlighted in a randomized, partially blinded dietary intervention trial conducted on 43 healthy nonsmokers who were provided a diet containing 600 g of fruits and vegetables per day or a diet devoid of fruits and vegetables but supplemented with vitamin and mineral pills corresponding to the micronutrient content provided by the 600 g of fruits and vegetables.[46] At the end of the 25-day intervention, participants on the fruit and vegetable diet showed significant increases in resistance of plasma lipoproteins to oxidation and erythrocyte glutathione peroxidase activity as compared to participants in the supplement arm. On the basis of the data, the research team hypothesized that the observed effects were the result of compounds within fruit and vegetable matrices working synergistically with vitamin and mineral micronutrients to influence oxidative homeostasis. Collectively, scientific data suggest that isolation and supplementation of compounds may not effectively capture the scope of functional foods. With this in mind, overly reductionist approaches to evaluating the diet–disease relationship may hinder the progress of science aimed at evaluating bioactive compounds in functional foods.

BROADENING THE NUTRITION PERSPECTIVE IN FUNCTIONAL FOOD TESTING

As biological entities, plant and animal foods are the result of a vast array of complex processes involving hundreds of bioactive compounds. Given the dynamic nature of these processes, food matrices represent a continuous, structurally diverse medium of nutrients and non-nutrients interacting physically and chemically.[47] Whether interactions are synergistic, inhibitory, or neutralizing, physicochemical properties have been shown to influence the release, digestibility, stability, and, ultimately, bioavailability of the compounds within.[48]

According to the Food and Drug Administration (FDA), bioavailability is defined as the rate and extent to which the active or therapeutic moieties of a compound are absorbed and become available at the intended site of action.[49] In consideration of matrix effects on BFCs, some compounds are more bioavailable in food form as compared to others that are more bioavailable when consumed as supplements. For example, the bioavailability of lutein in eggs and iron in red meat is much greater than from isolated or compounded supplements.[50,51] Likewise, soluble fiber within foods has been shown to increase the bioavailability of several minerals, including calcium and magnesium, such that the trophic effects of soluble fiber may be responsible for lowering intestinal pH, ionizing these minerals, and increasing their permeability across the intestinal lumen.[52] This type of fiber is different from phytates in fiber-rich foods, which have been shown to interfere with mineral absorption. In contrast, it should be acknowledged that some nutrients are more bioavailable in their isolated supplemental form due to negative interactions within the food matrix that limit their availability. A classic example of a compound that is more bioavailable in the supplemental form is folic acid whereas beta-carotene can be absorbed similarly from both food or supplement as long as it is provided within a lipid matrix.[53–55]

By understanding compound interactions within food matrices, functional foods can be designed to enhance the bioavailability of BFCs. For example, many new foods are being developed with structurally designed matrices that protect compounds of interest and assist in delivering them to the intended site of action within the body.[56] Proponents of structurally designed matrices advocate for thorough evaluation of bioactive compounds in their original food matrix so as to learn from and guide the design of matrices for improving compound bioavailability and protecting the active form of the compounds through the harsh environments of food processing and digestion.[47] Given the multiplicity of compound interactions and the sheer number of BFCs of interest, additional research is needed to evaluate these compounds in their natural matrices. Such research will inevitably be beneficial in guiding research and development of novel functional foods.

SUBSTANTIATING THE EFFICACY OF FUNCTIONAL FOODS

Given the current state of the science, it has become increasingly apparent that food-first nutrient acquisition should be the primary message communicated by health care professionals until such time as sufficient data from clinical trials support the use of nutritive and non-nutritive BFC supplements for lowering risks of chronic disease. Currently, scientists from numerous disciplines, including food science, nutrition science, biochemistry, and nutrigenomics, are partnering to address shared challenges in methodology and study design for evaluating bioactive compounds in functional foods.[57] Such partnerships are critical to comprehensively studying the putatively positive and negative effects of BFCs and foods termed "functional."

In addition to multidisciplinary collaborations, several guiding processes should be considered in evaluating the efficacy and safety of functional foods. For example, an expert panel commissioned by the Institute of Food Technologists outlined a seven-step process for addressing critical aspects in the design, development, and marketing of functional foods (Figure 4.2).[58] As would be expected, specific factors within each step would need to be undertaken and/or tailored in order to thoroughly evaluate different categories of bioactive compounds. Another exemplary resource for scientifically substantiating the efficacy and safety of functional foods is the specific criteria proposed by Hill in 1971.[59] Such criteria for evaluating research data include the strength of the association, consistency of the observed association, specificity of the association, temporal relationship of the observed

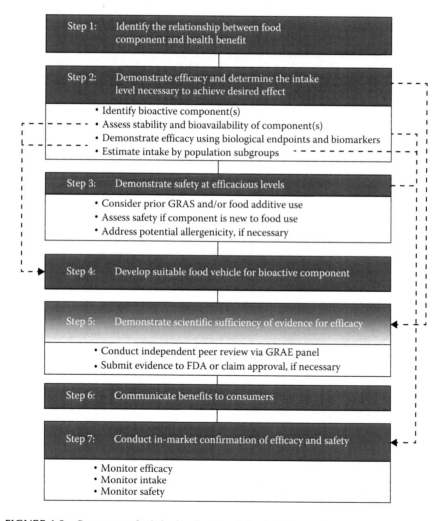

FIGURE 4.2 Seven steps for bringing functional foods to the market.

association, dose–response relationship, biological plausibility, and the coherence of the evidence. Unfortunately, in the case of functional foods, several of these criteria may be overlooked or omitted prior to marketing due to time and financial constraints within academia and industry. Such a lack of rigorous examination and questioning of data impedes the science and can potentially negatively impact human health and consumer belief in BFCs and functional foods.

To further complicate the process of scientifically substantiating functional foods, it must be acknowledged that BFC concentrations in natural plant and animal matrices vary based on agricultural production region and growing or feeding practices. For this reason, the science and potential impact of functional foods may be better advanced by evaluating the original matrix housing BFCs of interest and developing functional foods with standard concentrations of BFCs in a matrix suitable for protecting compound stability and enhancing compound bioavailability.

REGULATION OF FUNCTIONAL FOODS

The Japanese Ministry of Health, Labor, and Welfare was the first regulatory agency to recognize functional foods as a unique food category.[1] Since then, Japan has been the leader in the regulation of functional foods.[60] Japan's Food for Specified Health Uses (FOSHU) program began in 1991 and was the first to use scientific evidence to allow health claims for functional foods. FOSHU-approved products are allowed to use the FOSHU seal of approval on their product labels.[61]

In the United States, foods are regulated under the Federal Food, Drug, and Cosmetic Act of 1938, which does not make a provision for a definition of functional foods.[12] This is because functional foods are covered under regulations concerning the use of food ingredients that are adequate to cover functional food ingredients.[12,36,62] According to the FDA,[2,12] the main determinant for regulatory status is the intended use of a food. Products determined to be foods are regulated as food in conventional form, which includes functional foods and foods for special dietary use.[12] The Nutritional Labeling and Education Act of 1990 includes both conventional foods and foods for special dietary use.[12] Food manufacturers currently can use four categories of label claims to communicate health information to consumers: nutrient content claims, structure/function claims, health claims, and qualified health claims. All four types of claims are allowed on functional food labels as long as the claim meets the defined criteria outlined.[39] More information about types of claims that can be used on functional foods in the United States can be found on the FDA website.[63]

Nutrient content claims imply or describe the level of a nutrient in the food such as "high fiber" or "contains 100 calories" whereas structure function claims describe the role or mechanism of a dietary ingredient or nutrient to maintain or affect normal body structure or function such as "contains calcium for bone health" or "fiber promotes digestive health."[64] According to the Nutritional Labeling and Education Act, a product is allowed to bear a health claim after extensive review of the scientific evidence submitted to the FDA. Such claims are authorized based on significant scientific agreement or on an authoritative statement from a scientific body of the U.S. government or the National Academy of Sciences. Acceptable health claims are summarized on the FDA website.[65] Qualified health claims are intended to provide information about diet–disease relationships when the scientific support has not reached the highest level of scientific evidence.[66]

SUMMARY

Science and technology advances have facilitated functional food market growth, and, as a result, the number of functional food products continues to expand exponentially. At the same time, consumer interest in the health benefits of foods and food components is high and will likely continue to grow, thereby increasing the consumption of functional foods. The entrance of functional foods into the consumer market triggers the need for health professionals to update their knowledge base on functional foods and bioactive food compounds to be able to adequately counsel patients and clients.

REFERENCES

1. International Life Sciences Institute. Perspectives on ILSI's international activities on functional foods. http://www.ilsi.org/Europe/Publications/O2009Perspectives.pdf. May 2009. Accessed January 29, 2014.
2. Food and Drug Administration. Labeling and nutrition. http://www.fda.gov/Food/IngredientsPackagingLabeling/LabelingNutrition/default.htm. Updated November 6, 2013. Accessed January 29, 2014.
3. Henry CJ. Functional foods [editorial]. *Eur J Clin Nutr.* 2010;64(7):657–659.
4. Institute of Food Technologists. Functional foods: Opportunities and challenges. Expert Report. http://www.ift.org/knowledge-center/read-ift-publications/science-reports/scientific-status-summaries/~/media/Knowledge%20Center/Science%20Reports/Expert%20Reports/Functional%20Foods/Functionalfoods_expertreport_full.pdf. March 2005. Accessed January 29, 2014.
5. Crowe KM, Francis C. Position of the academy of nutrition and dietetics: Functional foods. *J Acad Nutr Diet.* 2013;113(8):1096–1103.
6. International Food Information Council. Functional foods. http://www.foodinsight.org/Content/3842/Final%20Functional%20Foods%20Backgrounder.pdf. Published July 2011. Accessed January 29, 2014.
7. International Life Sciences Institute Europe Functional Food Task Force. Functional foods—Scientific and global perspectives. http://www.ilsi.org/Europe/Publications/R2002Func_Food.pdf. Published June 2002. Accessed January 29, 2014.
8. Stein AJ, Rodriguez-Cerezo E (Eds.). Functional foods in the European Union (2008). http://ftp.jrc.es/EURdoc/JRC43851.pdf. Accessed January 29, 2014.
9. Health Canada. Policy paper—Nutraceuticals/functional foods and health claims on foods. http://www.hc-sc.gc.ca/fn-an/label-etiquet/claims-reclam/nutra-funct_foods-nutra-fonct_aliment-eng.php. Published November 1998. Accessed January 29, 2014.
10. Japan Ministry of Health, Labour, and Welfare. Food for specialized health uses. http://www.mhlw.go.jp/english/topics/foodsafety/fhc/02.html. Accessed January 29, 2014.
11. Codoñer-Franch P, Valls-Bellés V. Citrus as functional foods. *Curr Topics Nutraceut Res.* 2010;8(4):173–183.
12. Ross S. Functional foods: The food and drug administration perspective. *Am J Clin Nutr.* 2000;71(6 suppl.):1735S–1738S.
13. Basu A, Rhone M, Lyons T. Berries: Emerging impact on cardiovascular health. *Nutr Rev.* 2010;68:168–177.

14. Williamson G, Manach C. Bioavailability and bioefficacy of polyphenols in humans. II. Review of 93 intervention studies. *Am J Clin Nutr.* 2005;81:243S–255S.

15. Devore EE, Kang JH, Breteler MB, Grodstein F. Dietary intake of berries and flavonoids in relation to cognitive decline. *Ann Neurol.* 2012;72:135–143.

16. Sengupta A, Ghosh S, Bhattacharjee S. Allium vegetables in cancer prevention: An overview. *Asian Pacific J Cancer Prev.* 2004;5:237–245.

17. Liu K, Zhou R, Wang B et al. Effect of green tea on glucose control and insulin sensitivity: A meta-analysis of 17 randomized controlled trials. *Am J Clin Nutr.* 2013;98:340–348.

18. Butt MS, Sultan MT. Coffee and its consumption: Benefits and risks. *Crit Rev Food Sci Nutr.* 2011;51:363–373.

19. Rimbach G, Melchin M, Moehring J, Wagner AE. Polyphenols from cocoa and vascular health—A critical review. *Int J Mol Sci.* 2009;10:4290–4309.

20. Manchali S, Murthy KNC, Patil BS. Crucial facts about health benefits of popular cruciferous vegetables. *J Functional Foods.* 2012;4:94–106.

21. Tur JA, Bibiloni MM, Sureda A, Pons A. Dietary sources of omega 3 fatty acids: Public health risks and benefits. *Br J Nutr.* 2012;107(S2):S23–S52.

22. de Sousa VMC, dos Santos EF, Sgarbieri VC. The importance of prebiotics in functional foods and clinical practice. *Food Nutr Sci.* 2011;2:133–144.

23. Chauhan SV, Chorawala MR. Probiotics, prebiotics and synbiotics. *Int J Pharm Sci Res.* 2012;3(3):711–726.

24. Azadbakht L, Esmaillzadeh A. Soy intake and metabolic health: Beyond isoflavones. *Arch Iran Med.* 2012;15(8):460–461.

25. Taku K, Melby MK, Nishi N, Omori T, Kurzer MS. Soy isoflavones for osteoporosis: An evidence-based approach. *Maturitas.* 2011;70:333–338.

26. Mursu J, Robien K, Harnack LJ, Park K, Jacobs DR. Dietary supplements and mortality rate in older women: The Iowa Women's Health Study. *Arch Intern Med.* 2011;171(18):1625–1633.

27. Bjelakovic G, Nikolova D, Gluud LL, Simonetti RG, Gluud C. Mortality in randomized trials of antioxidant supplements for primary and secondary prevention. *JAMA.* 2007;297(8):842–857.

28. Hirvonen T, Pietinen P, Virtanen M. Intake of flavonols and flavones and risk of coronary heart disease in male smokers. *Epidemiology.* 2001;12:62–67.

29. Knekt P, Reunanen A, Jarvinen R, Seppanen R, Heliovaara M, Aromaa A. Antioxidant vitamin intake and coronary mortality in a longitudinal population study. *Am J Epidemiol.* 1994;139:1180–1189.

30. Fung TT, Willet WC, Stampfer MJ, Manson JE, Hu FB. Dietary patterns and the risk of coronary heart disease in women. *Arch Intern Med.* 2001;161:1857–1862.

31. Joshipura KJ, Hu, FB, Manson JE. Effect of fruit and vegetable intake on risk for coronary heart disease. *Ann Intern Med.* 2001;134:1106–1114.

32. Helmersson J, Arnlov J, Larsson A, Basu S. Low dietary intake of beta-carotene, alpha-tocopherol, and ascorbic acid is associated with increased inflammatory and oxidative stress status in a Swedish cohort. *Br J Nutr.* 2009;101:1775–1782.

33. Holt EM, Steffen LM, Moran A, Basu S, Steinberger J, Ross JA, Hong C, Sinaiko AR. Fruit and vegetable consumption and its relation to markers of inflammation and oxidative stress in adolescents. *J Am Diet Assoc.* 2009;109(3):414–421.

34. U.S. Department of Agriculture and U.S. Department of Health and Human Services. *Dietary Guidelines for Americans 2010*, 7th edn. http://health.gov/dietaryguidelines/dga2010/DietaryGuidelines2010.pdf. Accessed October 1, 2013.

35. Schieber A. Functional foods and nutraceuticals [editorial]. *Food Res Int.* 2012;46(2):437.

36. Thompson AK, Moughan PJ. Innovation in the foods industry: Functional foods. *Innov Manag Policy Pract.* 2008;10(1):61–73.

37. Labrecque J, Charlebois S. Functional foods an empirical study on perceived health benefits in relation to pre-purchase intentions. *Nutr Food Sci.* 2011;41(5):308–318.

38. French S. Functional foods: The next phase. *Food Beverage Int.* 2006;5:19–20.

39. US General Accounting Office. Food safety: Improvements needed in overseeing the safety of dietary supplements and "functional foods." http://www.gao.gov/new.items/rc00156.pdf. Published July 2000. Accessed January 29, 2014.

40. Doyon M, Labrecque J. Functional foods: A conceptual definition. *Br Food J.* 2008;110(11):1133–1149.

41. Dent EB. The international model: An alternative to the direct cause and effect construct for mutually causal organizational phenomena. *Foundations Sci.* 2003;8:81–100.

42. Jeffery E. Component interactions for efficacy of functional foods. *J Nutr.* 2005;135:1223–1225.

43. Stanner SA, Hughes J, Kelly CNM, Buttriss J. A review of the epidemiological evidence for the "antioxidant hypothesis". *Public Health Nutr.* 2003;7:407–422.

44. Yusuf S, Dagenais G, Pogue J, Bosch J, Sleight P. Vitamin E supplementation and cardiovascular events in high-risk patients: The Heart Outcomes Prevention Evaluation Study Investigators. *New Engl J Med.* 2000;342(3):154–160.

45. Brown B, Zhao XQ, Chait A et al. Simvastatin and niacin, antioxidant vitamins, or the combination for the prevention of coronary disease. *New Engl J Med.* 2001;345(22):1583–1592.

46. Dragsted LO, Pedersen A, Hermetter A et al. The 6-a-day Study: Effects of fruit and vegetables on markers of oxidative stress and anti-oxidative defense in healthy nonsmokers. *Am J Clin Nutr.* 2004;79(6):1060–1072.

47. Crowe KM. Designing functional foods with bioactive polyphenols: Highlighting lessons learned from original plant matrices. *J Hum Nutr Food Sci.* 2013;1:1018–1019.

48. Aguilera JM. Why food microstructure? *J Food Eng.* 2005;67:3–11.

49. Bioavailability and bioequivalence requirements: General. 21CFR320.1 (2012).

50. Chung HY, Rasmussen HM, Johnson EJ. Lutein bioavailability is higher from lutein-enriched eggs than from supplements and spinach in men. *J Nutr.* 2004;134:1887–1893.

51. Milman N, Pedersen AN, Ovesen L, Schroll M. Iron status in 358 apparently healthy 80-year-old Danish men and women: Relation to food composition and dietary and supplemental iron intake. *Ann Hematol.* 2004;83:423–429.

52. Greger JL. Nondigestible carbohydrates and mineral bioavailability. *J Nutr.* 1999;129:1434S–1435S.

53. Hannon-Fletcher MP, Armstrong NC, Scott JM et al. Determining bioavailability of food folates in a controlled intervention study. *Am J Clin Nutr.* 2004;80:911–918.

54. Sanderson P, McNulty H, Mastroiacovo P et al. Folate bioavailability: UK Food Standards Agency Workshop Report. *Br J Nutr.* 2003;90:473–479.

55. Donhowe E, Flores F, Kerr W, Wicker L, Kong F. Characterization and in vitro bioavailability of beta-carotene: Effects of microencapsulation method and food matrix. *LWT Food Sci Technol.* 2014;57:42–48.

56. McClements DJ, Decker EA, Park Y, Weiss J. Structural design principles for delivery of bioactive components in nutraceuticals and functional foods. *Crit Rev Food Sci Nutr.* 2009;49:577–606.

57. Crowe KM, Allison DB. Evaluating bioactive food components in obesity and cancer prevention. *Crit Rev Food Sci Nutr.* 2015;55:732–734.

58. The Institute of Food Technologists. IFT Expert Report on Functional Foods: Opportunities and Challenges. http://www.ift.org/Knowledge-Center/Read-IFT-Publications/Science-Reports/Scientific-Status-Summaries/Functional-Foods.aspx. Released March 2005. Accessed January 22, 2014.

59. Hill AB. Statistical evidence and inference. In: *Principles of Medical Statistics*, 9th edn. New York: Oxford University Press, 1971, pp. 309–323.

60. Yamada K, Sato-Mito N, Nagata J, Umegaki K. Health claim evidence requirements in Japan. *J Nutr.* 2008;138(6):1192S–1198S.

61. Shimizu M, Hachimura S. Gut as a target for functional food. *Trends Food Sci Technol.* 2011;22(12):646–650.

62. Functional food industry: Market research report, statistics and analysis. Report Linker website. http://reportlinker.com/ci02036/Functional-Food.html. Accessed January 29, 2014.

63. US Food and Drug Administration. Claims that can be made for conventional foods and dietary supplements. http://www.fda.gov/food/ingredientspackaginglabeling/labelingnutrition/ucm111447.htm. Published September 2003. Accessed January 29, 2014.

64. Food and Drug Administration. Guidance for industry: A food labeling guide (8. Claims). http://www.fda.gov/Food/GuidanceRegulation/GuidanceDocumentsRegulatory Information/LabelingNutrition/ucm064908.htm. Published January 2013. Accessed April 28, 2014.

65. Food and Drug Administration. Guidance for industry: A food labeling guide,_http://www.fda.gov/food/guidanceregulation/guidancedocumentsregulatoryinformation/labelingnutrition/ucm064919.htm. Published January 2013. Accessed January 29, 2014.

66. Food and Drug Administration. Guidance for industry: FDA's implementation of "Qualified Health Claims": Questions and answers; Final guidance. http://www.fda.gov/Food/GuidanceRegulation/GuidanceDocumentsRegulatoryInformation/LabelingNutrition/ucm053843.htm. Published May 2006. Accessed January 29, 2014.

5 Integrative Nutrition *Supplements*

Jennifer Doley, MBA, RD, CNSC, FAND

CONTENTS

INTRODUCTION

A "dietary supplement" is officially defined in the Dietary Supplement Health Education Act (DSHEA) as (1) a product intended to supplement the diet that contains at least one of the following: vitamin, mineral, herb, or other botanical or amino acid; (2) a dietary substance for use to supplement the diet by increasing the total dietary intake; and (3) a concentrate, metabolite, constituent, extract, or any combination of any of the previously described ingredients (DSHEA, 1994).

The use of dietary supplements has increased significantly in recent years, with approximately 50% of the U.S. population taking at least one supplement daily, according to 2003–2006 NHANES data (National Health and Nutrition Examination Survey). A large percentage of these supplements are multivitamins, with and without added minerals, which are used by approximately one-third of the U.S. population (Bailey et al., 2011a).

Dietary supplement use is more prevalent in non-Hispanic whites, individuals with higher educational accomplishments and those considered to be of normal weight (Bailey et al., 2011a). Research also shows that those individuals most likely to take a multivitamin have a higher dietary consumption of many vitamins and minerals than those who are least likely to take a multivitamin; paradoxically, it appears that individuals who might benefit the most from a multivitamin supplement are the least likely to take them (Bailey et al., 2011b, 2012).

REGULATION

The principal federal legislative act which addresses the production, marketing, and sale of dietary supplements is the DSHEA, which became law in 1994. In addition to providing a definition for dietary supplements, the DSHEA also defined the regulatory role of the Food and Drug Administration (FDA) in regard to product safety and labeling, established specific guidelines and requirements for labeling, authorized the FDA to establish Good Manufacturing Practices for dietary supplements, and established the Office of Dietary Supplements (ODS) (FDA, 2013).

Because dietary supplements are not classified as medications, they are not subject to the same strict regulations and approval from the FDA that is required of drugs. The DSHEA specifies that supplement manufacturers are responsible for providing safe and properly labeled products; however, the FDA must first prove that a supplement is unsafe or mislabeled before it can issue a public recall or ban the sale of a product. As a result, supplement manufacturers do not need to prove either safety or effectiveness before marketing and selling their products (FDA, 2013).

The exception to this rule is products that contain a "new dietary ingredient" (NDI), or a substance that meets the definition of a dietary supplement, but has not been sold in the United States before October 15, 1994. Manufacturers must provide the FDA evidence that a product with an NDI is "reasonably expected to be safe" at least 75 days prior to marketing. Several trade associations compiled lists, available on the FDA website, of dietary ingredients in use prior to October 15, 1994; however, it is acknowledged that these lists are not necessarily all inclusive. Ultimately, the manufacturer alone is responsible for determining if the ingredient qualifies as "new" (FDA, 2013).

In addition to safety, the DSHEA also defines the role of the FDA in the labeling of dietary supplements. FDA regulations require that labels contain the following: (1) a descriptive name of the product stating that it is a "supplement," (2) a name and place of business of the manufacturer, packager or distributor, and (3) a complete list of ingredients. However, the FDA does not analyze supplements to determine if the

---

TABLE 5.1

Information Required on the "Supplement Facts" Panel

Appropriate serving size

Directions for use

Quantity and % Daily Value of 14 nutrients and any other added nutrients

Amount per serving for ingredients with no established Reference Daily Intakes

For products with a proprietary blend, the total amount of the blend

All ingredients, listed by common name, in descending order by weight

---

list of posted ingredients is accurate. Labels are also required to carry a Supplement Facts panel. See Table 5.1 for required information on the Supplement Facts panel (FDA, 2013).

Product manufacturers by law cannot claim that their products treat or cure a specific disease or condition; however, supplement labels can include health claims, structure/function claims, and nutrient content claims. Health claims are those that describe a relationship between a food component and a reduced risk of a disease or health-related condition. The FDA has defined qualified health claims; these are listed on the FDA website with specific requirements a product must meet to make the claim. Structure/function claims are statements that describe the intended benefit of the ingredient on normal structure or function of the human body; for example, a label can state the product "builds strong bones," but cannot claim that the product "treats osteoporosis." Any supplement making structure/function claims must include the following statement on the label: "This statement has not been evaluated by the Food and Drug Administration. This product is not intended to diagnose, treat, cure, or prevent any disease" (FDA, 2013).

Current Good Manufacturing Practices (CGMPs) were established for dietary supplements in 2007, and implementation for all manufacturing companies was required by June 2010. The CGMPs are intended to ensure that all dietary products are processed in a consistent manner and meet quality standards. The CGMPs include provisions related to the design and construction of the physical plant, cleaning, manufacturing procedures, quality control practices, testing of products, handling customer complaints, and maintaining records (FDA, 2013).

The ODS was established in 1995 and is part of the National Institutes of Health. The purpose of the ODS is to explore the potential role of dietary supplements in improving healthcare in the United States; to promote, conduct, and coordinate research relating to dietary supplements; to collect and compile results of scientific research on dietary supplements; and to serve as an advisor to various government health agencies. The ODS provides a wide variety of resources on dietary supplements for researchers, other health professionals, and the public (ODSa, 2013).

BOTANICALS

Herbal or botanical products are generally defined as any part of a plant, including leaves, stems, flowers, roots, seeds, or some combination thereof. Some commercial herbal preparations may also contain animal products and minerals. Botanicals can be sold in their raw form, or as an extract, in which a solvent is used to release the biologically active compounds in the plant; the resulting liquid can then be used to form powders or pastes. Extracts can have a number of organic compounds, and it is often difficult to determine which ones have a therapeutic effect. Environmental factors such as soil, temperature, rainfall, and sunlight exposure can also change the concentration of organic compounds in individual plants; thus, standardization in preparing commercial mixtures poses challenges (Bent, 2004). See Table 5.2 for a list of select botanicals and their commonly intended use (Fragakis and Thompson, 2012).

CINNAMON

Cinnamon is a spice obtained from the inner bark of trees of the genus *Cinnamomum*; the most commonly used species are *C. zeylanicum* (also known as *C. verum* or "true" cinnamon) from Sri Lanka and *C. aromaticum* (also known as *C. cassia*) from China. Both varieties have been studied for their effects on blood glucose control in diabetes.

In vitro studies on the effect of *C. zeylanicum* on blood glucose control demonstrated reduction of glucose absorption via inhibition of the enzymes maltase, sucrase, and pancreatic alpha-amylase; increased adipocyte uptake of glucose; and increased insulin release. In vivo rat studies have also shown positive effects, including reductions in fasting blood glucose, A1C, LDL, and an increase in HDL. It has been hypothesized that its beneficial effects on serum lipid levels are due in part to increases in serum insulin and antioxidant effects on lipid metabolism (Ranasinghe et al., 2012).

Short-term supplementation (less than 4 months) of *C. aromaticum* has been studied in humans; in a review of six randomized controlled trials conducted since 2000, researchers concluded that supplementation of 1–6 g of cinnamon daily resulted in significant reductions of fasting blood glucose and A1C levels. Of the studies analyzed, some did not show significant improvements in these parameters; however, in those cases the patients studied had well controlled diabetes with baseline A1C levels ranging from 6.8% to 7.1%. In the two studies that did show a significant reduction in both parameters, the average baseline A1C of the subjects was 8.2%, suggesting that cinnamon may be of benefit for those patients with less than ideal blood glucose control (Akilen et al., 2012).

Cinnamon has largely been found to be safe for consumption; however, some agencies advocate for the use of *C. zeylanicum* instead of *C. aromaticum* because of its much lower content of coumarins; coumarins have anticoagulant, carcinogenic, and hepatotoxic properties which may limit the long-term use of *C. aromaticum* because of safety concerns (Ranasinghe et al., 2012).

Cinnamon is available in capsules or as a liquid extract; it is unclear which form is ideal, as the amount of active compounds will vary from product to product. Similarly, an optimal dosage is also unknown; recent study doses range from 1 to 6 g daily, although larger doses have also been studied (Akilen et al., 2012).

TABLE 5.2
Intended/Commonly Advertised Use of Select Botanicals

Botanical	Common Use
Black cohosh	Reduce premenstrual and menopausal symptoms
Cinnamon	Lower blood glucose in diabetes
CoEnzyme Q-10	Improve health of people with hypertension and heart disease, improve exercise performance, reduce cancer risk, improve immune function in HIV infection, help with neurological disorders, prevent migraine
Cranberry	Prevent and treat urinary tract infections
Echinacea	Enhance immune function, prevent and treat the common cold and upper respiratory infections
Feverfew	Prevent migraine
Garlic	Reduce blood pressure and cholesterol, improve circulation, enhance immune function, reduce cancer risk
Ginger	Treat nausea associated with pregnancy, chemotherapy, and postsurgery
Ginkgo biloba	Improve memory, improve symptoms of Alzheimer's disease, relieve tinnitus, prevent altitude sickness, improve symptoms of reduced circulation in intermittent claudication
Ginseng	Improve mood, energy, cognition, exercise performance, improve sexual function, reduce cancer risk, control blood glucose in diabetes
Glucosamine	Relieve joint pain from osteoarthritis
Grape seed extract	Antioxidant, improve cardiovascular health, reduce cancer risk, treat hyperpigmentation of the skin
Green tea extract	Antioxidant, improve cardiovascular health, prevent cancer, promote weight loss through increased energy expenditure
β-Hydroxy β-methyl butyrate (HMB)	Increase muscle strength, reduce exercise-induced muscle damage, increase lean mass, reduce fat mass, treat HIV or cancer-related wasting
Lutein	Treat age-related macular degeneration and cataracts, treat retinitis pigmentosa, prevent cancer
Lycopene	Reduce prostate cancer risk, prevent other cancers, reduce symptoms of exercise-induced asthma, prevent atherosclerosis
Melatonin	Regulate sleep/wake cycles, reduce jet lag, reduce cancer risk, prevent and treat migraine, enhance sex drive
Milk thistle	Reduce liver damage in alcoholic liver disease, treat viral hepatitis, improve overall liver health, prevent cancer
Red yeast rice	Treat hypercholesterolemia and dyslipidemia related to HIV therapy
S-adenosylmethionine	Reduce symptoms of arthritis, fibromyalgia, and depression, improve liver and gall bladder health
St. John's wort	Treat depression, promote emotional well-being
Saw palmetto	Improve symptoms of enlarged prostate, prevent prostate cancer, prevent male pattern baldness
Valerian	Enhance sleep, reduce stress and anxiety

Echinacea

Echinacea is a group of nine species of flowering plants; the species most commonly researched and used in herbal medicine is *E. purpurea*; however, *E. angustifolia* and *E. pallida* have also been studied. Echinacea is largely used to ward off infectious illnesses, such as the common cold, via its function as an immune system stimulator; however, researchers now believe "immune modulator" to be a more accurate term to describe its properties. Echinacea's organic compounds include caffeic acid derivatives, polysaccharides, and alkylamides; however, it is unclear which of its organic compounds have beneficial effects; this issue is further complicated by the wide variations in concentration of these compounds in commercial products, due to differences in species, the part of the plant used, and the method of extraction (Hudson, 2012).

Echinacea's immunologic effects appear to be multifactorial and include direct antiviral and antimicrobial properties, as well as immune enhancements such as stimulation of the phagocytic activity of macrophages and suppression of proinflammatory responses of epithelial cells exposed to viruses or bacteria (Hudson, 2012). In vitro studies have demonstrated echinacea's strong antiviral actions against influenza viruses, rhinoviruses, coronavirus, and respiratory syncytial virus (Hudson et al., 2005; Vimalanathan et al., 2005; Pleschka et al., 2009). In vitro studies have also shown that echinacea is effective against some bacteria, most notably *Clostridium difficile*, *Streptococcus pyogenes*, and *Haemophilus influenzae* (Hudson, 2012).

While in vitro studies show clear benefits, in vivo studies are less conclusive, due in part to common problems seen in herbal research, which include small sample sizes, differences in the type, dose, and duration of supplementation, and heterogeneous patient populations. However, a Cochrane review published in 2006 concluded that early use of *Echinacea purpurea* is effective in reducing the duration and severity of cold symptoms, although it is not effective in preventing colds (Linde et al., 2006).

There are no specific guidelines regarding dosing of echinacea; commercial echinacea preparations come in a variety of forms including tablets, juice, tinctures, and teas. In recent years, echinacea has become more commonly used in over-the-counter cold remedies that contain a variety of nonbotanical medications to treat cold symptoms. However, because of limited evidence, it is unclear what the most effective dose is and from which part of the plant the compounds should be extracted (Hudson, 2012).

Because of its immune-modulating effects, echinacea should be avoided in patients with autoimmune disorders, including lupus, HIV, and multiple sclerosis. Echinacea should not be used in patients who are taking immunosuppressive medications such as cyclosporine, azathioprine, basiliximab, tacrolimus, prednisone, and other corticosteroids (Fragakis and Thompson, 2012).

Garlic

Allium sativum, commonly known as garlic, is a member of the onion family and has been used for culinary and medicinal purposes for thousands of years. Garlic's most common medicinal use is in lowering serum lipid levels, but has also been investigated for its potential effect on infections, cancer, blood pressure, and circulation. Its biologically active compounds include S-allyl cysteine, S-allyl mercaptocysteine, allicin, alliin, and diallyl polysulfides (Fragakis and Thompson, 2012).

Garlic does appear to be effective in lowering lipids levels, although study results are variable. In several randomized, double-blind placebo-controlled trials, garlic was no more effective than placebo in reducing lipid levels in subjects with hypercholesterolemia (Isaacsohn et al., 1998; Satitvipawee et al., 2003). However, in other trials, subjects taking garlic had significant reductions in total cholesterol and LDL, and increases in HDL (Steiner et al., 1996; Sobenin et al., 2008). In a recently published meta-analysis, the authors concluded that garlic successfully treated dyslipidemia; however, it was most effective if supplementation was long term and subjects had higher baseline total cholesterol levels (Zeng et al., 2012).

It has been hypothesized that the conflicting results may be due in part to differences in the type and preparation methods of the supplemented garlic used in the studies. Further, differences in study subjects, including baseline cholesterol levels and diet, and the duration of supplementation may also contribute to the confounding results. In a recent review, authors concluded that garlic may be used in conjunction with a traditional lipid-lowering medication, but it is not effective enough to be used as a primary therapy (Qidwai and Ashfaq, 2013).

Garlic also appears to have a beneficial effect on blood pressure in hypertensive subjects. In two recent meta-analyses, the authors concluded that garlic supplementation resulted in statistically significant decreases in both systolic and diastolic blood pressure as compared to placebo for hypertensive subjects, but not normotensive subjects (Reinhart et al., 2008; Ried et al., 2008). As blood pressure reductions were mild (~7–8 mmHg), this suggests that garlic may be used as an adjunctive, rather than primary, therapy in treating hypertension.

Some research suggests garlic may have a chemoprotective effect on humans, but results are mixed and most research is from epidemiologic, observational, animal, and in vitro studies; long-term randomized control trials are necessary to more fully understand garlic's role as a potential anticancer agent (Li et al., 2013).

Garlic is said to be beneficial in fighting infections. In one small study, subjects receiving a daily garlic supplement developed fewer colds than participants taking a placebo (Josling, 2001). Several animal and cell studies suggest that garlic may be effective in reducing viral and bacterial growth; however, too little evidence exists at present to determine garlic's full effect on infectious pathogens and the immune system (Fragakis, 2012).

Garlic is available raw, or can be purchased as a capsule with powder or oil. It is safe for consumption, with few side effects except mild gastrointestinal (GI) upset and undesirable body odor; however, odor-free preparations are also available. Garlic does interact with some medications; it should be used with caution in patients taking anticoagulants or other herbal medicines with known blood-thinning properties. Garlic may also reduce the effectiveness of saquinavir and oral contraceptives, as well as a number of other classes of medications; any patients taking prescription medications should consult a pharmacist prior to starting garlic supplementation (Fragakis and Thompson, 2012).

GINGER

Ginger, *Zingiber officinale*, has been used medicinally for centuries. The most pharmacologically active compounds of ginger, gingerols and shogaols, are found in the plant's rhizome, a structure similar to a root, but botanically considered a stem. Ginger is commonly taken for GI ailments, particularly nausea and vomiting (N/V); it is thought that ginger's compounds work directly on the GI tract, and not through the central nervous system like antinausea medications (Fragakis and Thompson, 2012).

While traditional antinausea medications are effective in many cases of N/V, they are associated with significant side effects that may limit their long-term use. In cases with protracted or refractory N/V related to pregnancy, ginger may be of benefit. Several studies have shown that ginger was more effective than placebo in both prevention and treatment of N/V. It appears that ginger consumption is safe in pregnancy, as no difference in fetal outcomes were noted (Palatty et al., 2013).

The results of some preliminary animal studies indicate that ginger may be effective in treating chemotherapy-induced N/V; however, human study results have been mixed. While some study outcomes suggest that ginger is as effective as metoclopramide in reducing late phase chemotherapy-induced N/V, a more recent study showed ginger to be of no benefit (Manusirivithaya et al., 2004; Zick et al., 2009). Ginger has also been investigated as a treatment for N/V related to motion sickness, radiation, and surgery, although these studies yielded mixed results as well; thus, no specific recommendations can be made for the use of ginger in these cases (Palatty et al., 2013).

While most research focuses on GI disorders, in vitro and animal studies have been conducted to assess ginger's potential effects as an antioxidant and anti-inflammatory agent, and its possible use in treating diabetes and cancer. Further research is needed in these areas, as sufficient evidence is lacking to recommend the use of ginger in these conditions (Mashhadi et al., 2013).

Ginger is available commercially in a number of forms including fresh, dried, pickled, powdered, and candied. Ginger is also used in a number of commercially prepared foods and beverages; however, it is unlikely that the quantity used is sufficient to produce any pharmacological benefits. While optimal dose recommendations have not been established, amounts used in studies on N/V related to pregnancy range from 250 to 1000 mg/day, often given in divided doses. Ginger has been deemed GRAS status by the FDA and has few side effects; however, it may interact with some medications, specifically anticoagulants, so it should be used with caution in these patients (Fragakis and Thompson, 2012).

GINKGO BILOBA

Ginkgo biloba is a tree, the leaves of which are used to extract the ginkgo used medicinally, which contains the flavonoid glycosides myricetin and quercetin, as well as the terpenoids ginkgolides and bilobalides. Ginkgo is most commonly used to enhance memory and treat dementia, and its proposed mechanisms include an increased production of nitrous oxide in blood vessels and inhibition of a platelet-activating factor, which help in both cerebral and peripheral blood flow. Ginkgo is also thought to protect against free radical damage and is an inhibitor of monoamine oxidase A, norepinephrine, and amyloid-β neurotoxicity (Brondino et al., 2013).

In a recent review of four placebo-controlled trials on the use of ginkgo biloba extract (EGb 761®) in patients with Alzheimer's or vascular dementia with neuropsychiatric features, the authors concluded that the extract was significantly more effective than placebo or donepezil in improving cognitive performance and behavioral symptoms. Patients were treated with 240 mg of extract daily for 22–24 weeks (Ihl, 2013). However, ginkgo does not appear to be effective in preventing or delaying the onset of Alzheimer's disease (Vellas et al., 2012).

A typical dose of ginkgo biloba is 80–240 mg/day, divided into two to three doses per day, although up to 720 mg/day has been safely used in studies examining its effects on dementia, memory, and circulatory disorders. It has been suggested that ginkgo must be taken for 4–6 weeks before positive effects are seen for disorders in memory, mood, or physiologic function, although the studied duration of supplementation varied (Diamond and Bailey, 2013). However, risks of long-term use (i.e., years) should be considered when prescribing ginkgo, as mouse and rat studies have suggested that long-term use of ginkgo biloba may increase the incidence of liver and thyroid tumors (Dunnick and Nyska, 2013).

Because of ginkgo's effects on blood flow, there is a potential risk of bleeding, and several case reports have been published implicating ginkgo as a potential causative factor in bleeding abnormalities, including postoperative bleeding. Therefore, caution should be used in recommending ginkgo use in patients taking aspirin, anticoagulants, nonsteroidal anti-inflammatory medications, and other drugs which exhibit antiplatelet activity. Ginkgo may further interact with warfarin by increasing its bioavailability and reducing clearance (Diamond and Bailey, 2013).

Grape Seed Extract

Grape seed extract (GSE), a by-product of the wine and grape juice industries, is produced from the seeds of red grapes and is a strong antioxidant, and purported to play a role in chemoprevention and cardiac health. The key biologically active compounds of GSEs are proanthocyanidins, a subclass of flavonoids (Fragakis and Thompson, 2012).

The relationship between GSE and cancer development has largely been conducted via animal and in vitro studies. While further research on humans is needed, these preliminary studies yielded promising results, suggesting GSE may act as a chemoprotective agent for skin, prostate, colon, and breast cancers. In addition to its antioxidant properties, GSE appears to have several other mechanisms, including increased apoptosis, decreased cell growth, and inhibition of several enzymes and metabolic pathways (Kaur et al., 2009).

In a meta-analysis of nine randomized controlled trials assessing the potential cardioprotective effects of GSE, the authors concluded that the compound may help reduce systolic blood pressure and heart rate, although reductions in blood pressure were small and significantly less than seen with the administration of traditional antihypertensive medications. No effects on lipid or C-reactive protein levels were noted (Feringa et al., 2011).

At this time, GSE is considered safe, with no known side effects or drug inter-actions. It is available in capsule, tablet, or liquid form and suggested doses are 100–300 mg/day, although further research is needed to establish an optimal dose (Fragakis and Thompson, 2012).

Green Tea

Tea, one of the most commonly consumed beverages in the world, is produced from the plant *Camellia sinensis*, and although green, black, and oolong teas are all derived from the same species, the production process is different for each. Green tea is produced by steaming and drying the leaves, which helps retain the polyphenol content; the processes for producing black and oolong teas are different, thus they have less polyphenols. The biologically active polyphenols in green tea are epigal-locatechin gallate (EGCG), epicatechin (EC), and epicatechin gallate (ECG), all of which act as antioxidants (Fragakis and Thompson, 2012).

Green tea is widely recognized for its antioxidant properties, which include reducing free radical DNA damage, lipid peroxidation, and free radical generation. Because of these properties, its use in prevention of diseases, particularly cancer, has been studied. It has been suggested that green tea may have a protective effect against lung cancer in nonsmokers, and GI and breast cancers, although the research is difficult to interpret due to the variety of confounding factors, including the type of study, doses given, and differences in studied populations (Yuan et al., 2011; Fitz et al., 2013; Yiannakopoulou, 2013).

Green tea extract is also said to increase energy expenditure and is frequently a component of multi-ingredient supplements sold as weight loss aids. However, there is insufficient evidence of its efficacy in weight loss; further research in this area is needed (Fragakis and Thompson, 2012).

Hot brewed green tea has the highest concentration of polyphenols, about 100–200 mg/cup. Decaffeinated varieties are available; the decaffeination process does reduce the concentration of polyphenols, but likely not to a significant degree. Commercially prepared ready-to-drink green tea beverages and iced teas have sig-nificantly lower polyphenol content, although amounts will vary depending on the concentration of tea solids present (Fragakis and Thompson, 2012).

Green tea extract is also available in the form of capsules containing 100–600 mg of polyphenols, and doses of up to 1200 mg of EGCG per day appear to be safe, although there have been some reports of hepatotoxicity. Green tea may reduce nonheme iron absorption, although this effect can likely be mitigated in part by concomitant consumption of a food or beverage rich in vitamin C (Fragakis and Thompson, 2012).

Milk Thistle

Milk thistle, or *Silybum marianum*, is a plant whose ripe seeds contain the com-pound silymarin, a complex of flavonolignans that include silibinin, the compound most commonly used in milk thistle research and treatment. Silibinin has antioxidant and hepatoprotective effects, and thus is often used to treat hepatotoxic conditions, including amanita mushroom poisoning, hepatitis, and chemotherapy-induced liver dysfunction. Preliminary animal studies have also been conducted on milk thistle's effect on cancer, particularly of the prostate and colon, although much more research is needed to fully elucidate its effect on the disease (Siegel and Stebbing, 2013).

Milk thistle is most commonly taken to treat or prevent hepatic disease or its complications. While most research on silymarin and silibinin has been conducted on this patient population, results are inconclusive, due in large part to the quality of studies conducted; there are differences in both dosage amounts and forms given, duration of treatment, patient demographics and type and severity of hepatic disease; small sample size is also a common drawback. In 2005, the Cochrane Review Group concluded that milk thistle did not appear to have an effect on the course of the disease in patients with hepatitis B or C. Although studies defined as low quality showed significant reductions in liver-related mortality, this effect was not seen in high-quality studies. More research is needed to fully assess milk thistle's effects on liver disease (Rambaldi et al., 2005).

Use of milk thistle in cancer patients is common, as it is thought to act as a hepatoprotective agent, assisting in the hepatic clearance of multiple drugs and in the metabolism of products released from tumors treated with chemotherapy and/or radiation (Lougercio and Festi, 2011). In a study of children with acute lymphoblastic leukemia and chemotherapy-induced hepatotoxicity, supplementation with silymarin for 30 days resulted in a significant decrease in aspartate aminotransferase compared to controls (Ladas et al., 2010). Overall, however, few studies have been conducted in humans on the effect of milk thistle's potential hepatoprotective effects in patients receiving chemotherapy.

Silymarins antioxidant effects are due to its ability to bind and inhibit formation of free radicals, interfere with lipid peroxidation in cell membranes, and chelate iron. Its iron-chelating function makes it an effective treatment for iron overload, commonly seen in thalassemia, an inherited form of anemia in which too little hemoglobin and red blood cells are produced. In a recent study, thalassemia patients given silymarin with desferrioxamine, an iron chelating agent, for 9 months had significant reductions in serum ferritin and iron compared to controls receiving only desferrioxamine (Moayedi et al., 2013).

While there is no established recommended dose for milk thistle, most research on its effect on hepatic disorders used 200–400 mg given daily in divided doses. Milk thistle can be given in a variety of forms, including liquid extracts, soft gels, capsules, whole seeds, and cut herbs. It should be noted that in a recent study, a significant percentage of both the whole seed and cut herb forms were contaminated with a variety of potentially toxigenic molds, including *Aspergillus flavus*, an aflatoxin; thus, the other forms of milk thistle should be recommended (Tournas et al., 2013).

RESVERATROL

Resveratrol is polyphenolic flavonoid compound that has drawn the interest of the health community in the last few decades as a potential agent to prevent diseases associated with aging because of its anti-inflammatory, antioxidant, and anticarcinogenic actions. The compound is found in berries, peanuts, and the skins of grapes; red wine is also a significant source of resveratrol (Fragakis and Thompson, 2012).

Resveratrol has been studied extensively in the rat model and has been shown to be effective in increasing vasodilation, and reducing blood pressure and atherosclerotic lesions. It has been suggested that the compound also provides a protective effect in myocardial and cerebral ischemic injury, however, sufficient human studies are lacking (Xu and Si, 2012).

While a few rat studies have demonstrated reductions in serum lipid levels, these results have not been replicated in humans; in a recent meta-analysis of seven studies totaling 282 subjects, no significant change in serum lipid levels were seen in treatment vs. control groups. The author concluded that lipid lowering was likely not the mechanism of action with regard to resveratrol's apparent cardioprotective effects (Sahebkar, 2013).

Some trial results have also indicated that resveratrol may be a potentially effective agent in the fight against obesity and diabetes. In several trials, obese rats or rats fed a high-fat diet and supplemented with resveratrol showed reductions in body weight gain and insulin resistance compared to controls. However, neither have other studies shown these benefits nor have these results been reproduced in humans (Xu and Si, 2012).

Resveratrol is thought to exert anticancer effects via an increase in apoptosis in cancer cells, and reductions in tumor growth were seen in gastric and pancreatic cancer cell lines; however, human studies are lacking, thus no conclusions can yet be drawn regarding resveratrol's role in chemoprevention (Fragakis and Thompson, 2012).

Resveratrol can be consumed as a supplement and is usually found in doses of 250–500 mg; however, an optimal dose is unknown. Further, while the limited numbers of human studies have not reported significant side effects of supplementation, not enough evidence exists as yet to determine the risks of supplementation (Fragakis and Thompson, 2012).

St. John's Wort

St. John's wort, or *Hypericum perforatum*, is widely used to treat mild, moderate, and severe depression. It contains the bioactive compounds hyperforin and hypericin, which are thought to provide the therapeutic benefits, although it contains a number of other biological compounds. Although the method of action is unknown, it is hypothesized that St. John's wort may increase serotonin levels, and inhibit reuptake of monoamines, dopamine noradrenaline, and some neurotransmitters (Fragakis and Thompson, 2012).

Some studies indicate that St. John's wort is as effective as standard antidepressant medications, has fewer side effects, and is more effective than placebo (Linde et al., 2008). Others suggest that St. John's wort was no more effective than antidepressants and placebo; however, these results may be due to smaller supplemental doses. Research also indicates that patients taking St. John's wort had lower depression relapse rates and a longer duration of effect than standard antidepressants and placebo (Kasper et al., 2006).

Studied doses of St. John's wort vary, but 900 mg of hypericum extract appears to be both safe and effective. The extract most commonly used is called WS 5570, which comes in 300 mg tablets and which can be given three times daily. Side effects may include phototoxic rash, serotonin syndrome, and induced mania. Because of the neurological side effects, it is suggested that those with bipolar disorder or dementia avoid St. John's wort (Qureshi and Al-Bedah, 2013).

St. John's wort has been shown to significantly interact with many medications, including antiepileptics, beta blockers, antidepressives, benzodiazepines, anti-inflammatories, and oral contraceptives (Qureshi and Al-Bedah, 2013). Evidence suggests that the safety information provided by most hypericum extract manufacturers is inadequate, so healthcare providers should be sure to discuss potential side effects when prescribing or recommending the herb to patients and clients (Clauson et al., 2008).

BIOLOGIC SUBSTANCES

Fish Oil

Because most epidemiological studies show that increased fish consumption is associated with lower incidence of coronary heart disease, fish oil supplementation has been studied for its effect on heart disease. Fish oil is an excellent source of the omega-3 fatty acids eicosapentaenoic acid (EPA) and docosahexaenoic acid (DHA), the precursors to eicosanoids, which have strong anti-inflammatory and antiatherogenic effects. The effect of fish oil supplementation has also been investigated for its effects on blood pressure, atrial fibrillation, inflammatory bowel disease, and rheumatoid arthritis (RA) (Fragakis and Thompson, 2012).

Several large randomized placebo-controlled trials have demonstrated reductions in cardiovascular morbidity and mortality in subjects receiving fish oil supplements, although baseline cardiovascular risk and the dose and type of fish oil supplement varied among studies (Burr et al., 1989; GISSI, 1999; Yokoyama et al., 2007). Fish oil supplementation has also been shown to reduce plasma triglycerides, especially in those with hypertriglyceridemia, and mildly increase low-density lipoprotein (LDL) cholesterol; it has been suggested that this increase in LDL is not accompanied by an elevated risk of CHD due to the other mitigating effects of the fish oil (Fragakis and Thomson, 2012).

The strength of the evidence is such that the American Heart Association recommends individuals with coronary heart disease consume 1 g of EPA and DHA daily, preferably through dietary fish intake, or through fish oil supplementation if necessary, and individuals with hypertriglyceridemia consume 2–4 g of EPA and DHA daily, which can only be achieved through supplementation (AHA et al., 2006).

Some research suggests that fish oil in high doses may result in small decreases in blood pressure; however, the effectiveness of other interventions and the high dose required make fish oil supplements impractical therapeutic agents in the treatment of hypertension (Kris-Etherton et al., 2002). While some studies have shown fish oil to be beneficial in the prevention of postoperative and recurrent atrial fibrillation, the bulk of evidence suggests that it is not, thus it is not recommended for this purpose (Xin et al., 2013).

Because of its anti-inflammatory effects, it has been postulated that fish oil may be of benefit in inflammatory conditions such as RA and inflammatory bowel disease. Evidence suggests that supplementation in those with RA may effect mild reductions in joint stiffness and tenderness. Supplementation in ulcerative colitis and Crohn's disease has been shown to reduce relapse rates and corticosteroid requirements, and improve weight gain. However, further research in these areas is needed (Fragakis and Thompson, 2012).

Dietary intake of EPA and DHA is almost exclusively from fish; fattier fishes such as mackerel, herring, salmon, and tuna have larger amounts. Eggs from hens fed flaxseed contain small amounts of DHA; flaxseed and walnuts are good sources of alpha-linolenic acid, which is a precursor to EPA and DHA. Supplementation of fish oil can be achieved in the form of cod liver oil or commercial supplements in soft gel capsule form (Fragakis and Thompson, 2012).

Recommended doses vary widely; AHA guidelines should be followed for individuals with CHD; however, studied doses for other conditions range from 1 to 9 g daily. Fish oil has been deemed generally recognized as safe (GRAS) by the FDA in doses up to 3 g daily. EPA has been shown to increase clotting times; thus, it is recommended that fish oil supplements be withheld 1–2 weeks before surgery, and used with caution in individuals taking other medications affecting blood coagulation. While most commercial fish oil supplements do not contain vitamin A, some fish oils contain large amounts of the vitamin, which can have teratogenic effects and thus should be avoided by pregnant women (Fragakis and Thompson, 2012).

S-Adenosylmethionine

S-adenosylmethionine, or SAM-e, is a derivative of methionine produced in all living cells; it functions in a variety of metabolic reactions by transferring its methyl group to various substrates, transforming it to S-adenosylhomocysteine, which can then be converted back to methionine, SAM-e, cysteine, or glutathione. SAM-e became available as a supplement in the United States in 1999 and is most frequently used in the treatment of depression, osteoarthritis, and liver disease.

The potential effect of SAM-e on depression is not fully understood, but it has been hypothesized that it may increase the production of the neurotransmitters serotonin, norepinephrine, and dopamine (Fragakis and Thompson, 2012). A 2002 meta-analysis of 11 studies examining the use of SAM-e as a monotherapy in treating depression suggested the supplement may be as effective as standard antidepressants, although many of these studies were not placebo controlled, and thus could not conclusively demonstrate efficacy. Further, of the 11 studies, 7 used a parenteral form of SAM-e, as a stable oral form was not readily available when the studies were conducted (Hardy et al., 2003).

In a placebo-controlled double-blind study of SAM-e supplementation, patients considered nonresponsive to traditional serotonin reuptake inhibitors for major depression were given 800 mg of SAM-e twice daily as an adjunctive therapy. The treatment group had statistically significant improvements in depression symptoms compared to the placebo group (Papakostas et al., 2010). In a later study of patients with major depressive disorder, subjects received either 1600–3200 mg of SAM-e, 10–20 mg of escitalopram or placebo. Contrary to the earlier study, researchers found no significant difference in response or relapse rates between the three groups (Mischoulon et al., 2014).

Because of its suspected neurological effects, and the fact that those with Alzheimer's disease (AD) have significantly lower levels of SAM-e in their cerebrospinal fluid, SAM-e has been proposed as a potential therapy in the treatment of dementia (Linnebank et al., 2010). Although SAM-e supplementation in dementia has not been extensively studied, some initial animal studies have yielded results that merit further investigation. For example, supplementation of SAM-e for 1 month resulted in an 80% reduction in amyloid-β deposition in the brains of mice predisposed to AD, and a 24% reduction after 3 months of supplementation, suggesting that SAM-e may modulate the onset or progression of AD (Lee et al., 2012).

SAM-e has also been shown to be effective in the treatment of osteoarthritis; researchers hypothesize that the compound has both a protective and regenerative effect on joint cartilage. Early studies showed SAM-e to be as effective, and with fewer side effects, as nonsteroidal anti-inflammatory drugs in the treatment of pain related to osteoarthritis (Lopez, 2012). Further, another study showed SAM-e to be as effective as celecoxib (Celebrex) in reducing pain and improving joint function, although SAM-e had a slower onset of action (Najm et al., 2004). Because of safety concerns regarding the long-term use of celecoxib, SAM-e may prove to be a viable treatment alternative.

SAM-e supplementation may have a positive effect on liver injury through its ability to protect hepatocytes from apoptosis, raise glutathione levels, and suppress cytokine expression; however, these effects have only been demonstrated in animal models; there is insufficient research on SAM-e supplementation in human liver injury. In a 2006 Cochrane review of nine clinical trials, no benefit for SAM-e supplementation in alcoholic liver injury was seen (Rambaldi and Gluud, 2006). However, one placebo-controlled double-blind study in patients with alcoholic liver injury demonstrated a reduction in mortality and liver transplantation rates in patients supplemented with 1200 mg SAM-e daily for 2 years, but only when the patients with the most advanced liver disease were excluded from analysis (Mato et al., 1999).

SAM-e is available in a variety of forms, and while parenteral forms are more bioavailable, for practical use enteric-coated oral tablets are available for purchase over the counter in the United States. Recommended doses vary based on manufacturer, but 800 mg twice daily was most often used by researchers in depression trials, and 1200 mg daily in osteoarthritis trials. SAM-e appears to be well tolerated, with no more side effects than placebo in most trials. However, because of the role of B_6, B_{12}, and folate in the metabolism of SAM-e, deficiencies of these vitamins may result in elevated homocysteine levels, which have been associated with an increased incidence of cardiovascular diseases. Although this effect has not been proven by research, it may be prudent to recommend B vitamin supplements for individuals taking SAM-e (Halsted, 2013).

VITAMINS

Vitamins are organic compounds that are required in limited amounts, of which the body cannot produce sufficient quantities, thus they must be obtained from the diet. Some vitamins are actually groups of related compounds called vitamers; for example, the term vitamin A includes the substances retinol, retinal, retinoic acid, retinyl esters, and the carotenoids—beta-carotene, alpha-carotene, and beta-cryptoxanthin. Vitamins serve in a wide variety of biochemical functions; they are antioxidants, function as cofactors for a number of enzymes necessary for metabolism, and serve as regulators of mineral metabolism. Table 5.3 lists the common functions of vitamins.

At present, there are 13 compounds recognized as vitamins. These include the fat-soluble vitamins A, D, E, and K; the water-soluble vitamins B_1 (thiamin), B_2 (riboflavin), B_3 (niacin), B_5 (pantothenic acid), B_6 (pyridoxine), B_{12} (cyanocobalamin), biotin, and folic acid; and vitamin C (ascorbic acid). The USDA has established a Recommended Dietary Allowance (RDA), or the amount of a nutrient sufficient to meet the needs of 97%–98% of the population, divided into age and gender categories. Table 5.4 lists the RDAs of vitamins.

While vitamins make up a significant portion of dietary supplements taken worldwide, there is limited evidence to suggest that supplementation in the absence of deficiency is beneficial to health, and in some cases may actually be harmful. However, even in developed countries, insufficient intake of many vitamins is common due to poor-quality diets, and some individuals develop vitamin deficiencies. A vitamin

---

TABLE 5.3
Vitamin Functions

Vitamin	Function
A	Vision, reproduction, bone development, immune function, epithelial cell function
D	Bone development and maintenance, calcium absorption, neuromuscular function
E	Protects the integrity of cell membranes, prevention of red blood cell (RBC) lysis, protects vitamin A, antioxidant
K	Production of prothrombin used in normal blood clotting
C (ascorbic acid)	Maintains capillary integrity, promotes healing, aids in tooth and bone formation, increases iron absorption, collagen formation
B_1 (thiamin)	Carbohydrate metabolism, nerve cell membrane function
B_2 (riboflavin)	Carbohydrate, protein, and fat metabolism
B_3 (niacin)	Carbohydrate metabolism
B_6 (pyridoxine)	Protein metabolism, converts tryptophan to niacin, synthesis of hemoglobin, central nervous system integrity
B_{12} (cobalamin)	RBC maturation, body cell function, especially central nervous system, gastrointestinal and bone marrow
Folic acid	DNA synthesis, RBC synthesis, and maturation
Pantothenic acid	Carbohydrate, protein, and fat metabolism, hormone, and hemoglobin synthesis
Biotin	Carbohydrate metabolism, fatty acid synthesis

TABLE 5.4
Adult RDAs for Vitamins

Vitamin	Men	Women
Vitamin A	900 µg/day	700 µg/day
Vitamin D	15 µg/day	15 µg/day
	20 µg/day > 70 years	20 µg/day > 70 years
Vitamin E	15 mg/day	15 mg/day
Vitamin K	120 µg/day[a]	90 µg/day[a]
Vitamin C	90 mg/day	75 mg/day
Thiamin	1.2 mg/day	1.1 mg/day
Riboflavin	1.3 mg/day	1.1 mg/day
Niacin	16 mg/day	14 mg/day
Vitamin B_6	1.3 mg/day	1.3 mg/day
	1.7 mg/day > 50 years	1.5 mg/day > 50 years
Folate	400 µg/day	400 µg/day
Vitamin B_{12}	2.4 µg/day	2.4 µg/day

[a] Adequate intake.

deficiency may be primary, meaning it is caused by inadequate intake, or secondary, caused by a disease or medical condition that interferes with the absorption or metabolism of the vitamin.

Insufficient scientific knowledge on vitamin needs complicates the issue of supplementation. Controversy exists regarding not only the ideal intake of some vitamins, but also the way in which deficiency is diagnosed. Although new research continues to shed light on micronutrient needs, it is recognized that requirements may vary significantly depending on age, gender, disease condition, and a number of other factors; therefore, it is important that supplementation decisions be discussed with a qualified healthcare provider who can assess these factors to determine the need and proper dose and duration of supplementation. See Table 5.5 for common risk factors and signs and symptoms of vitamin deficiencies.

B VITAMINS

B vitamins are water soluble and include thiamin (B_1), riboflavin (B_2), niacin (B_3), pyridoxine (B_6), cobalamin (B_{12}), folic acid, pantothenic acid, and biotin. Because most B vitamins are found in a wide variety of foods, including meats, whole grains, and other plant-based foods, and in enriched foods such as cereals and other grain products, deficiency is relatively rare. It can occur, however, in those that are severely malnourished, usually as a result of significant nutrient malabsorption, starvation, or severe alcohol abuse. B vitamins have a wide variety of functions in the body, but most notably are necessary for carbohydrate, protein, and fat metabolism.

TABLE 5.5
Vitamin Deficiencies—Risk Factors and Signs/Symptoms

Vitamin	Risk Factors	Signs/Symptoms
A	Fat malabsorption, severe malnutrition, alcohol abuse, severe zinc deficiency	Night blindness, Bitot's spots (keratin build up on conjunctiva of the eye), conjunctival dryness, hyperkeratosis, anorexia, phrynoderma (dry pigmented papules around hair follicles), reduced T-helper cell activity, reduced mucus secretion
D	Limited sunlight exposure, poor vitamin D intake (dairy free, vegan), fat malabsorption, reduced cutaneous production (elderly, dark skinned individuals), increased sequestration (obesity)	Rickets (in children), osteomalacia, tissue calcification caused by hypercalcemia/hypercalciuria
E	Fat malabsorption	Increased platelet aggregation, reduced RBC survival, hemolytic anemia, neuron degeneration, reduced serum creatinine
K	Fat malabsorption	Abnormal bleeding and bruising
C (ascorbic Acid)	Inadequate intake, acute illness and inflammation reduce levels	Mild: anorexia, muscle pain, increased susceptibility to infection; severe: scurvy—anemia, bleeding gums, petechiae (tiny flat red spots on the skin), perifollicular hemorrhage, impaired wound healing, weakened collagen in bone, teeth and connective tissue
B_1 (thiamin)	Alcohol abuse, long-term parenteral nutrition, refeeding syndrome, malabsorption, dialysis, hyperemesis, bariatric surgery	Dry beriberi: paresthesia, anesthesia, weakness; Wet beriberi: cardiac failure, dyspnea, hepatomegaly, tachycardia, oliguria; Wernicke's encephalopathy: confusion, ataxia, nystagmus, coma
B_2 (riboflavin)	Alcohol abuse, malabsorption; usually accompanied by other B vitamin deficiencies	Sore throat, red eyes, edema of pharyngeal and oral mucosa, cheilosis (scaling and fissures at the corners of the mouth), glossitis, seborrheic dermatitis, visual impairment, anemia
B_3 (niacin)	Alcohol abuse, malabsorption (rare—can be synthesized from tryptophan)	Pellagra: dermatitis, memory loss, apathy, depression, headache, fatigue, diarrhea
B_6 (pyridoxine)	Alcohol abuse, malabsorption; usually accompanied by folate and/or B_{12} deficiency	Seborrheic dermatitis, microcytic anemia, convulsions, confusion, depression, angular stomatitis, glossitis, cheilosis

(Continued)

TABLE 5.5 (*Continued*)
Vitamin Deficiencies—Risk Factors and Signs/Symptoms

Vitamin	Risk Factors	Signs/Symptoms
B_{12} (cobalamin)	Alcohol abuse, reduced intake (vegetarian/vegan), decreased absorption (gastrectomy, gastric bypass, Crohn's disease, ileal resection, *H. pylori* overgrowth, chronic use of proton pump inhibitors), increased excretion (liver and renal disease)	Megaloblastic anemia, leukopenia, thrombocytopenia, glossitis, paresthesias of feet and hands, unsteadiness, confusion, depression, memory loss
Folic acid	Alcohol abuse, prolonged poor intake, malabsorption, medication use (phenytoin, cholestyramine, sulfasalazine, metformin)	Megaloblastic anemia, diarrhea, smooth and sore tongue, weight loss, decreased cell-mediated immunity, nervous irritability, dementia, neural tube defects with maternal deficiency
Pantothenic acid	Rare, associated with other B vitamin deficiencies and severe malnutrition	Paresthesias in toes and soles of the feet, burning sensation in feet, depression, fatigue, insomnia, weakness
Biotin	Rare, associated with other B vitamin deficiencies and severe malnutrition	Stomatitis, hair loss, dermatitis, glossitis, anorexia, nausea, depression, hepatic steatosis, hypercholesterolemia

B vitamin supplements are widely available, and often grouped together as a B-complex, as deficiency of one B vitamin is often accompanied by another. Of particular note is folic acid, which can be supplemented separately, or taken as part of a prenatal multivitamin, usually in doses of 400 µg. Adequate folic acid status is necessary to prevent neural tube defects and other birth complications; thus, it is recommended that all women capable of getting pregnant consume at least 400 µg of folic acid from supplements or fortified foods daily. Caution should be taken with folic acid supplementation; excess folic acid can mask the symptoms of B_{12} deficiency, thus it is recommended that intake from supplements and fortified foods not exceed 1000 µg/day (ODSb, 2013).

Perhaps the most common B vitamin deficiency is B_{12}. Sufficient gastric production of intrinsic factor is required for B_{12} absorption in the ileum; thus, those individuals with total or partial gastric and/or ileal resection are at high risk for deficiency, even if oral intake is adequate. Other gastric disorders can also impair B_{12} absorption, including atrophic gastritis, a condition in which hydrochloric acid production is insufficient. In the event of impaired absorption, B_{12} can be supplemented with nasal sprays; however, monthly intramuscular injections are often necessary. B_{12} is also one of the few B vitamins not found naturally in plant foods, so vegetarians and vegans are at higher risk for deficiency; in these cases, oral supplementation is usually sufficient to treat deficiency (ODSb, 2013).

Vitamin C

Vitamin C, or ascorbic acid, is a vitamin found in fruits and vegetables, with citrus fruits, strawberries, kiwifruit, tomatoes, sweet peppers, Brussels sprouts, and potatoes being the best sources of the vitamin. Vitamin C not only is a necessary component for the synthesis of collagen, L-carnitine, and some neurotransmitters, but also functions as a potent antioxidant, plays a role in immunity, and increases the absorption of nonheme iron. The RDA for adult women is 75 mg/day, adult men 90 mg/day, and an additional 35 mg/day is recommended for smokers (ODSb, 2013).

Vitamin C deficiency, or scurvy, is uncommon in developed countries, and typically only occurs in individuals consuming less than 10 mg/day of vitamin C for about a month. Symptoms of scurvy include fatigue, swollen, and bleeding gums, and as the disease progresses, petechiae, ecchymoses, purpura, joint pain, poor wound healing, hyperkeratosis, and corkscrew hairs are frequently seen (ODSb, 2013).

Vitamin C inadequacy is more common and is caused by a consistent intake of vitamin C above 10 mg/day, but less than the RDA. Those groups at risk for vitamin C inadequacy include smokers, individuals with very poor fruit and vegetable intake, and those with significant malabsorptive diseases. Low ascorbic acid levels have also been reported in patients with chronic kidney disease on hemodialysis (ODSb, 2013).

Vitamin C is frequently taken as a supplement due to its antioxidant properties, to boost the immune system, especially in an effort to reduce the incidence and duration of the common cold, and as a potential preventative or treatment agent for cancer and age-related macular degeneration (ODSb, 2013).

Vitamin C, used for decades in the prevention and treatment of the common cold, is a regular component of most anticold medications. In a recent Cochrane Review of 29 placebo-controlled trials of vitamin C supplementation of ≥200 mg of vitamin C daily, encompassing a total of over 11,000 participants, researchers concluded that vitamin C was ineffective in reducing the incidence of the common cold in the general population. However, results of five studies showed that participants supplemented with vitamin C and subjected to extremes in physical endurance, such as running a marathon, reduced their risk of developing a cold by half (Hemila and Chalker, 2013).

While vitamin C does not appear to reduce the risk of the common cold for the general population, based on results of a recent meta-analysis of 31 studies and nearly 10,000 cold episodes, vitamin C supplementation does appear to result in modest reductions in the duration of cold symptoms (Hemila and Chalker, 2013).

Some studies have also examined therapeutic vitamin C supplementation, for example, supplementation started only after the onset of cold symptoms. While an early trial of 8 g of ascorbic acid daily did appear to reduce the duration of cold symptoms, these results have not been replicated, and later studies showed no benefit of therapeutic vitamin C supplementation (Hemila and Chalker, 2013).

Vitamin C has also been studied in the prevention of cancer; in large epidemiologic studies, participants with the highest intake of fruits and vegetables had a lower incidence of many types of cancer, theoretically due in part to a higher intake of vitamin C. However, prospective cohort study results have varied; the Nurse's Health Study of over 82,000 participants showed a higher intake of vitamin C was correlated with a 63% lower incidence of breast cancer in women with a family history of the disease, whereas other studies have not shown such benefits. As pointed out in a review of the literature, however, in the studies showing no differences in cancer risk, the groups with the lowest intake still consumed vitamin C at levels above the RDA (ODSb, 2013). This suggests that perhaps cancer risk increases with insufficient intake of vitamin C, but intakes significantly higher than the RDA do not reduce cancer risk.

In vitamin C and cancer risk research, participants are also frequently supplemented with other antioxidant nutrients including selenium, zinc, molybdenum, vitamin E, and beta-carotene; no positive results were seen in most of these studies (Taylor et al., 1994; Gaziano et al., 2009; Lin et al., 2009). Again, this suggests that perhaps vitamin C intake significantly above the RDA has no effect on cancer risk. Limitations of these studies include the variety of doses provided, the differences in other nutrients supplemented, and the lack of measured vitamin C levels before and after supplementation. At this time, data does not support the recommendation for vitamin C intake above RDA levels for the prevention of cancer.

The use of vitamin C in the treatment of cancer is more controversial. In vitro studies show ascorbic acid's ability to function as a pro-oxidant at pharmacological doses, increasing oxidative damage to cellular components, thus impairing function and viability of cancer cells; this effect appears to target tumor cells, rather than healthy cells, because of their lower concentration of antioxidant enzymes. Studies have shown significantly reduced growth rates of ovarian, pancreatic, and glioblastoma tumors in rats given high-dose intravenous (IV) vitamin C. Although several case reports have been published detailing the use of high-dose IV vitamin C in the treatment of various cancers, information provided was limited and no large placebo-controlled trials on vitamin C as a single treatment for cancer have been conducted (Park, 2013).

Vitamin C, given both orally and by IV, appears to be well tolerated with little side effects besides nausea, diarrhea, and abdominal cramps at high doses. However, the use of vitamin C and other antioxidants during traditional cancer treatments, namely, chemotherapy and radiation, is controversial. While some data suggests that antioxidants may actually protect cancer cells from the desired effects of chemotherapy and radiation, other data indicates that antioxidants protect healthy cells from the same effects, as well as enhance the efficacy of these conventional treatments. While it seems likely that oral vitamin C supplementation, especially in doses not exceeding the tolerable upper limit of 2 g daily, will not result in serum levels high enough to cause these unwanted effects, it would be wise for individuals with cancer to consult their oncologist before starting antioxidant supplementation (ODSb, 2013).

Age-related macular degeneration (AMD) is a leading cause of vision loss in older adults. Several epidemiological studies have shown a correlation between vitamin C, as well as other antioxidants, and lower rates of AMD; however, other studies have not demonstrated this correlation. While there is insufficient evidence to support vitamin C supplementation to prevent the development of AMD, some studies suggest that antioxidant supplementation slows the progression of the disease. In the Age-Related Eye Disease Study (AREDS), participants with intermediate AMD had a 28% lower rate of progression to advanced AMD when supplemented with high-dose antioxidants, including 500 mg of vitamin C (AREDS Research Group, 2001).

Vitamin D

Vitamin D is a fat-soluble vitamin produced endogenously in skin exposed to ultraviolet radiation and is also found in fish and fortified foods such as milk and cereal. Vitamin D functions to maintain serum calcium and phosphorus equilibrium by enhancing calcium absorption in the gut and is required for bone remodeling and growth; it also has immune and neuromuscular functions. The RDA for vitamin D is 600 IU/day for adults up to the age of 70; 800 IU/day is recommended for adults older than 70. Although sun exposure can often produce sufficient levels of vitamin D, the RDAs have been set on the basis of minimal sun exposure (ODSb, 2013).

In recent years, scientists have noted an increased prevalence of vitamin D insufficiency and deficiency in the general population. At particular risk are individuals who receive minimal sun exposure, such as those living in northern latitudes and residents of long-term care facilities. Populations with reduced ability to produce vitamin D from sun exposure include dark-skinned individuals and the elderly. Insufficient intake may also contribute, most commonly seen in vegans and those with lactose intolerance; individuals with significant fat malabsorption, including those who have undergone gastric bypass surgery; and infants who are exclusively breast fed for prolonged periods. Last, those individuals with a body mass index greater than 30 may require more vitamin D, as greater amounts of the vitamin produced in the skin are sequestered in subcutaneous fat stores, resulting in reductions of circulating serum levels (ODSb, 2013).

Vitamin D status can be assessed by checking serum 25OH-hydroxyvitamin D levels; however, some disagreement exists regarding what level is optimal for maintenance of bone health, as well as other purported benefits. The classic sign of deficiency is rickets in children and osteomalacia in adults (ODSb, 2013).

As a supplement, vitamin D is available in two forms: ergocalciferol (D_2) and cholecalciferol (D_3). Both are considered approximately equivalent in terms of potency, although in high doses D_3 may be preferred. Vitamin D supplements can be found in a variety of doses, and the vitamin is sometimes combined with calcium supplements to enhance absorption of the mineral; these supplements are routinely used in individuals with osteomalacia or osteoporosis.

There are no benefits to supplementation if deficiency or insufficiency is not present; however, high-risk individuals may need to consume vitamin D supplements routinely to maintain optimal serum levels (ODSb, 2013). The Endocrine Society recently published clinical practice guidelines on the prevention and treatment of vitamin D deficiency. For deficient adults, 50,000 IU of either D_2 or D_3 weekly for 8 weeks or 6,000 IU daily is recommended, followed by a maintenance dose of 1,500–2,000 IU daily (Pramyothin and Holick, 2012).

Maintenance of optimal 25OH-hydroxyvitamin D levels appears to have health benefits beyond that of preservation of bone density. A number of studies suggest that vitamin D has antineoplastic effects, especially for colorectal cancer. While the Women's Health Initiative study of over 36,000 women did not show a reduction in colon cancer rates in those women supplemented with 400 IU of vitamin D and 1,000 mg of calcium daily compared to controls, it has been argued that perhaps the dose of vitamin D was too low to see any effects. Epidemiological evidence also suggests that vitamin D plays a role in breast and prostate cancer. Further research is needed to determine optimal serum levels as well as the most beneficial supplemental dose of vitamin D; authors of a recent review suggest a minimum of 800 IU of vitamin D daily be used in future research (Leyssens et al., 2013).

VITAMIN E

The term vitamin E is sometimes used to describe all tocopherols and tocotrienol derivatives; however, only alpha and gamma tocopherol have vitamin E activity; alpha tocopherol is the most abundant and active form of the two. Rich dietary sources of vitamin E include vegetable oils, nuts, sunflower seeds, fortified cereals, whole grains, leafy vegetables, and egg yolks. The RDA for vitamin E is 15 mg/day for both men and women. Its primary function is to act as an antioxidant, and thus its effects on heart disease, cancer, immune function, and cognition have been studied (ODSb, 2013).

Because vitamin E is fat soluble, its deficiency is relatively rare, most commonly occurring in individuals with medical conditions that result in fat malabsorption, such as short bowel syndrome, exocrine pancreatic insufficiency, and cystic fibrosis. Symptoms of deficiency include hemolytic anemia, peripheral neuropathy, skeletal muscle lesions, ataxia, and retinopathy. In conjunction with a physical exam and diet history, deficiency can be diagnosed by measuring serum alpha-tocopherol (ODSb, 2013).

Several large epidemiological cohort studies showed an inverse relationship between vitamin E intake and incidence of coronary heart disease (Riemersma et al., 1991; Rimm et al., 1993); thus randomized controlled trials were conducted to further examine this relationship. In a 2004 analysis, researchers found no positive effect of vitamin E supplementation on heart disease in six of seven studies (Eidelman et al., 2004); other research has similarly failed to show positive results (Fragakis and Thompson, 2012).

Detrimental effects of vitamin E supplementation have been noted in some studies. In the Heart Outcomes Prevention Evaluation (HOPE) study, long-term vitamin E supplementation of ≥400 IU daily resulted in an increased relative incidence of heart failure and hospitalizations for heart failure (Lonn et al., 2002). In a large analysis of 19 clinical trials, pooled all-cause mortality was significantly higher in participants taking ≥250 IU of vitamin E daily (Miller et al., 2005).

The HOPE study also examined cancer incidence with vitamin E supplementation; over the 7-year duration of the study, supplementation of vitamin E was not associated with incidence of cancer (Lonn et al., 2002). The U.S. Cancer Prevention Study II prospectively followed for 16 years over 991,000 patients; those with a self-reported consumption of vitamin E supplements for at least 10 years had a 40% lower incidence of bladder cancer (Jacobs et al., 2002). Research has been conducted on other types of cancers, most notably prostate cancer, and while some studies have shown promising results, others have not. Further research in this area is needed (Fragakis and Thompson, 2012).

Some evidence suggests that free radical damage influences the degree of cognitive impairment in patients with Alzheimer's disease (AD); thus, vitamin E has been proposed as a potential treatment. In a recent Cochrane review, only two studies on vitamin E and AD met the author's inclusion criteria. One small study reported that fewer AD patients supplemented with vitamin E reached negative end points (death, institutionalization, worsening of clinical dementia scores, or loss of two activities of daily living) than those not supplemented with vitamin E. The second study did not find any differences in cognition between AD patients supplemented and not supplemented with vitamin E. Because of these limited results, the authors concluded that vitamin E cannot be recommended as a therapy for AD (Farina et al., 2012).

Vitamin E supplements come in both natural and synthetic forms in a variety of doses; recent studies have suggested that natural vitamin E is more biologically active and more readily absorbed. At pharmacological doses (200 mg) absorption decreases significantly. For many supplements, doses of vitamin E are expressed as international units (IU); to convert to mg, multiply the dose in IU with 0.67 for natural forms, and with 0.45 for synthetic forms (Fragakis and Thompson, 2012).

While some study results are contradictory, others suggest that vitamin E supplementation be avoided in those taking anticoagulant therapy, as it may increase risk of bleeding. It has also been shown to reduce the efficacy of some chemotherapy medications, thus should be avoided in this patient population (Fragakis and Thompson, 2012).

MINERALS

Dietary minerals are not technically minerals but chemical elements that enter the food chain via plants that absorb them from the soil. Aside from the four basic elements that serve organic functions (hydrogen, carbon, nitrogen, and oxygen), the following chemical elements are known to be necessary for humans, those elements that are found in larger quantities in the body: sodium, magnesium, phosphorus, chloride, potassium, and calcium, and trace elements zinc, iron, manganese, copper, iodine, selenium, and molybdenum. Table 5.6 lists the RDAs of select minerals.

Some elements, such as potassium and sodium, function primarily as electrolytes, whereas others serve a structural function, such as calcium. Many are necessary for the production and function of a wide variety of enzymes necessary for normal metabolic reactions. Other functions include hormone synthesis, antioxidant activity, cell signaling, and energy production. See Table 5.7 for a list of mineral functions.

Additional elements such as nickel, cobalt, chromium, boron, and fluorine are present in even smaller amounts in the body; although some research has been conducted on these ultra-trace elements, there is currently insufficient data to suggest that they are essential for human life, and no RDAs have been set for them.

TABLE 5.6
Adult RDAs for Minerals

Mineral	Men	Women
Calcium	1000 mg/day	1000 mg/day
	1200 mg/day > 70 years	1200 mg/day > 50 years
Copper	900 µg/day	900 µg/day
Iodine	150 µg/day	150 µg/day
Iron	8 mg/day	18 mg/day ≤ 50 years
		8 mg/day > 50 years
Magnesium	400 mg/day ≤ 30 years	310 mg/day ≤ 30 years
	420 mg/day > 30 years	320 mg/day > 30 years
Molybdenum	45 µg/day	45 µg/day
Phosphorus	700 mg/day	700 mg/day
Selenium	55 µg/day	55 µg/day
Zinc	11 mg/day	8 mg/day

TABLE 5.7
Mineral Functions

Mineral	Function
Calcium	Structural foundation of bones and teeth, nerve transmission, vasoconstriction and vasodilation, muscle function, intracellular signaling, hormone synthesis
Copper	Red blood cell formation, iron utilization, energy production, antioxidant, synthesis of connective tissue
Iodine	Component of thyroid hormones
Iron	Formation of hemoglobin and myoglobin, component of enzyme necessary for ATP production, immune, and cognitive function
Magnesium	Cofactor for enzymes responsible for protein, glucose, and DNA metabolism, neuromuscular transmission, muscle contraction, cardiovascular excitability
Molybdenum	Cofactor for enzymes
Phosphorus	Structural foundation of bones and teeth; formation of DNA, RNA, ATP, and phospholipids; acid base regulation; glucose metabolism
Selenium	Cofactor for glutathione, iodine, and thyroid metabolism
Zinc	Protein and DNA synthesis, immune function, wound healing, growth

CALCIUM

Calcium is the most abundant mineral in the body, the bulk of it stored in bones and teeth. Aside from its structural function in bone, calcium is also necessary for vasoconstriction and vasodilation, muscle function, nerve transmission, intracellular signaling, and hormone synthesis. The best dietary sources of calcium are dairy products and sardines, but lesser amounts can be found in dark leafy greens and broccoli; foods commonly fortified with calcium include soy milk, tofu, orange juice, and cereals. The RDA for calcium varies depending on age and gender, ranging from 1000 to 1300 mg/day for adults (ODSb, 2013).

Calcium deficiency cannot be diagnosed with a blood test; the body maintains serum calcium levels by pulling calcium from bones if intake is insufficient. Because the hallmark of calcium deficiency is osteomalacia, bone mineral density tests are most indicative of total body calcium status, and should be conducted regularly in high-risk individuals. Those individuals most at risk for deficiency are women with reduced estrogen levels, including postmenopausal women and women with amenorrhea due to anorexia nervosa or excessive exercise, as calcium absorption is reduced and urine calcium excretion is increased. Another significant risk factor is insufficient calcium intake, most commonly seen in those with lactose intolerance, milk protein allergy, or vegans (ODSb, 2013).

In addition to its role in bone health, calcium has also been associated with cancer risk. Although some evidence is conflicting, it appears that calcium supplementation may reduce the risk of colorectal cancer; however, because colon cancer generally develops and advances slowly, more long-term studies are needed before calcium supplementation can be recommended as a preventative agent for this disease.

It has been suggested that calcium supplementation actually increases the risk of prostate cancer, as several epidemiologic studies have demonstrated a significant correlation between calcium intakes of greater than 1500–2000 mg daily and higher rates of prostate cancer. However, other studies have not seen these results, so further research is needed; there is insufficient evidence to suggest that men with osteomalacia or osteoporosis avoid calcium supplementation (ODSb, 2013).

Calcium in recent years has been touted as a weight loss aid. Although a few earlier studies indicated that increased intake of calcium or dairy products resulted in reduced weight gain or lower body weight over time, later clinical trials did not shown any correlation. A recent meta-analysis of 29 studies concluded that calcium intake had no influence on body weight (Trowman et al., 2006).

Calcium is available in a variety of forms; citrate and carbonate are most commonly used for calcium supplements; however, lactate, gluconate, and phosphate are also available. The amount of calcium absorbed varies based on the type consumed, but the amount of elemental calcium provided must be included on the supplement fact label so that consumers can determine how much they need to take. Calcium carbonate is more efficiently absorbed when taken with food, whereas calcium citrate can be taken either with or without food. The supplements themselves also come in a variety of forms, including chewable tablets and pills, and are often paired with vitamin D to increase absorption (ODSb, 2013).

A potential risk of calcium supplementation is increased incidence of kidney stones, although this effect appears to be modest (Prentice et al., 2013). Some scientific literature has suggested calcium supplementation may increase risk of cardiovascular events such as myocardial infarction; however, most analyses of this data indicate that there is no correlation, or that the data is inconclusive (Lutsey and Michos, 2013). Calcium supplementation not in excess of the tolerable upper limit appears to be safe and is effective in the treatment of osteoporosis.

Magnesium

Magnesium is stored primarily in bone, but is also found in muscles, intra- and extracellular fluids, and soft tissues. It is necessary for many biochemical functions, including protein, glucose, and DNA metabolism, neuromuscular transmission, muscle contraction, cardiovascular excitability, parathyroid hormone and vitamin D production, and calcium homeostasis. Green vegetables, unrefined grains, legumes, nuts, and seeds are good sources of dietary magnesium (Langley, 2012). The RDA for magnesium for adults 31 years and older is 420 and 320 mg/day, for men and women, respectively (USDA, 2013).

Research has suggested that diets rich in magnesium may reduce the incidence of hypertension; in a prospective study of over 28,000 women over the age of 45, researchers found that dietary magnesium intake was inversely associated with the risk of developing hypertension (Song et al., 2006a). The effect of magnesium supplementation on hypertension has also been investigated; however, although some results suggests a positive effect, there is insufficient data to recommend routine magnesium supplementation for the prevention or treatment of hypertension, as many of the studies have been conducted on normotensive subjects with small sample sizes (Rosanoff, 2010).

Magnesium has a multifactorial effect on bone health, as it is necessary for osteoblast function, and parathyroid hormone and vitamin D metabolism. Research suggests that magnesium supplementation may suppress bone turnover in some populations, (Dimai et al., 1998; Aydin et al., 2010) and higher intakes of magnesium are associated with increased bone mineral density (Tucker et al., 1999). While it is clear that adequate amounts of magnesium are important for bone health, further research is needed to understand the effect of magnesium supplementation on the prevention and treatment of osteoporosis.

Magnesium also appears to play a role in both the development and treatment of diabetes. In a large study of over 85,000 women aged 30–55 and over 42,000 men aged 40–75, subjects' diets were analyzed and followed for 18 and 12 years, for the women's and men's groups, respectively. Researchers discovered an inverse relationship between magnesium intake and risk of diabetes (Lopez-Ridaura et al., 2004).

Magnesium deficiency impairs blood glucose control in those with diabetes; research has shown improved glucose control with magnesium supplementation, but only in subjects with low serum magnesium levels at baseline (Song et al., 2006b). The American Diabetes Association does not recommend routine magnesium supplementation for individuals with diabetes; however, it acknowledges that micronutrient deficiencies are common when the disease is poorly controlled, and deficiencies should be treated with healthful diet and supplementation when necessary (Evert et al., 2013).

Hypomagnesemia may be caused by inadequate intake or absorption, increased excretion, or redistribution from extracellular to intracellular fluid. Deficiency may also be precipitated by medications, including certain diuretic, antineoplastic, and antibiotic medications, which either increase excretion or decrease absorption of magnesium. Medical conditions in which magnesium deficiency is common include malabsorptive GI diseases, alcoholism, and poorly controlled diabetes. See Table 5.8 for risk factors and signs and symptoms of mineral deficiencies.

Symptoms of deficiency include loss of appetite, nausea, vomiting, and weakness; in more severe cases, numbness and tingling, muscle cramps, cardiac arrhythmias, and seizures can occur. Serum magnesium does not necessarily correlate with whole body magnesium stores; long-term deficiency may be present and cannot be determined by the measurement of serum magnesium alone.

Magnesium should only be supplemented in those that have deficiency; recommended dosage will vary based on the cause and severity of the deficiency, comorbid conditions, and the form of supplement. Oral supplements are available in a variety of forms, including magnesium oxide, carbonate, hydroxide, citrate, lactate, chloride, and sulfate; the amount of elemental magnesium should be considered when choosing a supplement. Magnesium oxide is most well absorbed.

Common side effects of magnesium supplementation include nausea and diarrhea; magnesium can be given intravenously; however, this is typically only done in the acute care setting. Individuals with chronic kidney disease are unlikely to be deficient in magnesium, as the mineral is primarily excreted by the kidneys; if supplementation is necessary, it should be given cautiously in this population.

IRON

Iron is an important component of numerous proteins and enzymes, thus is required for many metabolic reactions, including cell growth and differentiation. Most notably, iron is a vital component of hemoglobin, which is necessary for oxygen transport in the blood; insufficient iron stores result in reduced tissue oxygenation, causing fatigue and decreased immune function. The RDA for iron is 8 mg daily for adults, except for women aged 18–50 years, who should consume 18 mg of iron daily, and pregnant women, who should consume 27 mg daily (ODSb, 2013).

Dietary iron is found in two forms; animal sources provide heme iron and plant-based sources provide nonheme iron. Heme iron is more readily absorbed than nonheme; intake of phytates, tannins, calcium, and polyphenols reduces nonheme iron absorption, although concomitant intake of vitamin C can help enhance absorption. Liver, oysters, red meat, and dark poultry meat are the best animal-based iron sources, whereas fortified cereals, beans, lentils, tofu, spinach, raisins, and molasses are good nonheme sources (ODSb, 2013).

Those most at risk for iron deficiency are vegetarians, vegans, menstruating women, pregnant women, infants exclusively breast fed past 6 months of age, preterm infants, individuals on hemodialysis, and those with malabsorption syndromes. Symptoms of iron deficiency include anemia, fatigue, weakness, decreased school and work performance, decreased immune function, and difficulty maintaining body temperature. Signs include pallor, koilonychia, or spoon-shaped nails, and glossitis. Diagnosis of iron deficiency should include laboratory analysis, physical assessment, and dietary intake assessment. See Table 5.9 for laboratory tests used to diagnose iron deficiency (ODSb, 2013).

Iron should be supplemented in cases of symptomatic deficiency, as well as deficiency in which needs cannot be met with food consumption, especially in cases of

TABLE 5.8
Mineral Deficiency—Risk Factors and Signs/Symptoms

Mineral	Risk Factors	Signs/Symptoms
Calcium	Chronic: Insufficient intake related to lactose intolerance, milk protein allergy, veganism	Chronic: Osteomalacia, osteoporosis
	Acute: hyperphosphatemia, decreased parathyroid hormone activity, massive blood transfusions, some medications	Acute hypocalcemia: hypotension, decreased myocardial contractility, paresthesias, muscle cramps, seizures
Copper	Uncommon; increased GI losses, malabsorption, excess zinc or iron administration	Spasticity and paresthesias to extremities, leukopenia, neutropenia, increased red blood cell turnover, hypercholesterolemia
Iodine	Rare—insufficient intake	Nodular goiter, weight loss, tachycardia, muscle weakness, skin warmth
Iron	Blood loss, malabsorption, reduced gastric acidity, insufficient intake most commonly seen in vegetarians/vegans, menstruating or pregnant women, preterm infants, infants exclusively breast fed past 6 months of age	Microcytic, hypochromic anemia; tachycardia, poor capillary refill, fatigue, anorexia, nausea, pallor, reduced work/intellectual performance, inability to maintain body temperature in cold environments, decreased immunity, koilonychia, glossitis
Magnesium	Chronic: insufficient intake, malabsorption Acute: reduced absorption or increased excretion, usually caused by medications such as diuretics; alcoholism, poorly controlled diabetes	Acute hypomagnesemia: Poor appetite, N/V, weakness, numbness and tingling, muscle cramps, cardiac arrhythmias, seizures
Phosphorus	Chronic: insufficient intake, malabsorption Acute: alcoholism, critical illness, respiratory and metabolic alkalosis, over administration of phosphorus binding medications	Acute hypophosphatemia: Ataxia, confusion, paresthesias, weakness, myalgia, cardiac or respiratory failure
Selenium	Chronic: insufficient intake, typically seen in areas of the world with low soil selenium levels, HIV disease, malabsorption Acute: Critical illness, burn injury, cholesterol-lowering statin medications interfere with selenoprotein synthesis	Altered thyroid hormone metabolism, increased oxidative injury, increased plasma glutathione levels, Keshan disease (cardiomyopathy)
Zinc	Decreased absorption, most commonly seen with GI disease and administration of other mineral supplements; burn injury, trauma, increased GI losses, sickle cell disease, alcoholism	Fatigue, skin lesions, alopecia, taste and smell changes, impaired immune function and wound healing

TABLE 5.9

Diagnosis of Iron Deficiency

Test	Normal Range[a]	Indication of deficiency
Serum iron[b]	50–170 μg/L (males)	↓
	28–160 μg/L (females)	
Ferritin[c] (storage protein)	11–307 ng/mL	↓
Transferrin saturation	20%–50%	↓
Transferrin[b] (transport protein)	170–340 mg/dL	↑
Total iron binding capacity	261–478 μg/dL	↑

[a] Normal range values will vary by laboratory.
[b] Low in inflammation.
[c] High in inflammation.

malabsorption and/or excessive losses. Supplements are available in ferrous forms including fumarate, sulfate, and gluconate. Ferrous fumarate is most well absorbed, although the elemental amount, or amount that will be absorbed, must be listed on the supplement label. The recommended dose to treat deficiency is 150–200 mg of elemental iron daily, ideally separated into two or three divided doses, as absorption is reduced at higher doses. The Centers for Disease Control and Prevention (CDC) recommends low-dose supplementation of 30 mg of iron for all pregnant women. Iron can be supplemented intramuscularly or intravenously, although this is generally only done in a hospital setting (ODSb, 2013).

Iron supplements can cause GI side effects including nausea, vomiting, diarrhea, constipation, and dark stools. Supplementation is otherwise considered safe, except for individuals with hemochromatosis, a genetic condition in which iron is very efficiently absorbed, resulting in excess iron being deposited in tissues and organs (ODSb, 2013).

ZINC

Zinc is widely distributed in all cells of the body and plays a role in immune function, wound healing, protein and DNA synthesis, and growth. Zinc is found in a wide variety of foods, including meat, poultry, nuts, seeds, beans, whole grains, and fortified cereals; oysters in particular are extremely high in zinc. The RDA for zinc is 11 and 8 mg/day for adult men and women, respectively (ODSb, 2013).

Zinc has been recognized as a necessary nutrient for a healthy immune system, and deficiency is associated with impaired immune function. The effect of zinc supplementation on immune function has been studied, and while results have shown improved immune parameters, many studies were small, with the supplementation of zinc varying by type, amount, and duration; thus, it is difficult to make recommendations for zinc supplementation specifically for immune health. In many of the studies, participants were zinc deficient at baseline, suggesting that zinc supplementation may not benefit those that are not deficient (Boukaiba et al., 1993; Prasad et al., 2007).

Zinc is commonly found in many over-the-counter cold remedies. In a Cochrane review of 18 placebo-controlled trials with a total of over 1700 healthy subjects, researchers determined that zinc supplementation taken within 24 h of the onset of cold symptoms was effective in reducing the duration of colds. However, there is insufficient evidence to recommend routine zinc supplementation for the prevention of the common cold (Singh and Das, 2013).

Zinc is necessary for the formation of healthy granulation tissue, and thus is important for wound healing; deficiency has been shown to delay healing. In studies of zinc supplementation and wound healing, the type of wounds, heterogeneity of subjects, amount and duration of zinc supplementation, and small sample sizes make it challenging to make specific recommendations for zinc supplementation in healing (ODSb, 2013). Further, in many studies, zinc is often not supplemented alone; some research has indicated that zinc, when given with additional arginine and vitamin C, may have a positive effect on wound healing when compared to controls (Heyman et al., 2008; Cereda et al., 2009). While these results are promising, sufficient evidence is lacking to recommend zinc supplementation for wound healing in those that are not zinc deficient.

Several trials have examined the effect of zinc supplementation on AMD. A recent meta-analysis analyzing 11 studies concluded that while there was insufficient evidence to suggest that zinc intake was correlated with the development of AMD, supplementation does appear to help prevent progression to advanced AMD in those that already have the disease (Vishwanathan et al., 2013).

Conditions that increase the risk for zinc deficiency include celiac disease, inflammatory bowel disease, short bowel syndrome, bariatric surgery, chronic kidney disease, excessive GI fluid losses such as high-output GI fistulas and diarrhea, excessive alcohol intake, sickle cell disease, and burns. Signs and symptoms of deficiency include fatigue, skin lesions, alopecia, taste and smell alterations, and impaired immune function and wound healing. Diagnosis of zinc deficiency can be challenging; serum zinc is often not reflective of true zinc status, and zinc levels decrease in acute illness and inflammation. Risk factors, physical signs and symptoms, and nutrition intake should also be assessed when screening for deficiency (ODSb, 2013).

Zinc is most commonly supplemented as sulfate or gluconate and can be found in a variety of forms including tablets, oral sprays, lozenges, and intravenous doses. The standard oral dose for treatment of deficiency is 220 mg twice daily; if given parenterally, typical doses are between 5 and 20 mg/day and should be limited to no more than 40 mg/day. Supplemental zinc at levels above the RDA should only be supplemented for 10–14 days, and then zinc status reassessed; only cases of chronic losses should receive prolonged zinc supplementation. It is necessary to limit the dose and duration of supplementation, as excessive zinc administration may cause nausea and diarrhea, interfere with copper and iron absorption, and impair wound healing (ODSb, 2013).

SELENIUM

Selenium is a trace element that is essential for immune and thyroid function and also acts as an antioxidant. The RDA for selenium is 55 μg/day for adult men and women (USDA, 2013). Selenium is found in a wide variety of foods; however, the amount in plant sources will vary depending on the selenium concentration of the soil in which the plant was grown, and the amount in animal sources will depend on the selenium content of the animals' feed. Low soil selenium levels have been identified in some areas of the world, including parts of China, Northern Europe, New Zealand, and Russia; however, most Americans consume adequate amounts of selenium via their usual diets (Combs, 2001; Boosalis, 2008).

Selenium is needed for the activation, proliferation, and differentiation of many immune cells, and thus has been investigated for its role in immune-related diseases. Serum selenium levels decrease significantly in many HIV-infected individuals, which is associated with increased mortality. Research suggests selenium supplementation in this population may result in fewer hospitalizations, reduced viral load, and increased CD4 T-cell counts; however, selenium supplementation has also led to increases in viral shedding in some studies (Stone et al., 2010).

Much of the research on supplementation in HIV has been conducted on subjects in the latter stages of the disease; however, a recent double-blind placebo-controlled study was conducted by Baum et al. on HIV-positive individuals in an earlier stage of the disease (CD4 count of >350/μL, not on antiretroviral therapy). Groups were randomized to receive a multivitamin alone, selenium alone, a combination of both multivitamin and selenium, or a placebo for up to 2 years; the multivitamin with selenium group was the only treatment group that had a significantly lower risk of deteriorating immune function (CD4 count of < 250/μL) compared to controls (Baum et al., 2013).

The effect of selenium supplementation on critically ill patients with systemic inflammatory response syndrome has also been investigated, and some results have shown generally positive effects, including reduced mortality, infection rates, and disease severity. However, trial interventions and results were not consistent, so further research in this area is needed (Forceville et al., 2007; Manzanares et al., 2011; Valenta et al., 2011).

Selenium's effect on other immune parameters has also been examined. Some trials have shown improvements in both cellular and humoral immune response to an administered vaccine in subjects supplemented with 100 μg/day of selenium (Girodon et al., 1999; Broome et al., 2004). However, it should be noted that most of the subjects in these studies were selenium deficient at baseline; there is no evidence to suggest that selenium supplementation provides immunologic benefits in those with adequate selenium stores.

Because of its antioxidant properties, selenium has been investigated as a chemopreventative agent. In the Nutrition Prevention of Cancer Trial (NPC), subjects were supplemented with 200 μg/day of selenium; no effects on the study's primary outcome measure, incidence of skin cancer, were seen; however, the intervention group had lower mortality from all cancers, and a lower incidence of prostate cancer (Duffield-Lillico et al., 2002). In the Selenium and Vitamin E Cancer Prevention Trial (SELECT), researchers supplemented men with 200 μg/day of selenium, 400 IU/day of vitamin E, or both, and found that vitamin E actually increased the risk of prostate cancer, while selenium had no effect (Klein et al., 2011).

Participants' baseline selenium levels were significantly lower in the NPC study compared to the SELECT study (114 vs. 136 μg/L); this may account for the conflicting results. Researchers have postulated that perhaps serum selenium levels are more important than selenium intake in decreasing cancer risk, and some have recommended maintaining serum selenium levels at 120–160 μg/L, which in most cases can be accomplished by consuming a healthful diet without selenium supplementation (Rocourt and Cheng, 2013). Additional research on the link between selenium and prostate cancer risk has yielded conflicting results, thus selenium supplementation is not recommended at this time unless deficiency is present (Jiang et al., 2010; Kristal et al., 2010; Penney et al., 2010).

Individuals most at risk for selenium deficiency are those who live in an area of the world with low soil selenium levels; deficiency is also seen in malabsorptive GI diseases, high-output chylous fistula, HIV infection, and provision of long-term parenteral nutrition without adequate selenium. Selenium deficiency may cause Keshan's disease, a form of cardiomyopathy, and altered thyroid metabolism. Serum selenium is an indicator of short-term selenium status; however, it should be noted that serum levels decrease during acute and inflammatory illnesses. Erythrocyte selenium levels may also be measured to assess long-term selenium status (Clark, 2012; ODSb, 2013).

Selenium supplementation dosage depends on the degree of deficiency and comorbidities; there are no specific guidelines available. The tolerable upper limit is 400 μg/day, and frequently studied doses range from 100 to 200 μg/day. A concern with selenium supplementation is a possible link between higher serum selenium levels and increased risk of type 2 diabetes. Researchers in the NPC trial noted a higher incidence of type 2 diabetes in those subjects with the highest serum selenium concentrations; however, these results were not seen in the SELECT trial. Some scientists have suggested that the relationship between selenium and type 2 diabetes is U-shaped, with an increased risk of diabetes at both the lowest and highest levels of serum selenium; however, further research in this area is needed (Rayman and Stranges, 2013).

REFERENCES

Age-Related Eye Disease Study Research Group. 2001. A randomized, placebo-controlled, clinical trial of high-dose supplementation with vitamins C and E, beta carotene, and zinc for age-related macular degeneration and vision loss: AREDS report no. 8. *Arch Ophthalmol* 119:1417–1436.

Akilen R, Tsiami A, Devendra D, Robinson N. 2012. Cinnamon in glycaemic control: Systematic review and metaanalysis. *Clin Nutr* 31(5):609–615.

American Heart Association Nutrition Committee, Lichtenstein AH, Appel LJ et al. 2006. Diet and lifestyle recommendations revision 2006: A scientific statement from the American Heart Association Nutrition Committee. *Circulation* 114:82–96.

Aydin H, Deyneli O, Yavuz D et al. 2010. Short-term oral magnesium supplementation suppresses bone turnover in postmenopausal osteoporotic women. *Biol Trace Elem Res* 133:136–143.

Bailey RL, Fulgoni VL 3rd, Keast DR, Dwyer JT. 2011b. Dietary supplement use is associated with higher intakes of minerals from food sources. *Am J Clin Nutr* 94(5):1376–1381.

Bailey RL, Fulgoni VL 3rd, Keast DR, Dwyer JT. 2012. Examination of vitamin intakes among US adults by dietary supplement use. *J Acad Nutr Diet* 112(5):657–663.

Bailey RL, Gahche JJ, Lentino CV et al. 2011a. Dietary supplement use in the United States, 2003–2006. *J Nutr* 141(2):261–266.

Baum MK, Campa A, Lai S et al. 2013. Effect of micronutrient supplementation on disease progression in asymptomatic antiretroviral-naïve, HIV-infected adults in Botswana. *JAMA* 310(20):2154–2163.

Bent S, Ko R. 2004. Commonly used herbal medicines used in the United States: A review. *Am J Med* 116(7):478–485.

Boosalis MG. 2008. The role of selenium in chronic disease. *Nutr Clin Pract* 23:152–160.

Boukaiba N, Flament C, Acher S et al. 1993. A physiological amount of zinc supplementation: Effects on nutritional, lipid, and thymic status in an elderly population. *Am J Clin Nutr* 57:566–572.

Brondino N, De Silvestri A, Re S et al. 2013. A systematic review and meta-analysis of Ginkgo biloba in neuropsychiatric disorders: From ancient tradition to modern-day medicine. *Evid Based Complement Altern Med* 2013:915691. Epub May 28, 2013.

Broome CS, McArdle F, Kyle JAM et al. 2004. An increase in selenium intake improves immune function and poliovirus handling in adults with marginal selenium status. *Am J Clin Nutr* 80:154–162.

Burr ML, Fehily AM, Gilbert JF et al. 1989. Effects of changes in fat, fish, and fibre intakes on death and myocardial reinfarction: Diet and reinfarction trial (DART). *Lancet* 2:757–761.

Cereda E, Gini A, Pedrolli C, Vanotti A. 2009. Disease-specific, versus standard, nutritional support for the treatment of pressure ulcers in institutionalized older adults: A randomized controlled trial. *J Am Geriatr Soc* 57:1395–1402.

Clark SF. 2012. Chapter 8—Vitamins and trace elements. In: Mueller, C.M. (ed.). *The ASPEN Adult Nutrition Support Core Curriculum*, 2nd edn. American Society for Parenteral and Enteral Nutrition, Silver Spring, MD, pp. 121–151.

Clauson KA, Santamarina ML, Rutledge JC. 2008. Clinically relevant safety issues associated with St John's wort product labels. *BMC Complement Altern Med* 8:42–57.

Combs GF. 2001. Selenium in global food systems. *Br J Nutr* 85:517–547.

Diamond BJ, Bailey MR. 2013. Ginkgo biloba: Indications, mechanisms and safety. *Psychiatr Clin N Am* 36:73–83.

Dietary Supplement Health and Education Act of 1994 (DSHEA). Public law No. 103–417, 108 Stat. http://www.health.gov/dietsupp/ch1.htm.

Dimai HP, Porta S, Wirnsberger G et al. 1998. Daily oral magnesium supplementation suppresses bone turnover in young adult males. *J Clin Endocrinol Metab* 83: 2742–2748.

Duffield-Lillico AJ, Reid ME, Turnbull BW et al. 2002. Baseline characteristics and the effect of selenium supplementation on cancer incidence in a randomized clinical trial: A summary report of the Nutritional Prevention of Cancer Trial. *Cancer Epidemiol Biomarkers Prev* 11:630–639.

Dunnick JK, Nyska A. 2013. The toxicity and pathology of selected dietary herbal medicines. *Toxicol Pathol* 41(2):374–386.

Eidelman RS, Hollar D, Hebert PR et al. 2004. Randomized trials of vitamin E in the treatment and prevention of cardiovascular disease. *Arch Intern Med* 164:1552–1556.

Evert AB, Boucher JL, Cypress M et al. 2013. Nutrition therapy recommendations for the management of adults with diabetes. *Diab Care* 36:3821–3842.

Farina N, Isaac MGEKN, Clark AR et al. 2012. Vitamin E for Alzheimer's dementia and mild cognitive impairment (review). *Cochrane Database Syst Rev*, 11:Art. No.: CD002854.

Feringa HH, Laskey DA, Dickson JE, Coleman CI. 2011. The effect of grape seed extract on cardiovascular risk markers: A meta-analysis of randomized controlled trials. *J Am Diet Assoc* 111(8):1173–1181.

Fitz H, Seely D, Kennedy DA et al. 2013. Green tea and lung cancer: A systematic review. *Integr Cancer Ther* 12(1):7–24.

Food and Drug Administration (FDA). Q & A on dietary supplements. Accessed September 2013. http://www.fda.gov/Food/DietarySupplements/QADietarySupplements/default.htm

Forceville X, Laviolle B, Annane D et al. 2007. Effects of high doses of selenium, as sodium selenite, in septic shock: A placebo-controlled, randomized, double-blind, phase II study. *Crit Care* 11:R73.

Fragakis AS, Thompson C. 2012. *The Health Professional's Guide to Popular Dietary Supplements*, 3rd edn. Academy of Nutrition and Dietetics.

Gaziano JM, Glynn RJ, Christen WG et al. 2009. Vitamins E and C in the prevention of prostate and total cancer in men: The Physicians' Health Study II randomized controlled trial. *JAMA* 301:52–62.

Girodon F, Galan P, Monget AL et al. 1999. Impact of trace elements and vitamin supplementation on immunity and infections in institutionalized elderly patients: A randomized controlled trial. *Arch Intern Med* 159:748–754.

GISSI-Prevenzione Investigators. 1999. Dietary supplementation with n-3 polyunsaturated fatty acids and vitamin E after myocardial infarction: Results of the GISSI-Prevenzione trial. *Lancet* 354:447–455.

Halsted CH. 2013. B-Vitamin dependent methionine metabolism and alcoholic liver disease. *Clin Chem Lab Med* 51(3):457–465.

Hardy M, Coulter I, Morton SC et al. 2003. *S*-adenosyl-L-methionine for treatment of depression, osteoarthritis, and liver disease. *Evid Rep Technol Assess* (Summ). (64):1–3

Hemila H, Chalker E. January 31, 2013. Vitamin C for preventing and treating the common cold. *Cochrane Database Syst Rev* 1:CD000980.

Heyman H, Van De Looverbosch DE, Meijer EP, Schols JM. 2008. Benefits of an oral nutritional supplement on pressure ulcer healing in long-term care residents. *J Wound Care* 17:476–478, 480.

Hudson JB. 2012. Applications of the phytomedicine Echinacea purpurea (Purple Coneflower) in infectious diseases. *J Biomed Biotechnol* 2012:769896. Epub 2011 Oct 26.

Hudson JB, Vimalanathan S, Kang L et al. 2005. Characterization of antiviral activities in Echinacea root preparations. *Pharm Biol* 43(9):790–796.

Ihl R. 2013. Effects of Ginkgo biloba extract EGb 761® in dementia with neuropsychiatric features: Review of recently completed randomised, controlled trials. *Int J Psychiatry Clin Pract* 17(Suppl 1):8–14.

Isaachsohn JL, Moser M, Stein EA et al. 1998. Garlic powder and plasma lipids and lipoproteins: A multicenter, randomized, placebo-controlled trial. *Arch Intern Med* 158:1189–1194.

Jacobs EJ, Henion AK, Briggs PJ et al. 2002. Vitamin C and vitamin E supplement use and bladder cancer mortality in a large cohort of US men and women. *Am J Epidemiol.* 156:1002–1010.

Jiang L, Yang KH, Tian JH et al. 2010. Efficacy of antioxidant vitamins and selenium supplement in prostate cancer prevention: A meta-analysis of randomized controlled trials. *Nutr Cancer* 62:719–727.

Josling P. 2001. Preventing the common cold with a garlic supplement: A double-blind, placebo-controlled survey. *Adv Ther* 18:189–193.

Kasper S, Anghelescu IG, Szegedi A et al. 2006. Superior efficacy of St John's wort extract WS 5570 compared to placebo in patients with major depression: A randomized, double-blind, placebo-controlled, multi-center trial. *BMC Med* 4:14–37.

Kaur M, Agarwal C, Agarwal R. 2009. Anticancer and cancer chemopreventive potential of grape seed extract and other grape-based products. *J Nutr* 139(9):1806S–1812S.

Klein EA, Thompson IM, Tangen CM et al. 2011. Vitamin E and the risk of prostate cancer: The selenium and vitamin E cancer prevention trial (SELECT). *JAMA* 306:1549–1556.

Kris-Etherton PM, Harris WS, Appel LJ. 2002. Fish consumption, fish oil, omega 3 fatty acids, and cardiovascular disease. *Circulation* 106:2747–2757.

Kristal AR, Arnold KB, Neuhouser ML et al. 2010. Diet, supplement use, and prostate cancer risk: Results from the prostate cancer prevention trial. *Am J Epidemiol* 172:566–577.

Ladas EJ, Kroll DJ, Oberlies NH et al. 2010. A randomized, controlled, double-blind, pilot study of milk thistle for the treatment of hepatotoxicity in childhood acute lymphoblastic leukemia (ALL). *Cancer* 116:506–513.

Langley G. 2012. Chapter 7—Fluids, electrolytes and acid-base disorders. In: Mueller CM (ed.). *The ASPEN Adult Nutrition Support Core Curriculum*, 2nd edn. American Society for Parenteral and Enteral Nutrition, Silver Spring, MD, pp. 98–120.

Lee S, Lemere CA, Frost JL, Shea TB. 2012. Dietary supplementation with *S*-adenosyl methionine delayed amyloid-β and tau pathology in 3xTg-AD mice. *J Alzheimers Dis* 28(2):423–431.

Leyssens C, Verlinden L, Verstuyf A. 2013. Antineoplastic effects of 1,25(OH)2D3 and its analogs in breast, prostate and colorectal cancer. *Endocr Relat Cancer* 22(2):R31–R47.

Li L, Sun T, Tian J et al. 2013. Garlic in clinical practice: An evidence-based overview. *Crit Rev Food Sci Nutr* 53(7):670–681.

Lin J, Cook NR, Albert C et al. 2009. Vitamins C and E and beta carotene supplementation and cancer risk: A randomized controlled trial. *J Natl Cancer Inst* 101:14–23.

Linde K, Barrett B, Wölkart K et al. 2006. *Echinacea* for preventing and treating the common cold. *Cochrane Database Syst Rev* 2006 Jan 25;(1):CD000530.

Linde K, Berner MM, Kriston L. 2008. St John's wort for major depression. In Linde, Klaus. *Cochrane Database Syst Rev* (4):CD000448.

Linnebank M, Popp J, Smulders Y et al. 2010. *S*-adenosylmethionine is decreased in the cerebrospinal fluid of patients with Alzheimer's disease. *Neurodegener Dis* 7(6):373–378.

Loguercio C, Festi D. 2011. Silybin and the liver: From basic research to clinical practice. *World J Gastroenterol* 17(18):2288–2301.

Lonn E, Yusuf S, Hoogwerf B et al. 2002. Effects of vitamin E on cardiovascular and microvascular outcomes in high-risk patients with diabetes: Results of the HOPE study and MICRO-HOPE substudy. *Diabetes Care* 25:1919–1927.

Lopez HL. 2012. Nutritional interventions to prevent and treat osteoarthritis. Part II: Focus on micronutrients and supportive nutraceuticals. *PMR* 4(5 Suppl):S155–S68.

Lopez-Ridaura R, Willett WC, Rimm EB et al. 2004. Magnesium intake and risk of type 2 diabetes in men and women. *Diabetes Care* 27:134–140.

Lutsey PL, Michos ED. 2013. Vitamin D, calcium, and atherosclerotic risk: Evidence from serum levels and supplementation studies. *Curr Atheroscler Res* 15:293.

Manusirivithaya S, Sripramote M, Tangjitgamol S et al. 2004. Antiemetic effect of ginger in gynecologic oncology patients receiving cisplatin. *Int J Gynecol Cancer* 14(6):1063–1069.

Manzanares W, Biestro A, Galusso F et al. 2011. Serum selenium and glutathione peroxidase-3 activity: Biomarkers of systemic inflammation in the critically ill? *Intensive Care Med* 35:882–889.

Mashhadi NS, Ghiasvand R, Askari G et al. 2013. Anti-oxidative and anti-inflammatory effects of ginger in health and physical activity: Review of current evidence. *Int J Prev Med* 4(Suppl 1):S36–S42.

Mato JM, Camara J, Fernandez de Paz J et al. 1999. *S*-adenosylmethionine in alcoholic liver cirrhosis: A randomized, placebo-controlled double-blind, multicenter trial. *J Hepatol* 30:1081–1089.

Miller ER 3rd, Pastor-Barriuso R, Dalal D et al. 2005. Meta-analysis: High-dosage vitamin E supplementation may increase all-cause mortality. *Ann Intern Med* 142:37–46.

Mischoulon D, Price LH, Carpenter LL et al. 2014. A double-blind, randomized, placebo-controlled clinical trial of *S*-adenosyl-L-methionine (SAMe) versus escitalopram in major depressive disorder. *J Clin Psychiatry*, 75(4):370–376.

Moayedi B, Gharagozloo M, Esmaeil N et al. 2013. A randomized double-blind, placebo-controlled study of therapeutic effects of silymarin in β-thalassemia major patients receiving desferrioxamine. *Eur J Haematol* 90(3):202–209.

Najm WI, Reinsch S, Hoehler F et al. 2004. *S*-adenosyl methionine (SAMe) versus celecoxib for the treatment of osteoarthritis symptoms: A double-blind cross-over trial. *BMC Musculoskelet Disord* 5:6.

Office of Dietary Supplements (ODSa). Mission, origin and mandate. Accessed September 1, 2013. http://ods.od.nih.gov/About/MissionOriginMandate.aspx

Office of Dietary Supplements (ODSb). Dietary supplement fact sheets. Accessed October 2013. http://ods.od.nih.gov/factsheets/list-all/.

Palatty PL, Haniadka R, Valder B et al. 2013. Ginger in the prevention of nausea and vomiting: A review. *Crit Rev Food Sci Nutr* 53(7):659–669.

Papakostas GI, Mischoulon D, Shyu I et al. 2010. *S*-adenosyl methionine (SAMe) augmentation of serotonin reuptake inhibitors for antidepressant nonresponders with major depressive disorder: A double-blind, randomized clinical trial. *Am J Psychiatry* 167(8):942–948.

Park C. 2013. The effects of high concentrations of vitamin C on cancer cells. *Nutrients* 5(9):3496–3505.

Penney KL, Schumacher FR, Li H et al. 2010. A large prospective study of SEP15 genetic variation, interaction with plasma selenium levels, and prostate cancer risk and survival. *Cancer Prev Res* 3:604–610.

Pleschka S, Stein M, Schoop R, Hudson JB. 2009. Anti-viral properties and mode of action of standardized Echinacea purpurea extract against highly pathogenic avian influenza virus (H5N1, H7N7) and swine-origin H1N1 (S-OIV). *Virol J* 6:197.

Pramyothin P, Holick MF. 2012. Vitamin D supplementation: Guidelines and evidence for subclinical deficiency. *Curr Opin Gastroenterol* 28(2):139–150.

Prasad AS, Beck FWJ, Bao B et al. 2007. Zinc supplementation decreases incidence of infections in the elderly: Effect of zinc on generation of cytokines and oxidative stress. *Am J Clin Nutr* 85:837–844.

Prentice RL, Pettinger MB, Jackson RD et al. 2013. Health risks and benefits from calcium and vitamin D supplementation: Women's Health Initiative clinical trial and cohort study. *Osteoporos Int* 24:567–580.

Qidwai W, Ashfaq T. 2013. Role of garlic usage in cardiovascular disease prevention: An evidence-based approach. *Evid Based Complement Altern Med* 2013:125649. Epub April 17, 2013.

Qureshi NA, Al-Bedah AM. 2013. Mood disorders and complementary and alternative medicine: A literature review. *Neuropsychiatr Dis Treat* 9:639–658.

Rambaldi A, Gluud C. 2006. *S*-adenosyl-L-methionine for alcoholic liver diseases. *Cochrane Database Syst Rev* 2006 Apr 19;(2):CD002235.

Rambaldi A, Jacobs BP, Iaquinto G, Gluud C. 2005. Milk thistle for alcoholic and/or hepatitis B or C liver diseases—A systematic cochrane hepato-biliary group review with meta-analyses of randomized clinical trials. *Am J Gastroenterol* 100(11):2583–2591.

Ranasinghe P, Jayawardana R, Galappaththy P et al. 2012. Efficacy and safety of 'true' cinnamon (Cinnamomum zeylanicum) as a pharmaceutical agent in diabetes: A systematic review and meta-analysis. *Diabet Med* 29(12):1480–1492.

Rayman MP, Stranges S. 2013. Epidemiology of selenium and type 2 diabetes: Can we make sense of it? *Free Radic Biol Med* 65:1557–1564.

Reinhart KM, Coleman CI, Teevan C et al. 2008. Effects of garlic on blood pressure in patients with and without systolic hypertension: A meta-analysis. *Ann Pharmacother* 42(12):1766–1771.

Ried K, Frank OR, Stocks NP et al. 2008. Effect of garlic on blood pressure: A systematic review and meta-analysis. *BMC Cardiovasc Disord* 8:13.

Riemersma RA, Wood DA, Macintyre CC et al. 1991. Risk of angina pectoris and plasma concentrations of vitamins A, C, and E and carotene. *Lancet* 337:1–5.

Rimm EB, Stampfer MJ, Ascherio A et al. 1993. Vitamin E consumption and the risk of coronary heart disease in men. *N Engl J Med* 328:1450–1456.

Rocourt CRB, Cheng W-H. 2013. Selenium supranutrition: Are the potential benefits of chemoprevention outweighed by the promotion of diabetes and insulin resistance? *Nutrition* 5:1349–1365.

Rosanoff A. 2010. Magnesium supplements may enhance the effect of antihypertensive medications in stage 1 hypertensive subjects. *Magnes Res* 23:27–40.

Sahebkar A. 2013. Effects of resveratrol supplementation on plasma lipids: A systematic review and meta-analysis of randomized controlled trials. *Nutr Rev* 71(12):822–835.

Satitvipawee P, Rawdaree P, Indrabhakti S et al. 2003. No effect of garlic extract supplement on serum lipid levels in hypercholesterolemic subjects. *J Med Assoc Thai* 86:750–757.

Siegel AB, Stebbing J. 2013. Milk thistle: Early seeds of potential. *Lancet Oncol* 14(10):929–930.

Singh M, Das RR. 2013. Zinc for the common cold. *Cochrane Database Syst Rev* 18(6):CD001364.

Sobenin IA, Andrianova IV, Demidova ON et al. 2008. Lipid-lowering effects of time-released garlic powder tablets in double-blinded placebo-controlled randomized study. *J Atheroscler Thromb* 15(6):334–338.

Song Y, He K, Levitan EB, Manson JE, Liu S. 2006b. Effects of oral magnesium supplementation on glycaemic control in Type 2 diabetes: A meta-analysis of randomized double-blind controlled trials. *Diabet Med* 23:1050–1056.

Song Y, Sesso HD, Manson JE et al. 2006a. Dietary magnesium intake and risk of incident hypertension among middle-aged and older US women in a 10-year follow-up study. *Am J Cardiol* 98:1616–1621.

Steiner M, Khan AH, Holbert D, Lin RIS. 1996. A double-blind crossover study in moderately hypercholesterolemic men that compared the effect of aged garlic extract and placebo administration on blood lipids. *Am J Clin Nutr* 64(6):866–870.

Stone CA, Kawai K, Kupka R, Fawzi WW. 2010. Role of selenium in HIV infection. *Nutr Rev* 68:671–681.

Taylor PR, Li B, Dawsey SM et al. 1994. Prevention of esophageal cancer: The nutrition intervention trials in Linxian, China. Linxian Nutrition Intervention Trials Study Group. *Cancer Res* 54(7 Suppl):2029s–2031s.

Tournas VH, Rivera Calo J, Sapp C. 2013. Fungal profiles in various milk thistle botanicals from US retail. *Int J Food Microbiol* 164(1):87–91.

Trowman R, Dumville JC, Hahn S, Torgerson DJ. 2006. A systematic review of the effects of calcium supplementation on body weight. *Br J Nutr* 95:1033–1038.

Tucker KL, Hannan MT, Chen H et al. 1999. Potassium, magnesium, and fruit and vegetable intakes are associated with greater bone mineral density in elderly men and women. *Am J Clin Nutr* 69:727–736.

USDA United States Department of Agriculture: National Agricultural Library. Dietary Reference Intakes: RDA and AI for Vitamins and Elements. Accessed online at http://iom.edu/Activities/Nutrition/SummaryDRIs/~/media/Files/Activity%20Files/Nutrition/DRIs/RDA%20and%20AIs_Vitamin%20and%20Elements.pdf on November 11, 2013.

Valenta J, Brodska H, Drabek T et al. 2011. High-dose selenium substitution in sepsis: A prospective randomized clinical trial. *Intensive Care Med* 37:808–815.

Vellas B, Coley N, Ousset P et al. 2012. Long-term use of standardised ginkgo biloba extract for the prevention of Alzheimer's disease (GuidAge): A randomised placebo-controlled trial. *Lancet Neurol* 11:851–859.

Vimalanathan S, Kang L, Amiguet VT et al. 2005. Echinacea purpurea aerial parts contain multiple antiviral compounds. *Pharm Biol* 43(9):740–745.

Vishwanathan R, Chung M, Johnson EJ. 2013. A systematic review on zinc for the prevention and treatment of age-related macular degeneration. *Invest Ophthalmol Vis Sci* 54:3985–3998.

Xin W, Wei W, Lin Z et al. 2013. Fish oil and atrial fibrillation after cardiac surgery: A meta-analysis of randomized controlled trials. *PLoS One* 8(9):e72913.

Xu Q, Si L-Y. 2012. Resveratrol role in cardiovascular and metabolic health and potential mechanisms of action. *Nutr Res* 32(9):648–658.

Yiannakopoulou EC. 2013. Effect of green tea catechins on breast carcinogenesis: A systematic review of in-vitro and in-vivo experimental studies. *Eur J Cancer Prev* 23(2):84–89.

Yokoyama M, Origasa H, Matsuzaki M et al. 2007. Japan EPA lipid intervention study (JELIS) Investigators: Effects of eicosapentaenoic acid on major coronary events in hypercholesterolaemic patients (JELIS): A randomized open-label, blinded endpoint analysis. *Lancet* 369:1090–1098.

Yuan J-M, Sun C, Butler LM. 2011. Tea and cancer prevention: Epidemiologic studies. *Pharmacol Res* 64(2):123–135.

Zeng T, Guo FF, Zhang CL et al. 2012. A meta-analysis of randomized, double-blind, placebo-controlled trials for the effects of garlic on serum lipid profiles. *J Sci Food Agric* 92(9):1892–1902.

Zick SM, Ruffin MT, Lee J et al. 2009. Phase II trial of encapsulated ginger as a treatment for chemotherapy-induced nausea and vomiting. *Support Care Cancer* 17(5):563–572.

6 Integrative Approach to Nutrition in Infants, Children, and Adolescents

Hilary H. McClafferty, MD, FAAP

CONTENTS

INTRODUCTION

In an integrative medicine, model nutrition is one important predictor of health. Other important predictors include: regular physical activity, limits on-screen time, free play, time in nature, avoidance of environmental toxins, positive social relationships, opportunities for reflection and personal growth, and adequate sleep, all habits that children can pattern from an early age (Ostbye et al. 2013). Figure 6.1 shows the pediatric integrative medicine model.

NUTRITION AS PREVENTION

Ideally, nutrition would be emphasized at every pediatric visit as a foundation of preventative health. However, nutrition historically receives little emphasis in conventional medical training, especially the Mediterranean or anti-inflammatory diet often recommended in integrative medicine. Compounding this teaching deficit, practitioners and caretakers face "serious" competition from the food and beverage industries, whose sophisticated campaigns often directly target children, even newborns. For example, 66% of hospitals surveyed in the CDC National Survey of Maternity Practices in Infant Nutrition and Care distributed discharge packs to breastfeeding mothers that contained commercial infant formula (Centers for

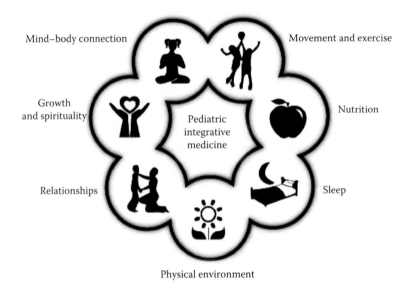

FIGURE 6.1 Pediatric integrative medicine model.

Disease Control and Prevention 2008). A total of $4.2 billion was spent on fast food marketing and advertising in 2009 alone, using advertising in television markets, and social media such as Facebook, Twitter, YouTube, mobile website banner ads, smartphone applications, and text message advertising, all specifically designed to engage children (Harris et al. 2010).

In contrast, the USDA's agency the Center for Nutrition Policy and Promotion has an average annual operating budget of only $6.5 million, representing "a contrast of" ~0.1% on the part of the USDA for every $1 spent by the marketing industry (United States Department of Agriculture 2010).

As a result of these educational and financial disparities, practitioners may fail to make the "crucial" connection between their patients' diet and illness. Although studies exist demonstrating that providers trained in nutrition counseling have increased confidence and success in teaching nutrition topics (Willis et al. 2013), they may still miss important opportunities for early intervention. Providers may also underestimate their ability to educate families about nutrition, "or may be reluctant to jeopardize the professional relationship for fear of insulting parents."

The sheer amount of information available on nutrition, and the field's many pockets of specialization are additional obstacles faced by practitioners trying to educate families about this important area of children's health.

To balance some of these challenges, the intent of this chapter is to lay a solid foundation by focusing on selected themes in children's nutrition rather than attempting an exhaustive review. These themes include maintenance of healthy weight, understanding the building blocks of nutrition, integration of nutrition in the pediatric treatment plan, the Mediterranean or anti-inflammatory diet, environmental exposures, common dietary supplements, and food sensitivities.

MAINTENANCE OF HEALTHY WEIGHT

Maintenance of healthy weight is important in both healthy children and in those living with chronic illnesses. While obesity, underweight, and failure-to-thrive are serious conditions, these topics exceed the scope of this chapter.

The maintenance of ideal weight in infancy and childhood is a key factor in obesity prevention in adolescence and adulthood (Dhuper et al. 2013; The et al. 2010). Yet a 2011 Institute of Medicine report on early childhood obesity prevention policies indicated that almost 10% of infants and toddlers and 20% of children between the ages of 2 and 5 years already meet criteria for overweight or obesity. Data from the 2007 National Health and Nutrition Examination Survey (NHANES) indicate that nearly half of American children qualify as either overweight or obese with more than half of those children overweight by age 2 years, and for many even by age 3 months (Harrington et al. 2010; The et al. 2010).

This is of concern, because the duration of obesity (from childhood through adulthood) has been correlated with progressively increased risk of comorbidities such as type 2 diabetes, the metabolic syndrome, and NAFLD (Merten 2010), and of serious cardiovascular risk factors such as hypertension, and thickening or carotid and abdominal aortal vascular wall thickening, mimicking adult cardiovascular disease (Dawson et al. 2009; Yücel et al. 2013). Large population studies have also shown that overweight and obesity place children and adolescents at high risk for depression, bullying, body image concerns, low self-esteem, social isolation, ADHD, learning disability, eating disorders, conduct disorder, and missed school days (Frisco et al. 2013; Halfon et al. 2013).

Healthy Weight: Early Programming

It is now understood that healthy weight in children is programmed early, even influenced in utero by maternal prenatal body mass index (BMI) and by maternal weight gain during pregnancy. Paternal BMI has also been identified as a risk factor (Linabery 2013; Weng et al. 2012; Weng et al. 2013). Accordingly, it is a research priority to identify time windows in infant development where nutrition interventions and counseling to prevent or counteract obesity will be most effective (Zhang et al. 2012; Zhang et al. 2013).

One of these critical windows occurs at birth as parents make the important decision about the infant's nutrition. Breastfeeding is strongly endorsed by the World Health Organization and the Institute of Medicine, and in a 2012 revision of the AAP policy, breastfeeding is described as a medical priority for infants rather than a lifestyle choice by the parent. The AAP recommends exclusive breastfeeding for about 6 months, and continued use of breast milk in conjunction with solid foods after they are introduced.

According to the AAP report, obesity is significantly less prevalent in breastfed infants. Risk of overweight is inversely correlated with duration of breastfeeding, with each month of breastfeeding associated with an estimated 4% risk reduction of overweight. In fact, a 15%–30% reduction in adolescent and adult obesity rates has been documented if any breastfeeding occurred in infancy compared to no breastfeeding in infancy. An important point to convey to parents is that while breast milk delivered in any form is preferable to commercial formula, babies who nurse self-regulate milk intake and have lower rates of obesity compared to those receiving bottle-fed breast milk. In addition to its beneficial effect on weight, breast milk contains many important immune modulatory factors and has been shown to be protective against a diverse range of illnesses, including otitis media and upper respiratory infections, gastrointestinal infections, necrotizing enterocolitis, sudden infant death syndrome, allergic disease, celiac disease, inflammatory bowel disease, type 1 diabetes, childhood leukemia and lymphoma, and in neurodevelopmental outcomes. Other components in breast milk linked to healthy weight are vitamin D and omega-3 fatty acids in the form of docosahexaenoic acid (DHA). An overview of these two dietary supplements is provided in the supplements section of the chapter.

Healthy Weight: Parental Resistance

It has been reported that parents are often unaware of their infant or child's risk for obesity, usually due to perception of what constitutes a healthy weight in infants and children (Warschburger and Kröller 2009). Other studies have shown that parents may be unwilling to institute preventative measures until their child reaches the 97th percentile for weight due to a lack of recognition or willingness to acknowledge the health risks associated with their child's excess weight. These issues can challenge the practitioner reluctant to alienate the family by suggesting their infant is overweight (Warschburger and Kröller 2012).

HEALTHY WEIGHT: STRATEGIES FOR PREVENTION

Although the U.S. dietary guidelines for Americans do not currently include nutrition recommendations for children under age 2 years (United States Department of Agriculture 2013), recommendations of the IOM committee (Institute of Medicine 2002) do include guidelines to measure and record growth parameters at every well visit, and suggest early discussion and intervention in children with growth measurements at or above the 85th percentile for age, rapid rate of weight gain, and in parents who are overweight or obese. Since September 2010, consensus from the AAP and CDC recommends use of the WHO growth curves for all children younger than 24 months, because they more accurately reflect growth of healthy breastfed infants and more accurately identify overweight and obese infants (American Academy of Pediatrics 2012). Parents may be more receptive to counseling about their infant's weight if policy changes focused on children below 24 months are more widely publicized and adopted.

Key concepts in maintenance of healthy weight

- Obesity is programmed early, often in infancy.
- Obesity tracks through childhood and adolescence into adult life.
- Overweight and obesity puts children and adolescents at risk for serious mental and physical comorbidities.
- Breastfeeding is protective against overweight.
- Early intervention in well visits is important for the prevention of overweight.
- Nutrition counseling should be accompanied by education on healthy lifestyle measures starting before age 2 years.

INTEGRATING NUTRITION INTO THE TREATMENT PLAN

Table 6.1 offers an example of a systematic approach to incorporating nutrition into a child's health plan. This approach may be used for healthy children and modified for those with health conditions.

STEP 1: EXPANDING THE NUTRITIONAL HISTORY

A good understanding of the child's nutritional baseline is important. Sample questions include

- What is the child eating on a typical day (breakfast, lunch, dinner, snacks)?
- What is the family dynamic around mealtimes? Typically enjoyable or stressful?
- Who is the person responsible for food shopping and cooking?
- Is the child involved in meal planning or preparation?
- Are there specific family obstacles to address?
- What is going well? Are there strengths to work from?

TABLE 6.1

Incorporating Nutrition into a Child's Health Plan

Six Basic Steps

1. Expand the nutritional history.
2. Determine BMI for age and daily energy budget.
3. Evenly distribute the daily energy (calorie) budget.
4. Understand ratios and proportions: carbohydrates, proteins, and fats.
5. Correlate the energy budget with healthy foods.
6. Fill nutrition gaps with judicious use of dietary supplements if indicated.

Research shows that children in families that eat together have improved intake of fruits and vegetables, reduced intake of fried foods, lower intake of trans and saturated fats, intake of foods with a lower glycemic load (GL), more fiber, and improved micronutrient intake (Gillman et al. 2000). For example, a large population-based study in 4746 middle-school adolescents found that an increased frequency of family meals per week was positively associated with intake of fruits, vegetables, grains, calcium-rich foods, fiber, diversity of micronutrients, and was negatively associated with soft drink consumption (Neumark-Sztainer et al. 2003).

STEP 2: DETERMINE BMI-FOR-AGE AND DAILY ENERGY BUDGET

BMI-for-Age

BMI is the most common measurement used to assess relative body fatness. In children, the percentile indicates the relative position of the child's BMI number among children of the same sex and age, and is therefore called BMI-for-age. Table 6.2 shows BMI categories in children. A useful resource to tailor individual caloric intake and to track growth parameters is the website of the Children's Nutritional Research Center, a joint project of the U.S. Department of Agricultural Research and Baylor College of Medicine, one of six USDA/Agricultural Research Service Human Nutrition Centers in the United States. The website includes well-designed online tools and resources such as a children's energy needs calculator that provides individualized guides to portion sizes and daily energy needs based on the child's BMI-for-age and daily activity levels, which can be found at: http://www.bcm.edu/cnrc/.

Another BMI-for-age calculator resource that is adjustable to exact age can be found on the CDC website: http://apps.nccd.cdc.gov/dnpabmi/.

Daily Energy Budget

Many practitioners lack familiarity with the average daily energy needs of children. Tables 6.3 and 6.4 are a resource adapted from the Dietary Guidelines for Americans 2010. Data analysis from large pediatric studies suggest that even a small daily average of positive energy intake (excess calories) adds up over time,

TABLE 6.2
BMI Categories in Children

Weight Status Category	Percentile Range
Underweight	Less than the 5th percentile
Healthy weight	5th percentile to less than the 85th percentile
Overweight	85th to less than the 95th percentile
Obese	Equal to or greater than the 95th percentile

Source: Adapted from Centers for Disease Control, Healthy weight: About BMI for children and teens, http://www.cdc.gov/ healthyweight/assessing/bmi/childrens_bmi/about_childrens_ bmi.html.

TABLE 6.3
Daily Energy Needs (in Calories per Day) for Boys

Boys (Years)	Not Active	Somewhat Active	Very Active
2–3	1000–1200	1000–1400	1000–1400
4–8	1200–1400	1400–1600	1600–2000
9–13	1600–2000	2400–2800	2800–3200
14–18	2000–2400	2400–2800	2800–3200

Sources: United States Department of Agriculture, Guidelines for Americans, http://www.cnpp.usda.gov/DietaryGuidelines. htm, 2010; National Institutes of Health, Parent tips: Calories needed each day, http://www.nhlbi.nih.gov/health/public/ heart/obesity/wecan/downloads/calreqtips.pdf, 2010.

TABLE 6.4
Daily Energy Needs (in Calories per Day) for Girls

Girls (Years)	Not Active	Somewhat Active	Very Active
2–3	1000	1000–1200	1000–1400
4–8	1200–1600	1600–2000	1400–1800
9–13	1400–1600	1600–2000	1800–2200
14–18	1800	2000	2400

Sources: United States Department of Agriculture, Guidelines for Americans, http://www.cnpp.usda.gov/DietaryGuidelines. htm, 2010; National Institutes of Health, Parent tips: Calories needed each day, http://www.nhlbi.nih.gov/health/public/ heart/obesity/wecan/downloads/calreqtips.pdf, 2010.

and relatively small changes in eating behaviors, on average a deficit of only 70–160 kcal/day, in addition to appropriate physical activity, may be enough to prevent continued weight gain in overweight children. This range (70–160 kcal/day) is the energy contained in a small pack of commercial potato chips or two average-sized cookies (Pereira et al. 2013).

STEP 3: EVEN DISTRIBUTION OF THE DAILY ENERGY BUDGET

Regular spacing of nutrients throughout the day is important in obesity prevention, maintenance of blood glucose levels, and improved school performance. A well-balanced breakfast is especially important for children (Cooper et al. 2011; Merten et al. 2009; Overby et al. 2013; Pereira et al. 2013; Smeets and Westerterp-Plantenga 2008). A useful rule of thumb is three approximately equal-sized meals and two snacks per day, for example, breakfast, midmorning snack, lunch, midafternoon snack, and dinner. Table 6.5 shows an example of the distribution of a 1800 cal daily energy budget.

STEP 4: NUTRITIONAL BUILDING BLOCKS AND PROPORTIONS: CARBOHYDRATES, PROTEINS, AND FATS

Carbohydrates

An understanding of carbohydrates is important because of their prevalence in the pediatric diet. There are several forms of carbohydrates, including monosaccharides, disaccharides and oligosaccharides, and polysaccharides. The digestible forms of carbohydrates are starches and simple sugars, while nondigestible forms make up the various types of fibers. Carbohydrates vary in their effects on blood glucose levels and can be compared using the glycemic index, which reflects the potency of foods to raise blood glucose and rates of glucose clearance.

(Glycemic index is defined as the incremental area under the blood glucose response curve [AUC] within a 2 h period elicited by a portion of food containing 50 g of available carbohydrate, relative to the AUC elicited by 50 g glucose.)

TABLE 6.5
Distribution of a Child's Daily Energy Budget of 1800 cal

Daily Energy Budget

Breakfast	500 cal
Snack	100 cal
Lunch	500 cal
Snack	100 cal
Dinner	500 cal
Total	**1800 cal**

Foods with more dense carbohydrate structures are absorbed more slowly, causing less rapid increase in postprandial blood glucose levels. These are therefore classified as low glycemic index foods. Examples include steel cut oatmeal and whole grain bread. Other starchy foods, such as baked potatoes and corn flakes, are less dense and therefore more rapidly digested to glucose, producing faster increases in blood glucose levels and subsequently increased insulin levels. These foods are therefore high on the glycemic index (Jenkins et al. 1981).

GL has also been used to define the quality of carbohydrates. GL is defined as glycemic index × w/100, where w is the value in grams of available carbohydrate contained in the amount of food consumed. GL is more accurate than glycemic index at estimating the functional impact of carbohydrates on insulin levels, insulin sensitivity, and inflammatory markers (Salmerón et al. 1997).

Multiple clinical trials have found that subjects consuming low glycemic index or low GL meals have improved glycemic control and improved lipid profiles and lower circulating levels of inflammatory biomarkers (Solomon et al. 2010). The quality of carbohydrate foods consumed by an individual has a major impact on their long-term health. Specifically, consuming diets that favor slowly digested carbohydrates has been associated with a reduced risk of coronary heart disease and type 2 diabetes (Chiu et al. 2011).

Fructose

One carbohydrate that deserves special mention is fructose. Many individuals, especially children, adolescents, African-American adults, and Hispanic adults, are ingesting as much as 30% of their diet as fructose and other added sugars, far exceeding the U.S. mean of 74 g/day, equivalent to 2.5 sugary soft drinks (Johnson et al. 2010).

The consumption of soft drinks containing high fructose corn syrup has been identified as an independent risk factor for metabolic syndrome as fat accumulates in the liver due to increased lipogenesis (Nseir et al. 2010). Fructose metabolism within liver cells is complex and has been shown to generate multiple harmful compounds, such as triglycerides, uric acid, and free radicals. Triglycerides accumulate in liver cells and disrupt normal liver function, leading to nonalcoholic fatty liver disease (NAFLD), and, in severe cases, cirrhosis. Free radicals can damage cell structure, disrupt enzymes, and even interfere with gene expression. More specifically, NAFLD is characterized by two steps of liver injury: intrahepatic lipid accumulation (hepatic steatosis), and inflammatory progression to nonalcoholic steatohepatitis (NASH) (Lim et al. 2010). This form of liver injury carries a 20%–50% risk for progressive fibrosis, 30% risk for cirrhosis, and 5% risk for hepatocellular carcinoma (Bugianesi et al. 2002). NAFLD has become staggeringly prevalent in the pediatric population, now affecting nearly 11% of adolescents and upward of 50% of obese males (Welsh et al. 2013).

Here are some examples of high-fructose foods:

- Soda
- Fruit juice blends

- Breakfast cereals of all types
- Yogurt with fruit flavor
- Salad dressings/condiments
- Breads and baked goods including whole wheat (as opposed to whole grain)
- Candy
- Nutrition and energy bars
- Meal supplement drinks
- Agave syrup

Fats

Fats play multiple roles in the body: they provide efficient energy; influence cell membrane structure and function; are integral to brain and nervous system health; support function of fat-soluble vitamins such as vitamins A, D, E, and K; are building blocks and regulators of many hormones; impact skin health and help regulate body temperature; protect and support internal organs; and function as immune system modulators (Katz 2008).

When considering the different types of fats, in general, form dictates function.

Saturated fat is solid at room temperature. It is used primarily as a food energy source, and has been consistently shown to raise cholesterol. The lack of double bonds in the saturated fatty acid chain makes them stiffer and less susceptible to oxidation. Common sources of saturated fats are red meat, dairy fat, and tropical oils.

Monounsaturated fats contain one double bond in their long fatty acid carbon chains. Oils rich in monounsaturated fat are typically liquid at room temperature but get cloudy and thick when refrigerated. The most common monounsaturated fatty acid in food is oleic acid. Olive oil and canola oil are common sources of oleic acid.

Polyunsaturated fats contain two or more double bonds in their long fatty acid carbon chains. Oils rich in polyunsaturated fat are liquid at room temperature. Polyunsaturated fatty acids add flexibility to the phospholipid bilayer of cell membranes. Examples of polyunsaturated fatty acids include omega-3 and omega-6 fatty acids.

Trans fatty acid can be natural or artificial. Small amounts of trans fats occur naturally in beef and some dairy foods. Artificial trans fats are created when hydrogen gas reacts with oil. An estimated 80% of trans fats in the U.S. diet comes from artificially produced, partially hydrogenated vegetable oil that has been modified for the commercial purpose of increasing food shelf life. Trans fats have been conclusively linked to coronary artery disease, increase in total cholesterol, and lowering of HDL cholesterol. Foods containing trans fats include margarine, icing, many commercial baked goods, and many brands of potato chips (Katz 2008).

Protein

The building blocks of proteins are amino acids. Proteins are important in muscle cells, collagen, and cartilage. They catalyze biochemical reactions as enzymes, and serve as transport and storage sources for molecules such as ferritin, among many other functions in the body. They supply energy at 4 kcal/g. The typical American diet generally provides more than enough protein for healthy children (Katz 2008).

RATIOS AND PROPORTIONS: CARBOHYDRATES, PROTEINS, AND FATS

In addition to total calorie intake and calorie distribution, correct proportions of food groups are important. Table 6.6 shows the current USDA Guidelines of ratios and proportions per meal.

In children without disqualifying medical conditions (malabsorption, failure to thrive, or other serious illness), intake of total fat can be safely limited to 30% of total calories, saturated fat limited to 7%–10% of total calories, and dietary cholesterol limited to 300 mg/day. The remaining 20% of the daily fat budget should be a mixture of monounsaturated and polyunsaturated fats. Trans fats should be avoided.

To date, there are few studies in children examining the relationship between various fatty acids (saturated, polyunsaturated, and monounsaturated) and dietary lipids. One study by Sanchez-Bayle in 673 6-year-olds found that children with the highest saturated fat consumption had significantly higher mean levels of total cholesterol, LDL cholesterol, and lower HDL cholesterol, while children with the highest monounsaturated fat consumption had significantly higher mean levels of HDL cholesterol, and lower total cholesterol, and LDL cholesterol and apolipoprotein B. No statistically significant relationships between polyunsaturated fats and lipid levels were seen in this study group. More studies in this area are needed in children (Sanchez-Bayle et al. 2008).

In practice, the challenge is to maintain this approximate ratio of nutrient distribution (carbohydrate, healthy fats, and protein) at each meal and snack each day, as diagramed in Figure 6.2. The importance of consistent distribution of fats,

---

TABLE 6.6
USDA Guidelines of Ratio and Proportions per Meal

Building Block	Proportion (%)
Carbohydrates	50–60
Protein	25–30
Healthy fats	25–35
Saturated fats[a]	10

Source: United States Department of Agriculture, Guidelines for Americans, http://www.cnpp.usda.gov/DietaryGuidelines.htm, 2010.

[a] Fat percentages may be higher for children 12 months and younger depending on growth velocity and weight.

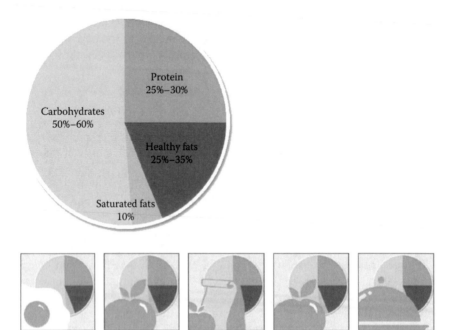

FIGURE 6.2   Maintaining ratios at each meal and snack.

carbohydrates, and proteins throughout the day is one of the primary messages of the new MyPlate.gov (n.d.) website that provides many online tools for children and their families and can be found at: http://www.choosemyplate.gov/index.html.

STEP 5: CORRELATE THE ENERGY BUDGET WITH HEALTHY FOODS

Once a basic understanding of the child's daily energy needs and appropriate ratios of nutritional building blocks are established, it may still seem *daunting* to translate that information into a healthy meal plan. One approach that has been correlated with significant health benefits in adults, and more recently in children and adolescents, is the Mediterranean or anti-inflammatory diet pattern. This approach minimizes intake of processed foods and includes a high consumption of vegetables and fruits, olive oil as the principal source of fat, high-quality grains, low consumption of meat and poultry, moderate use of low-fat dairy products, regular fish intake, and (in adults) moderate consumption of wine.

Education about the Mediterranean diet pattern can help families to navigate more confidently around the processed food and sugary beverages in the marketplace and simplify meal planning by emphasizing fresh whole foods. Ideally this dietary pattern would be introduced to children at the earliest opportunity, preferably with the introduction of solid foods. An important benefit of increased consumption of vegetables and fruits are phytonutrients, natural chemical compounds that confer protective health effects through their potent antioxidant properties. Flavonoids and carotenoids are two major classes of phytochemicals (Katz 2008).

The Mediterranean or inflammatory diet pattern has been shown to be of particular benefit in inflammatory mediated illnesses. For example, multiple large studies confirm reduction of cardiovascular disease in adults (Hoevenaar-Blom et al. 2012; Martínez-González et al. 2012; Sofi et al. 2008; Tognon et al. 2013b), and recent studies support its role in lowering of cardiovascular risk in children (Giannini et al. 2013; Lydakis et al. 2012; Tognon et al. 2013a). The Mediterranean diet pattern has also been linked to the prevention and treatment of obesity in children (Kontogianni et al. 2010) and adults (Bonaccio et al. 2013). Recent research suggests correlation with *decreased cancer risk* (Jafri and Mills 2013; Merendino et al. 2013) and a reduction in the prevalence of allergy and asthma symptoms in patients following a Mediterranean diet (Arvaniti et al. 2011). It is encouraging that national initiatives are under way to educate children and families about the importance of fresh whole foods, and to bring about substantial improvement in the food quality in the public school system (Centers for Disease Control and Prevention 2011; Huang et al. 2013).

STEP 6: FILL NUTRITION GAPS WITH JUDICIOUS USE OF DIETARY SUPPLEMENTS IF INDICATED

Ideally, children would have their nutritional needs met through the intake of healthy foods.

Often this is not realistic, and children may benefit from a high-quality, age-appropriate multivitamin to ensure adequate daily intake of important micronutrients. Omega-3 fatty acids and vitamin D are two other supplements often lacking in the diet that play critical roles throughout the pediatric lifecycle. The following provides an overview of these two supplements.

Omega-3 Fatty Acids

The omega fatty acids are essential fatty acids: the body is unable to synthesize them.

They are polyunsaturated fats and fall into two main categories: omega-3 fatty acids and omega-6 fatty acids. Broadly speaking, omega-3 fatty acids have an anti-inflammatory effect, while omega-6 are associated with a more pro-inflammatory effect. Both these acids are key components of biomembranes and play important roles in cell integrity, development, maintenance, and function. In general, the very high ratio of omega-6 to omega-3 fatty acid found in a typical Western diet is associated with higher incidence of cardiovascular disease, cancer, and inflammatory and autoimmune illness, whereas a lower ratio has been found to be protective. It is now known that the omega-3 fatty acids have regulatory roles in at least three hepatic transcription networks, lending new insight into the complexity of their metabolic interactions and shedding light on how the omega-3 fatty acids confer their protective effect against cardiovascular, metabolic, immunologic, and neurologic illnesses.

Fatty acids in the diet have a substantial impact on

- Cell signaling
- Gene expression

- Circulating inflammatory markers
- Lipoproteins levels
- Adipose tissue synthesis

Eicosapentaenoic acid (EPA) and DHA are the primary active omega-3 fatty acids. The highest concentrations of EPA/DHA are in fish (especially fatty cold water fish such as wild caught salmon, cod, mackerel, tuna, sardines, and herring), fresh seaweed, marine mammals and other seafood, *nonruminant muscle and organ meats,* and *enriched eggs.*

DHA has a critical role in physiology throughout the life-span. Brain accumulation of DHA starts in utero and is present in significant amounts in brain gray matter, neurons, and synapses. It is also prevalent in sperm and testicles and in the rods and cones of the retina. DHA may play a key role in the coordination of metabolic networks that promote the efficient use of dietary protein, stimulating muscle protein synthesis (Innis et al. 2013; Mozaffaria and Wu 2011; Mozaffarian and Wu 2012).

DHA in Pregnancy

The metabolic demand for DHA is increased during pregnancy because of the extra needs of the fetus, expanded maternal cell mass, and placental growth. Maternal stores of DHA can reduce 50% during pregnancy and not return to prepregnancy levels until 6 months postpartum. While the optimal intake/dose of DHA during pregnancy is not known, large-scale trials assessing marine oil supplementation with large doses indicate that DHA supplementation in pregnancy is safe (da Rocha and Kac 2012; Ellsworth-Bowers and Corwin 2012). A significant association with prolonging gestation and reducing the risk of preterm delivery at less than 34 weeks gestation has been shown with DHA in both low-risk and high-risk pregnancies (Mozurkewich and Klemens 2012). DHA is vital for normal brain and nervous system development for the rapid synthesis of cell membranes, particularly neural cells. There is growing evidence that omega-3 consumption during pregnancy enhances infant neurodevelopment (Mozurkewich and Klemens 2012).

Postmortem studies have indicated that the developing fetus accumulates approximately 70 mg/day primarily as DHA in the last trimester when the developing brain experiences significant growth (Makrides 2012).

There is some suggestive evidence that maternal consumption of omega-3 fatty acids during and postpregnancy has been associated with lowered allergen-specific Th2 responses and elevated Th1 responses with the potential to be protective against allergy (D'Vaz et al. 2012).

Maternal omega-3 fatty acid supplementation may also decrease the risk of food allergy and IgE-associated eczema during the first year of life in infants with a family history of allergic disease when 1.6 g EPA + 1.1 g DHA are taken by the mother from the 25th week of pregnancy through the third month of breastfeeding (Furuhjelm et al. 2009).

DHA is passed from mother to infant in the breast milk, and DHA levels in breast milk have been shown to correlate with maternal DHA stores. The current minimum recommended DHA supplement dose for pregnant and lactating women according to the International Society for the Study of Fatty Acids and Lipids is 200 mg/day (International Society for the Study of Fatty Acids and Lipids 1999).

Prior to 2002 in the United States, formula-fed infants did not receive these fatty acids and relied solely on endogenous conversion of the dietary essential *omega-3 and omega-6 fatty acids, ALA and linoleic acids, to DHA and AA*, respectively. Synthetic DHA has become an integral ingredient in infant formula to promote healthy brain development. However, despite significant research interest in this area, claims of improvement in visual, neural, or developmental outcomes in infants receiving DHA supplementation either through breast milk or through formula enhanced with DHA have not been consistently demonstrated. Further research is underway (Campoy et al. 2012; Drover et al. 2012; D'Vaz et al. 2012; Hoffman et al. 2009; Makrides 2012).

Low levels of omega-3 fatty acids have been identified in certain mental health conditions. A recent study examining red blood cell fatty acid profiles in a case-controlled study of depressed adolescents (n = 150) and controls (n = 161) found a reduced omega-3 fatty acid content in depressed patients' red blood cell fatty acid profiles, concluding a need for randomized controlled studies (Pottala et al. 2012).

The Institute of Medicine has set an acceptable macronutrient distribution range (AMDR) for total omega-3 fatty acid intake at 0.6–1.2 g/day for ages 1 and up. However, IOM admits that data are lacking in this area, and these may be conservative figures. For cardiovascular health, most experts recommend 1–2 g of EPA + DHA per day. For elevated triglycerides, the dose is 4 g EPA + DHA per day (Institute of Medicine 2002; Melanson et al. 2005).

Omega-3 supplements (both vegetarian and nonvegetarian) available in the United States are relatively free of detectable levels of mercury, polychlorinated biphenyls (PCBs), and organochlorine (OC) pesticides and come in liquid, capsule, and chewable forms.

Vitamin D

Vitamin D is a fat-soluble vitamin. It is also technically considered a hormone, because it can be synthesized in the body, has specific target tissues, and does not have to be supplied by the diet.

Vitamin D3 (cholecalciferol) can be produced in the skin after exposure to UVB in sunlight, or be obtained in the diet.

Vitamin D2 (ergocalciferol) is produced by plants and has activity in people. Vitamin D2 is most commonly used to fortify foods in the United States.

After being synthesized in the skin or ingested, the vitamins D3 and D2 are transported to the liver, where they are hydroxylated to form calcitriol or 25-hydroxyvitamin D [25(OH)D], which is the major circulating form of vitamin D. Increased sun exposure or increased intake of vitamin D increases serum concentrations of 25(OH)D. This is the most common blood test used to check vitamin D status. PTH and calcium absorption are not optimized until serum 25(OH)D levels reach approximately 80 nmol/L (32 ng/mL). From the liver, the calcitriol or 25-hydroxyvitamin D [25(OH)D] is sent to the kidney, where a second hydroxylation takes place, creating

1 alpha, 25-dihydroxyvitamin D [1,25(OH)2D]—the most potent form of vitamin D. The primary effects of vitamin D are related to the activity of this compound, 1, 25(OH)2D (Holick 2005).

The functions of vitamin D are as follows:

- Maintains normal calcium and phosphorus blood metabolism
- Helps the uptake of calcium and phosphorous from the GI tract
- Works with parathyroid hormone and estrogen to regulate bone metabolism
- Increases renal tubular absorption of calcium and phosphorous
- Is critical for many cellular processes, including nerve function, immune health, and bone growth and calcification of the bones

Metabolic functions affected by insufficient vitamin D include (Holick 2005)

- Insulin resistance
- Cardiac disease
- Allergic and atopic disease
- Asthma
- Depression
- Cancer
- Diabetes
- Immune function

Fortified foods provide most of the vitamin D in U.S. diets, because very few foods are naturally high in vitamin D. Fatty fish such as salmon, tuna, and mackerel are among the best natural sources. Beef liver, cheese, and egg yolks provide small amounts. Mushrooms provide some vitamin D. Almost all of the U.S. milk supply is fortified with 400 IU of vitamin D per quart. Foods made from milk, like cheese and ice cream, are usually not fortified. In the United States, vitamin D is added to breakfast cereals and to some brands of orange juice, yogurt, margarine, and soy beverages.

Risk factors for low vitamin D include (Thacher and Clarke 2011)

- Fat malabsorption syndromes (cystic fibrosis, pancreatitis, celiac disease, short gut syndrome)
- Obesity (vitamin D is stored in fat cells)
- Vegan or strict vegetarian diet, unless getting enough sun exposure
- Exclusive breastfeeding

Insufficient vitamin D impairs calcium absorption, causing the parathyroid glands to increase parathyroid hormone secretion to mobilize calcium from bone. In severe cases of insufficient vitamin D, this can lead to rickets in children (weight-bearing limbs begin to bow) and osteomalacia in adults due to poor mineralization of the collagen matrix (Holick and Chen 2008). Vitamin D receptors have been discovered in many tissues including pancreas and muscle. Vitamin D has been shown to influence immune system macrophages, monocytes, T and B cell lymphocytes regulating cytokine synthesis, monocyte maturation, and macrophage activity (Prietl et al. 2013). Vitamin D also appears to have a beneficial effect on the action of insulin. An inverse correlation between vitamin D and insulin resistance has been established in adults. In children, the relationship between insulin resistance and vitamin D seems to be modified by puberty when more of an adult pattern emerges (Khadgawat et al. 2012; Office of Dietary Supplements, National Institutes of Health 2011).

Exclusively breastfed infants are at high risk of vitamin D deficiency, especially if they have increased skin pigmentation or receive little sun exposure. Breast milk generally provides 25 IU of vitamin D per liter, which is insufficient for an infant if this is the sole source of nutrition. Older infants and toddlers exclusively fed milk substitutes, and weaning foods that are not vitamin D fortified are also at an increased risk of vitamin D deficiency. The American Academy of Pediatrics recommends that all infants that are not consuming at least 500 mL (16 ounces) of vitamin D–fortified formula or milk be given a vitamin D supplement of 400 IU/day (American Academy of Pediatrics).

Children in the United States have almost universally low vitamin D levels (Mansbach et al. 2009); therefore, attention to serum levels in children is important, because low vitamin D is an independent predictor of insulin resistance and the metabolic syndrome in children, especially in obese children (Misra et al. 2008; Reis et al. 2009), and is associated with older age, puberty, higher percentage of body fat, presence of acanthosis nigricans (at risk for type 2 DM), and increased insulin resistance (Garanty-Bogacka et al. 2011). Small preliminary studies show that correcting vitamin D improves insulin sensitivity in obese adolescents. Research is active in this area (Belenchia et al. 2013).

Data from supplementation studies indicates that vitamin D intakes of at least 800–1000 IU/day are required by adults living in temperate latitudes to achieve serum 25 (OH)D levels of at least 32 ng/mL. Difficulty in reaching or maintaining adequate levels in a child or adolescent should prompt endocrine consult. Table 6.7 shows lifetime daily reference intakes for vitamin D.

TABLE 6.7
Daily Reference Intakes for Vitamin D

Life Stage Group	Estimated Average Requirement (IU/day)	Recommended Dietary Allowance (IU/day)	Upper-Level Intake
Infants 0–6 months	a	a	1000
Infants 6–12 months	a	a	1500
1–3 years old	400	600	2500
4–8 years old	400	600	3000
14–70 years old	400	600	4000
Over 79 years old	400	800	4000

Source: Linus Pauling Institute/Vitamin D, http://lpi.oregonstate.edu/infocenter/vitamins/vitaminD/.

[a] For infants, adequate intake is 400 IU/day for 0–6 months of age and 400 IU/day for 6–12 months of age.

The key concepts in integrating nutrition into the pediatric treatment plan are as follows:

- Expand the nutritional history: know the child's nutritional baseline.
- Understand the child's daily energy budget and BMI-for-age.
- Distribute the daily energy (approximate calories) budget evenly.
- Recall the nutritional building blocks (carbohydrates, fats, and proteins)
- Be familiar with ratios and proportions of carbohydrates, proteins, and fats.
- Limit processed foods and sugary beverages. Discourage use of food as a reward.
- Correlate the energy budget with healthy foods and beverages—emphasize the Mediterranean or anti-inflammatory diet pattern
- Fill nutrition gaps with judicious use of dietary supplements if indicated.

ENVIRONMENTAL CONCERNS

Pesticide residues are commonly found on U.S. conventional produce. Although USDA recommendations stress the importance of eating fruits and vegetables of any kind for their health benefits, one or more pesticides were identified on 70% of the samples tested in the most recent USDA tests. The CDC's national biomonitoring program has identified pesticides in blood and urine samples in 95.6% of more than 5000 Americans age 6 and up (Centers for Disease Control and Prevention 2009; United States Department of Agriculture 2009).

It has been clearly established that dietary intake is the primary source of pesticide load in children (Forman and Silverstein 2012, 1406–1415; Lu et al. 2008), although debate is ongoing regarding the overall benefit of organic foods in children and adults (Smith-Spangler et al. 2012, 358–366).

While the American Academy of Pediatrics has not developed a conclusive policy statement endorsing the benefits of organic foods for children, ample evidence has accumulated about the link between pesticides and neurodevelopmental disorders such as ADHD (Bellinger 2012; Polańska et al. 2013; Roberts and Karr 2012; Xu et al. 2011), and to thyroid disorders, Parkinson-like disorders, reproductive problems, and cancer in adults (Centers for Disease Control and Prevention 2009).

Research is also active examining possible causative links between certain classes of pesticides and obesity in children and adults (Twum and Wei 2011; Wei et al. 2013).

An excellent resource for consumers is the *Environmental Working Group Shopper's Pesticide Guide to Produce*, which gives up-to-date and practical information about pesticide load in various fruits and vegetables to help guide purchasing decisions (Environmental Working Group 2013).

BISPHENOL-A

Bisphenol-A is another toxin of significant concern in the food supply, primarily due to its endocrine-disrupting properties. Controversy and questions surround the specifics of tolerable dose and exposure in vulnerable populations such as infants and pregnant women. BPA has been used by industry since the 1940s to make rigid polycarbonate and epoxy resins. It remains one of the highest volume industrial chemicals produced with approximately seven billion pounds manufactured annually. BPA has been estimated to be present in 93% of people in the United States, with concentrations highest in infants and children. In 2007, it was recognized that every major manufacturer of infant formula in the United States used BPA to line the metal portions of their cans (vom Saal et al. 2007).

Primary exposure sources of BPA have historically been hard plastic (polycarbonate) beverage and food containers, including baby bottles and water bottles. It is also found in the liners of most cans, and in dental sealants, hard plastics used in healthcare, and in thermal paper receipts. BPA exposure has been linked to a variety of medical conditions, including polycystic ovarian syndrome, allergic asthma, diabetes and the metabolic syndrome, and low sperm count (Fenichel et al. 2013; Kandaraki et al. 2011; Vaidya and Kulkarni 2012).

Research is active examining links of BPA to obesity in children and adults. For example, elevated levels of urinary BPA above the mean in a group of 1326 students in grades 4–12 were associated with a more than two-fold risk of weight greater than the 90th percentile in girls in a large study in children in Shanghai, China (Li et al. 2013; Trasande et al. 2012).

Education about practical steps to reduce BPA and other important environmental toxin exposures is available through these resources:

- Environmental Working Group: www.ewg.org.
- The Good Guide: www.goodguide.com.

FOOD SENSITIVITY

There are special populations in children where certain foods may trigger disease symptoms. Celiac disease is a good example. In celiac disease, diagnosis is possible through *well*-validated testing such as endomysial antibodies, (EMA-IgA), which are *very* specific in most patients, or by small bowel biopsy. In other illnesses, such as irritable bowel disease, gluten sensitivity, or ADHD, food triggers may be less straightforward and diagnostic criteria less *concrete*. This can lead to confusion and frustration if symptoms persist, especially because food allergy testing can be unreliable or correlate poorly with clinical symptoms in children. A recent study estimates that food allergy in total affects 5% of children under the age of 5 years and 4% of teens and adults. Food allergy prevalence appears to be on the increase (Branum and Lukacs 2009).

MOST COMMON FOOD ALLERGIES

Common foods that cause allergies are

- Eggs
- Milk
- Peanuts
- Soy
- Wheat
- Crustacean shellfish
- Fish

Long-term health problems associated with food allergies can encompass chronic diseases such as asthma, eosinophilic gastrointestinal diseases (Boyce et al. 2011; Wolfe and Aceves 2011), atopic dermatitis, and allergic rhinitis. There are multiple methods for diagnosing food allergies that include skin prick tests, serum IgE levels and double-blind, placebo-controlled food challenge; however, these tests can be expensive, are not always accurate, or well tolerated in children (Sapone et al. 2010). Elimination diets with systematic reintroduction of suspected trigger foods may be a preferable option (for non-life-threatening allergy only). Referral to an allergist can help assist in differentiating those who can participate in elimination diet. There are many ways to approach elimination diets, including eliminating one substance at a time or by groups. The following example offers one approach.

SAMPLE ELIMINATION DIET

> *Step one*: Six-food elimination diet that excludes cow's milk, soy, wheat, egg, peanuts/tree nuts, and seafood. Wheat, dairy, and soy are quite pervasive in packaged food, so close attention to packaged food ingredients is required. Additional foods may be eliminated depending on specific patient symptoms and any previous allergy testing.
> Maintain a food diary looking at multiple areas of quality of life through the course of the day including gut symptoms, behavior, pain, headaches, mood, sleep, and energy level.
> *Step two*: Reintroduce foods after 2 weeks, if symptoms have improved, reintroduce foods that were eliminated, and continue to document symptoms in the food diary. Foods can be introduced one at time or in groups every 3 days. Introduce food or group of foods and observe symptoms for 2 days. If a symptom is not triggered, it is unlikely to be a problem food. Even so, wait until the whole trial is complete to start eating again this particular food again. Continue systematically until all suspected foods have been reintroduced.

Of note, prolonged elimination diets that omit multiple foods have been reported to induce nutrient deficiencies and are not recommended in children (Christie et al. 2002).

SUMMARY

Nutrition in pediatrics is a very broad topic with many areas of specialization. The purpose of this chapter was to raise awareness of common themes in children's nutrition, such as: maintenance of healthy weight, understanding of BMI-for-age and daily energy intake, building blocks of nutrition (carbohydrates, fats, and proteins), benefits of the anti-inflammatory of Mediterranean diet pattern, environmental concerns, key dietary supplements, and food sensitivities. Challenges in promoting healthy nutrition are significant, and include competition from well-funded food industry advertising and marketing campaigns, lack of physician training and time, parental resistance, lack of family mealtime, changeable dietary recommendations, lack of access to healthy foods, and financial considerations for many families. However, reasons to promote healthy nutrition in children are compelling, perhaps, the most important being a focus on preventative health across the life-span.

REFERENCES

American Academy of Pediatrics. 2012. Policy statement 2012. *Pediatrics* (March) 129: e827–e841. http://pediatrics.aappublications.org/content/129/3/e827.full#sec-30.

American Academy of Pediatrics. Breastfeeding initiatives. http://www2.aap.org/breastfeeding/. Accessed December 5, 2013.

Arvaniti F, Priftis KN, Papadimitriou A, Papadopoulos M, Roma E, Kapsokefalou M, Anthracopoulos MB, and Panagiotakos DB. 2011. Adherence to the Mediterranean type of diet is associated with lower prevalence of asthma symptoms, among 10–12 years old children: The PANACEA study. *Pediatr Allergy Immunol* (May) 22(3): 283–289.

Belenchia AM, Tosh AK, Hillman LS, and Peterson CA. 2013. Correcting vitamin D insufficiency improves insulin sensitivity in obese adolescents: A randomized controlled trial. *Am J Clin Nutr* (April) 97(4): 774–781.

Bellinger DC. 2012. Comparing the population neurodevelopmental burdens associated with children's exposures to environmental chemicals and other risk factors. *Neurotoxicology* (August) 33(4): 641–643.

Bonaccio M, Di Castelnuovo A, Costanzo S, De Lucia F, Olivieri M, Donati MB, de Gaetano G, Iacoviello L, and Bonanni A. 2013. Nutrition knowledge is associated with higher adherence to Mediterranean diet and lower prevalence of obesity. Results from the Moli-sani study. *Appetite* (September) 68: 139–146.

Boyce JA, Assa'ad A, Burks AW, Jones SM, Sampson HA, Wood RA, Plaut M et al. 2011. Guidelines for the diagnosis and management of food allergy in the United States: Summary of the NIAID-sponsored expert panel report. *Nutr Res* (January) 31(1): 61–75.

Branum AM and Lukacs SL. 2009. Food allergy among children in the United States. *Pediatrics* (December) 124(6): 1549–1555.

Buganesi E, Leone N, Vanni E, Marchesini G, Brunello F, Carucci P, Musso A et al. 2002. Expanding the natural history of nonalcoholic steatohepatitis: From cryptogenic cirrhosis to hepatocellular carcinoma. *Gastroenterology* (July) 123(1): 134–140.

Campoy C, Escolano-Margarit MV, Anjos T, Szajewska H, and Uauy R. 2012. Omega 3 fatty acids on child growth, visual acuity and neurodevelopment. *Br J Nutr* (June) 107(Suppl. 2): S85–S106.

Centers for Disease Control and Prevention. 2008. Breastfeeding-related maternity practices at hospitals and birth centers—United States, 2007. *Morb Mortal Wkly Rep* (June) 57(23): 621–625.

Centers for Disease Control and Prevention. 2009. Fourth National Report on human exposure to environmental chemicals. Department of Health and Human Services. http://www.cdc.gov/exposurereport/pdf/FourthReport.pdf. Accessed December 5, 2013.

Centers for Disease Control and Prevention. 2011. School health guidelines to promote healthy eating and physical activity. *MMWR Recomm Rep* (September 16) 60(RR-5): 1–76.

Chiu CJ, Liu S, Willett WC, Wolever TM, Brand-Miller JC, Barclay AW, and Taylor A. 2011. Informing food choices and health outcomes by use of the dietary glycemic index. *Nutr Rev* (April) 69(4): 231–242.

Christie L, Hine RJ, Parker JG, and Burks W. 2002. Food allergies in children affect nutrient intake and growth. *J Am Diet Assoc* (November) 102(11): 1648–1651.

Cooper SB, Bandelow S, and Nevill ME. 2011. Breakfast consumption and cognitive function in adolescent schoolchildren. *Physiol Behav* (July) 103(5): 431–439.

da Rocha CM and Kac G. 2012. High dietary ratio of omega-6 to omega-3 polyunsaturated acids during pregnancy and prevalence of post-partum depression. *Matern Child Nutr* (January) 8(1): 36–48.

Dawson JD, Sonka M, Blecha MB, Lin W, and Davis PH. 2009. Risk factors associated with aortic and carotid intima-media thickness in adolescents and young adults: The Muscatine Offspring Study. *J Am Coll Cardiol* (June) 53(24): 2273–2279.

Dhuper S, Buddhe S, and Patel S. 2013. An aging cardiovascular risk in overweight children and adolescents. *Paediatr Drugs* (June) 15(3): 181–190.

Drover JR, Felius J, Hoffman DR, Castañeda YS, Garfield S, Wheaton DH, and Birch EE. 2012. A randomized trial of DHA intake during infancy: School readiness and receptive vocabulary at 2–3.5 years of age. *Early Hum Dev* (July) 88(11): 885–891.

D'Vaz N, Meldrum SJ, Dunstan JA, Lee-Pullen TF, Metcalfe J, Holt BJ, Serralha M, Tulic MK, Mori TA, and Prescott SL. 2012. Fish oil supplementation in early infancy modulates developing infant immune responses. *Clin Exp Allergy* (August) 42(8): 1206–1216.

Ellsworth-Bowers ER and Corwin EJ. 2012. Nutrition and the psychoneuroimmunology of postpartum depression. *Nutr Res Rev* (June) 25(1): 180–192.

Environmental Working Group. 2013. Environmental working group shopper's pesticide guide to produce. http://www.ewg.org/foodnews/summary.php. Accessed December 5, 2013.

Fenichel P, Chevalier N, and Brucker-Davis F. 2013. Bisphenol A: An endocrine and metabolic disruptor. *Ann Endocrinol* (July) 74(3): 211–220.

Forman J and Silverstein J. 2012. Organic foods: Health and environmental advantages and disadvantages. *Pediatrics* (November) 130(5): e1406–e1415.

Frisco ML, Houle JN, and Lippert AM. 2013. Weight change and depression among US young women during the transition to adulthood. *Am J Epidemiol* (July) 178(1): 22–30. Epub June 9, 2013.

Furuhjelm C, Warstedt K, Larsson J, Fredriksson M, Böttcher MF, Fälth-Magnusson K, and Duchén K. 2009. Fish oil supplementation in pregnancy and lactation may decrease the risk of infant allergy. *Acta Paediatr* (September) 98(9): 1461–1467.

Garanty-Bogacka B, Syrenicz M, Goral J, Krupa B, Syrenicz J, Walczak M, and Syrenicz A. 2011. Serum 25-hydroxyvitamin D (25-OH-D) in obese adolescents. *Endokrynol Pol* 62(6): 506–511.

Giannini C, Diesse L, D'Adamo E, Chiavaroli V, de Giorgis T, Di Iorio C, Chiarelli F, and Mohn A. 2013. Influence of the Mediterranean diet on carotid intima-media thickness in hypercholesterolaemic children: A 12-month intervention study. *Nutr Metab Cardiovasc Dis* (June) pii: S0939–S4753(13)00093-8.

Gillman MW, Rifas-Shiman SL, Frazier AL, Rockett HR, Camargo CA Jr, Field AE, Berkey CS, and Colditz GA. 2000. Family dinner and diet quality among older children and adolescents. *Arch Fam Med* (March) 9(3): 235–240.

Halfon N, Larson K, and Slusser W. 2013. Associations between obesity and comorbid mental health, developmental, and physical health conditions in a nationally representative sample of US children aged 10 to 17. *Acad Pediatr* (January–February) 13(1): 6–13.

Harrington JW, Nguyen VQ, Paulson JF, Garland R, Pasquinelli L, and Lewis D. 2010. Identifying the tipping point age for overweight pediatric patients. *Clin Pediatr* (July) 49(7): 638–643.

Harris JL, Schwartz MB, and Brownell KD. 2010. Evaluating fast food nutrition and marketing to youth. Yale Rudd Center for Food Policy and Obesity. http://www.yaleruddcenter.org. Accessed December 5, 2013.

Hoevenaar-Blom MP, Nooyens AC, Kromhout D, Spijkerman AM, Beulens JW, van der Schouw YT, Bueno-de-Mesquita B, and Verschuren WM. 2012. Mediterranean style diet and 12-year incidence of cardiovascular diseases: The EPIC-NL Cohort Study. *PLoS One* 7(9): e45458.

Hoffman DR, Boettcher JA, and Diersen-Schade DA. 2009. Toward optimizing vision and cognition in term infants by dietary docosahexaenoic and arachidonic acid supplementation: A review of randomized controlled trials. *Prostaglandins Leukot Essent Fatty Acids* (August–December) 81(2–3): 151–158.

Holick MF. 2005. The vitamin D epidemic and its health consequences. *J Nutr* (November) 135(11): 2739S–2748S.

Holick MF and Chen TC. 2008. Vitamin D deficiency: A worldwide problem with health consequences. Neonates born to mothers with low vitamin D had significantly lower bone mineral content that may continue into childhood. *Am J Clin Nutr* (April) 87(4): 1080S–1086S.

Huang TT, Sorensen D, Davis S, Frerichs L, Brittin J, Celentano J, Callahan K, and Trowbridge MJ. 2013. Healthy eating design guidelines for school architecture. *Prev Chronic Dis* (February) 10: E27.

Innis SM, Novak EM, and Keller BO. 2013. Long chain omega-3 fatty acids: Micronutrients in disguise. *Prostaglandins Leukot Essent Fatty Acids* (January) 88(1): 91–95.

Institute of Medicine. 2002. Dietary reference intakes for energy, carbohydrate, fiber, fat, fatty acids, cholesterol, protein, and amino acids. http://www.iom.edu/Activities/Nutrition/DRIMacronutrients.aspx. Accessed December 5, 2013.

International Society for the Study of Fatty Acids and Lipids. 1999. Workshop on the essentiality of and recommended dietary intakes for (RDI) for omega-6 and omega-3 fatty acids. http://www.issfal.org/statements/adequate-intakes-recommendation-table.   Accessed December 5, 2013.

Jafri SH and Mills G. 2013. Lifestyle modification in colorectal cancer patients: An integrative oncology approach. *Future Oncol* (February) 9(2): 207–218.

Jenkins DJ, Wolever TM, Taylor RH, Barker H, Fielden H, Baldwin JM, Bowling AC, Newman HC, Jenkins AL, and Goff DV. 1981. Glycemic index of foods: A physiological basis for carbohydrate exchange. *Am J Clin Nutr* (March) 34(3): 362–366.

Johnson RJ, Sanchez-Lozada LG, and Nakagawa T. 2010. The effect of fructose on renal biology and disease. *J Am Soc Nephrol* (December) 21(12): 2036–2039.

Kandaraki E, Chatzigeorgiou A, Livadas S, Palioura E, Economou F, Koutsilieris M, Palimeri S, Panidis D, and Diamanti-Kandarakis E. 2011. Endocrine disruptors and polycystic ovary syndrome (PCOS): Elevated serum levels of bisphenol A in women with PCOS. *J Clin Endocrinol Metab* (March) 96(3): E480–E484.

Katz D. 2008. *Nutrition in Clinical Practice*, 2nd edn. (Lippincott, Williams, & Wilkins, Philadelphia, PA, 2008).

Khadgawat R, Thomas T, Gahlot M, Tandon N, Tangpricha V, Khandelwal D, and Gupta N. 2012. The effect of puberty on interaction between vitamin D status and insulin resistance in Obese Asian-Indian children. *Int J Endocrinol* 2012: 173581.

Kontogianni MD, Farmaki AE, Vidra N, Sofrona S, Magkanari F, and Yannakoulia M. 2010. Associations between lifestyle patterns and body mass index in a sample of Greek children and adolescents. *J Am Diet Assoc* (February) 110(2): 215–221.

Li DK, Miao M, Zhou Z, Wu C, Shi H, Liu X, Wang S, and Yuan W. 2013. Urine bisphenol-a level in relation to obesity and overweight in school-age children. *PLoS One* (June) 8(6): e65399.

Lim JS, Mietus-Snyder M, Valente A, Schwarz JM, and Lustig RH. 2010. The role of fructose in the pathogenesis of NAFLD and the metabolic syndrome. *Nat Rev Gastroenterol Hepatol* (May) 7(5): 251–264.

Linabery AM, Nahhas RW, Johnson W, Choh AC, Towne B, Odegaard AO, Czerwinski SA, and Demerath EW. 2013. Stronger influence of maternal than paternal obesity on infant and early childhood body mass index: The Fels Longitudinal Study. *Pediatr Obes* (June) 8(3): 159–169.

Lu C, Barr DB, Pearson MA, and Waller LA. 2008. Dietary intake and its contribution to longitudinal organophosphorus pesticide exposure in urban/suburban children. *Environ Health Perspect* (April) 116(4): 537–542.

Lydakis C, Stefanaki E, Stefanaki S, Thalassinos E, Kavousanaki M, and Lydaki D. 2012. Correlation of blood pressure, obesity, and adherence to the Mediterranean diet with indices of arterial stiffness in children. *Eur J Pediatr* (September) 171(9): 1373–1382.

Makrides M. 2012. DHA supplementation during the perinatal period and neurodevelopment: Do some babies benefit more than others. *Prostaglandins Leukot Essent Fatty Acids* (June) 88(1): 87–90.

Mansbach JM, Ginde AA, and Camargo CA. 2009. Serum 25-hydroxyvitamin D levels among US children aged 1 to 11 years: Do children need more vitamin D? *Pediatrics* (November) 124(5): 1404–1410.

Martínez-González MA, Guillén-Grima F, De Irala J, Ruíz-Canela M, Bes-Rastrollo M, Beunza JJ, López del Burgo C, Toledo E, Carlos S, and Sánchez-Villegas A. 2012. The Mediterranean diet is associated with a reduction in premature mortality among middle-aged adults. *J Nutr* (September) 142(9): 1672–1678.

Melanson SF, Lewandrowski EL, Flood JG, and Lewandrowski KB. 2005. Measurement of organochlorines in commercial over-the-counter fish oil preparations: Implications for dietary and therapeutic recommendations for omega-3 fatty acids and a review of the literature. *Arch Pathol Labor Med* (January) 129(1): 74–77.

Merendino N, Costantini L, Manzi L, Molinari R, D'Eliseo D, and Velotti F. 2013. Dietary ω-3 polyunsaturated fatty acid DHA: A potential adjuvant in the treatment of cancer. *Biomed Res Int* 2013: 310186.

Merten MJ. 2010. Weight status continuity and change from adolescence to young adulthood: Examining disease and health risk conditions. *Obesity* (July) 18(7): 1423–1428. Epub October 22, 2009.

Merten MJ, Williams AL, and Shriver LH. 2009. Breakfast consumption in adolescence and young adulthood: Parental presence, community context, and obesity. *J Am Diet Assoc* (August) 109(8): 1384–1391.

Misra M, Pacaud D, Petryk A, Collett-Solberg PF, Kappy M, and Drug and Therapeutics Committee of the Lawson Wilkins Pediatric Endocrine Society. 2008. Vitamin D deficiency in children and its management: Review of current knowledge and recommendations. *Pediatrics* 122: 398–417.

Mozaffarian D and Wu JH. 2011. Omega-3 fatty acids and cardiovascular disease: Effects on risk factors, molecular pathways, and clinical events. *J Am Coll Cardiol* (November) 58(20): 2047–2067.

Mozaffarian D and Wu JH. 2012. (n-3) fatty acids and cardiovascular health: Are effects of EPA and DHA shared or complementary? *J Nutr* (March) 142(3): 614S–625S.

Mozurkewich EL and Klemens C. 2012. Omega-3 fatty acids and pregnancy: Current implications for practice. *Curr Opin Obstet Gynecol* (March) 24(2): 72–77.

My Plate.gov. (n.d.). United States Department of Agriculture, Alexandria, VA. http://www.choosemyplate.gov. Accessed December 5, 2013.

Neumark-Sztainer D, Hannan PJ, Story M, Croll J, and Perry C. 2003. Family meal patterns: Associations with sociodemographic characteristics and improved dietary intake among adolescents. *J Am Diet Assoc* (March) 103(3): 317–322.

Nseir W, Nassar F, and Assy N. 2010. Soft drinks consumption and nonalcoholic fatty liver disease. *World J Gastroenterol* (June) 16(21): 2579–2588.

Office of Dietary Supplements, National Institutes of Health. 2011. Dietary supplement fact sheet: Vitamin D. http://ods.od.nih.gov/factsheets/VitaminD-HealthProfessional/. Accessed December 5, 2013.

Ostbye T, Malhotra R, Stroo M, Lovelady C, Brouwer R, Zucker N, and Fuemmeler B. 2013. The effect of the home environment on physical activity and dietary intake in preschool children. *Int J Obes Lond* (May) 20.

Overby NC, Lüdemann E, and Høigaard R. 2013. Self-reported learning difficulties and dietary intake in Norwegian adolescents. *Scand J Public Health* (May) 41(7): 754–760.

Pereira HR, Bobbio TG, Antonio MA, and Barros Filho AD. 2013. Childhood and adolescent obesity: How many extra calories are responsible for excess of weight? *Rev Paul Pediatr* (June) 31(2): 252–257.

Polańska K, Jurewicz J, and Hanke W. 2013. Review of current evidence on the impact of pesticides, polychlorinated biphenyls and selected metals on attention deficit/hyperactivity disorder in children. *Int J Occup Med Environ Health* (March) 26(1): 16–38.

Pottala JV, Talley JA, Churchill SW, Lynch DA, von Schacky C, and Harris WS. 2012. Red blood cell fatty acids are associated with depression in a case-control study of adolescents. *Prostaglandins Leukot Essent Fatty Acids* (April) 86(4–5): 161–165.

Prietl B, Treiber G, Pieber TR, and Amrein K. 2013. Vitamin D and immune function. *Nutrients* (July) 5(7): 2502–2521.

Reis JP, von Muchlen D, and Miller RE. 2009. Vitamin D status and cardio metabolic risk factors in the United States adolescent population. *Pediatrics* 124: e371–e379.

Roberts JR and Karr CJ. 2012 Pesticide exposure in children. *Pediatrics* (December) 130(6): e1765–e1788.

Salmerón J, Manson JE, Stampfer MJ, Colditz GA, Wing AL, and Willett WC. 1997. Dietary fiber, glycemic load, and risk of non-insulin-dependent diabetes mellitus in women. *JAMA* (February 12); 277(6): 472–477.

Sanchez-Bayle M, Gonzalez-Requejo A, Pelaez MJ, Morales MT, Asensio-Anton J, and Anton-Pacheco E. 2008. A cross-sectional study of dietary habits and lipid profiles. The Rivas-Vaciamadrid study. *Eur J Pediatr* (February) 167(2): 149–154.

Sapone A, Lammers KM, Mazzarella G, Mikhailenko I, Cartenì M, Casolaro V, and Fasano A. 2010. Differential mucosal IL-17 expression in two gliadin-induced disorders: Gluten sensitivity and the autoimmune enteropathy celiac disease. *Int Arch Allergy Immunol* 152(1): 75–80.

Smeets AJ and Westerterp-Plantenga MS. 2008. Acute effects on metabolism and appetite profile of one meal difference in the lower range of meal frequency. *Br J Nutr* (June) 99(6): 1316–1321.

Smith-Spangler C, Brandeau ML, Hunter GE, Bavinger JC, Pearson M, Eschbach PJ, Sundaram V et al. 2012. Are organic foods safer or healthier than conventional alternatives?: A systematic review. *Ann Intern Med* (September) 157(5): 348–366.

Sofi F, Cesari F, Abbate R, Gensini GF, and Casini A. 2008. Adherence to Mediterranean diet and health status: Meta-analysis. *BMJ* (September) 337: a1344.

Solomon TP, Haus JM, Kelly KR, Cook MD, Filion J, Rocco M, Kashyap SR, Watanabe RM, Barkoukis H, and Kirwan JP. 2010. A low-glycemic index diet combined with exercise reduces insulin resistance, postprandial hyperinsulinemia, and glucose-dependent insulinotropic polypeptide responses in obese, prediabetic humans. *Am J Clin Nutr* (December) 92(6): 1359–1368.

Thacher TD, Clarke BL. 2011. Vitamin D insufficiency. *Mayo Clin Proc* (January) 86(1): 50–60.

The NS, Suchindran C, North KE, Popkin BM, and Gordon-Larsen P. 2010. Association of adolescent obesity with risk of severe obesity in adulthood. *JAMA* (November 10) 304(18): 2042–2047.

Tognon G, Hebestreit A, Lanfer A, Moreno LA, Pala V, Siani A, Tornaritis M et al. 2013a. Mediterranean diet, overweight and body composition in children from eight European countries: Cross-sectional and prospective results from the IDEFICS study. *Nutr Metab Cardiovasc Dis* (July) pii: S0939–S4753(13)00115-4.

Tognon G, Lissner L, Sæbye D, Walker KZ, and Heitmann BL. 2013b. The Mediterranean diet in relation to mortality and CVD: A Danish cohort study. *Br J Nutr* (July) 3: 1–9.

Trasande L, Attina TM, and Blustein J. 2012. Association between urinary bisphenol A concentration and obesity prevalence in children and adolescents. *JAMA* (September) 308(11): 1113–1121.

Twum C and Wei Y. 2011. The association between urinary concentrations of dichlorophenol pesticides and obesity in children. *Rev Environ Health* 26(3): 215–219.

United States Department of Agriculture. 2009. Pesticide data program: Annual summary. http://www.ams.usda.gov/AMSv1.0/getfile?dDocName = STELPRDC509105.5. Accessed December 5, 2013.

United States Department of Agriculture. 2010. Guidelines for Americans. http://www.cnpp.usda.gov/DietaryGuidelines.htm. Accessed December 5, 2013.

United States Department of Agriculture. 2013. Diet quality of children age 2–17 years as measured by the healthy eating index-2010. Last modified July 2013. http://www.cnpp.usda.gov/Publications/NutritionInsights/Insight52.pdf.

Vaidya SV and Kulkarni H. 2012. Association of urinary bisphenol A concentration with allergic asthma: Results from the National Health and Nutrition Examination Survey 2005–2006. *J Asthma* (October) 49(8): 800–806.

vom Saal FS, Akingbemi BT, Belcher SM, Birnbaum LS, Crain DA, Eriksen M, Farabollini F et al. 2007. Chapel Hill bisphenol A expert panel consensus statement: Integration of mechanisms, effects in animals and potential to impact human health at current levels of exposure. *Reprod Toxicol* (August–September) 24(2): 131–138.

Warschburger P and Kröller K. 2009. Maternal perception of weight status and health risks associated with obesity in children. *Pediatrics* (July) 124(1): e60–e68.

Warschburger P and Kröller K. 2012. Childhood overweight and obesity: Maternal perceptions of the time for engaging in child weight management. *BMC Public Health* (April 20) 12: 295.

Wei Y, Zhu J, and Nguyen A. 2013. Urinary concentrations of dichlorophenol pesticides and obesity among adult participants in the U.S. National Health and Nutrition Examination Survey (NHANES) 2005–2008. *Int J Hyg Environ Health* (July) pii: S1438–S4639(13)00096-5.

Welsh JA, Karpen S, and Vos MB. 2013. Increasing prevalence of nonalcoholic fatty liver disease among United States adolescents, 1988–1994 to 2007–2010. *J Pediatr* (March) 162(3): 496–500.e1.

Weng SF, Redsell SA, Nathan D, Swift JA, Yang M, and Glazebrook C. 2013 Estimating overweight risk in childhood from predictors during infancy. *Pediatrics* (July) 132(2): e414–e421.

Weng SF, Redsell SA, Swift JA, Yang M, and Glazebrook CP. 2012. Systematic review and meta-analyses of risk factors for childhood overweight identifiable during infancy. *Arch Dis Child* (December) 97(12): 1019–1026.

Willis TA, George J, Hunt C, Roberts KP, Evans CE, Brown RD, and Rudolf MC. 2013. Combating child obesity: Impact of HENRY on parenting and family lifestyle. *Pediatr Obes* (July) 9(5): 339–350.

Wolfe JL and Aceves SS. 2011. Gastrointestinal manifestations of food allergies. *Pediatr Clin North Am* (April) 58(2): 389–405, x.

Xu X, Nembhard WN, Kan H, Kearney G, Zhang ZJ, and Talbott EO. 2011. Urinary trichlorophenol levels and increased risk of attention deficit hyperactivity disorder among US school-aged children. *Occup Environ Med* (August) 68(8): 557–561.

Yücel O, Cevik H, Kinik ST, Tokel K, Aka S, and Dinc F. 2013 Abdominal aorta intima media thickness in obese children. *J Pediatr Endocrinol Metab* (May) 10: 1–7.

Zhang J, Himes JH, Guo Y, Jiang J, Yang L, Lu Q, Ruan H, and Shi S. 2013. Birth weight, growth and feeding pattern in early infancy predict overweight/obesity status at two years of age: A birth cohort study of Chinese infants. *PLoS One* (June) 8(6): e64542.

Zhang J, Jiang J, Himes JH, Zhang J, Liu G, Huang X, Guo Y, Shi J, and Shi S. 2012. Determinants of high weight gain and high BMI status in the first three months in urban Chinese infants. *Am J Hum Biol* (September–October) 24(5): 633–639.

7 Women's Health and Nutrition

Laurie Tansman, MS, RD, CDN

CONTENTS

INTRODUCTION

That men and women are different is no big secret. And, while it is true that when we think of women's health, we tend to first think of issues related to the reproductive life cycle (e.g., pregnancy, menopause), when we think of men's health, testicular health is not the number one thought that comes to mind, but rather cardiovascular health. Yet, cardiovascular health is just as important for women as it is for men. That is because heart disease strikes and kills more women than breast cancer, which by the way is not exclusively a women's disease. In fact, since 1984, more women have died each year from heart disease than men [1].

In 1990, the Office of Research on Women's Health (ORWH), established within the National Institutes of Health (NIH), was the first public health office dedicated specifically to women's health [2]. In 1991, the Office on Women's Health (OWH) was established within the U.S. Department of Health and Human Services (HHS) to be followed in 1994 with the establishment of the Office of Women's Health (OWH) within the Food and Drug Administration (FDA) [3,4]. While the mission of each of these offices may slightly differ, they all are committed to addressing women's health.

This chapter will present current nutrition recommendations on topics of concern as it relates to women's health. The chapter begins with weight, because it is a risk factor, ranging from pregnancy complications to diabetes, heart disease, and breast cancer. In fact, weight, especially overweight/obesity, is the common thread throughout most of the sections in this chapter.

WEIGHT

Weight Assessment

There is variation in how weight is assessed and that includes not only the actual body weight but also the distribution of weight. Three are discussed as follows:

> To assess ideal body weight (IBW), a *quick rule of thumb* known as the Hamwi Equation is often used and that takes into account a person's gender. For women, IBW is assessed by [5]:
> 100 pounds (lb) for the first 5 ft of height. For each inch above this, add 5 lb. For each inch under 5 ft, there is inconsistency; some will subtract 5 lb for each inch under 5 ft, while others will use a lesser amount.
> Next is the body mass index (BMI) that is used to identify the degree of adiposity [6,7]. Table 7.1 provides the classification of the BMI. While this is considered the standard for assessing adiposity, it is not without faults [8].
> Finally, measurement of the waist circumference is used to assess abdominal adiposity, which can be a separate risk factor for type 2 diabetes, hypertension, and cardiovascular disease (CVD), even if the BMI is assessed as normal [6,7]. For women, disease risk increases for those with a waist circumference greater than 35 in. (88 cm).

TABLE 7.1
BMI Classification

BMI (kg/m²)	Assessment of Weight
<18.5	Underweight
18.5–24.9	Normal weight
25–29.9	Overweight
30–34.9	Class 1 obesity
35–39.9	Class 2 obesity
≥40	Class 3 extreme obesity

Source: National Institutes of Health, *The Practical Guide, Identification, Evaluation, and Treatment of Overweight and Obesity in Adults,* National Institutes of Health, NIH Publication No. 02-4084, Bethesda, MD, Originally printed 2000, Reprinted January 2002.

OVERWEIGHT/OBESITY

Data released in October 2013 from the National Center for Health Statistics (NCHS) for the prevalence of obesity in adults, 2011–2012, show that while the trajectory of obesity has abated, more than one-third of U.S. adults were obese [9]. A close look at the data indicates except for those who are middle aged (40–59 years of age), more adult women are obese compared to adult men, especially those 60 and over [9]. As per that NCHS data: "The only difference by sex was found among non-Hispanic black adults: 56.6% of non-Hispanic black women were obese compared with 37.1% of non-Hispanic black men" [9].

What is further disconcerting about obesity rates for American women is that the prevalence of class 3 extreme obesity has been estimated to be approximately 50% higher than for men [10].

Among the factors that may contribute to the incidence of overweight/obesity in women are cultural/ethnic/racial attitudes. For example, white males appear to have a preference for thinner women compared to black men [11]. The pressure to lose weight is not as great among black women compared to their white counterparts [12]. This is probably a reason why black women who are overweight have a more positive attitude about their size compared to white women [13,14]. In some cultures, female obesity is a positive attribute for marriage and fertility. Taking this to an extreme is the force-feeding that continues to be practiced among young women in Mauritania [15].

EATING DISORDERS

While there are many reasons for the incidence of anorexia and bulimia, it is especially predominant among females because of the desire/societal pressure to be thin [16,17]. After all, it was not a man who said "you can never be too rich or too thin" [18]. Just flipping through the pages of most mainstream fashion magazines shows female models are mostly thin, whereas the men are of a more normal weight.

Compounding the pressure to be thin is the discrimination especially experienced by obese women [19].

McCarthy proposed that a "women's pursuit of thinness" may be a key factor that explains the parallel of eating disorders and depression in women [16].

REPRODUCTIVE LIFE CYCLE

MENSTRUATION

Menstruation is a milestone in the life-span as it represents the female transition into womanhood, preparing the body for childbearing. Yet this milestone can present itself with multiple challenges that for some can disrupt daily routine, in particular, dysmenorrhea. More commonly referred to as menstrual cramps, this is reportedly the most common gynecological disorder in women, affecting up to 90% of reproductive-aged women [20]. It is reported that this is the most common reason for work as well as school absenteeism in adolescents. In fact, there are countries where a woman may take a "menstrual leave." This concept originated in Japan almost a century ago and while few countries support this, it has continued to be addressed in some countries up to the present time [21].

There has been limited research to address relief from dysmenorrhea. Thiamine, magnesium, vitamin E, and omega-3 polyunsaturated fatty acids (PUFAs) supplementation have been reviewed. Studies have not demonstrated that supplementation with magnesium and thiamine could be recommended for relief of pain, but there may be some possibility of relief with vitamin E and omega-3 PUFAs [20].

However, two of the most important nutrition-related issues to consider for the menstruating female are iron deficiency and premenstrual syndrome (PMS).

Iron deficiency remains a global concern [22]. Its incidence is greatest in young children and women during their reproductive years, especially those who are pregnant [23]. The reason for this high incidence in women is related to menstrual blood loss, thus one of the reasons for the higher Recommended Dietary Allowance (RDA) for iron for females [24]. Table 7.2 identifies the RDA for the female throughout her reproductive

---

TABLE 7.2
RDA for Iron during Female Reproductive Years

Life Stage (Years)	RDA (mg/day)	RDA for Pregnancy (mg/day)	RDA for Lactation (mg/day)
14–18	15	27	10
19–30	18	27	9
31–50	18	27	9

Source: Food and Nutrition Board, Institute of Medicine, *Dietary Reference Intakes for Vitamin A, Vitamin K, Arsenic, Boron, Chromium, Copper, Iodine, Iron, Manganese, Molybdenum, Nickel, Silicon, Vanadium, and Zinc*, National Academies Press, Washington, DC, 2001.

life-span. The RDA only differs from males for 14–50 years of age and during pregnancy and lactation. During those years, the RDA for iron for males is 8 mg/day [24].

For a woman who has a *heavy* menstrual flow and where there is a concern for iron deficiency, a good way to optimize dietary iron intake is daily intake of an iron-fortified cold cereal, not only as a meal with milk but also dry as a snack. If you live in New York City, like this author, it is not uncommon to see a young mother giving her toddler a snack bag of cold cereal while riding the bus or subway. So why should not a woman do the very same for herself instead of snacking on empty calories such as chips or candy? An additional benefit of having a cold iron-fortified cereal is that most are fortified with a host of other vitamins and minerals, especially folic acid (See the section "Preconception").

PMS is a wide constellation of symptoms that present as physical, psychological, and emotional generally occurring during the second half—the luteal phase—of the menstrual cycle [25,26]. Symptoms range from breast tenderness, irritability, and insomnia to bloating, headache, mood swings, and food cravings [25,26].

In a review by Verma and colleagues, the following changes in dietary habits may provide some relief [26]:

- Increasing tryptophan intake, an indispensable amino acid, may reduce mood symptoms.
- Reducing sodium and sugar intake may reduce symptoms of fluid retention.
- Reducing intake of methylxanthines (from coffee, tea, colas, and chocolate) may help in reducing breast discomfort.
- Soy intake may reduce cramps and fluid retention.

While these strategies may be helpful, this author doubts that a chocolate lover with food cravings probably will not want to decrease her chocolate intake.

Other diet strategies have looked at vitamins and minerals. In a study based upon data from the Nurses' Health Study II looking at dietary and supplemental mineral intake, high intake of nonheme iron and possibly zinc may be associated with a lower risk of PMS, whereas a high potassium intake may be associated with an increased risk for PMS [26]. However, the overall health benefits of a high dietary potassium intake should not be neglected in considering reducing intake, because it *might* provide a reduced risk for PMS. And, for a woman taking potassium supplementation, it first needs to be considered if that woman is taking it because of a potassium-depleting medication such as the loop and thiazide diuretics.

Finally, two natural remedies that have been suggested to reduce PMS symptoms, as addressed by the National Center for Complementary and Alternative Medicine (NCCAM) of NIH, are evening primrose oil and chasteberry [27,28]. Both have demonstrated in a few studies to show some relief of symptoms, although data for chasteberry appears more reliable and promising [27].

POLYCYSTIC OVARY SYNDROME

Polycystic ovary syndrome (PCOS) is an endocrine disorder that affects women during their child-bearing years [29]. It is characterized by menstrual irregularities, enlarged ovaries with multiple cysts, infertility, and insulin resistance. The clinical presentation includes acne, hirsutism, and obesity, especially abdominal adiposity [29,30]. According to the 2013 Clinical Practice Guideline from The Endocrine Society for the diagnosis and treatment of PCOS, while weight loss is a recommended therapy for the overweight/obese woman, especially as it may be beneficial to address other health risks, "the role of weight loss in improving PCOS status per se, is uncertain" [30].

Preconception

Research has provided much information, including nutrition-related information, to help a woman prepare for a healthy pregnancy. However, because many pregnancies are unintended, 49% in the United States during 2006, all women in their reproductive years (especially those who are sexually active) should consider the following nutrition-related recommendations as prescribed by the Centers for Disease Control and Prevention (CDC) [31]:

- 400 µg of folic acid daily.
- Maintain a healthy diet and weight.
- Abstain from alcohol.

Because of the higher incidence of unplanned pregnancy, women should also be careful of taking preformed vitamin A supplements as epidemiological data point to the possibility of teratogenic effects, particularly during the first trimester when a woman may not yet know she is pregnant, especially because the pregnancy may be unintended [24,32].

Something of interest to note is the fortification of foods with folic acid that became mandatory in the United States by January 1, 1998. This FDA requirement made the fortification of only enriched cereal-grain products mandatory, not all cereal-grain products. Thus, whole grain products may or may not be fortified with folic acid. The intended purpose of this requirement was to assure optimal folate intake by women during their child-bearing years to reduce the incidence of neural tube defects (NTDs), one of the most common birth defects. However, what is interesting is that the 1995 Dietary Guidelines for Americans (DGA) (as well as subsequent guidelines) encourages the consumption of whole grains. Therefore, theoretically, the female for whom this fortification law was intended and who consumes only whole grains that may not be fortified with folic acid may not be getting adequate folate intake. Furthermore, this mandatory law is not without controversy, especially because of the concern that high intakes of folic may mask a vitamin B_{12} deficiency [33]. In fact, while there are many nations that do have this mandatory requirement, none in the European Union have mandated this public health initiative although the United Kingdom has been strongly considering this during 2014.

Pregnancy

It was not that long ago that pregnancy was relatively "straightforward" unless a woman had health problems and/or problems during the course of the pregnancy that ranged from hyperemesis gravidarum to an unfortunate fetal demise. But with the increased incidence in obesity as well as more women having their first pregnancy at an older age and because of increased technologies, especially in vitro fertilization (IVF), pregnancy has become very complicated.

Weight and Weight Gain

Since this chapter began with weight, this is a good starting point. The literature is filled with information about the impact of obesity on a healthy pregnancy because of the obesity pandemic [34–38]. Being obese puts a woman at increased risk for gestational diabetes mellitus (GDM), thromboembolic events, and hypertensive disorders, especially preeclampsia, a life-threatening condition that is often only resolved with delivery, and increased incidence for a cesarean section. And if an obese woman has a cesarean section, there is the concern of postsurgical wound healing. Then there is the impact of obesity on the unborn fetus that ranges from increased incidence of NTDs and other birth defects including multiple congenital anomalies to intrauterine growth restriction (IUGR), duration of pregnancy, fetal death, and stillbirth [34–36,38–40]. Maternal obesity also puts the newborn at increased risk for infant death [39]. Last, maternal obesity can also be a determinant of offspring long-term health including mortality from cardiovascular events in the adult offspring [35,36,39,41]. The offspring becomes a *victim* of their mother's obesity.

On the other hand, maternal underweight brings its own risks that can lead to problems, including IUGR [40].

All these reasons make it important to achieve a healthy weight prior to planning a pregnancy.

When considering gestational weight gain, many of the concerns identified with obese mothers can also occur in the normal weight mother who gains too much weight, especially GDM and preeclampsia.

In 2009, the Institute of Medicine (IOM) of the National Academies released updated guidelines for maternal weight gain for a singleton pregnancy (Table 7.3) [42].

The weight gain guidelines are intended for all women, regardless of stature, racial/ethnic background, and age. For a twin pregnancy, provisional guidelines were recommended (Table 7.4) [42].

For women pregnant with three or more fetuses, the IOM has not released weight gain guidelines. At the very least, the upper end of the weight gain range for twins

---

TABLE 7.3

IOM Recommendations for Maternal Weight Gain for a Singleton Pregnancy

Pregravid Weight	BMI	Recommended Range of Total Weight Gain (lb)
Underweight	<18.5	28–40
Normal Weight	18.5–24.9	25–35
Overweight	25–29.9	15–25
Obese (all classes)	≥30	11–20

TABLE 7.4

IOM Recommendations for Maternal Weight Gain for a Twin Pregnancy

Pregravid Weight	BMI	Recommended Range of Total Weight Gain (lb)
Normal weight	18.5–24.9	37–54
Overweight	25–29.9	31–50
Obese (all classes)	≥30	25–42

should be achieved. Probably the best guideline in such circumstances will be the ultrasound growth scan that identifies the estimated fetal weight (EFW) along with the growth percentile.

Nutrition Needs

Calorie and protein needs: In 2005, the IOM released the Dietary Reference Intakes (DRIs) for calories and macronutrients and that included recommendations for pregnancy and lactation. The RDAs for calorie and protein needs above usual needs for a singleton pregnancy are summarized in Table 7.5 [43].

Additional calories and protein needs for twin pregnancies have been updated most recently by Goodnight and Newman from earlier published work by Luke [44,45].

Micronutrient needs: Each release of the DRIs has included recommendations for pregnancy and lactation based upon a singleton pregnancy. Table 7.6 provides a summary of the RDAs for calcium, folate, and iron.

Calcium needs do not change during pregnancy [46]. Folate needs do increase by 50% [47]. Although there is mandatory folic acid fortification of enriched grain products in the United States, most prenatal vitamins contain the RDA for folate as folic acid. For iron, there is a likewise increased need. Iron is often included in standard prenatal vitamin preparations [24].

For twins, the needs for several micronutrients have been estimated by Goodnight and Newman [44].

TABLE 7.5

RDA for Additional Calorie and Protein Needs for a Singleton Pregnancy

Trimester	Additional Daily Calories	Additional Daily Protein (g)
First	None	None
Second	340	25
Third	452	25

TABLE 7.6
Select RDAs for Micronutrients for a Singleton Pregnancy

Life Stage (Years)	Calcium (mg/day)	Folate (µg/day)[a]	Iron (mg/day)
14–18	1300	600	27
19–30	1000	600	27
31–30	1000	600	27

Sources: Food and Nutrition Board, Institute of Medicine, *Dietary Reference Intakes for Vitamin A, Vitamin K, Arsenic, Boron, Chromium, Copper, Iodine, Iron, Manganese, Molybdenum, Nickel, Silicon, Vanadium, and Zinc*, National Academies Press, Washington, DC, 2001; Food and Nutrition Board, Institute of Medicine, *Dietary Reference Intakes for Calcium and Vitamin D*, National Academies Press, Washington, DC, 2010; Food and Nutrition Board, Institute of Medicine, *Dietary Reference Intakes for Thiamin, Riboflavin, Niacin, Vitamin B$_6$, Folate, Vitamin B$_{12}$, Pantothenic Acid, Biotin, and Choline*, National Academies Press, Washington, DC, 1998.

[a] As dietary folate equivalents.

Food Safety

The FDA has an excellent tool that summarizes food safety for the pregnant woman [48]. The three specific food-borne risks addressed by the FDA are

1. *Listeria*: A bacteria that can grow in refrigerated ready-to-eat foods as well as unpasteurized milk and milk products. A pregnant woman should not consume unpasteurized dairy products. To prevent listeriosis, the label of the cheese product must indicate that it was made with pasteurized milk. Smoked seafood such as salmon, trout, and whitefish should not be eaten unless it has been cooked such as part of a casserole. Hot dogs and luncheon meats should not be eaten unless they are reheated until, what the FDA says is, steaming hot. Last, refrigerated pates or meat spreads should not be eaten.

2. *Methylmercury*: The fish that should be avoided are king mackerel, shark, swordfish, and tilefish. All other fish can be safely consumed but limited to 12 oz weekly. The exception to this is white albacore tuna that should be limited to 6 oz weekly. Five of the most commonly eaten fish that are low in mercury as per the FDA include shrimp, canned light tuna, salmon, pollack, and catfish.

3. *Toxoplasma*: A parasite that can cause toxoplasmosis. In the food supply, it can be found in raw and undercooked meat as well as unwashed fruits and vegetables. Careful cleaning and handling of these foods as well as the proper cooking of meats should be employed.

The FDA, in collaboration with the Environmental Protection Agency (EPA), recently released a draft of updated advice on fish consumption that encourages the consumption of eating fish for women planning a pregnancy, pregnant women, lactating women, and young children within the limits as described above [49].

Common Reported Nutrition-Related Complaints

Constipation: During pregnancy, movement through the gut is slowed to allow
for optimal nutrient absorption. The positioning of the fetus(es) against the
gut can also contribute to constipation as does the often necessary requirement for an iron and/or calcium supplement. However, there are nutrition
strategies that the pregnant woman can consider. First, avoid constipating
foods such as bananas [50]. In this reference by Müller-Lissner, it should
also be noted that chocolate was thought to be constipating in the population studied. Second, eat plenty of other washed raw fruits and vegetables as
well as high-fiber cereals. Third, if all else fails, a laxative, recommended
by a healthcare provider, will usually provide relief.

Gastroesophageal reflux (GERD) aka heartburn: Sitting up while eating can
be helpful as well as not eating anything for a couple of hours prior to going
to sleep. Other strategies include avoiding foods that normally are contraindicated in GERD (see Chapter 14). Sometimes it will be necessary to take a
medication recommended by a healthcare provider.

Nausea and vomiting: Affecting at least half of all pregnant women, this can
range from early morning nausea and possible vomiting for a few weeks
to its extreme form known as hyperemesis gravidarum [51,52]. For women
who have "morning sickness," having a few dry crackers upon awakening
and a very late breakfast may successfully address this problem. Some
may need to undertake more additional strategies such as avoiding cooking odors, eating only foods that are cold or at room temperature, and
avoiding high fat foods. Also, a vitamin B6 supplement may be helpful
[51]. Crystallized ginger or "flat" ginger ale may be helpful too. A ginger
dietary supplement may be helpful but should be limited to small doses
[52,53]. For those women who require more intense treatment, an antiemetic will be prescribed by the healthcare provider. In cases where relief
is not provided by oral anti-emetics, a woman may need to be hospitalized and started on intravenous (IV) anti-emetics with the possibility for
her to be discharged home on an IV anti-emetic regimen. In extreme circumstances, where there is continued intolerance to eating accompanied
by weight loss, nutrition support will need to be considered [51].

Finally, another pregnancy challenge for which nutrition is involved is where there is
concern for premature delivery. Some healthcare providers will understandably try a
variety of strategies, the two most popular nutrition interventions are

Artificially sweetened beverages and foods: There has been a controversy in
the literature about the impact of artificial sweeteners and preterm delivery
[54–57]. However, there are many healthcare providers who none-the-less
will advise such patients to avoid artificial sweeteners. For the pregnant
woman with GDM, this can be a "big deal" if her regular intake includes
artificially sweetened soda along with other artificially sweetened foods.

Fish oil supplementation: There have been a number of studies that have shown
a positive correlation with such supplementation and greater gestational

duration [58]. Supplementation with fish oil may result in greater gestational duration in women with previous pregnancy complications and who
did not have a high fish intake. And a more recent study showed that supplementation with only docosahexaenoic acid (DHA) during the latter half of
pregnancy resulted in greater gestational duration [59].

Before leaving this section, it would be remiss to not mention the importance of alcohol avoidance during pregnancy. It is well known that pregnant women need to avoid
alcohol; this avoidance has been dealt with even in television, movie, and play scripts
when an actress is portraying a pregnant woman. There is always a scene where
the actress intentionally avoids an alcoholic beverage, because she is pregnant. Yet,
it is estimated that one in nine women drink alcohol during pregnancy [60]. And,
every now and then an article surfaces in the professional literature that says that
some degree of alcohol intake may not have adverse effects. Most recently, this was
reported in late 2013 [61]. Nevertheless, the recommendations have not changed and
pregnant women should abstain from alcohol intake during pregnancy. As stated by
Waterman and coauthors, "Fetal alcohol exposure is the leading preventable cause of
birth and developmental defects in the United States" [60].

LACTATION

Breastfeeding exclusively is undisputedly the preferred way to feed an infant [62].
For women who are unable to breastfeed, availability and use of donor breast milk
has increased [63]. As per recent available data in the United States, 75% of mothers
are attempting breastfeeding with the rate falling to 43% at the end of 6 months [64].
For those who do not breastfeed, the reasons are multiple and include poor family
and social support, social norms, embarrassment as well as employment and child
care. There are also mothers who cannot breastfeed for medical reasons. First is
illness, particularly women with HIV [65]. Breastfeeding is not advocated for the
HIV-infected mother, because HIV can be transmitted through breast milk. Second
is medication that can be transferred in breast milk. Sometimes the medication may
only be temporary, such as completing a course of antibiotics. Under such circumstances, the mother should begin pumping and discard her milk until it is deemed
safe to give the milk to her baby.

The advantages of breastfeeding are not exclusively for the infant but for the
mother too. Exclusively breastfeeding promotes gestational weight loss [66]. For the
woman with GDM, breastfeeding ≥3 months can reduce the risk for type 2 diabetes
and delay its development [67].

The nutrition needs to support breastfeeding for one infant is an additional 330 cal
daily for the first 6 months and 600 additional calories daily thereafter. Protein needs
are an additional 25 g daily [43]. For twins, a few recommendations are suggested by
Goodnight and Newman [44].

MENOPAUSE

Menopause represents a new chapter in the female life-span. It can occur naturally as a result of the aging process or it can be caused by surgery as well as the

TABLE 7.7

RDAs for Calcium and Vitamin D for the Postmenopausal Years

Life Stage (Years)	Calcium (mg/day)	Vitamin D (µg/day)
51–70	1200	15
>70	1200	20

Source: Food and Nutrition Board, Institute of Medicine, *Dietary Reference Intakes for Calcium and Vitamin D*. National Academies Press, Washington, DC, 2010.

treatment for illness. As with PMS, there are a range of symptoms that a woman can experience, and that includes a time span of several years during this transition to menopause [68]. Probably the two most common menopausal symptoms are hot flashes and night sweats. To address these symptoms, women may turn to alternative therapies including soy isoflavones and black cohosh [68,69]. However, use of these supplements is controversial and the risks verses benefits issue needs to be addressed.

There are, however, important nutrition issues that a woman needs to be proactive in pursuing as she arrives at menopause and that she might not readily recognize as she may be more concerned with relief of the previously mentioned symptoms. Because of the decreased production in estrogen, incidence of osteoporosis and CVD in women increases. Nutrition strategies to reduce the risk for these are important and addressed further in this chapter.

Before leaving this section, overweight and obesity need to be readdressed. As mentioned earlier, more women are obese compared to men, especially those 60 and over. As will be mentioned further in this chapter, overweight/obesity not only increases the risk for CVD but especially for breast cancer in the postmenopausal woman.

So what are the best nutrition strategies for a woman who is entering menopause and beyond? Eat a well-balanced diet that is consistent with guidelines to reduce CVD risk and that includes maintaining a healthy weight as well as being sure to get adequate dietary calcium and vitamin D intake (Table 7.7) [46,70].

CHRONIC DISEASE

CARDIOVASCULAR DISEASE

In 2002, the Red Dress pin became the symbol for women and heart disease awareness in the United States. The following year, the National Heart, Lung and Blood Institute collaborated with the American Heart Association (AHA) to further increase awareness of heart disease as the number one killer of woman. This led to National Wear Red Day annually observed on the first Friday of February.

When it comes to diet, the basic guidelines for CVD risk reduction as recommended by the AHA do not differ for men or women except as follows:

Sugar: In August, 2009, the AHA released a Scientific Statement recommending a reduction in sugar intake because of the concern about the adverse effects of excess sugar consumption, obesity, and that increases CVD risk. For women, the recommendation was not to exceed 100 kcals/day (i.e., 25 g which is approximately 6.2 teaspoons of sugar) of added sugar [71].

In the AHA Guideline–2011 Update for cardiovascular disease prevention in women, specific recommendations were made [72]:

Fish: Pregnant women should be counseled to avoid high-mercury fish: king mackerel, shark, swordfish, and tilefish.
Alcohol: ≤1 serving weekly.

But, the first strategy that a woman should undertake to reduce her risk of CVD is to maintain a healthy weight. Given that overweight/obesity is more prevalent in women, this is probably that much more important in reducing the statistics for the reduction of CVD in women.

A last note: The AHA/American Stroke Association (ASA) has recently released guidelines for the prevention of stroke in women [73]. Within these guidelines, a dietary recommendation was made for the prevention of preeclampsia, a hypertensive disorder in pregnancy: calcium supplementation of ≥1 g/day should be considered for women who consume <600 mg/day of dietary calcium.

BREAST DISEASE

Fibrocystic Breasts

Fibrocystic breast (sometimes referred to as fibrocystic breast disease, fibrocystic breast condition) is a benign condition in which the breast(s) are lumpy and often swollen and/or painful. For years, it was thought that high fat or high caffeine intake may cause/increase risk for fibrocystic breasts. However, the data has not been compelling to demonstrate a link and further research to identify a diet-related link has not been actively pursued [74,75].

Breast Cancer

Breast cancer is probably the most feared and dreaded of all cancers for women. Yet, it is neither number one in the incidence of all cancers by site nor the number one cause of cancer deaths in American women. According to the most recently released facts and figures from the American Cancer Society (ACS), excluding cancers of the skin, while breast cancer accounts for 29% of all newly diagnosed cancers, cancers of the lung and bronchus are the number one site of cancer mortality in women [76]. Worldwide the statistics differs depending upon the country for breast cancer incidence and mortality in the female population. But what is of concern from this most recent statistics released from the International Agency for Research on Cancer of the World Health Organization in December, 2013, is since 2008, breast cancer incidence has increased by greater than 20% and mortality by 14% [77].

The plethora of research seeking the breast cancer–diet connection has for the most part been contradictory just as it has been for many other cancers, except for two consistently positive connections: weight and alcohol intake.

Weight

Overweight and obesity appears to increase a woman's risk for breast cancer, especially in the postmenopausal years. However, in the premenopausal population, increasing adiposity has been associated with decreased breast cancer risk [78]. But for the overweight/obese young woman, this should not be misunderstood as a reason or excuse to not pursue weight loss.

Alcohol Intake

It is now regarded as a fact that alcohol intake increases a woman's risk for breast cancer. In the current recommendations from the ACS, women should limit their alcohol intake to no more than one drink daily [78]. It is further indicated that only a few drinks per week may contribute to a slightly higher breast cancer risk [79]. This is something to strongly consider for the woman who may already have other breast cancer risk factors and that may not be modifiable.

Soy Intake

Research continues to be published about the soy–breast cancer connection, a connection that was originally identified in the Asian female population where soy intake is greater compared to Western countries and breast cancer incidence is significantly lower [80]. The research is not only focused on breast cancer incidence but also breast cancer recurrence [81–83]. The understanding of this connection at least in part centers around the phytochemicals in soy, soy isoflavones, that have a weak estrogenic effect. Compounding the understanding of this link is the age at which soy intake appears to be most beneficial, namely, early in life. The most current research links the potential benefit for breast cancer risk to women with specific polymorphisms in genes associated with breast cancer [81]. Soy intake may also be beneficial in reducing recurrence in the postmenopausal woman with breast cancer positive for estrogen and progesterone receptors [83].

What is key to understanding the potential benefit of soy consumption is that it should be a food source and not an isolated supplement. In the most current recommendations by the ACS, there are no specific dietary recommendations made for soy intake.

OVARIAN AND UTERINE (ENDOMETRIAL) CANCER

Weight

Excess weight continues to be a factor linked to increased cancer risk. In more recent years, an increased BMI is now being correlated with ovarian and uterine cancers [84,85]. Thus, another reason for women to maintain a healthy weight.

Dairy Intake and Ovarian Cancer

There has been some limited research attempting to demonstrate a link between dairy and ovarian cancer, but data is inconclusive [86,87]. The bottom line here is a woman should not stop consuming high-calcium dairy sources because of a questionable link that *might* be correlated to ovarian cancer.

In the most recently published review trying to establish a link between diet and ovarian cancer, no specific components of the diet have been consistently shown to impact ovarian cancer risk [88].

CERVICAL CANCER

While certain subtypes of human papilloma virus (HPV) are the primary cause of most cervical cancers, there are some steps that a woman can take to increase the possibility that the virus will resolve rather than cause progressive cervical changes that result in cervical cancer.

With regard to diet, folate and its relation to cervical changes dates back almost 50 years. Research continues to surface attempting to correlate a protective effect of one or more of the B vitamins with cervical dysplasia, especially in those infected with HPV. The research has, not surprisingly, been conflicting [89–91].

So what diet strategies can a woman follow to reduce her risk for any cancer? Follow the recommendations of the ACS [76] (Box 7.1).

DIABETES

According to the CDC, from data collected for 2010, the incidence of diabetes is greater for men than for women [92]. Yet, although the incidence is greatest in men, women with diabetes tend to be sicker and their risk for other chronic illnesses, especially for CVD, increases more than it does for men.

BOX 7.1 SUMMARY OF DIET RECOMMENDATIONS FROM THE AMERICAN CANCER SOCIETY

- Achieve and maintain a healthy weight.
- Consume a healthy diet with an emphasis on plant foods.
  Choose foods and beverages in amounts that help to achieve and maintain a healthy weight.
  Limit consumption of processed meat and red meat.
  Eat at least 2½ cups of vegetables and fruits each day.
  Choose whole grains instead of refined-grain products.
- If you drink alcoholic beverages, limit consumption. (For women, limit intake to no more than one drink per day.)

Source: American Cancer Society, *Cancer Facts & Figures 2013*, American Cancer Society, Atlanta, GA, 2013.

When it comes to risk factors for diabetes, the one risk factor that is unique to females is prior history of GDM. As diabetes is addressed elsewhere (see Chapter 12), this section will focus exclusively on GDM. Risk factors for GDM include advanced maternal age, obesity, and family history of diabetes [93]. Prior history of GDM is, of course, a risk factor too. While GDM often resolves following delivery, 5%–10% are found to have type 2 diabetes [92]. However, just because diabetes usually resolves following delivery does not imply that a woman's risk of diabetes is the same as if she had not had GDM. Therefore, lifelong screening for the diagnosis of prediabetes/diabetes is recommended at least every 3 years [94].

The most current recommendation for detection and diagnosis of GDM is [94]

- *First prenatal visit*: Screen for type 2 diabetes in the woman with risk factors.
- *Week 24–28 weeks gestation*: Screen for GDM in women not known to have diabetes.

The diagnosis and treatment of GDM is important, because such women are at increased risk for maternal and fetal complications including preeclampsia, fetal macrosomia (large-for-gestational age), and neonatal hypoglycemia [93]. For the woman with diabetes prior to pregnancy, optimal glycemic control is also important because of the increased risk for fetal malformations [95–97].

So what is the one modifiable risk factor for GDM? Obesity, of course!

Once a woman has been diagnosed with GDM, because of the need for glycemic control, diet compliance is critical. As stated by Cheung, "It is generally accepted that dietary therapy is the cornerstone of treatment of GDM" [97]. While control for the amount and distribution of carbohydrate throughout the day is an important component of medical nutrition therapy [96], it is recognized by the 2014 Standards of Medical Care by the American Diabetes Association that "macronutrient distribution should be based on individualized assessment of current eating patterns, preferences and metabolic goals" [94]. Individualization of diet therapy is key to helping a woman cope with the diagnosis of GDM and can vary from one or two simple dietary adjustments to addressing carbohydrate counting.

OSTEOPOROSIS

Based upon 2005–2006 National Health and Nutrition Examination Survey (NHANES) data, at last 80% of those with osteoporosis are women [98]. For females, what is key is that peak bone mass be achieved, usually by age 20, to assure optimal bone mass throughout adult life [99]. Decline in bone mass in the aging population increases the risk for osteoporosis. This decline in women usually begins at the time of menopause and once was a reason for treating women with hormone replacement therapy (estrogen with/without progesterone).

Adequate dietary intake of several micronutrients is critical, especially for calcium and vitamin D. To maintain optimal bone mass in the postmenopausal population, the RDA for calcium in the 51–70-year-old female population is 1200 mg/day. For men of the same age range, the RDA is 1000 mg/day (increasing to 1200 mg/day after age 70) [46]. This is the *only* life stage group for which there is a difference between females and males for the RDA for calcium.

Of concern is that females more than males do not consistently meet the RDA for calcium [100]. This may be a reason why females rely so heavily on calcium supplements. In fact, many of the calcium supplements have been targeted toward the female population. For a woman who is counting her calories, it may be a lot more desirable to slowly enjoy the yummy taste of a 20–30 kcal chocolate-flavored candy-like calcium supplement with added vitamin D and K than to get the equivalent amount of calcium from milk or yogurt.

However, the safety of calcium supplements versus dietary calcium has been questioned with the results of a data review from the Women's Health Initiative (WHI). That landmark paper by Bolland et al. increased attention on the relationship between calcium supplementation and risk of cardiovascular events, questioning the use of calcium supplementation in addressing osteoporosis [101]. While prior to that 2011 paper, there had been papers published regarding the same concerns, it was that paper that put the spotlight on calcium supplementation and cardiovascular risk. Since then, the number of publications seems without end in addressing this issue and has even expanded to looking at CVD risk and calcium supplementation in males. In addressing CVD risk associated with calcium supplementation, it may be that the total amount of calcium consumed exceeded the 2000 mg/day upper limit (UL) for calcium intake as established by the IOM [46]. This is a realistic concern when you think about how easily the UL can be exceeded with just a few candy-like calcium supplements.

In one review article, Dr. Robert Heaney and his coauthors expressed the opinion that the research at the time of that publication did not support a change in the IOM's recommendation that encourages the use of calcium supplementation to promote optimal bone health in those who are unable to achieve the RDA for calcium intake by diet [102].

EPIDEMIOLOGICAL STUDIES

One of the criticisms of medicine is that most of the studies to identify risk factors, as well as to diagnose and treat most medical problems, has been concentrated in the male population. However, women have not been totally left out of the picture. More than 65 years ago when the well-known Framingham Heart Study to identify the risks associated with CVD began, the initial recruits included women [103]. Those original recruits are still being followed and in 2002, a third generation was recruited, the grandchildren of that original cohort. However, women are not without that own epidemiological studies. Two of the most well-known examples are discussed here.

NURSES' HEALTH STUDY

Initially established in 1976, this study enrolled 121,700 female nurses. (*Note*: the Physicians' Health Study, an all male cohort, was not established until 1980.) The Nurses' Health Study II was established in 1989 with an enrollment of 116,000 female nurses. A third cohort of 100,000 females is now being recruited. Over the years, this immense study has provided much knowledge, in particular, about cancer and CVD in the female population. Some of the highlights of the nutrition issues are [104]

Obesity
- Increased breast cancer risk in postmenopausal women. Weight loss after menopause is associated with a reduced breast cancer risk.
- Increased colon cancer risk.
- Strong positive relationship between weight (BMI) and risk of CVD.
- Protection against hip fracture related to "extra padding" around the hips.

Alcohol
- One or more daily drinks increases breast cancer risk.
- Moderate alcohol intake reduces the risk of coronary heart disease.

Diet
- Fish intake reduces stoke risk.
- Nut and whole grains reduces CVD risk.
- Higher intake of folate, vitamin B6, calcium, and vitamin D reduces colon cancer risk. High intake of red and processed meats increases colon cancer risk.
- Calcium supplementation in those with low dietary calcium intake reduces risk for hip fracture.

WOMEN'S HEALTH INITIATIVE

A 15-year study enrolled 161,808 postmenopausal women to study heart disease, breast and colorectal cancer, and osteoporotic fractures. There were three parts to the study: a randomized clinical trial (CT), an observational study (OS), and a community prevention study (CPS) [105].

There were three components to the clinical trial: Hormone Therapy Trial (HT), Dietary Modification Trial (DM), and the Calcium/Vitamin D Trial (CaD).

The OS looked at the relationship between lifestyle, health, and risk factors with specific disease outcomes.

Some of the nutrition-related results published to date are as follows:

Ovarian cancer *risk* was reduced by 40% in those who decreased the amount of dietary fat consumed by at least 4 years. A statistically significant difference was neither noted for breast and colorectal cancer nor heart disease risk [106].

A low fat diet does not necessarily lead to weight gain [107].

Results from the CaD trial are not included here, because there is controversy about its design. That is, women who had previously been taking calcium supplements with/without vitamin D were permitted to continue to do so prior to randomization. Therefore, a woman in the control group could theoretically have as high or possibly higher intake of calcium and vitamin D compared to a woman enrolled in the intervention group.

CASE STUDY

JB is a 23-year-old female with a BMI of 35. She already has two children and is thinking abouvt getting pregnant again. However, she is very concerned about the FDA fish advisory for pregnant and lactating women. She has a family history of heart disease and is very conscientious about getting adequate fish intake because of recommendations made by the AHA. The problem is that the only fish she eats is white meat albacore tuna. Her concern is that if she cuts back on her tuna intake while pregnant she may be increasing her risk for heart disease during that time frame. You advise her to

1. Try light meat tuna
2. Not to worry and recommend fish oil supplements while she is pregnant
3. Attempt a slow weight loss of about two pounds per week
4. Other _____

INTERESTING OBSERVATIONS

Should the Physicians' Health Study be renamed to indicate an all male cohort? The reason this is being questioned is because as of 2012 data, 30.2% of physicians with an active license to practice medicine in the United States were women [108].

During the final editing of this chapter, the author came across an article by the distinguished Martijn Katan and colleagues, reflecting on the greatest nutrition discoveries and challenges from 1976 to 2006 identified by attendees at a symposium in Wageningen, the Netherlands. There were 15 nutrition discoveries identified, 2 in the top 10 were female focused: number 1 was folic acid, which prevents birth defects, and number 8 was alcohol, which causes breast cancer [109].

REFERENCES

1. American Heart Association. Heart disease statistics at a glance–Go red for women. Available at: https://www.goredforwomen.org/about-heart-disease/facts_about_heart_disease_in_women-sub-category/statistics-at-a-glance/. Accessed September 14, 2014.
2. National Institutes of Health. History and mission—Office of Research on Women's Health (ORWH). Available at: http://orwh.od.nih.gov/about/mission.asp. Accessed August 11, 2014.
3. U.S. Department of Health and Human Services. Office on women's health. Vision, mission, history. Available at: http://www.womenshealth.gov/about-us/mission-history-goals/index.html#history. Accessed August 11, 2014.
4. U.S. Food and Drug Administration. FDA for women. Available at: http://www.fda.gov/ForConsumers/ByAudience/ForWomen/default.htm. Accessed August 11, 2014.

5. Hammond KA, Demarest LM. Clinical: Inflammation, physical, and functional assessments. In *Krause's Food and the Nutrition Care Process*, 13th edn., LK Mahan, S Escott-Stump, and JL Raymond (Eds.). Saunders, St. Louis, MO, 2012.

6. NIH. *The Practical Guide, Identification, Evaluation, and Treatment of Overweight and Obesity in Adults*. National Institutes of Health. NIH Publication No. 02-4084, Bethesda, MD, Originally printed 2000, Reprinted January 2002.

7. American College of Cardiology/American Heart Association Task Force on Practice Guidelines, Obesity Expert Panel, 2013. Executive Summary: Guidelines (2013) for the management of overweight and obesity in adults: A report of the American College of Cardiology/American Heart Association Task Force on Practice Guidelines and the Obesity Society published by the Obesity Society and American College of Cardiology/American Heart Association Task Force on Practice Guidelines. Based on a systematic review from The Obesity Expert Panel, 2013. *Obesity*. 2014; 22(Suppl. 2):S5–S39.

8. Rothman KJ. BMI-related errors in the measurement of obesity. *Int J Obes*. 2008;32:S56–S59.

9. Ogden CL, Carroll MD, Kit BK, Flegal KM. Prevalence of obesity among adults. United States, 2011–2012. NCHS Data Brief, No. 131, National Center for Health Statistics, Hyattsville, MD, 2013.

10. Sturm R, Hatton A. Morbid obesity rates continue to rise rapidly in the United States. *Int J Obes*. 2013;37:889–891.

11. Greenberg DR, LaPorte DJ. Racial differences in body type preferences of men for women. *Int J Eat Disord*. 1996;19:275–278.

12. Striegel-Moore RH, Wilfley DE, Caldwell MB, Needham ML, Brownell KD. Weight-related attitudes and behaviors of women who diet to lose weight: A comparison of black dieters and white dieters. *Obes Res*. 1996;4:109–116.

13. Shoneye C, Johnson F, Steptoe A, Wardle J. A qualitative analysis of black and white British women's attitudes to weight and weight control. *J Hum Nutr Diet*. 2011;24:536–542.

14. Powell AD, Kahn AS. Racial differences in women's desires to be thin. *Int J Eat Disord*. 1995;17:191–195.

15. Ouldzeidoune N, Keating J, Bertrand J, Rice J. A description of female genital mutilation and force-feeding practices in Mauritania: Implications for the protection of child rights and health. *PLoS One*. April 9, 2013;8:e60594.

16. McCarthy MM. The thin ideal, depression and eating disorders in women. *Behav Res Ther*. 1990;28:205–215.

17. Farley D. Eating disorders. When thinness becomes an obsession. In *Current Issues in Women's Health*, 2nd edn. An FDA Consumer Special Report, Food and Drug Administration, Rockville, MD, 1994.

18. A quote attributed to the late Wallis Simpson, Duchess of Windsor. Available at: http://en.wikipedia.org/wiki/Wallis_Simpson. Accessed August 11, 2014.

19. Puhl RM, Andreyeva T, Brownell, KD. Perceptions of weight discrimination: Prevalence and comparison to race and gender discrimination in America. *Int J Obes*. 2008;32:992–1001.

20. Lloyd KB, Hornsby LB. Complementary and alternative medications for women's health issues. *Nutr Clin Pract*. 2009;24:589–608.

21. Dan AJ. The law and women's bodies: The case of menstruation leave in Japan. *Health Care Women Int*. 1986;7:1–14.

22. Stoltzfus RJ. Iron deficiency: Global prevalence and consequences. *Food Nutr Bull*. 2003;24(Suppl. 4):S99–S103.

23. Centers for Disease Control and Prevention. Recommendations to prevent and control iron deficiency in the United States. *MMWR*. 1998;47(No. RR-3):1–36.

24. Food and Nutrition Board, Institute of Medicine. *Dietary Reference Intakes for Vitamin A, Vitamin K, Arsenic, Boron, Chromium, Copper, Iodine, Iron, Manganese, Molybdenum, Nickel, Silicon, Vanadium, and Zinc.* National Academies Press, Washington, DC, 2001.

25. Chocano-Bedoya PO, Manson JE, Hankinson SE et al. Intake of selected minerals and risk of premenstrual syndrome. *Am J Epidemiol.* 2013;177:1118–1127.

26. Verma RK, Chellappan DK, Pandy AK. Review on treatment of premenstrual syndrome: From conventional to alternative approach. *J Basic Clin Physiol Pharmacol.* 2014;25(4):319–327.

27. National Center for Complementary and Alternative Medicine. National Institutes of Health. Herbs at a glance. Chasteberry. Available at: http://nccam.nih.gov/sites/nccam.nih.gov/files/Herbs_At_A_Glance_Chasteberry_06-13-2012_0.pdf. Accessed August 11, 2014.

28. National Center for Complementary and Alternative Medicine. National Institutes of Health. Herbs at a glance. Evening primrose oil. Available at: http://nccam.nih.gov/sites/nccam.nih.gov/files/Herbs_At_A_Glance_Evening_Primrose_Oil_06-14-2012_0.pdf. Accessed August 11, 2014.

29. Farshchi H, Rane A, Love, Kennedy RL. Diet and nutrition in polycystic ovary syndrome (PCOS): Pointers for nutritional management. *J Obstet Gynaecol.* 2007;27:762–773.

30. Legro RS, Aarslanian SA, Ehrmann DA et al. Diagnosis and treatment of polycystic ovary syndrome: An endocrine society clinical practice guideline. *J Clin Endocrinol Metab.* 2013;8:4565–4592.

31. Centers for Disease Control and Prevention. Reproductive Health. Unintended pregnancy prevention. Available at: http://www.cdc.gov/reproductivehealth/UnintendedPregnancy/index.htm. Accessed August 11, 2014.

32. Rothman KJ, Moore LL, Singer MR, Nguyen US, Mannino S, Milunsky A. Teratogenicity of high vitamn A intake. *N Engl J Med.* 1995;333:1369–1373.

33. European Food Safety Authority. Folic acid: An update on scientific developments. 2010. Available at: http://www.efsa.europa.eu/en/home/publication/efsafolicacid.pdf. Accessed August 11, 2014.

34. Correa A, Marcinkevage J. Prepregnancy obesity and the risk of birth defects: An update. *Nutr Rev.* 2013;71(Suppl. 1):S68–S77.

35. Frias AE, Grove KL. Obesity: A transgenerational problem linked to nutrition during pregnancy. *Semina Reprod Med.* 2012;30:472–478.

36. Kett MM, Denton KM. Maternal obesity. Bad for baby's future. *Hypertension.* 2013;62:457–458.

37. Lee CYW, Koren G. Maternal obesity: Effects on pregnancy and the role of preconception counselling. *J Obstet Gynaecol.* 2013;30:101–106.

38. Public Affairs Committee of the Teratology Society. Teratology public affairs committee position paper: Maternal obesity and pregnancy. *Birth Defects Res (Part A).* 2006;76:73–77.

39. Aune D, Saugstad OD, Henriksen T, Tonstad S. Maternal body mass index and the risk of fetal death, stillbirth, and infant death. *JAMA.* 2014;311:1536–1546.

40. Cetin II, Mando C, Calabrese S. Maternal predictors of intrauterine growth restriction. *Curr Opin Clin Nutr Metab Care.* 2013;16:310–319.

41. Poston L. Maternal obesity, gestational weight gain and diet as determinants of offspring long term health. *Best Pract Res Clin Endocrinol Metab.* 2012;26:627–639.

42. Kathleen M. Rasmussen and Ann L. Yaktine (eds.), *Weight Gain during Pregnancy: Reexamining the Guidelines*, Committee to Reexamine IOM Pregnancy Weight Guidelines, Food and Nutrition Board and Board on Children, Youth, and Families. National Academies Press, Washington, DC, 2009.

43. Food and Nutrition Board, Institute of Medicine. *Dietary Reference Intakes for Energy, Carbohydrate, Fiber, Fat, Fatty Acids, Cholesterol, Protein, and Amino Acids (Macronutrients)*. National Academies Press, Washington, DC, 2005.

44. Goodnight W, Newman R. Optimal nutrition for improved twin pregnancy outcome. *Obstet Gynecol.* 2009;114:1121–1134.

45. Luke B. Nutrition and multiple gestation. *Semin Perinatol.* 2005;29:349–354.

46. Food and Nutrition Board, Institute of Medicine. *Dietary Reference Intakes for Calcium and Vitamin D.* National Academies Press, Washington, DC, 2010.

47. Food and Nutrition Board, Institute of Medicine. *Dietary Reference Intakes for Thiamin, Riboflavin, Niacin, Vitamin B_6, Folate, Vitamin B_{12}, Pantothenic Acid, Biotin, and Choline.* National Academies Press, Washington, DC, 1998.

48. U.S. Food and Drug Administration. Food safety for moms-to-be. Available at: http://www.fda.gov/Food/ResourcesForYou/HealthEducators/ucm083308.html. Accessed August 20, 2014.

49. U.S. Food and Drug Administration. Fish: What pregnant women and parents should know. Draft update advice by FDA and EPA. June, 2014. Available at: http://www.fda.gov/downloads/Food/FoodborneIllnessContaminants/Metals/UCM400358.pdf. Accessed August 20, 2014.

50. Müller-Lissner SA, Kaatz V, Brandt W, Keller J, Layer P. The perceived effect of various foods and beverages on stool consistency. *Eur J Gastroenterol Hepatol.* 2005;17(1):109–112.

51. Niebyl JR. Nausea and vomiting in pregnancy. *N Engl J Med.* 2010;363:1544–1550.

52. Niebyl JR, Briggs GG. The pharmacologic management of nausea and vomiting of pregnancy. *J Fam Pract.* 2014;63(Suppl. 2):S31–S37.

53. National Center for Complementary and Alternative Medicine. National Institutes of Health. Herbs at a glance. Ginger. Available at: http://nccam.nih.gov/sites/nccam.nih.gov/files/Herbs_At_A_Glance_Ginger_06-15-2012_0.pdf. Accessed August 20, 2014.

54. Halldorsson TI, Storm M, Olsen SF. Intake of artificially sweetened soft drinks and risk of preterm delivery: A prospective cohort study in 59, 334 Danish pregnant women. *Am J Clin Nutr.* 2010;92:626–633.

55. Bursey RG, Watson ML. Intake of artificially sweetened soft drinks and risk of preterm delivery. *Am J Clin Nutr.* 2010;92:1277–1278.

56. La Vecchia C. Intake of artificially sweetened soft drinks and risk of preterm delivery. *Am J Clin Nutr.* 2010;92:1540.

57. Englund-Ögge L, Brantsœter AL, Haugen M et al. Association between intake of artificially sweetened and sugar-sweetened beverages and preterm delivery: A large prospective cohort study. *Am J Clin Nutr.* 2012;96:552–559.

58. Olsen SF, Østerdal ML, Salvig JD, Weber T, Tabor A, Secher NJ. Duration of pregnancy in relation to fish oil supplementation and habitual fish intake: A randomized clinical trial with fish oil. *Eur J Nutr.* 2007;61:976–985.

59. Carlson SE, Colombo J, Gajewski BJ et al. DHA supplementation and pregnancy outcomes. *Am J Clin Nutr.* 2013;97:808–815.

60. Waterman EH, Pruett D, Caughey AB. Reducing fetal alcohol exposure in the United States. *Obstet Gynecol Surv.* 2013;68:367–378.

61. McCarthy FP, O'Keefe LM, Khashan AS et al. Association between maternal alcohol consumption in early pregnancy and pregnancy outcomes. *Obstet Gynecol.* 2013;122:830–837.

62. The New York City Department of Health and Mental Hygiene. Encouraging and supporting breastfeeding. April 2009. Available at: http://www.nyc.gov/html/doh/downloads/pdf/chi/chi28-suppl1.pdf. Accessed August 11, 2014.

63. Brent N. The risks and benefits of human donor breast milk. *Pediatr Ann.* 2013;42:84–89.

64. US Department of Health and Human Services. *Executive Summary: The Surgeon General's Call to Action to Support Breastfeeding.* US Department of Health and Human Services, Office of the Surgeon General, Washington, DC, January 20, 2011.

65. Committee on Pediatric AIDS. American Academy of Pediatrics. Policy Statement: Infant feeding and transmission of human immunodeficiency virus in the United States. *Pediatrics.* 2013;11:391–396.

66. Sámano R, Martinez-Rojano H, Godinez Martinez E et al. Effects of breast feeding on weight loss and recovery of pregestational weight in adolescent and adult mothers. *Food Nutr Bull.* 2013;34:123–130.

67. Much D, Beyerlein A, Roßbauer M, Hummel S, Ziegler AG. Beneficial effects of breast-feeding in women with gestational diabetes mellitus. *Mol Metab.* 2014;3:284–292.

68. National Center for Complementary and Alternative Medicine. National Institutes of Health. Get the facts. Menopausal symptoms and complimentary health practices. Available at: http://nccam.nih.gov/health/menopause. Accessed August 11, 2014.

69. Hajirahimkhan A, Dietz BM, Bolton JL. Botanical modulation of menopausal symptoms: Mechanisms of action. *Planta Med.* 2013;79:S38–S53.

70. Rao SR, Singh M, Parkar M, Sugarmaran R. Health maintenance for postmenopausal women. *Am Fam Phys.* 2008;78:583–591.

71. Johnson RK, Appel LJ, Brands M et al; on behalf of American Heart Association Nutrition Committee of the Council on Nutrition, Physical Activity, and Metabolism and the Council on Epidemiology and Prevention. Dietary sugars intake and cardiovascular health: A scientific statement from the American Heart Association. *Circulation.* 2009;120:1011–1020.

72. Mosca L, Benjamin EJ, Berra K et al. Effectiveness-based guidelines for the prevention of disease in women—2011 Update. A guideline from the American Heart Association. *Circulation.* 2011;123:1243–1262.

73. Bushnell C, McCullough LD, Awad IA et al.; on behalf of the American Heart Association Stroke Council, Council on Cardiovascular and Stroke Nursing, Council on Clinical Cardiology, Council on Epidemiology and Prevention, and Council for High Blood Pressure Research. Guidelines for the prevention of stroke in women. A statement for healthcare professionals from the American Heart Association/American Stroke Association. Epub February 6, 2014. Available at: http://stroke.ahajournals.org/content/early/2014/02/06/01.str.0000442009.06663.48.full.pdf+html. Accessed August 20, 2014.

74. Horner NK, Lampe JW. Potential mechanisms of diet therapy for fibriocyctic breast conditions show inadequate evidence of effectiveness. *J Am Diet Assoc.* 2000;100:1368–1380.

75. Leinson W, Dunn PM. Nonassociation of caffeine and fibrocystic breast disease. *Arch Intern Med.* 1986;146:1773–1775.

76. American Cancer Society. *Cancer Facts & Figures 2013.* American Cancer Society, Atlanta, GA, 2013.

77. International Agency for Research on Cancer. World Health Organization. Globocan 2012: Estimated cancer incidence, mortality and prevalence worldwide in 2012. Available at: http://globocan.iarc.fr/Pages/fact_sheets_cancer.aspx. Accessed September 14, 2014.

78. American Cancer Society. *Breast Cancer Facts & Figures 2013–2014.* American Cancer Society, Inc., Atlanta, GA, 2013.

79. Chen WY, Rosner B, Hankinson SE, Colditz GA, Willett WC. Moderate alcohol consumption during adult life, drinking patterns, and breast cancer risk. *JAMA.* 2011;306:1884–1890.

80. Messina M, Wu AH. Perspectives on the soy-breast cancer relation. *Am J Clin Nutr.* 2009;89(Suppl.):1673S–1679S.

81. Hilakivi-Clarke L, Andrade JE, Helferich W. Is soy consumption good or bad for the breast. *J Nutr.* 2010;140:2326S–2334S.

82. Magee PJ, Rowland I. Soy products in the management of breast cancer. *Curr Opin Clin Nutr Metab Care.* 2012;15:586–591.

83. Kang X, Zhang Q, Wang S, Huang X, Jin S. Effect of soy isoflavones on breast cancer recurrence and death for patients receiving adjuvant endocrine therapy. *CMAJ.* 2010;182(17):1857–1862.

84. Leitzmann MF, Koebnick C, Danforth KN et al. Body mass index and risk of ovarian cancer. *Cancer.* 2009;115:812–822.

85. Ward KK, Roncancio AM, Shah NR et al. The risk of uterine malignancy is linearly associated with body mass index in a cohort of US women. *Am J Obstet Gynecol.* 2013;209:579.e1–579.e5.

86. Faber MT, Jensen A, Sogaard M et al. Use of dairy products, lactose, and calcium and risk of ovarian cancer—Results from a Danish case-control study. *Acta Oncol.* 2012;51:454–464.

87. Merritt MA, Cramer DW, Vitonis AF, Titus LJ, Terry KL. Dairy foods in relation to risk of ovarian cancer and major histological subtypes. *Int J Cancer.* 2013;132:1114–1124.

88. Crane TE, Khulpateea BR, Alberts DS, Basen-Enqquist K, Thomson CA. Dietary intake and ovarian cancer risk: A systematic review. *Cancer Epidemiol Biomarkers Prev.* 2014;23:255–273.

89. Hernandez BY, McDuffie K, Wilkens LR, Kamemoto L, Goodman MT. Diet and premalignant lesions of the cervix: Evidence of a protective role for folate, riboflavin, thiamin, and vitamin B_{12}. *Cancer Causes Control.* 2003;14:859–870.

90. Hwang JH, Kim MK, Lee JK. Dietary supplements reduce the risk of cervical intraepithelial neoplasia. *Int J Gynecol Cancer.* 2010;20:398–403.

91. Chih HJ, Lee AH, Colville L, Binns CW, Xu D. A review of dietary prevention of human papillomavirus-related infection of the cervix and cervical intraepithelial neoplasia. *Nutr Cancer.* 2013;65:317–328.

92. Centers for Disease Control and Prevention. National diabetes statistics report, 2014. Available at: http://www.cdc.gov/diabetes/pubs/statsreport14/national-diabetes-report-web.pdfhttp://www.cdc.gov/diabetes/pubs/statsreport14/national-diabetes-report-web.pdf. Accessed August 20, 2014.

93. Gilmartin AB, Ural SH, Repke JT. Gestational diabetes mellitus. *Rev Obstet Gynecol.* 2008;1:129–134.

94. American Diabetes Association. Executive summary: Standards of medical care 2014. *Diabetes Care.* 2014;37(Suppl. 1):S5–S13.

95. Wender-Ozegowska E, Wróblewska K, Zawiejska A, Pietryga M, Szczapa J, Biczysko R. Threshold values of maternal blood glucose in early diabetic pregnancy–prediction of fetal malformations. *Acta Obstet Gynecol Scand.* 2005;84:17–25.

96. Blumer I, Hadar E, Hadden DR et al. Diabetes and pregnancy: An Endocrine Society Clinical Practice Guideline. *J Clin Endocrinol Metab.* 2013;98:4227–4249.

97. Cheung NW. The management of gestational diabetes. *Vasc Health Risk Manage.* 2009;5:153–164.

98. Centers for Disease Control and Prevention. FastStats. Osteoporosis. Available at: http://www.cdc.gov/nchs/fastats/osteoporosis.htm. Accessed August 11, 2014.

99. Centers for Disease Control and Prevention. Nutrition for everyone. Calcium and bone health. Available at: http://www.cdc.gov/nutrition/everyone/basics/vitamins/calcium.html. Accessed August 20, 2014.

100. National Institutes of Health. Calcium. Dietary supplement fact sheet. Available at: http://ods.od.nih.gov/factsheets/Calcium-HealthProfessional/. Accessed August 20, 2014.

101. Bolland MJ, Grey A, Avenell A, Gamble GD, Reid IR. Calcium supplements with or without vitamin D and risk of cardiovascular events: Reanalysis of the Women's Health Initiative limited access dataset and meta-analysis. *BMJ.* 2011;342:d2040.

102. Heaney RP, Kopecky KC, Hatcock J, MacKay D, Wallace TC. A review of calcium supplements and cardiovascular disease risk. *Adv Nutr.* 2012;3:763–771.

103. Framingham Heart Study. History of the Framingham Heart Study. Available at: http://www.framinghamheartstudy.org/about-fhs/history.php. Accessed August 11, 2014.

104. The Nurses' Health Study. Findings: Some highlights. Available at: http://www.channing.harvard.edu/nhs/?page_id=197. Accessed August 11, 2014.

105. National Institutes of Health. Women's health initiative. WWHI background. Available at: https://www.nhlbi.nih.gov/whi/backgroundapaperbyKatanandcolleagues.htm. Accessed August 20, 2014.

106. Prentice RL, Thomson CA, Caan B et al. Low-fat dietary pattern and cancer incidence in the women's Health Initiative dietary modification randomized controlled trial. *J Natl Cancer Inst.* 2007;99:1534–1543.

107. Howard BV, Manson JE, Stefanick ML et al. Low-fat dietary pattern and weight change over 7 years. The Women's Health Initiative dietary modification trial. *JAMA.* 2006;295(1):39–49.

108. Young A, Chaudhry HJ, Thomas JV, Dugan M. A consensus of actively licensed physicians in the United States, 2012. *J Med Regul.* 2013;99:11–24.

109. Katan MB, Borkschoten MV, Connor WE et al. Which are the greatest discoveries and the future challenges in nutrition? *Eur J Clin Nutr.* 2009;63:2–10.

8 Integrative Nutritional Therapy for Cardiovascular Disease

Mimi Guarneri, MD, FACC
and Ryan Bradley, ND, MPH

CONTENTS

INTRODUCTION

Nutrition: Most of us get to decide what we eat each day—a luxury compared to our humble beginnings gathering local green leafy vegetables, harvesting seeds one at a time, and trying to eat meat that ran away. We were once subject to the forces of weather and geography, of natural supply and demand. The foods available in our environment provided the necessary nutrition to reach reproductive age, and the risks of infection and trauma allowed few to live far beyond early adulthood. Malnutrition was more common than diseases of abundance and obesity. Few people had the access to the opulence that allowed for type 2 diabetes and ischemic heart disease.

In contrast, now many suffer from diet and nutrition-related chronic diseases, that is, cardiovascular disease (CVD) and type 2 diabetes. The "standard American diet" (SAD)—a dietary pattern rich in refined carbohydrates, animal-based protein and fats, heavily cooked foods, and few fresh fruits and vegetables—is considered a contributor [1–4]. Yet, we are also blessed with access to the Mediterranean diet deep in the Midwest of the United States, where the fountain of everlasting youth is captured in 1.5 gal jugs of extra virgin olive oil available in neighborhood "big box" stores! Organic vegetables have made it prime time, and wild salmon can be shipped anywhere in the world within 24 h of reaching an Alaskan port! With abundant access to many healthful foods, and the many knowledge advances that have resulted from nutritional science, why have we not prevented CVD?

We are confused. Advertisements tempt us with vivid images of bacon sizzling in a pan, tickling our limbic cravings for fat and salt. We are mortally cursed with infinite access to foods we are programmed to desire, and yet intuitively know will harm us. Making the confusion worse, some authors and experts claim that fried, highly glycated, peroxidized, chemically processed, hormone- and antibiotic-laden pork is better for us than whole grains, while others claim grain is the only noble path to nirvana. Despite our individual and mutual efforts within cardiology, nutrition, and integrative medicine to increase public awareness of healthy dietary patterns, we are also confused, and confuse each other by looking through varying lenses of "nutrition" and making overarching statements about the "right" diet.

Nutritional epidemiology also has limitations [5–8]. Although excess "fat," "carbohydrates," and "cholesterol" are commonly implicated macronutrients for heart disease, this overly general system lacks precision in the classification of nutritional "exposures." For example, types of fat, for example, short-chain saturated fats versus long-chain saturated fats, and carbohydrates, for example, high- versus low-glycemic index, are not always differentiated, and differences in cooking methods, which can impact the inflammatory response of foods [9], are rarely considered even for common exposures, for example, boiled eggs versus fried eggs [10–13]. Adding additional challenges to the interpretation of nutritional epidemiological studies, the commonly used tools for assessing nutritional exposures, including nutritional biomarkers, are fraught with limitations [6–8]. Few cohort studies measure nutritional variables using "gold-standard" measurement methods, and relay on self-reported frequency of intake of certain foods. Despite the "validation" of food frequency questionnaires and other measurement tools, people commonly over-report intake of healthful foods and underreport intake of foods thought to be "bad." Various statistical methods, for example, principal component analysis and reduced rank regression, are used to manufacture dietary patterns statistically, but still do not reflect the totality of what people actually eat. Furthermore, it is shockingly difficult to determine what foods are actually "good for us" versus foods that just are not "bad for us," that is, foods/nutrients actually preserve or extend function versus those that substitute for the "bad" stuff but have a neutral direct effect on outcome. The unfortunate bottom line is that despite a few decades of nutritional science and the advent of more sophisticated thinkers and techniques to study "nutrition," we still have very limited knowledge.

Adding further complexity to "nutritional therapies" for CVD is the important differentiation between "food," "nutrients" (or bioactives), and "nutritional supplements." Grapes may be an important source of polyphenolic "antioxidants," for example, resveratrol, but bench research findings on the mechanisms of resveratrol in cell culture (or animal models) do not necessarily apply to grapes, should not be immediately extrapolated as in vivo effects in humans. Similar mismatch occurs between nutritional epidemiology and experimental nutritional cardiology. For example, observational research demonstrating increased serum concentrations of carotenoids and slower progression of atherosclerosis [14] did not translate into the prevention of atherosclerosis from the use of β-carotene supplements [15]. Thus, it is important not to translate observational evidence into clinical practice prematurely.

The limitations in our knowledge lead to patient frustration, many of whom have multiple overlapping chronic diseases for which different dietary patterns may be technically indicated. Imagine the person with heart disease, diabetes, *and* chronic kidney disease trying to follow a low-fat, low-carb, low-protein diet! Water and air may provide a healthful short-term cleanse, but obviously do not provide a sustainable dietary pattern!

The good news is we do have a considerable base of observational and experimental data that allows the sophisticated clinician to evaluate patients' diet and provide them with healthful recommendations that can modify their risk for heart disease across the entire continuum of risk, from primordial prevention through tertiary prevention. Of course in many cases, no matter how precise our dietary prescription may be based on nutritional status and current risk, patients' adherence to our plan adds an additional challenge! Thus, applying nutritional strategies for CVD effectively requires both the knowledge and the development of a mutual trusting therapeutic relationship.

The intention behind this chapter is to summarize some of the knowledge we have collected regarding diet and nutritional approaches to reduce risk for CVD, focusing mostly on the human experimental evidence.

DIET PATTERNS AND PLANS

Maintaining excellent cardiovascular health through diet requires adopting a dietary pattern that is balanced with protein, fats, and carbohydrates, as well as plant-based nutrients, polyphenolic compounds, fiber, and other nutrients. The exact macro/micronutrient composition may vary according to specific clinical goals, but the core features of most heart health-promoting dietary patterns are as follows [16–21]:

- They are plant-based, including a foundation of vegetables and fruits, supplemented with whole grains and legumes.
- They include animal protein in small portions, and typically lean sources like seafood and poultry; they are high in viscous fibers.
- They are less dependent on salt as a seasoning and often include other herbs and spices.
- They are typically low in fat and may emphasize intake of mono- and poly-unsaturated fats (MUFAs and PUFAs, respectively) from olive oil, nuts, seeds, and fish.

Some specific examples of dietary patterns with established cardiovascular benefits include the Dietary Approach to Stop Hypertension (DASH) diet, the Portfolio diet, the Ornish diet, and the Mediterranean diet. The dietary patterns covered in this section are also summarized as Table 8.1.

"Low-Fat" Diets

Although following a "low-fat" diet is a familiar recommendation for improving lipid profiles and cardiovascular health, this generic recommendation does not have robust evidence for affecting cardiovascular outcomes. For example, the Women's Health Initiative implemented a low-fat diet in women at risk for cardiovascular events targeting fat intake less than 20% of total calories per day [22]. Participants were encouraged to eat five servings of fruits and vegetables per day and six servings of whole grains per day. The intervention group reduced intakes of saturated, MUFAs, and PUFAs by 2.9%, 3.3%, and 1.5%, respectively. After a mean period of 8.1 years, there was no significant reduction in cardiovascular events in the low fat intervention group, although there was a trend for reduced events in women who had the greatest reductions in saturated and *trans* fats, and higher intakes of vegetables. The results of the Women's Health Initiative demonstrate the lack of precision in the recommendation to follow a "low-fat diet" and can lead to patients removing all sources of fat from their diets, including MUFAs and PUFAs, which often involves the elimination or restriction of foods that contain healthful fats. Limiting dietary intake of saturated fat remains a good idea for most patients. Saturated fat is known to cause rapid changes in endothelial function, and increases

TABLE 8.1
Dietary Patterns for the Reduction of Cardiovascular Disease Risk

Dietary Pattern	Description	Effects/Outcomes[a]
DASH	• Plant-based • Whole grains emphasized • Lean meats • Total sodium 1.5–3 g	The combination of the DASH diet and a low level of sodium lowered systolic blood pressure by • 11.5 mmHg in participants with hypertension • 12.6 mmHg for blacks • 9.5 mmHg for others • 7.1 mmHg in participants without hypertension • 7.2 mmHg for blacks • 6.9 mmHg for others • 6.8 mmHg in men • 10.5 mmHg in women
Portfolio	• Starts with AHA step 2 diet • Almonds (22.5 g/1000 kcal) • Soy protein (22.5 g/1000 kcal) • Viscous fibers (10 g/1000 kcal) • Plant sterols (1.0 g/1000 kcal)	• 28.6% reduction in LDL • 28.2% reduction in CRP. Respective reductions in systolic and diastolic blood pressure at 1 year were: • −4.2 ± 1.3 mmHg • −2.3 ± 0.7 mmHg
Ornish	• Vegan diet <20% total fat	• 7.9% reduction in coronary artery stenosis diameter • 60% relative risk reduction for CVD event
Mediterranean	• Foundation of fruits/vegetables and whole grains • Lean meats • High MUFA and PUFA intake as olive oil, nut/seed oils, and seafood • High *Allium* intake • Low intake of red meats and sweets	• 30% relative risk reduction for major CVD events • 52% reduced incidence of type 2 diabetes and metabolic syndrome

[a] See main text for citations.

in circulating biomarkers of oxidative stress in the post-prandial period in persons with and without metabolic disease [23,24]. Current guidelines recommend saturated fat intake to not exceed 7% of total calories. Despite significant background research and mechanistic plausibility, some experts still argue the scientific evidence for replacing saturated fat for PUFA remains underwhelming [25].

However, it is important to consider the effects of replacing saturated fats with other sources of calories. Review studies demonstrate differential effects on risk factors from replacing saturated fat with other fats, compared to replacing fat with carbohydrates. Notably, replacing saturated fats with MUFAs and PUFAs tends to lower low-density lipoprotein (LDL) and improve the LDL to high-density lipoprotein

(HDL) ratio [26], whereas replacing saturated fat with carbohydrates tends to lower both LDL and HDL, without affecting their ratio, and tends to increase triglycerides, which can actually raise risk (especially in women) [27]. Studies evaluating palm oil (PO) as a substitute for *trans* fats reported that PO's effects were similar to *trans* fats, specifically a worsening LDL by 12%–16% compared to PUFA-dense soybean and canola oils, respectively, without affecting HDL [28].

Of course, no discussion of dietary fats is complete without villainizing *trans* fats, produced by the partial hydrogenation of MUFA- and PUFA-rich vegetable oils. Although debate continues regarding a potentially differential effect of *trans*-oleic acid versus *trans*-linoleic acid, the best general rule of thumb remains to avoid them both. *Trans* fats are known to reduce HDL, increase vascular inflammation including C-reactive protein (CRP), promote endothelial dysfunction, and increase the risk for cardiovascular events, including sudden death [29–32].

LOW-CARBOHYDRATE DIETS

Increasingly popular for weight loss, high-protein and low-carbohydrate diets have mixed evidence for health effects. Numerous short-term benefits have been measured for CVD risk factors, including improved blood pressure, reduced waist circumference, increased insulin sensitivity, reduced total cholesterol, LDL and triglycerides, and increasing HDL [33–35]. Low-carb diets can decrease triglycerides by 8%–21%, and may increase HDL up to 15%, compared to a calorically matched high-carbohydrate diet. Mechanistically, many of the observed benefits could result from weight loss and improved insulin sensitivity alone [36,37]. Low-carbohydrate diets have the added benefit of being easier to maintain, that is, adhere to, long-term compared to low-fat diets or the Mediterranean diet pattern [38].

However, despite these seemingly positive health effects, meta-analyses of low-carbohydrate dietary patterns suggest an *increase* in all-cause mortality in those groups following low-carbohydrate dietary patterns [39]. This increase does not appear to be due to increased cardiovascular incidence or mortality, and remains unexplained. One theoretical concern of a low carbohydrate diet is the relative increase in protein intake, which may lead to renal impairment. However, short-term studies evaluating renal function from clinical trials of a low-carb diet for low weight found no evidence of renal compromise [40].

It may be less important which foods are reduced, that is, carbohydrates, than which foods fill the void that is created! For example, as described earlier, replacing saturated fats with MUFAs and PUFAs from plant sources appears to offer cardiovascular benefits, while replacing them with carbohydrates may increase triglycerides and lower HDL, especially in patients with insulin resistance. Yet, replacing carbohydrates with animal sources of saturated fat may increase frank atherosclerosis, even if there may be apparent benefit in insulin sensitivity.

DASH DIET

The Dietary Approach to Stop Hypertension, commonly known as the DASH diet, is a comprehensive dietary approach developed with the specific goal of helping to reduce blood pressure. It emphasizes fruits and vegetables, whole grains, low-fat dairy and lean meats, and very little salt and saturated fat. Compared to a SAD, eating the DASH diet for 30 days was been shown to reduce blood pressure by up to 11 mmHg in 412 patients with hypertension [41], and also appears to have a side benefit of improving total cholesterol and LDL values [42]. Notably, the clinical trial support for the DASH diet demonstrated even the high sodium intake version of the diet (i.e., ~3 g/day) and still demonstrated blood pressure lowering effects relative to the SAD; however, the blood pressure benefits of the DASH diet did increase linearly with sodium reduction down to 1500 mg/day. These results suggest a potent, and generalizable, benefit of sodium lowering, in addition to the benefits of a lower-fat, plant-based diet.

PORTFOLIO DIET

The Portfolio diet was specifically designed to incorporate foods known to help lower LDL cholesterol. The diet follows the American Heart Association Step 2 diet low in saturated fat and higher in fiber and vegetables plus specific supplemental foods and food ingredients including almonds (22.5 g/1000 kcal), plant sterols (1.0 g/1000 kcal), soy protein (22.5 g/1000 kcal), and viscous fibers (10 g/1000 kcal, present in foods like psyllium, oat bran, okra, and eggplant). Following the Portfolio pattern for just three months resulted in a 28.6% reduction of LDL lipoproteins and a reduction in CRP of 28.2% [43]. Following 66 participants over 1 year under "real-world" conditions, the individuals that most closely adhered to the dietary recommendations were able to lower their cholesterol by up to 20%—a rate comparable to that achieved by the use of statin drugs [18]. Just as the DASH diet helped to lower cholesterol, the Portfolio diet also reduced blood pressure [17].

ORNISH LIFESTYLE HEART DIET

Several studies have demonstrated the possibility of reversing or halting the progression of heart disease through intensive nutritional intervention. The most famous of these studies was that performed by Dr. Dean Ornish. His Lifestyle Heart Trial found that individuals with heart disease who ate a very low 10% fat vegetarian diet including plentiful amounts of fruits, vegetables, soybean products, and legumes for at least 1 year significantly slowed progression of atherosclerotic plaque and suggested some improvement in luminal diameter in the coronary arteries [44]. It is important to note that this experimental group also had ongoing social support, performed aerobic exercise for 1 h/day, and practiced stress management practices (e.g., guided imagery, breathing exercises, meditation, and yoga) for at least 1 h/day. A control group did not follow this regimen followed the American Heart Association Step 2 diet, and had increased stenosis diameter after 1 year, compared to the reduced stenosis diameter in the intensive treatment group.

MEDITERRANEAN DIET

Ideally, a dietary pattern would protect against both CVD and metabolic disease, and although modified low-fat dietary patterns can be designed for reducing individual risk factors, that is, DASH for hypertension, Portfolio for LDL, etc., the ideal pattern would also emphasize the importance of substituting MUFAs and PUFAs for carbohydrates, emphasize fruits and vegetables, and include lean sources of protein from a wide variety of plant and animal sources. This idealistic image exists as the Mediterranean diet.

The Mediterranean diet, based on the traditional foods of people living around the Mediterranean Sea, has long been viewed as a dietary pattern worthy of emulation. This traditional diet is rich in legumes, vegetables, fruits, nuts, and fish with moderate mealtime red wine and minimal refined sugars, dairy, and red or processed meat, and most of the fat coming from olive oil.

Although earlier data have supported the cardiovascular benefits of the Mediterranean diet for many decades, including the Lyon Heart Study demonstrating improved survival following first myocardial infarction (MI) from the Mediterranean diet [45], the evidence for the Mediterranean diet was heavily buttressed in 2013 by the results of the PREDIMED trial [20]. PREDIMED was a multi-site clinical trial conducted in Spain that randomized 7447 people at risk for cardiovascular events to either a Mediterranean diet supplemented with walnuts, supplemented with extra-virgin olive oil, or a control diet with advice to lower dietary fat intake. After a median follow-up period of 4.8 years, those participants randomized to the Mediterranean diet arms had an approximate 30% reduction in first cardiovascular event. Several other large studies of the Mediterranean diet including a meta-analysis cumulatively evaluating follow-up of 1.5 million people from between 3 and 18 years [46] found that even modestly greater adherence (increasing 2 points on a 10-point scale) to a Mediterranean diet led to an overall 9% reduction in deaths from heart disease. Similar to the Lyon Heart Study but much smaller, Tuttle et al. examined about 200 people after their first heart attack, and found that individuals receiving counseling on either a low-fat or a Mediterranean diet had better long-term survival than individuals receiving usual post-hospitalization care [47].

The studies cited earlier are only a few of the many available that document the cardiovascular and other health benefits of the Mediterranean diet pattern including protection against the metabolic syndrome [48–50], obesity [51,52], endothelial dysfunction [53,54], and some cancers [55,56]. The mechanisms for these benefits are under scrutiny, but are known to include anti-inflammatory effects [57–59], protection of DNA from oxidative stress [60], and mediation of gene-nutrient interactions [57,61–63].

DIETARY PATTERN IN THE CONTEXT OF CLINICAL GOALS

Dietary patterns can be flexible and modified to reach clinical goals. A nutritional approach to CVD treatment would be different from a model targeting prevention. Both approaches would need to consider factors beyond macronutrient composition, including current risk, degree of vascular disease, metabolic status, current nutritional status, and short- and long-term therapeutic goals. For example, a very low-carbohydrate diet may be appropriate to achieve short-term weight loss and improvement in metabolic status, but long-term substitution of high saturated-fat animal products for carbohydrates will have inflammatory, lipid-, and potentially renal-related consequences in most patients. These effects may be direct effects due to directly imparting cumulative endothelial dysfunction [23] and/or indirect effects due to a negative impact on the gut microbiota [64]. Similarly, a patient in their 70s who strives to "reverse" their coronary artery disease without medications will require stricter guidelines for an anti-inflammatory diet than in patients in their 60s without coronary disease interested in continuing to delay or prevent disease.

Fortunately, dietary patterns known to be heart healthful, like the Mediterranean diet, are available to form an excellent structure from which macronutrient composition can be manipulated. For example, a low carbohydrate Mediterranean diet pattern can be created by replacing several servings of grain with increased intake of nuts, seeds, olive oil, low-fat yoghurt, additional vegetables, and other lean proteins. A low fat Mediterranean diet pattern can be created by replacing animal sources of protein with more legumes, whole grains, additional vegetables, and vegetable proteins. In both of these scenarios, the core benefits of the Mediterranean diet remain intact—largely plant-based, high-fiber, high vegetable, lean proteins, and an emphasis on MUFAs and PUFAs.

INDIVIDUAL FOODS AND BEVERAGES

Despite the preceding discussion about the virtues of various macronutrients, people eat and drink actual foods during the day, and few stop to think in detail about their composition of proteins, carbs, and fats. Fortunately, many heart healthy foods are the finest tasting foods in the world! Unfortunately, with the exception of alcohol, the research on many individual foods remains focused on risk factor reduction, and not hard clinical cardiovascular events or mortality, and therefore, remains somewhat limited.

ALCOHOL

Alcohol, specifically in the forms of beer and wine, may offer cardiovascular benefits when consumed in small to moderate amounts [65,66]. Mechanistically, alcohol intake appears to shift the overall lipid density, preferentially increasing numbers of medium and large LDL and HDL particles [67]. Moderate intake of alcohol increases HDL-C by 5%–15%, though to be due to increased HDL turnover *in vivo* [68]. However, continued intake can lead to hypertension and increased risk of hemorrhagic stroke [69]. The question of "healthy" alcohol intake is further questioned by recent suggestions that even small amounts of alcohol intake may increase hormone-sensitive breast cancer risk in women [70], although the associations between alcohol intake and breast cancer risk have not been consistent [71]. Despite a suggestion of CV benefits in small doses, the potential for abuse remains high and few doctors feel comfortable recommending alcohol as treatment [72]. For patients who already drink, doctors should help survey patients for their intake and encourage limiting intake to one drink per day for women and two drinks per day for men.

Almonds

Almonds contain several constituents that may benefit cardiovascular health including fiber, polyphenols, and plant sterols. A few small, short-term clinical trials have focused on the potential for almonds to lower LDL cholesterol and raise HDL cholesterol. A meta-analysis of these trials found only very modest benefit to lipid profiles with between 1 and 6 oz of almonds daily [73], but further analysis suggested that nondiabetic participants with high cholesterol may benefit the most. However, confusing matters somewhat, this group was also at risk for HDL lowering secondary to almonds. This based on the available data, almonds may have a neutral effect on lipids, and should probably not be considered the cornerstone of treatment for high cholesterol. Despite this position, almonds have held a key role in the Portfolio dietary pattern for LDL lowering [43], and subsequent studies have not only confirmed an LDL-lowering effect of almond-supplemented diets [74], but have also demonstrated CRP lowering [75], and reduced LDL oxidation [76]. Additional cardiometabolic benefits of almond intake include reduced post-prandial blood glucose, that is, reducing the glycemic response of high carbohydrate-mixed meals [77].

Other Nuts

In addition to almonds, clinical trial results suggest cardiovascular benefits from intake of other nuts as well, including pistachios [78–80], walnuts [81], and pecans [82] for improving lipid ratios. Both walnuts and pistachios also improve endothelial function and pistachios appear to reduce LDL oxidation. Recent ancillary analyses from the PREDIMED Mediterranean diet trial demonstrated a 39% reduction in *total mortality* in those participants who consumed >3 servings of nuts per week [83]. Additional observational findings also support a benefit of nut intake for reduced mortality, especially from cardiovascular causes, including the Physicians Health Study [84] and the Iowa Women's Health Study [85].

Avocado

Avocado provides a rich dietary source of MUFAs, in addition to plant sterols, lutein, L-carnitine, reduced glutathione, and potassium. Several clinical studies have investigated the impact of adding avocado to the diet and evaluated the effects of lipid parameters. Although findings are mixed, most studies suggest that substituting avocados for saturated fats in the diet has a beneficial effect on lowering LDL and triglycerides without lowering HDL [86–90]. Additional benefits have been shown on the preservation of endothelial function when avocado is added to a high fat meal [91].

Garlic

For decades, clinical and basic science research has suggested garlic, and especially aged garlic, has potent antioxidant activity relevant to vascular function. Specifically, in 1993 Phelps et al. demonstrated a 34% reduction in the susceptibility of LDL cholesterol to oxidation after aged garlic supplementation (Kwai, 600 mg/day) was administered to 10 healthy adult participants for just 2 weeks [92]. In 1999, Ide and Lau reported that aged garlic extract specifically preserved antioxidant reserves in cultured endothelial cells, as well as reduced the accumulation of potent oxidants called peroxides in endothelial cell models [93]. The same research group also demonstrated that the observed activity appeared to be due to the action of S-allycysteine, a sulfur-based antioxidant formed exclusively during the aging of garlic [94]. Whether this antioxidant action was unique to aged garlic or could also be extended to other forms of garlic was explored a few years later by Munday et al. in a translational clinical study in which human participants were supplemented with either aged garlic (2.4 g/day), raw garlic (6 g/day), or vitamin E (0.8 g/day) for 7 days and LDL samples were collected and measured again for susceptibility to oxidation. Their results suggested that the aged garlic group, *but not the raw garlic group*, showed reduced susceptibility to oxidative stress when measured outside of the body, and that the degree of protection from peroxidation was similar in magnitude to vitamin E supplementation [95]. These four mechanistic studies were surprisingly consistent in their findings and clearly demonstrate a plausible mechanism of action for *aged* garlic as a protective agent for the cardiovascular system. However, despite the consistency of these findings, larger studies measuring clinically meaningful risk factors like cholesterol levels and blood pressure are also needed to fully understand how garlic may, or may not, fit into the clinical management of risk factors like cholesterol and blood pressure.

One of the earliest controlled clinical trials of garlic for cholesterol lowering was published in 1996 by Steiner et al. in which the group administered 7.2 g of aged garlic extract to 41 patients with elevated cholesterol and measured changes in their total cholesterol and LDL cholesterol after 6 months of treatment [96]. In this small clinical trial total cholesterol was reduced by ~6% compared to the changes in the placebo group of the study. Additionally, they also observed a 5.5 mmHg reduction in systolic blood pressure. Although these reductions were modest at best, the findings were significant and led to a series of follow-up trials to further test garlic preparations for cholesterol-lowering properties. Two subsequent clinical trials of garlic powder (standardized, nonaged garlic) and one trial of garlic oil went on to find that there was no effect of these garlic preparations for reducing cholesterol or LDL [97–99]. These conflicting studies led to controversy about the effectiveness of garlic for cholesterol lowering, and fortunately, led to a definitive study. In 2007, Gardner et al. published the results of a four-group, parallel-designed, placebo controlled trial of raw garlic versus aged garlic versus standardized garlic in a tablet versus placebo in 192 adults with moderately elevated total cholesterol [100]. All doses were designed to be equivalent to an averaged sized garlic clove, essentially eaten daily for 6 days/week for 6 months. Despite being designed to detect a 10% reduction in LDL lipoproteins no significant effect was measured for any of the garlic preparations tested.

Although the study by Gardner et al. is the most comprehensive clinical trial of garlic for reducing cholesterol to date, there are two additional studies that deserve discussion because they report contrasting results. In 2001, Kannar et al. published a very small clinical trial of an enteric-coated garlic preparation in which they treated 46 patients with elevated cholesterol for just 12 weeks; [101] at the end of the trial LDL cholesterol was reduced approximately 6.6%, although, interestingly, HDL cholesterol was also reduced in the active garlic treatment group compared to the placebo group. The findings are notable for two reasons. First, the comparison groups did not include the enteric coated garlic product used in the trial by Gardner et al., so although a neutral result, clinical questions remain regarding the possible effectiveness of enteric-coated products. Secondly, the Kannar study was performed in participants who had either "failed" or who were not adherent to other therapies, suggesting the potential clinical use of this product in situations where other therapies are not effective or preferred.

Adding further support for the potential of more slowly absorbed/time-released garlic for treating cholesterol was a second independent study published in 2008 by Sobenin et al. in which 46 men with elevated lipids were treated for with a nonaged, time-released garlic product (Allicor, 600 mg/day) [102]. At the end of the 12 weeks' study, LDL cholesterol was significantly lower in the active treatment group compared to the placebo group by 11.5% (p=0.002), and the difference in LDL from the start of the trial to the end of the trial in the active group was 13.8% (p=0.009). One key difference in this trial was that HDL cholesterol also improved, increasing by 11.5% (p=0.013). Although this study still needs to be replicated, ideally in larger study groups, an 11.5% reduction in LDL cholesterol, especially alongside an 11.5% increase in HDL cholesterol, is a clinically significant treatment affect that deserves additional research.

The potential role of garlic for blood pressure lowering was supported by a recent meta-analysis of 10 clinical trials by Reinhart et al. in which results from studies of various garlic preparations on blood pressure were combined and analyzed together [103]. This formal meta-analysis found that garlic appears to significantly lower blood pressure *in patients with hypertension* by approximately 16 and 9 mmHg in systolic and diastolic blood pressures, respectively. Since the publication of this meta-analysis, one additional clinical trial evaluated garlic for blood pressure lowering has been reported. In 2009, Sobenin et al. compared time-released garlic (600 mg/day) to placebo, and simultaneously compared aged garlic (Kwai 900 mg/day) to time-released garlic (Allicor 2400 mg/day) in 84 patients following 8 weeks of treatment [104]. The results of their clinical trial demonstrated Allicor resulted in a 7 mmHg reduction in both systolic and diastolic blood pressures, while Kwai resulted in the same reduction in systolic, but not diastolic, suggesting the slower release of the Allicor may be critical for optimal effects. Also notable, the increased dose of Allicor used in the study (2400 mg/day) had no additional effect beyond the lower dose (600 mg/day).

Despite the mixed findings on lipids and blood pressure, garlic seems to beneficially impact other parameters of cardiovascular health, including coagulation parameters and may have a direct effect on atherosclerosis (perhaps by reducing the oxidation of LDL). Garlic reduces blood coagulation similar to the effects of aspirin [105,106]. A randomized, double-blind, placebo-controlled clinical trial found that garlic powder reduced arteriosclerosis in both femoral and carotid arteries by 5%–18% in a group of subjects aged 50–80 years [107]. A small pilot study of 23 patients with atherosclerosis on statin therapy found that those treated with an aged garlic extract had less plaque growth over 1 year than those treated with placebo [108].

Clinically, care should be taken to reduce the risk for herb–drug interactions with garlic, as garlic is known to impact hepatic drug metabolism by altering cytochrome P450 (CYP) activity, including induction of CYP1A1/2 and CYP2B1/2 and possibly glutathione S-transferase (GST), but inhibition of CYP2E1, CYP2C9, and CYP2C19 [109]. Since garlic is most commonly used for dyslipidemia (despite the limited evidence supporting this use), one clinically significant interaction to be aware of is a possible interaction between garlic and atorvastatin, in which garlic increases the area under the atorvastatin concentration curve in rats, which may increase the risk of statin-related myopathy [110]. This interaction is curious as atorvastatin is metabolized mostly by CYP3A4, which was not affected by garlic in other studies [109]. Clinical monitoring and dose reduction may be necessary. Theoretical concern has been raised about garlic in relation to its anti-coagulation effects and possible interaction with the anticoagulant effects of warfarin, which could increase the risk of internal bleeding. This concern has been tempered by a recent trial showing that patients on warfarin did not have increased bleeding when given garlic over a 12-week time period [111].

Onions

Onions contain significant amounts of the antioxidant polyphenol quercetin, which may be cardioprotective, though evidence supporting their use is still preliminary. Eating onions does seem to decrease coagulation parameters, which may reduce risk [112,113]. Early studies also find that onions are useful for cholesterol lowering [114], which is supported by recent research in unstable angina and non-ST-elevation myocardial infarctions (STEMI) [115]. Quercetin supplementation by itself has demonstrated blood pressure-lowering properties in some patients with early hypertension [116].

Other Spices

Ginger (*Zingiber officinale*) is another common spice that may have heart-healthy benefits. Dyslipidemic patients receiving 3 g of ginger powder daily for 45 days had lower LDL and higher HDL levels than patients treated with placebo [117]. Ginger does increase bleeding times when co-administered with warfarin, so caution is warranted [118].

Turmeric (*Curcuma longa*) has a long use outside of cooking in Indian traditional herbal medicine. Laboratory studies suggest that it may lower cholesterol (possibly by reducing intestinal absorption), reduce oxidative damage to blood vessels, and decrease systemic inflammation [119,120]. Specifically, turmeric appears to protect fat against peroxidation (a form of oxidation) that occurs during cooking, reduce the oxidation of LDL cholesterol that occurs from eating peroxidated foods, and may protect the liver from the damaging effects of oxidized food as well. Clinical trials to determine turmeric's true medicinal value are anticipated by physicians already recommending this herb for patients with CVD. Given turmeric's relatively low cost and high safety profile, this may be a valuable addition to many patients' health regimen.

Soy-Based Foods

Foods based on the soybean—tofu, tempeh, soy milk, and soy proteins—provide a protein-rich alternative to animal products for many people without sensitivity. Clinical trials have looked at the effects of different types of soy food on lipids, and meta-analyses of these trials have lent support to the idea that 25–60 g of soy protein daily lowers LDL cholesterol by 5%–6% [121–123]. Effects on blood pressure have been less well-researched, though early trials are promising [124,125]. Part of any benefit may simply be related to a reduction in dietary saturated fats and cholesterol associated with the substitution, although some researchers believe that particular phytoestrogen isoflavones in soy may be responsible for the benefits observed.

Apples

Apples are an excellent dietary source of vitamin C, quercetin, pectin, and phytosterols. Clinical trials of apples are few, and demonstrate mixed results. In two small studies in healthy individuals and postmenopausal women, dried apple intake beneficially affected total cholesterol and lowered LDL, with some benefits on CRP and endothelial function [126,127]. Dried apple intake in postmenopausal women reduced LDL by 24% at 6 months of treatment! However, shorter-term studies in adults with hypercholesterolemia suggested no benefit of either high- or low-polyphenol dried apple powder on endothelial function [128]. Although an apple a day may keep the doctor away, it may be because apples are substituted for more inflammatory foods. More research is needed to determine the unique health effects of apples and consideration should be given to other characteristics of the apples used in future research, that is, fiber content, polyphenol content, and organic status.

Watermelon

Although often thought of mostly as a source of water and fiber, watermelon is a potent dietary source of lycopene, lutein, and the amino acid L-citrulline, which is a precursor to L-arginine, a precursor to nitric oxide, and thus a candidate vasodilator. L-citrulline in isolation has demonstrated improvement in left ventricular function [129]. Clinical research for watermelon is in its infancy, though several clinical trials have recently demonstrated blood pressure lowering and improved measures of arterial stiffness, likely due to improved nitric oxide availability and improved endothelial function [130–132].

Pomegranate

Pomegranate, a tree-born fruit that shines red like a faceted ruby, has long been cultivated throughout the Middle East, the Mediterranean, and the Indian subcontinent. Rich in antioxidant compounds, including ellagic acid, preliminary human studies suggest relatively small "doses" of pomegranate juice, that is, 2–6 oz/day, have cardiovascular health benefits, including blood pressure lowering, reducing LDL oxidation, lowered cholesterol, increasing coronary artery perfusion, and perhaps reducing carotid intima media thickness [133–138]. In the earliest trials, Aviram et al. evaluated pomegranate juice was investigated for blood pressure lowering properties and for reducing LDL oxidation. There early short-term results suggested pomegranate juice lowered systolic blood pressure via ACE inhibitor activity [133]. After 1 year of pomegranate juice, blood pressure was reduced 12%, LDL oxidation was reduced by 90%, carotid intima media thickness (IMT) reduced by 30% (compared to the control group which increased by 9%), and paraoxonase-1 (PON-1) activity, an enzyme that assists with reducing LDL oxidation, was increased by 83% [134]. Pomegranate juice has also been shown to reduce LDL-c in patients with diabetes, without negative effect on blood sugar [136]. Most post exciting, pomegranate juice consumed at 8 oz/day for just 3 months increased coronary perfusion measured by single-photon emission computed tomography (SPECT) testing in participants with established coronary artery disease [138].

Other Polyphenol-Rich Foods

Several other plant foods may also have significant benefits to cardiovascular health, primarily related to their polyphenol content, including black and green tea, grapes, chocolate, apples, and coffee. Technically, "polyphenol" is a classification of compounds that includes thousands of different chemicals including tannins, lignins, and flavonoids, each of which can be further subdivided into smaller groups.

A nutritional epidemiological study of 34,492 individuals who were initially free of CVD found that, over the long term, the ingestion of foods and beverages with high levels of catechins (a type of flavonoid, common in green tea and apples) was associated with a decreased risk of developing coronary artery disease [139]. A similar prospective cohort study of 806 men aged 65–84 years found that the consumption of catechins, primarily from chocolate, apples, and black tea, was inversely related to the risk of mortality from ischemic heart disease [140].

Short-term clinical trials have also sought to determine if foods rich in polyphenols might be beneficial to human health. Dark chocolate, grapes, and wine have all been shown to improve endothelial function [141–144], possibly inhibiting the development of atherosclerosis by inhibiting the oxidation of LDL. Dark chocolate, red wine, and olive oil all have demonstrable lipid-lowering effects [145–147]. Adding dark chocolate and/or cocoa-based flavones may also be beneficial for hypertension [148].

The grape-derived polyphenol resveratrol has been isolated and is heavily promoted for its cardioprotective effects. Several animal studies suggest that this compound may be the one involved in reducing atherosclerosis [149]. Human studies examining the effects of multiple grape compounds have found cardioprotective

TABLE 8.2

Select Foods with Evidence-Supported Cardiovascular Benefits

Food	Supported Cardiovascular Effects[a]
Alcohol	• Increased HDL
Almonds	• Reduced LDL, hsCRP, and LDL oxidation
Other nuts (pistachios, walnuts, pecans)	• Improved lipid profiles
Avocado	• Reduced triglycerides
Garlic	• Reduced blood pressure (aged or time-released)
	• Improved lipid profiles (*conflicting evidence*)
Onions	• Reduced platelet adhesion
Ginger	• Improved LDL:HDL
Turmeric	• Reduced LDL oxidation
Soy-based foods	• Reduced LDL
Apples	• Reduced LDL
Watermelon	• Reduced blood pressure
	• Reduced arterial stiffness
Pomegranate	• Reduced blood pressure
	• Improved coronary perfusion
Other polyphenol-rich foods:	• Reduced LDL oxidation
• Dark chocolate	• Reduced blood pressure
• Grapes	
• Red wine	

[a] See main text for citations.

effects, including reduced oxidation of LDL [150], improved endothelial function [142], reduced CRP (in smokers) [151], increased adiponectin, and reduced coagulation parameters in people with coronary disease [152] (Table 8.2).

INDIVIDUAL NUTRIENTS AND BIOACTIVE COMPOUNDS

A number of individual molecular compounds (fiber, fatty acids, amino acids, vitamins, minerals, and a few other compounds) have been researched for their possible benefits in heart disease. These molecules may be found in specific foods, but are also typically available as nutritional supplements. Similar to the research on specific foods, we have few randomized trials that have measured hard clinical events on which to base recommendations for nutritional/dietary supplements. The relatively sparse clinical trials of dietary supplements that have measured changes in cardiovascular risk factor are limited by their small size, short duration, emphasis on surrogate outcome measures, and are often conducted in samples with limited generalizability to the general population. Despite the limitations of small trials, several nutrients have multiple clinical trials supporting their use for risk factor reduction, improved function/performance, and/or improved quality of life, and when taken collectively provide some justification for their use, when the totality of evidence is considered collectively.

FIBER

Maintaining adequate dietary fiber intake remains one of the easiest, most important, though least exciting, ways to reduce dyslipidemia. Although maintaining adequate fiber intake occurs easily when following a mostly plant-based diet of raw and cooked vegetables, combining with legumes and whole grains when consumed, supplemental fiber may further assist in improving lipid parameters, as demonstrated in the clinical trials of the Portfolio diet plan [17,18,43]. Oat and psyllium fiber provide easy, inexpensive fiber supplements. Oat bran fiber—which contains beta-glucan, a polysaccharide-soluble fiber—reduced LDL-C by 26% when eaten consumed at 2.6 g/day for 2 months [153]. Psyllium fiber, consumed at 10–12 g/day for 2 months also reduced total cholesterol and LDL, but less than oat fiber, 3%–14% and 5%–10% for total and LDL, respectively [154,155]. Oat fiber may also reduce blood pressure [156–158].

ESSENTIAL FATTY ACIDS

Essential fatty acids include the omega-3 fatty acid, alpha-linolenic acid (ALNA), omega-6 fatty acid, and alpha-linoleic acid (ALA). From these, two unsaturated fatty acids and other critical PUFAs can be created. Of course, many clinicians are aware that there is considerable variance in the degree to which people can convert ALNA the more unsaturated docosapentaenoic acid (DHA) and eicosapentaenoic (EPA), that is, the PUFAs generically referred to as "fish oil." Factors including gender and dietary omega-3 to omega-6 ratio may also impact conversion; women appear to be able to convert ALNA to DHA at about twice that of men [159–161]. Dietary sources of ALNA include flax, pumpkin, hemp, perilla and canola seed oils, soybean oil, and walnut oil. Dietary sources of ALA include safflower, sunflower, evening primrose, borage, hemp, soy, walnut, sesame, and pistachio oils. Direct sources of DHA and EPA come from fish or dietary supplements. Cold-water fish from sustainable fisheries remains the healthiest of options for the consumption of wild fish. Unfortunately, it is increasingly difficult to recommend the intake of fresh fish, considering the contamination of fish with mercury and other chemicals, and the unhealthy state of the world's oceans and fisheries.

Fish oils are a known treatment for hypertriglyceridemia in doses of 3–5 g/day and prescription versions are available and covered by some insurers. Fish oil as a treatment for triglycerides has the added advantage of having modest beneficial effects on HDL [162].

PUFAs found in fish have been heavily investigated for their effects on the heart, and the results have been quite dramatic. Substantial evidence suggest omega-3 fatty acids reduce the risk of hypertension, MI, cardiac death, and recurrent cardiovascular events [163–165] (including one research measured toenail mercury concentration to adjust for any detrimental mercury intake may have had on their outcomes [166]). However, scientists rarely agree, and two recent high-profile meta-analyses did not support an overall benefit of fish oil in the prevention of cardiovascular events, or mortality [167,168]. One landmark supporting a benefit of fish oil for CVD was the GISSI-Prevenzione trial, which divided 11,324 heart attack survivors into groups receiving either omega-3, vitamin E, both, or placebo [169]. After a 3-year trial, participants receiving omega-3 supplementation had fewer heart attacks, strokes, or death. Other cardiovascular effects of fish oil are less clear. Fish oils do not seem to have a substantial effect on arrhythmias [170], whereas they may have a small beneficial effect on congestive heart failure [171].

In most cases, we continue to recommend adequate dietary intake of PUFAs from plant seed and nut oil sources, and from high quality fish oil supplements or wild fish where available. In the clinic, when dietary recalls and signs/symptoms of low omega-3 intake do not match, or if poor digestion or fat absorptions is suspected, it is prudent to order nutritional laboratory evaluations that measure the omega-3 content of red blood cells, and/or measure intermediates in DHA and EPA production in order to determine patients' individual needs for fish oil supplementation.

Typical doses for EPA and DHA are 1–2 g/day for general cardiovascular maintenance and 3–5 g/day for triglycerides.

Vitamins C and E

Because oxidative processes have a mediating role in atherosclerotic damage, the antioxidant vitamins C (ascorbic acid) and E (really a misnomer referring to four tocopherols and four tocotrienols) have received research attention as possible supplemental interventions to prevent heart attack and stroke. Early research found benefit from high levels of these vitamins in the diet, and there was some preliminary support for their supplemental use. However, the HOPE (Heart Outcomes Prevention Evaluation) trials looked specifically at whether long-term supplementation with α-tocopherol would help prevent CVD [172]. Following over 9000 patients for up to 7 years, researchers found no evidence that supplementation with α-tocopherol could help prevent CVD, and in fact, rates of congestive heart failure actually increased in the vitamin E supplement group. Skeptics suggest the results may have been null due to imbalanced vitamin C intake relative to vitamin E, that the form of vitamin E was incorrect, and that the dose used may have been too low. Supporting the possibility that the dose may have been too low, dose-finding studies of α-tocopherol by Roberts et al. suggest at least 1600–3200 IU/day is needed to reduce biomarkers of lipid peroxidation—the primary indication supplement with vitamin E [173]. Potentially refuting the argument that vitamin E may have worked better if co-administered with vitamin C, the Physician's Health Study II (PHS-II) studied 14,641 male physicians who were divided into groups taking either vitamin E (α-tocopherol) and vitamin C, either vitamin alone (with a placebo pill in place of the other vitamin), or two placebo pills. After a follow-up lasting almost 8 years, the study found no support for the use of these antioxidant vitamins in conjunction with standard medical management for the prevention of heart disease [174]. Because vitamin E occurs in food as a combination of eight slightly different molecular forms, the trials that used only supplemental α-tocopherol have been roundly criticized as not adequately addressing the interplay between different forms. It has been hypothesized that the negative studies seen with α-tocopherol are because it is suppressing the activity of the other forms of the molecule. A small trial published after HOPE and PHS-II found that volunteers given α-tocopherol with vitamin C did have suppressed blood levels of γ-tocopherol, lending credence to this hypothesis [175]. Until longer-term trials of mixed tocopherols are conducted, the best bet still seems to be getting antioxidant vitamins from regular consumption of fruits and vegetables [176].

Typical doses of vitamin C and E range between 250 mg and 1 g three times daily and 400–1600 IU of mixed tocopherols per day, respectively, with meals.

VITAMINS B2, B6, B12, AND FOLIC ACID

High blood levels of homocysteine, a breakdown product of protein, have been linked to the development of atherosclerosis and associated CVDs. Vitamins B6 (pyridoxine), B12 (cobalamin), and folic acid are all involved in the biochemical breakdown of homocysteine. Physicians and researchers have hoped that by identifying people with high levels of homocysteine and then treating them with this triple-vitamin combination, they could help prevent atherosclerosis, heart attack, and stroke. While research has consistently shown that treatment with these vitamins does reliably lower homocysteine levels, meta-analysis has not found a corresponding decrease in the rates of atherosclerosis, stroke, or heart attack [177,178].

Prior to the publication of these analyses, larger, longer-term trials were initiated to evaluate the impact of homocysteine-lowering on CVD events. One study included 3749 recent MI randomized to B6, B12, and folate and followed for 40 months; although homocysteine concentrations were lower in the supplemented group, no significant reduction in cardiovascular events occurred between the vitamin group and the placebo group [179]. Another study of 5442 women with cardiovascular risk factors found no benefit of B vitamin supplementation for over 7 years [84]. Although these studies do not support a major contribution of homocysteine for CVD risk, there remained some evidence that suggests homocysteine lowering may reduce the risk of stroke; however, recent studies similarly do not support the prevention of, or improvement in, stroke from B-vitamin treatment of hyper-homocysteinemia [180–182]. Notably, people with select polymorphisms of the methylenetetrahydrofolate reductase (MTHFR) enzyme may be more vulnerable to the vascular effects of homocysteine, as their homocysteine concentrations tend to be very high.

Although homocysteine-targeted supplements are available, and some cases of hyper-homocysteinemia are intractable to B-vitamin treatment, homocysteine is typically lowered by a typical B-complex vitamin. In unresponsive cases, MTHFR status measurement should be considered, which may require methylated forms of folate. In carriers of the C677 → T polymorphism, riboflavin (B2) may be required to lower homocysteine [183]. In fact, in people with hypertension and C677 → T polymorphisms, treatment with riboflavin was more effective at lowering blood pressure than anti-hypertensive therapy [184].

VITAMIN B3 (NIACIN)

Niacin has been suggested as a preventive therapy for CVD by lowering LDL and raising HDL levels [185]. Niacin is also one of few therapies that has clinical trial support for lowering Lp(a) [186]. Niacin is also increasingly being combined in mainstream medicine with statins. These combinations are extremely effective in improving the lipid profile in patients with heart disease [187]. However, recent research questions whether any additive benefit occurs when niacin is added to statin therapy, and has also led to questions about the value of HDL-targeted therapies [188]. The dose necessary for such benefits is 2 to 3g/day, which may cause glucose intolerance, increase uric acid, and increase liver enzymes in some individuals. It is important to use a timed-release or delayed-release formulation of niacin to reduce the common vasodilation ("flushing") that can occur; however, cases of fulminant hepatic failure requiring liver transplantation have been described. Flushing can also be avoided by taking aspirin prior to niacin, or by gradually increasing doses of the vitamin.

Typical therapeutic doses of niacin range from 500 to 2000 mg/day, although dose titration may take months for patients who are intolerant to the common flushing. Extended release preparations reduce the flushing effects, but have less flexibility for dividing doses and may increase the risk of fulminant hepatic failure [189].

Vitamin D

Vitamin D has been classically known for its importance in regulating calcium and magnesium levels, but over the past decade more work has focused on other important roles it plays in the body, including in helping to maintain cardiovascular health. The third National Health and Nutrition Examination Survey (NHANES-III) conducted a comprehensive health history of 16,603 Americans. After adjusting for traditional risk factors (lipids, blood pressure, etc.), an analysis of NHANES-III found that low vitamin D levels just may be an independent risk factor in CVD [190]. Additional evidence is emerging to link vitamin D to atherosclerosis, hyperlipidemia, and hypertension [191]. Vitamin D insufficiency may also play a role in atrial fibrillation and congestive heart failure [192,193]. Several other observational studies have tested relationships between vitamin D and cardiovascular health, each finding negative consequences for those with insufficiency or deficiency [194,195]. Although these studies have shown strong observational associations between vitamin D deficiency increasing risk for having a heart attack, heart failure, and stroke, these observational studies may be plagued by reverse causation, that is, poor health may have led to vitamin D insufficiency or deficiency rather than the converse. Also, very few clinical trials of vitamin D have been performed that evaluate cardiovascular outcomes, and thus there is very little evidence that suggests replacing vitamin D, or raising 25-hydroxycholecalciferol concentration above "normal" using supplements reduces risk or alters the course of CVD. Adding further challenge, experimental research has not established an optimal serum concentration to gain cardiovascular benefits (if they exist); most recommendations for optimal serum concentrations are based on conjecture from observational research.

One exception may for clinical research evaluating the effects of vitamin D on blood pressure. Although several small clinical trials suggest blood pressure lowering with vitamin D replacement, the findings are not consistent [196–200]. The effects of vitamin D replacement for blood pressure may depend on important covariates including type of vitamin D used, baseline 25-hydroxycholecalciferol and magnesium status, BMI, ethnicity, and menopausal status (to suggest a few!) [201].

The strength of the observational data for the detrimental health effects of vitamin D insufficiency and/or deficiency, combined with the high prevalence of vitamin D insufficiency in the public (and the essentiality of the vitamin to maintain normal calcium and magnesium status!), create a strong case for evaluating patients' 25-hydroxycholecalciferol status and replacing vitamin D as needed [202]. However, any cardiovascular specific health effects of repletion are unknown. Research on the health effects of vitamin D is happening at a rapid pace, and new guidelines and treatment recommendations will hopefully clarify these issues for the practicing clinician.

Recent research supports 10,000 IU/day for 3 months as an effective clinical method to replenishing vitamin D in deficiency or insufficiency in routine clinical populations [201].

OTHER FAT-SOLUBLE NUTRIENTS

DIETARY CAROTENOIDS

Carotenoids include the pigmented compounds that give fruits and vegetables their bright color, including beta-carotene, alpha-carotene, lycopene, lutein, zeaxanthin, and beta-cryptoxanthin. Serum carotenoid concentrations are established biomarkers of fruit and vegetable intake [203,204], and several longitudinal studies have measured inverse associations between serum concentrations of various carotenoid fractions (especially lutein and zeaxanthin) and biomarkers of endothelial dysfunction [205], risk of atherosclerosis [206], and slower progression of atherosclerosis [14]. However, as discussed in the introduction, biomarkers of dietary intake do not necessarily mean the biomarker itself is the cause of the association, that is, just because serum carotenoids increase with fruit and vegetable intake does not mean that carotenoids themselves are responsible for any observed benefits.

Several clinical trials have been performed evaluating carotenoid supplementation and various cardiovascular endpoints. Unfortunately, only the CARET trial, which only applied beta-carotene as an intervention and not mixed-carotenoids, has evaluated hard clinical endpoints and showed no reduction of cardiovascular events [15].

Because carotenoid concentration increases in LDL with supplementation (or increased intake of fruits and vegetables), much research has focused on the impact of carotenoids on the susceptibility of LDL to oxidation. Results have been mixed with some studies suggesting reduced resistance to oxidation with supplementation, while others have demonstrated neutral effects [207–209]. Additional research has focused exclusively on lycopene as a potential treatment for hypertension by reducing oxidative stress and improving endothelial dysfunction; again, findings are mixed with some trials suggesting benefits on LDL and HDL oxidation state, and improved endothelial function [210–213], while others have shown no benefit [214,215]. One recent promising study is a 6-month clinical trial performed by

Zhou et al. that evaluated 20 mg lutein combined with 20 mg lycopene/day for 1 year in participants with subclinical disease. After 1 year, carotid IMT was significantly reduced in the carotenoid supplemented group compared to placebo [216].

Unfortunately, many of the clinical trials of carotenoid fractions have been limited to very short durations, or acute administration, and have not been representative of the daily dietary intake of fruits and vegetables that demonstrates CVD risk protection in study after study. Until more clinical research is performed, the best advice regarding carotenoids remains to increase them through the dietary intake of fruits and vegetables to ensure all of the benefits of fruits and vegetables are realized.

Vitamin K

Vitamin K is a fat-soluble vitamin that occurs in most vegetables and is in particularly high concentrations in green, leafy vegetables. Vitamin K1 (i.e., hylloquinone, phytomenadione, or phytonadione) is found in plant foods, while animals convert K1 to vitamin K2 (menaquinone) for storage. Vitamin K has a critical role in the coagulation cascade, and also regulated vitamin D-mediated calcification [217,218]. Low vitamin K status has been attributed as the cause for the increase risk of vascular calcification in patients treated with warfarin [219]. Cardiovascular epidemiology is just beginning to evaluate associations between serum vitamin K concentration and cardiovascular endpoints, and so far vitamin K2 intake appears to be inversely associated with risk [220,221]. Although several in vitro and animal in vivo studies support vitamin K as a protective nutrient to reduce atherosclerosis and vascular calcification [219,222,223], no clinical trials are available that have evaluated effects in humans. Until more research is available, recommended high vitamin K dietary intake from green leafy vegetables and titrating warfarin doses *around a diet rich in vitamin K* remain prudent approaches to ensuring adequate intake of this important nutrient.

Minerals

In addition to the vitamins described earlier, several minerals are important to cardiovascular health, especially those that maintain the electrical rhythm of the heart. Although many providers routinely measure "lytes," how carefully are the results scrutinized, or even considered a nutritional biomarker? Serum magnesium, despite its limitations as a biomarker, is rarely included on electrolyte panels, yet is as important as calcium, sodium, and potassium.

Calcium channeling is critical for both cardiac contractility and vasomotor activity, yet "calcification" is also implicated in the development of atherosclerotic plaques. Thus, the topic of calcium supplementation to treat CVD remains controversial. Large trials have not found strong evidence that calcium has either positive or negative effects on CVD risk in postmenopausal women being supplemented for osteoporosis prevention [224,225]. One meta-analysis found that calcium had only a small beneficial effect in the treatment of high blood pressure, but the trials were all considered small and of relatively poor quality [226]. While lifetime intake is critically important to bone health, it remains unclear if calcium supplementation has any role in cardio protection.

Magnesium can be often thought of as the balancing of calcium in cells, for example, calcium influx is important for vasoconstriction and magnesium influx is helpful for vasodilation. Magnesium deficiency is considered common, and may also be exacerbated with diuretic use [227]. Epidemiologic data suggests a decreased incidence in heart disease among those with regular intake of magnesium [228]. However, because excellent dietary sources of magnesium include whole grains, legumes, tofu, green leafy vegetables, and seeds—very heart healthy foods—it is impossible to definitively know that *magnesium* itself is responsible for the reduced incidence.

Magnesium has been studied rather extensively for the treatment of CVD, including for hypertension, MI, and arrhythmia. Both a meta-analysis of trials and a Cochrane review concluded small reductions in blood pressure from magnesium supplementation, but noted that these effects were typically reported from small trials and, therefore, may not be reliable estimates of clinical effects [229,230]. Some benefits, including reduced arrhythmias during treatment and angioplasty, have been noted for intravenous magnesium as part of hospital-based MI treatment, but adverse effects also occurred, including hypotension and bradycardia [231–233]. Typical doses of magnesium range from 250 mg to 1.5 g/day depending on status and bowel tolerance.

Potassium regulates blood pressure, improves angina, and reduces the risk of heart failure, including congestive heart failure [234]. As with magnesium and calcium, literature reviews have been critical of the size and strength of trials using potassium to treat high blood pressure, though potassium supplementation (including substitution of sodium with potassium) is one of the few lifestyle strategies recommended for reduction of blood pressure [235]. In addition to frequently low dietary intake of potassium, digitalis and nonpotassium sparing diuretics also contribute significantly to low potassium status. Diuretic-induced potassium loss is also implicated in the link between diuretics and the development of diabetes [236].

Zinc deficiency has been implicated in hyperlipidemia, though supplementation may lower the levels of the beneficial HDLs [237]. Zinc deficiency has been noted in patients with congestive heart failure, and may be related to the progression of the disease [238]. Zinc administration requires proper balance with copper, as high intakes of zinc can induce copper deficiency, which may result in negative consequences on cardiovascular health [239–241].

Chromium, an essential mineral found in various meats, vegetables, and brewer's yeast, has been heavily studied for its effects on blood sugar. Given the links between diabetes and heart disease, there is preliminary interest in its use for cardiovascular health. Although epidemiologic studies suggest an overlap between chromium deficiency and cardiac risk, few strong trials have found substantial benefit for cardiovascular prevention or treatment [242].

Iron, a critical building block of heme, is an essential mineral for adequate red blood cell formation and thus oxygen delivery, however, excess iron in the blood can contribute to increased oxidative stress and endothelial dysfunction. Hemochromatosis, a genetic condition of iron overload characterized by significantly elevated serum ferritin, has been associated with the development of several specific cardiac diseases, including ventricular dysfunction, infiltrative cardiomyopathy, and sudden cardiac death (likely due to acute endothelial dysfunction and vasospasm) [243,244]; evidence for hemochromatosis increasing risk for ischemic heart disease is mixed [245,246]. Similarly, a review of studies linking body iron stores with CVD did not find consistent links between the two, suggesting that further research is needed to clarify this matter [247]. If discovered, the removal of extra iron is achievable with therapeutic phlebotomy or iron chelation therapy [248]. Supporting a contribution of relative iron excess to the cardiovascular risk profile of the metabolic syndrome, in the absence of hemochromatosis, therapeutic phlebotomy has been evaluated in people with the metabolic syndrome, and found to be effective at reducing blood pressure, glucose, HbA1c, and LDL to HDL ratio [249].

MITOCHONDRIAL-TARGETED THERAPY WITH L-CARNITINE, CoQ10, AND/OR D-RIBOSE

All muscle tissue requires functioning mitochondria to provide adequate ATP for contraction. Myocardial tissue is especially dependent on adequate ATP production in order to maintain adequate contractility and stroke volume. Coenzyme Q10, L-carnitine, and D-ribose are three dietary supplements that theoretically provide mitochondrial substrates for improved function.

Coenzyme-Q10 (aka, CoQ10 or ubiquinol) is critical for energy production in heart cells by serving as intermediate electron shuttle in the electron transport chain during the production of ATP. Additionally, CoQ10 has antioxidant properties that may help prevent the development of atherosclerosis and subsequent heart disease, in part due to its interaction with paraoxonase-1 (PON-1), which helps mediate HDL oxidation and function in reverse cholesterol transport [250]. Patients with some forms of heart disease, including congestive heart failure, have been found to have significantly lower serum concentrations of CoQ10 than healthy individuals [251], and a small trial in 39 patients demonstrated improved exercise tolerance and reduced shortness of breath and other symptoms in these patients [252]. CoQ10 has shown promising benefit in decreasing triglycerides in instances where conventional therapy and fish oils have failed [253]. CoQ10 may also be a valuable antihypertensive, and, according to a meta-analysis of several clinical trials, may lower blood pressure by as much as 17 mmHg systolic and 10 mmHg diastolic [254]. Small trials have also found CoQ10 to be useful in some arrhythmias and angina [255,256]. Notably, CoQ10 may reduce the risk of a second event [257].

CoQ10 is best known for the depletion caused by HMG-CoQ reductase, that is, "statin" drugs, a cornerstone of conventional treatment for atherosclerosis and CVD prevention. Statins block the biochemical pathways involved in both cholesterol synthesis and CoQ10 [258]. Statin use may also lead to memory loss, cognitive impairment, and fatigue, and these effects may be related to CoQ10 depletion (and corrected by supplementation) [259]. Supplementing with CoQ10 may reduce myalgias when they do occur secondary to statins, although general use of CoQ10 with statins may not reduce the rate of statin-induced myalgias in a general population [260].

In general, clinical research showing clear benefit of supplementation is still preliminary, despite the multitudes of mechanistic evidence that supports its use. However, given the excellent safety profile of CoQ10 [261], especially patients taking statin drugs may find this a valuable addition to their regimen. Admittedly, clinical trials that measured clinical events evaluating statin therapy with and without supplemental CoQ10 have not been performed. Typical CoQ10 doses in practice range from 30 mg (minimal dose to prevent statin-induced losses) up to 200 mg or higher (for anti-hypertensive effects and improvement in CHF).

The amino acid L-carnitine is used for many purposes in the body, including energy production in muscle from the metabolism of free fatty acids via beta-oxidation. Demonstrating its importance for normal myocardial function, researchers have linked a variety of heart disorders, such as cardiac myopathies, cardiac enlargement, congestive heart failure, and other disorders to L-carnitine deficiencies [262].

L-carnitine was found to help lower LDL cholesterol in patients with diabetes [263], and may help to lower blood pressure when combined with α-lipoid acid [264]. L-carnitine has also been shown to improve function and metabolism in patients with ischemic heart disease [265]. A study of 2500 patients found that L-carnitine administered for up to a year can improve angina symptoms and greater exercise capacity in patients with coronary artery disease and cardiomyopathy [266]. Carnitine also reduced the risk of heart failure and death in patients with a history of myocardial infarction [267]. In patients with CHF, L-carnitine supplementation may improve exercise capacity [268]. Research is still unearthing the full value of L-carnitine, but so far, this amino acid looks like it may be a valuable addition for those interested in the natural heart support. Typical doses of L-carnitine are 1–3 g/day.

Recent controversy related to L-carnitine involves its potential interactions with gut flora to produce a potentially pro-inflammatory intermediate called trimethylamine-N-oxide (TMAO), which is increased in the blood when L-carnitine is given to people who have TMAO-producing bacteria in the gut [269]. These findings are somewhat paradoxical given the many clinical benefits that have been measured in clinical trials of L-carnitine. This area of research is still emerging, but highlights the importance of treating CVD holistically and not as an isolated system, starting with the old naturopathic tenant of "treat the gut [and health will follow]."

Ribose, a five-carbon sugar also involved in muscle-cell energy production, is often added to regimens of carnitine and CoQ10 for cardiovascular support, though research on ribose alone is minimal [270]. In a very small study of 15 people with CHF, oral supplementation with ribose was shown to improve diastolic function, and quality-of-life compared to placebo [271]. D-ribose has also been shown to increase treadmill time and reduce activity-induced ST segment elevation in people with stable angina performing stress tests [272]. Typical doses of D-ribose are 5 g of ribose powder two to three times per day.

While many clinicians use CoQ10, L-carnitine, and D-ribose in combination, few clinical trials have evaluated this "cocktail" and the clinical results achieved by combining them remain mostly undocumented.

OTHER AMINO ACIDS

L-ARGININE

L-arginine is the primary nitrogen donor for the production of nitric oxide (NO) via the action of endothelial nitric oxide synthase (eNOS), and thus is critical to normal vasodilation. L-arginine also stimulates the release on insulin from the pancreas, and therefore, has indirect glucose-lowering effects. The combined actions of glucose-lowering and vasodilation have the potential to improve endothelial dysfunction. This fundamental action has led many to endorse supplementation with L-arginine as a method to combat endothelial dysfunction, reduce blood pressure, and improve angina. However, nitric oxide production is carefully regulated in vivo because excess nitric oxide in an inflammatory vascular environment, that is, endothelial dysfunction, can increase the production of reactive nitrogen species (RNS), including peroxynitrite, which is known to modify endothelial proteins, including functional receptors. Human physiology has endogenous mechanisms in place to regulate the production of NO, including its overproduction; one major mechanism is the production of asymmetric dimethylarginine (ADMA) from arginine, which then competes with arginine for binding sites on eNOS. It is possible to out compete ADMA for eNOS binding sites, but it requires very large concentrations to do so, and thus very large doses of supplemental L-arginine. Although ADMA has not been measured in most clinical trials of L-arginine, it may explain why many trials have used very large doses ranging from 3 to 9 g/day. Because it is possible to out compete ADMA without fundamentally changing the metabolic environment, it is important to interpret the research on L-arginine critically, for example, short-term changes in blood pressure due to overriding ADMA may not translate into long-term improvements in function, and theoretically could actually *worsen* endothelial function due to overproduction of RNS. In fact, clinical investigations of L-arginine supplementation in people with hypertension demonstrated increases in ADMA [273], which have been associated with worsened cardiovascular outcomes [274].

A few clinical trials of L-arginine have measured ADMA or related biomarkers of oxidative stress and have demonstrated benefits in glucose disposal, endothelial function, and/or blood pressure. Lucotti et al. evaluated 6.4 g of L-arginine per day in nondiabetic patients after coronary artery bypass graft (CABG) and demonstrated reduced ADMA, reduced ADMA: arginine ratio (which would be expected from increasing serum arginine alone), improved glucose disposal, and reduced biomarkers of immune activation associated with atherosclerosis [275]. Additional clinical studies suggest benefits from L-arginine supplements administered in 6 g/day doses for 10 days may improve endothelial function during a fatty meal challenge; however, the investigators did not find improvements in glutathione status, suggesting arginine improved vasodilation, but did not reduce oxidative stress [276]. Additional research has found L-arginine supplementation (administered in 9 g/day doses for 7 days) improves exercise tolerance and ejection fraction (but did not reduce oxidative stress) in New York Heart Association class II–III systolic heart failure [277], and 8 g/day for 2 months improved right-sided ejection fraction [278].

L-arginine may also increase exercise capacity in stable angina when administered in doses of 6 g/day for 3 days; no measures of oxidative stress were measured in this very short clinical study [279].

However, not all studies have demonstrated L-arginine. L-arginine does not appear to improve acute exercise tolerance in generally healthy patients with hyperlipidemia [280], and 6-month studies of L-arginine supplemented at 3 g/day for peripheral artery disease did not demonstrate benefit, and in fact demonstrated worse outcomes than placebo [281].

Mechanistically, if a clinician could change the inflammatory environment through dietary change, there would be lower risk that supplemental L-arginine would increase RNS. Alternatively, reducing oxidative stress through antioxidant supplementation could serve as a decoy (to superoxide free radicals), allowing supplemental L-arginine to be more effective. Evidence for this hypothesis is provided by BBB et al. who supplemented N-acetylcysteine (600 mg) with L-arginine (1.2 g) in people with type 2 diabetes for 6 months, and measured significant reductions in blood pressure, reduction in oxidative stress, and improvement in glutathione status [282].

L-arginine should be considered as an adjunctive therapy only when dietary changes have been made, and inflammatory biomarkers have been reduced. When possible, N-acetylcysteine or other superoxide and/or RNS scavenging antioxidants should be combined with L-arginine. To reduce the risk of hypotension, L-arginine should not be combined with nitroglycerine, other angina medications, or phosphodiesterase-5 (PDE-5) inhibitors. When prescribed, typical doses range from 1 to 9 g/day, often in divided doses. Sustained release preparations of L-arginine deserve rigorous clinical research for their benefits.

TAURINE

Taurine, technically a sulfonic acid and *not* an amino acid, has many amazing physiological functions [283–285], which appear to results in part improved osmoregulation of intracellular electrolytes—with implications for both improved myocardial function and nerve conduction. Taurine is also a major component of bile, and thus critical for the absorption of fat-soluble vitamins and nutrients (i.e., vitamin D, K2, and carotenoids). Lipid metabolism also requires taurine, which impacts the secretion of apoprotein B (ApoB), and thus the production of LDL by the liver.

Several observational studies have linked lower serum concentrations of taurine and/or increased elimination of taurine to increased CVD, including ischemic disease [286–288]. Clinical trials of taurine have demonstrated improvements in serum triglycerides, and non-HDL to HDL lipid ratios in overweight, nondiabetic patients [289]; improved left ventricular function and increased exercise tolerance in CHF [290,291]; and improved endothelial function in young adults with type 1 diabetes [292]. Notably, several trials have been performed combining taurine with mitochondrial-targeted therapies, including small clinical trials of MyoVive [293], containing CoQ10, taurine, and carnitine, demonstrating reduced end-diastolic volume in patients with left ventricular dysfunction, and of CoQ10 and taurine suggesting improved function post-MI [294]. Taurine appears to be very safe to supplement, and typical doses are 500 mg–1.5 g/day in divided doses.

SUMMARY AND CONCLUSIONS

"Nutritional" therapy for CVD prevention and treatment begins with the foundation of a plant-based diet, rich in actual fruits and vegetables, and sources of dietary fiber. There is no evidence that the use of dietary supplements offsets the risk of CVD that results from a poor-quality diet. Although diets high or low in particular macronutrients may offer particularly therapeutic benefits in the short term (e.g., a low-saturated-fat diet for LDL reduction, a low-carbohydrate diet for improved insulin sensitivity, etc.), patients need sustainable diets, and the balanced pattern represented by the Mediterranean diet provides the most evidence-based diet for the prevention of CVD (plus diabetes and cognitive decline!) and, therefore, provides an excellent framework to begin tailoring diets to the preferences and goals of individual patients. Individual foods may offer targeted diet-based therapies for individual risk factors (e.g., soy protein for LDL lowering, aged garlic for blood pressure lowering, pomegranate for oxidized LDL (oxLDL) lowering, etc.) and can be over-represented with the Mediterranean pattern to enhance clinical effects for certain individual risk factors. Research on dietary supplements remains in its infancy, and dietary supplements should not replace dietary quality. In most cases, research support for supplements is limited to short-term trials focused on surrogate outcomes. However, when selectively applied, dietary supplements can offer benefits including improved endothelial function, increased contractility, reduced LDL oxidation, etc. As with any clinical recommendation, providing patients with the knowledge of dietary approaches to the prevention and treatment of CVD is only part of the challenge—the art of practice requires developing a therapeutic relationship that helps the knowledge translate into action!

REFERENCES

1. Nettleton, J.A., Polak, J.F., Tracy, R., Burke, G.L., and Jacobs, D.R., Jr. 2009. Dietary patterns and incident cardiovascular disease in the multi-ethnic study of atherosclerosis. *Am J Clin Nutr* 90:647–654.
2. Nettleton, J.A., Steffen, L.M., Mayer-Davis, E.J., Jenny, N.S., Jiang, R., Herrington, D.M., and Jacobs, D.R., Jr. 2006. Dietary patterns are associated with biochemical markers of inflammation and endothelial activation in the multi-ethnic study of atherosclerosis (MESA). *Am J Clin Nutr* 83:1369–1379.
3. Diehr, P. and Beresford, S.A. 2003. The relation of dietary patterns to future survival, health, and cardiovascular events in older adults. *J Clin Epidemiol* 56:1224–1235.
4. Stampfer, M.J., Hu, F.B., Manson, J.E., Rimm, E.B., and Willett, W.C. 2000. Primary prevention of coronary heart disease in women through diet and lifestyle. *N Engl J Med* 343:16–22.
5. Mayne, S.T. 2003. Antioxidant nutrients and chronic disease: Use of biomarkers of exposure and oxidative stress status in epidemiologic research. *J Nutr* 133(Suppl 3): 933S–940S.
6. Kuhnle, G.G. 2012. Nutritional biomarkers for objective dietary assessment. *J Sci Food Agric* 92:1145–1149.

7. Jenab, M., Slimani, N., Bictash, M., Ferrari, P., and Bingham, S.A. 2009. Biomarkers in nutritional epidemiology: Applications, needs and new horizons. *Hum Genet* 125:507–525.

8. Hedrick, V.E., Dietrich, A.M., Estabrooks, P.A., Savla, J., Serrano, E., and Davy, B.M. 2012. Dietary biomarkers: Advances, limitations and future directions. *Nutr J* 11:109.

9. Poulsen, M.W., Hedegaard, R.V., Andersen, J.M., de Courten, B., Bugel, S., Nielsen, J., Skibsted, L.H., and Dragsted, L.O. 2013. Advanced glycation endproducts in food and their effects on health. *Food Chem Toxicol* 60:10–37.

10. Chagas, P., Caramori, P., Galdino, T.P., Barcellos Cda, S., Gomes, I., and Schwanke, C.H. 2013. Egg consumption and coronary atherosclerotic burden. *Atherosclerosis* 229:381–384.

11. Shin, J.Y., Xun, P., Nakamura, Y., and He, K. 2013. Egg consumption in relation to risk of cardiovascular disease and diabetes: A systematic review and meta-analysis. *Am J Clin Nutr* 98:146–159.

12. Li, Y., Zhou, C., Zhou, X., and Li, L. 2013. Egg consumption and risk of cardiovascular diseases and diabetes: A meta-analysis. *Atherosclerosis* 229:524–530.

13. Spence, J.D., Jenkins, D.J., and Davignon, J. 2012. Egg yolk consumption and carotid plaque. *Atherosclerosis* 224:469–473.

14. Dwyer, J.H., Paul-Labrador, M.J., Fan, J., Shircore, A.M., Merz, C.N., and Dwyer, K.M. 2004. Progression of carotid intima-media thickness and plasma antioxidants: The Los Angeles atherosclerosis study. *Arterioscler Thromb Vasc Biol* 24:313–319.

15. Goodman, G.E., Thornquist, M.D., Balmes, J., Cullen, M.R., Meyskens, F.L., Jr., Omenn, G.S., Valanis, B., and Williams, J.H., Jr. 2004. The beta-carotene and retinol efficacy trial: Incidence of lung cancer and cardiovascular disease mortality during 6-year follow-up after stopping beta-carotene and retinol supplements. *J Natl Cancer Inst* 96:1743–1750.

16. Ornish, D., Scherwitz, L.W., Billings, J.H., Brown, S.E., Gould, K.L., Merritt, T.A., Sparler, S., Armstrong, W.T., Ports, T.A., Kirkeeide, R.L. et al. 1998. Intensive lifestyle changes for reversal of coronary heart disease. *JAMA* 280:2001–2007.

17. Jenkins, D.J., Kendall, C.W., Faulkner, D.A., Kemp, T., Marchie, A., Nguyen, T.H., Wong, J.M., de Souza, R., Emam, A., Vidgen, E. et al. 2008. Long-term effects of a plant-based dietary portfolio of cholesterol-lowering foods on blood pressure. *Eur J Clin Nutr* 62:781–788.

18. Jenkins, D.J., Kendall, C.W., Faulkner, D.A., Nguyen, T., Kemp, T., Marchie, A., Wong, J.M., de Souza, R., Emam, A., Vidgen, E. et al. 2006. Assessment of the longer-term effects of a dietary portfolio of cholesterol-lowering foods in hypercholesterolemia. *Am J Clin Nutr* 83:582–591.

19. The DASH diet. Dietary approaches to stop hypertension. *Lippincotts Primary Care Practice* 1998;2:536–538.

20. Estruch, R., Ros, E., Salas-Salvado, J., Covas, M.I., Corella, D., Aros, F., Gomez-Gracia, E., Ruiz-Gutierrez, V., Fiol, M., Lapetra, J. et al. 2013. Primary prevention of cardiovascular disease with a Mediterranean diet. *N Engl J Med* 368:1279–1290.

21. Salas-Salvado, J., Bullo, M., Babio, N., Martinez-Gonzalez, M.A., Ibarrola-Jurado, N., Basora, J., Estruch, R., Covas, M.I., Corella, D., Aros, F. et al. 2011. Reduction in the incidence of type 2 diabetes with the Mediterranean diet: Results of the PREDIMED-Reus nutrition intervention randomized trial. *Diabetes Care* 34:14–19.

22. Howard, B.V., Van Horn, L., Hsia, J., Manson, J.E., Stefanick, M.L., Wassertheil-Smoller, S., Kuller, L.H., LaCroix, A.Z., Langer, R.D., Lasser, N.L. et al. 2006. Low-fat dietary pattern and risk of cardiovascular disease: The Women's Health Initiative Randomized Controlled Dietary Modification Trial. *JAMA* 295:655–666.

23. Ceriello, A., Taboga, C., Tonutti, L., Quagliaro, L., Piconi, L., Bais, B., Da Ros, R., and Motz, E. 2002. Evidence for an independent and cumulative effect of postprandial hypertriglyceridemia and hyperglycemia on endothelial dysfunction and oxidative stress generation: Effects of short- and long-term simvastatin treatment. *Circulation* 106:1211–1218.

24. Bloomer, R.J., Kabir, M.M., Marshall, K.E., Canale, R.E., and Farney, T.M. 2010. Postprandial oxidative stress in response to dextrose and lipid meals of differing size. *Lipids Health Dis* 9:79.

25. Chowdhury, R., Warnakula, S., Kunutsor, S., Crowe, F., Ward, H.A., Johnson, L., Franco, O.H., Butterworth, A.S., Forouhi, N.G., Thompson, S.G. et al. 2014. Association of dietary, circulating, and supplement fatty acids with coronary risk: A systematic review and meta-analysis. *Ann Intern Med* 160:398–406.

26. Kris-Etherton, P.M., Krummel, D., Russell, M.E., Dreon, D., Mackey, S., Borchers, J., and Wood, P.D. 1988. The effect of diet on plasma lipids, lipoproteins, and coronary heart disease. *J Am Diet Assoc* 88:1373–1400.

27. Sacks, F.M. and Katan, M. 2002. Randomized clinical trials on the effects of dietary fat and carbohydrate on plasma lipoproteins and cardiovascular disease. *Am J Med* 113(Suppl 9B):13S–24S.

28. Vega-Lopez, S., Ausman, L.M., Jalbert, S.M., Erkkila, A.T., and Lichtenstein, A.H. 2006. Palm and partially hydrogenated soybean oils adversely alter lipoprotein profiles compared with soybean and canola oils in moderately hyperlipidemic subjects. *Am J Clin Nutr* 84:54–62.

29. Lemaitre, R.N., King, I.B., Mozaffarian, D., Sotoodehnia, N., Rea, T.D., Kuller, L.H., Tracy, R.P., and Siscovick, D.S. 2006. Plasma phospholipid trans fatty acids, fatal ischemic heart disease, and sudden cardiac death in older adults: The cardiovascular health study. *Circulation* 114:209–215.

30. Lemaitre, R.N., King, I.B., Raghunathan, T.E., Pearce, R.M., Weinmann, S., Knopp, R.H., Copass, M.K., Cobb, L.A., and Siscovick, D.S. 2002. Cell membrane trans-fatty acids and the risk of primary cardiac arrest. *Circulation* 105:697–701.

31. Mozaffarian, D. 2006. Trans fatty acids—Effects on systemic inflammation and endothelial function. *Atheroscler Suppl* 7:29–32.

32. Mozaffarian, D., Katan, M.B., Ascherio, A., Stampfer, M.J., and Willett, W.C. 2006. Trans fatty acids and cardiovascular disease. *N Engl J Med* 354:1601–1613.

33. Hu, T. and Bazzano, L.A. 2014. The low-carbohydrate diet and cardiovascular risk factors: Evidence from epidemiologic studies. *Nutr Metab Cardiovasc Dis* 24:337–343.

34. Hu, T., Mills, K.T., Yao, L., Demanelis, K., Eloustaz, M., Yancy, W.S., Jr., Kelly, T.N., He, J., and Bazzano, L.A. 2012. Effects of low-carbohydrate diets versus low-fat diets on metabolic risk factors: A meta-analysis of randomized controlled clinical trials. *Am J Epidemiol* 176(Suppl 7):S44–S54.

35. Santos, F.L., Esteves, S.S., da Costa Pereira, A., Yancy, W.S., Jr., and Nunes, J.P. 2012. Systematic review and meta-analysis of clinical trials of the effects of low carbohydrate diets on cardiovascular risk factors. *Obes Rev* 13:1048–1066.

36. Ballard, K.D., Quann, E.E., Kupchak, B.R., Volk, B.M., Kawiecki, D.M., Fernandez, M.L., Seip, R.L., Maresh, C.M., Kraemer, W.J., and Volek, J.S. 2013. Dietary carbohydrate restriction improves insulin sensitivity, blood pressure, microvascular function, and cellular adhesion markers in individuals taking statins. *Nutr Res* 33:905–912.

37. Ruth, M.R., Port, A.M., Shah, M., Bourland, A.C., Istfan, N.W., Nelson, K.P., Gokce, N., and Apovian, C.M. 2013. Consuming a hypocaloric high fat low carbohydrate diet for 12 weeks lowers C-reactive protein, and raises serum adiponectin and high density lipoprotein-cholesterol in obese subjects. *Metabolism* 62:1779–1787.

38. Greenberg, I., Stampfer, M.J., Schwarzfuchs, D., and Shai, I. 2009. Adherence and success in long-term weight loss diets: The dietary intervention randomized controlled trial (DIRECT). *J Am Coll Nutr* 28:159–168.
39. Noto, H., Goto, A., Tsujimoto, T., and Noda, M. 2013. Low-carbohydrate diets and all-cause mortality: A systematic review and meta-analysis of observational studies. *PLoS One* 8:e55030.
40. Tirosh, A., Golan, R., Harman-Boehm, I., Henkin, Y., Schwarzfuchs, D., Rudich, A., Kovsan, J., Fiedler, G.M., Bluher, M., Stumvoll, M. et al. 2013. Renal function following three distinct weight loss dietary strategies during 2 years of a randomized controlled trial. *Diabetes Care* 36:2225–2232.
41. Sacks, F.M., Svetkey, L.P., Vollmer, W.M., Appel, L.J., Bray, G.A., Harsha, D., Obarzanek, E., Conlin, P.R., Miller, E.R., 3rd, Simons-Morton, D.G. et al. 2001. Effects on blood pressure of reduced dietary sodium and the dietary approaches to stop hypertension (DASH) diet. DASH-sodium collaborative research group. *N Engl J Med* 344:3–10.
42. Obarzanek, E., Sacks, F.M., Vollmer, W.M., Bray, G.A., Miller, E.R., 3rd, Lin, P.H., Karanja, N.M., Most-Windhauser, M.M., Moore, T.J., Swain, J.F. et al. 2001. Effects on blood lipids of a blood pressure-lowering diet: The dietary approaches to stop hypertension (DASH) Trial. *Am J Clin Nutr* 74:80–89.
43. Jenkins, D.J., Kendall, C.W., Marchie, A., Faulkner, D.A., Wong, J.M., de Souza, R., Emam, A., Parker, T.L., Vidgen, E., Lapsley, K.G. et al. 2003. Effects of a dietary portfolio of cholesterol-lowering foods vs lovastatin on serum lipids and C-reactive protein. *JAMA* 290:502–510.
44. Ornish, D., Brown, S.E., Scherwitz, L.W., Billings, J.H., Armstrong, W.T., Ports, T.A., McLanahan, S.M., Kirkeeide, R.L., Brand, R.J., and Gould, K.L. 1990. Can lifestyle changes reverse coronary heart disease? The lifestyle heart trial. *Lancet* 336:129–133.
45. de Lorgeril, M., Salen, P., Martin, J.L., Monjaud, I., Delaye, J., and Mamelle, N. 1999. Mediterranean diet, traditional risk factors, and the rate of cardiovascular complications after myocardial infarction: Final report of the Lyon Diet Heart Study. *Circulation* 99:779–785.
46. Sofi, F., Cesari, F., Abbate, R., Gensini, G.F., and Casini, A. 2008. Adherence to Mediterranean diet and health status: Meta-analysis. *BMJ* 337:A1344.
47. Tuttle, K.R., Shuler, L.A., Packard, D.P., Milton, J.E., Daratha, K.B., Bibus, D.M., and Short, R.A. 2008. Comparison of low-fat versus Mediterranean-style dietary intervention after first myocardial infarction (from The Heart Institute of Spokane Diet Intervention and Evaluation Trial). *Am J Cardiol* 101:1523–1530.
48. Babio, N., Bullo, M., Basora, J., Martinez-Gonzalez, M.A., Fernandez-Ballart, J., Marquez-Sandoval, F., Molina, C., and Salas-Salvado, J. 2009. Adherence to the Mediterranean diet and risk of metabolic syndrome and its components. *Nutr Metab Cardiovasc Dis* 19:563–570.
49. Di Daniele, N., Petramala, L., Di Renzo, L., Sarlo, F., Della Rocca, D.G., Rizzo, M., Fondacaro, V., Iacopino, L., Pepine, C.J., and De Lorenzo, A. 2013. Body composition changes and cardiometabolic benefits of a balanced Italian Mediterranean Diet in obese patients with metabolic syndrome. *Acta Diabetol* 50:409–416.
50. Kesse-Guyot, E., Ahluwalia, N., Lassale, C., Hercberg, S., Fezeu, L., and Lairon, D. 2013. Adherence to Mediterranean diet reduces the risk of metabolic syndrome: A 6-year prospective study. *Nutr Metab Cardiovasc Dis* 23:677–683.
51. Mendez, M.A., Popkin, B.M., Jakszyn, P., Berenguer, A., Tormo, M.J., Sanchez, M.J., Quiros, J.R., Pera, G., Navarro, C., Martinez, C. et al. 2006. Adherence to a Mediterranean diet is associated with reduced 3-year incidence of obesity. *J Nutr* 136:2934–2938.

52. Romaguera, D., Norat, T., Vergnaud, A.C., Mouw, T., May, A.M., Agudo, A., Buckland, G., Slimani, N., Rinaldi, S., Couto, E. et al. 2010. Mediterranean dietary patterns and prospective weight change in participants of the EPIC-PANACEA project. *Am J Clin Nutr* 92:912–921.

53. Karatzi, K., Papamichael, C., Karatzis, E., Papaioannou, T.G., Voidonikola, P.T., Vamvakou, G.D., Lekakis, J., and Zampelas, A. 2008. Postprandial improvement of endothelial function by red wine and olive oil antioxidants: A synergistic effect of components of the Mediterranean diet. *J Am Coll Nutr* 27:448–453.

54. Rallidis, L.S., Lekakis, J., Kolomvotsou, A., Zampelas, A., Vamvakou, G., Efstathiou, S., Dimitriadis, G., Raptis, S.A., and Kremastinos, D.T. 2009. Close adherence to a Mediterranean diet improves endothelial function in subjects with abdominal obesity. *Am J Clin Nutr* 90:263–268.

55. Couto, E., Boffetta, P., Lagiou, P., Ferrari, P., Buckland, G., Overvad, K., Dahm, C.C., Tjonneland, A., Olsen, A., Clavel-Chapelon, F. et al. 2011. Mediterranean dietary pattern and cancer risk in the EPIC cohort. *Br J Cancer* 104:1493–1499.

56. Bamia, C., Lagiou, P., Buckland, G., Grioni, S., Agnoli, C., Taylor, A.J., Dahm, C.C., Overvad, K., Olsen, A., Tjonneland, A. et al. 2013. Mediterranean diet and colorectal cancer risk: Results from a European cohort. *Eur J Epidemiol* 28:317–328.

57. Camargo, A., Delgado-Lista, J., Garcia-Rios, A., Cruz-Teno, C., Yubero-Serrano, E.M., Perez-Martinez, P., Gutierrez-Mariscal, F.M., Lora-Aguilar, P., Rodriguez-Cantalejo, F., Fuentes-Jimenez, F. et al. 2012. Expression of proinflammatory, pro-atherogenic genes is reduced by the Mediterranean diet in elderly people. *Br J Nutr* 108:500–508.

58. Mena, M.P., Sacanella, E., Vazquez-Agell, M., Morales, M., Fito, M., Escoda, R., Serrano-Martinez, M., Salas-Salvado, J., Benages, N., Casas, R., et al. 2009. Inhibition of circulating immune cell activation: A molecular antiinflammatory effect of the Mediterranean diet. *Am J Clin Nutr* 89:248–256.

59. Urpi-Sarda, M., Casas, R., Chiva-Blanch, G., Romero-Mamani, E.S., Valderas-Martinez, P., Salas-Salvado, J., Covas, M.I., Toledo, E., Andres-Lacueva, C., Llorach, R. et al. 2012. The Mediterranean diet pattern and its main components are associated with lower plasma concentrations of tumor necrosis factor receptor 60 in patients at high risk for cardiovascular disease. *J Nutr* 142:1019–1025.

60. Mitjavila, M.T., Fandos, M., Salas-Salvado, J., Covas, M.I., Borrego, S., Estruch, R., Lamuela-Raventos, R., Corella, D., Martinez-Gonzalez, M.A., Sanchez, J.M. et al. 2013. The Mediterranean diet improves the systemic lipid and DNA oxidative damage in metabolic syndrome individuals. A randomized, controlled, trial. *Clin Nutr* 32:172–178.

61. Garaulet, M., Esteban Tardido, A., Lee, Y.C., Smith, C.E., Parnell, L.D., and Ordovas, J.M. 2012. SIRT1 and CLOCK 3111T > C combined genotype is associated with evening preference and weight loss resistance in a behavioral therapy treatment for obesity. *Int J Obes (Lond)* 36:1436–1441.

62. Ortega-Azorin, C., Sorli, J.V., Asensio, E.M., Coltell, O., Martinez-Gonzalez, M.A., Salas-Salvado, J., Covas, M.I., Aros, F., Lapetra, J., Serra-Majem, L. et al. 2012. Associations of the FTO rs9939609 and the MC4R rs17782313 polymorphisms with type 2 diabetes are modulated by diet, being higher when adherence to the Mediterranean diet pattern is low. *Cardiovasc Diabetol* 11:137.

63. Konstantinidou, V., Covas, M.I., Sola, R., and Fito, M. 2013. Up-to date knowledge on the in vivo transcriptomic effect of the Mediterranean diet in humans. *Mol Nutr Food Res* 57:772–783.

64. Tuohy, K.M., Fava, F., and Viola, R. 2014. "The way to a man's heart is through his gut microbiota"—Dietary pro- and prebiotics for the management of cardiovascular risk. *Proc Nutr Soc* 73:172–185.

65. Arranz, S., Chiva-Blanch, G., Valderas-Martinez, P., Medina-Remon, A., Lamuela-Raventos, R.M., and Estruch, R. 2012. Wine, beer, alcohol and polyphenols on cardiovascular disease and cancer. *Nutrients* 4:759–781.

66. Movva, R. and Figueredo, V.M. 2013. Alcohol and the heart: To abstain or not to abstain? *Int J Cardiol* 164:267–276.

67. Brinton, E.A. 2012. Effects of ethanol intake on lipoproteins. *Curr Atheroscler Rep* 14:108–114.

68. De Oliveira, E.S.E.R., Foster, D., McGee Harper, M., Seidman, C.E., Smith, J.D., Breslow, J.L., and Brinton, E.A. 2000. Alcohol consumption raises HDL cholesterol levels by increasing the transport rate of apolipoproteins A-I and A-II. *Circulation* 102:2347–2352.

69. Goldstein, L.B., Bushnell, C.D., Adams, R.J., Appel, L.J., Braun, L.T., Chaturvedi, S., Creager, M.A., Culebras, A., Eckel, R.H., Hart, R.G. et al. 2011. Guidelines for the primary prevention of stroke: A guideline for healthcare professionals from the American Heart Association/American Stroke Association. *Stroke* 42:517–584.

70. Li, C.I., Chlebowski, R.T., Freiberg, M., Johnson, K.C., Kuller, L., Lane, D., Lessin, L., O'Sullivan, M.J., Wactawski-Wende, J., Yasmeen, S. et al. 2010. Alcohol consumption and risk of postmenopausal breast cancer by subtype: The women's health initiative observational study. *J Natl Cancer Inst* 102:1422–1431.

71. Scoccianti, C., Lauby-Secretan, B., Bello, P.Y., Chajes, V., and Romieu, I. 2014. Female breast cancer and alcohol consumption: A review of the literature. *Am J Prev Med* 46:S16–25.

72. Hansel, B., Kontush, A., and Bruckert, E. 2012. Is a cardioprotective action of alcohol a myth? *Curr Opin Cardiol* 27:550–555.

73. Phung, O.J., Makanji, S.S., White, C.M., and Coleman, C.I. 2009. Almonds have a neutral effect on serum lipid profiles: A meta-analysis of randomized trials. *J Am Diet Assoc* 109:865–873.

74. Damasceno, N.R., Perez-Heras, A., Serra, M., Cofan, M., Sala-Vila, A., Salas-Salvado, J., and Ros, E. 2011. Crossover study of diets enriched with virgin olive oil, walnuts or almonds. Effects on lipids and other cardiovascular risk markers. *Nutr Metab Cardiovasc Dis* 21(Suppl 1):S14–20.

75. Rajaram, S., Connell, K.M., and Sabate, J. 2010. Effect of almond-enriched high-mono-unsaturated fat diet on selected markers of inflammation: A randomised, controlled, crossover study. *Br J Nutr* 103:907–912.

76. Jalali-Khanabadi, B.A., Mozaffari-Khosravi, H., and Parsaeyan, N. 2010. Effects of almond dietary supplementation on coronary heart disease lipid risk factors and serum lipid oxidation parameters in men with mild hyperlipidemia. *J Altern Complement Med* 16:1279–1283.

77. Josse, A.R., Kendall, C.W., Augustin, L.S., Ellis, P.R., and Jenkins, D.J. 2007. Almonds and postprandial glycemia—A dose-response study. *Metabolism* 56:400–404.

78. Kocyigit, A., Koylu, A.A., and Keles, H. 2006. Effects of pistachio nuts consumption on plasma lipid profile and oxidative status in healthy volunteers. *Nutr Metab Cardiovasc Dis* 16:202–209.

79. Sari, I., Baltaci, Y., Bagci, C., Davutoglu, V., Erel, O., Celik, H., Ozer, O., Aksoy, N., and Aksoy, M. 2010. Effect of pistachio diet on lipid parameters, endothelial function, inflammation, and oxidative status: A prospective study. *Nutrition* 26:399–404.

80. Sheridan, M.J., Cooper, J.N., Erario, M., and Cheifetz, C.E. 2007. Pistachio nut consumption and serum lipid levels. *J Am Coll Nutr* 26:141–148.

81. Cortes, B., Nunez, I., Cofan, M., Gilabert, R., Perez-Heras, A., Casals, E., Deulofeu, R., and Ros, E. 2006. Acute effects of high-fat meals enriched with walnuts or olive oil on postprandial endothelial function. *J Am Coll Cardiol* 48:1666–1671.

82. Rajaram, S., Burke, K., Connell, B., Myint, T., and Sabate, J. 2001. A monounsaturated fatty acid-rich pecan-enriched diet favorably alters the serum lipid profile of healthy men and women. *J Nutr* 131:2275–2279.

83. Guasch-Ferre, M., Bullo, M., Martinez-Gonzalez, M.A., Ros, E., Corella, D., Estruch, R., Fito, M., Aros, F., Warnberg, J., Fiol, M. et al. 2013. Frequency of nut consumption and mortality risk in the PREDIMED nutrition intervention trial. *BMC Med* 11:164.

84. Albert, C.M., Cook, N.R., Gaziano, J.M., Zaharris, E., MacFadyen, J., Danielson, E., Buring, J.E., and Manson, J.E. 2008. Effect of folic acid and B vitamins on risk of cardiovascular events and total mortality among women at high risk for cardiovascular disease: A randomized trial. *JAMA* 299:2027–2036.

85. Ellsworth, J.L., Kushi, L.H., and Folsom, A.R. 2001. Frequent nut intake and risk of death from coronary heart disease and all causes in postmenopausal women: The Iowa Women's Health Study. *Nutr Metab Cardiovasc Dis* 11:372–377.

86. Alvizouri-Munoz, M., Carranza-Madrigal, J., Herrera-Abarca, J.E., Chavez-Carbajal, F., and Amezcua-Gastelum, J.L. 1992. Effects of avocado as a source of monounsaturated fatty acids on plasma lipid levels. *Arch Med Res* 23:163–167.

87. Carranza-Madrigal, J., Herrera-Abarca, J.E., Alvizouri-Munoz, M., Alvarado-Jimenez, M.R., and Chavez-Carbajal, F. 1997. Effects of a vegetarian diet vs. a vegetarian diet enriched with avocado in hypercholesterolemic patients. *Arch Med Res* 28:537–541.

88. Colquhoun, D.M., Moores, D., Somerset, S.M., and Humphries, J.A. 1992. Comparison of the effects on lipoproteins and apolipoproteins of a diet high in monounsaturated fatty acids, enriched with avocado, and a high-carbohydrate diet. *Am J Clin Nutr* 56:671–677.

89. Lerman-Garber, I., Ichazo-Cerro, S., Zamora-Gonzalez, J., Cardoso-Saldana, G., and Posadas-Romero, C. 1994. Effect of a high-monounsaturated fat diet enriched with avocado in NIDDM patients. *Diabetes Care* 17:311–315.

90. Pieterse, Z., Jerling, J.C., Oosthuizen, W., Kruger, H.S., Hanekom, S.M., Smuts, C.M., and Schutte, A.E. 2005. Substitution of high monounsaturated fatty acid avocado for mixed dietary fats during an energy-restricted diet: Effects on weight loss, serum lipids, fibrinogen, and vascular function. *Nutrition* 21:67–75.

91. Li, Z., Wong, A., Henning, S.M., Zhang, Y., Jones, A., Zerlin, A., Thames, G., Bowerman, S., Tseng, C.H., and Heber, D. 2013. Hass avocado modulates postprandial vascular reactivity and postprandial inflammatory responses to a hamburger meal in healthy volunteers. *Food Funct* 4:384–391.

92. Phelps, S. and Harris, W.S. 1993. Garlic supplementation and lipoprotein oxidation susceptibility. *Lipids* 28:475–477.

93. Ide, N. and Lau, B.H. 1999. Aged garlic extract attenuates intracellular oxidative stress. *Phytomedicine* 6:125–131.

94. Ide, N. and Lau, B.H. 1999. S-allylcysteine attenuates oxidative stress in endothelial cells. *Drug Dev Ind Pharm* 25:619–624.

95. Munday, J.S., James, K.A., Fray, L.M., Kirkwood, S.W., and Thompson, K.G. 1999. Daily supplementation with aged garlic extract, but not raw garlic, protects low density lipoprotein against in vitro oxidation. *Atherosclerosis* 143:399–404.

96. Steiner, M., Khan, A.H., Holbert, D., and Lin, R.I. 1996. A double-blind crossover study in moderately hypercholesterolemic men that compared the effect of aged garlic extract and placebo administration on blood lipids. *Am J Clin Nutr* 64:866–870.

97. Berthold, H.K., Sudhop, T., and von Bergmann, K. 1998. Effect of a garlic oil preparation on serum lipoproteins and cholesterol metabolism: A randomized controlled trial. *JAMA* 279:1900–1902.

98. Isaacsohn, J.L., Moser, M., Stein, E.A., Dudley, K., Davey, J.A., Liskov, E., and Black, H.R. 1998. Garlic powder and plasma lipids and lipoproteins: A multicenter, randomized, placebo-controlled trial. *Arch Intern Med* 158:1189–1194.

99. Superko, H.R. and Krauss, R.M. 2000. Garlic powder, effect on plasma lipids, postprandial lipemia, low-density lipoprotein particle size, high-density lipoprotein subclass distribution and lipoprotein(a). *J Am Coll Cardiol* 35:321–326.

100. Gardner, C.D., Lawson, L.D., Block, E., Chatterjee, L.M., Kiazand, A., Balise, R.R., and Kraemer, H.C. 2007. Effect of raw garlic vs. commercial garlic supplements on plasma lipid concentrations in adults with moderate hypercholesterolemia: A randomized clinical trial. *Arch Intern Med* 167:346–353.

101. Kannar, D., Wattanapenpaiboon, N., Savige, G.S., and Wahlqvist, M.L. 2001. Hypocholesterolemic effect of an enteric-coated garlic supplement. *J Am Coll Nutr* 20:225–231.

102. Sobenin, I.A., Andrianova, I.V., Demidova, O.N., Gorchakova, T., and Orekhov, A.N. 2008. Lipid-lowering effects of time-released garlic powder tablets in double-blinded placebo-controlled randomized study. *J Atheroscler Thromb* 15:334–338.

103. Reinhart, K.M., Coleman, C.I., Teevan, C., Vachhani, P., and White, C.M. 2008. Effects of garlic on blood pressure in patients with and without systolic hypertension: A meta-analysis. *Ann Pharmacother* 42:1766–1771.

104. Sobenin, I.A., Andrianova, I.V., Fomchenkov, I.V., Gorchakova, T.V., and Orekhov, A.N. 2009. Time-released garlic powder tablets lower systolic and diastolic blood pressure in men with mild and moderate arterial hypertension. *Hypertens Res* 32:433–437.

105. Ali, M. and Thomson, M. 1995. Consumption of a garlic clove a day could be beneficial in preventing thrombosis. *Prostaglandins Leukot Essent Fatty Acids* 53:211–212.

106. Kiesewetter, H., Jung, F., Pindur, G., Jung, E.M., Mrowietz, C., and Wenzel, E. 1991. Effect of garlic on thrombocyte aggregation, microcirculation, and other risk factors. *Int J Clin Pharmacol Ther Toxicol* 29:151–155.

107. Koscielny, J., Klussendorf, D., Latza, R., Schmitt, R., Radtke, H., Siegel, G., and Kiesewetter, H. 1999. The antiatherosclerotic effect of *Allium sativum*. *Atherosclerosis* 144:237–249.

108. Budoff, M.J., Takasu, J., Flores, F.R., Niihara, Y., Lu, B., Lau, B.H., Rosen, R.T., and Amagase, H. 2004. Inhibiting progression of coronary calcification using Aged Garlic Extract in patients receiving statin therapy: A preliminary study. *Prev Med* 39:985–991.

109. Hermann, R. and von Richter, O. 2012. Clinical evidence of herbal drugs as perpetrators of pharmacokinetic drug interactions. *Planta Med* 78:1458–1477.

110. Reddy, G.D., Reddy, A.G., Rao, G.S., and Kumar, M.V. 2012. Pharmacokinetic interaction of garlic and atorvastatin in dyslipidemic rats. *Indian J Pharmacol* 44:246–252.

111. Macan, H., Uykimpang, R., Alconcel, M., Takasu, J., Razon, R., Amagase, H., and Niihara, Y. 2006. Aged garlic extract may be safe for patients on warfarin therapy. *J Nutr* 136:793S–795S.

112. Baghurst, K.I., Raj, M.J., and Truswell, A.S. 1977. Onions and platelet aggregation. *Lancet* 1:101.

113. Hubbard, G.P., Wolffram, S., Lovegrove, J.A., and Gibbins, J.M. 2004. Ingestion of quercetin inhibits platelet aggregation and essential components of the collagen-stimulated platelet activation pathway in humans. *J Thromb Haemost* 2:2138–2145.

114. Bordia, A., Bansal, H.C., Arora, S.K., and Singh, S.V. 1975. Effect of the essential oils of garlic and onion on alimentary hyperlipemia. *Atherosclerosis* 21:15–19.

115. Liu, Y., Zhang, L., Liu, Y.F., Yan, F.F., and Zhao, Y.X. 2008. Effects of Bulbus allii macrostemi on clinical outcomes and oxidized low-density lipoprotein and plasminogen in unstable angina/non-ST-segment elevation myocardial infarction patients. *Phytother Res* 22:1539–1543.

116. Edwards, R.L., Lyon, T., Litwin, S.E., Rabovsky, A., Symons, J.D., and Jalili, T. 2007. Quercetin reduces blood pressure in hypertensive subjects. *J Nutr* 137:2405–2411.

117. Alizadeh-Navaei, R., Roozbeh, F., Saravi, M., Pouramir, M., Jalali, F., and Moghadamnia, A.A. 2008. Investigation of the effect of ginger on the lipid levels. A double blind controlled clinical trial. *Saudi Med J* 29:1280–1284.

118. Shalansky, S., Lynd, L., Richardson, K., Ingaszewski, A., and Kerr, C. 2007. Risk of warfarin-related bleeding events and supratherapeutic international normalized ratios associated with complementary and alternative medicine: A longitudinal analysis. *Pharmacotherapy* 27:1237–1247.

119. Miriyala, S., Panchatcharam, M., and Rengarajulu, P. 2007. Cardioprotective effects of curcumin. *Adv Exp Med Biol* 595:359–377.

120. Srivastava, G. and Mehta, J.L. 2009. Currying the heart: Curcumin and cardioprotection. *J Cardiovasc Pharmacol Ther* 14:22–27.

121. Harland, J.I. and Haffner, T.A. 2008. Systematic review, meta-analysis and regression of randomised controlled trials reporting an association between an intake of circa 25 g soya protein per day and blood cholesterol. *Atherosclerosis* 200:13–27.

122. Reynolds, K., Chin, A., Lees, K.A., Nguyen, A., Bujnowski, D., and He, J. 2006. A meta-analysis of the effect of soy protein supplementation on serum lipids. *Am J Cardiol* 98:633–640.

123. Taku, K., Umegaki, K., Sato, Y., Taki, Y., Endoh, K., and Watanabe, S. 2007. Soy isoflavones lower serum total and LDL cholesterol in humans: A meta-analysis of 11 randomized controlled trials. *Am J Clin Nutr* 85:1148–1156.

124. Kim, J.Y., Gum, S.N., Paik, J.K., Lim, H.H., Kim, K.C., Ogasawara, K., Inoue, K., Park, S., Jang, Y., and Lee, J.H. 2008. Effects of nattokinase on blood pressure: A randomized, controlled trial. *Hypertens Res* 31:1583–1588.

125. Welty, F.K., Lee, K.S., Lew, N.S., and Zhou, J.R. 2007. Effect of soy nuts on blood pressure and lipid levels in hypertensive, prehypertensive, and normotensive postmenopausal women. *Arch Intern Med* 167:1060–1067.

126. Bondonno, C.P., Yang, X., Croft, K.D., Considine, M.J., Ward, N.C., Rich, L., Puddey, I.B., Swinny, E., Mubarak, A., and Hodgson, J.M. 2012. Flavonoid-rich apples and nitrate-rich spinach augment nitric oxide status and improve endothelial function in healthy men and women: A randomized controlled trial. *Free Radic Biol Med* 52:95–102.

127. Chai, S.C., Hooshmand, S., Saadat, R.L., Payton, M.E., Brummel-Smith, K., and Arjmandi, B.H. 2012. Daily apple versus dried plum: Impact on cardiovascular disease risk factors in postmenopausal women. *J Acad Nutr Diet* 112:1158–1168.

128. Auclair, S., Chironi, G., Milenkovic, D., Hollman, P.C., Renard, C.M., Megnien, J.L., Gariepy, J., Paul, J.L., Simon, A., and Scalbert, A. 2010. The regular consumption of a polyphenol-rich apple does not influence endothelial function: A randomised double-blind trial in hypercholesterolemic adults. *Eur J Clin Nutr* 64:1158–1165.

129. Balderas-Munoz, K., Castillo-Martinez, L., Orea-Tejeda, A., Infante-Vazquez, O., Utrera-Lagunas, M., Martinez-Memije, R., Keirns-Davis, C., Becerra-Luna, B., and Sanchez-Vidal, G. 2012. Improvement of ventricular function in systolic heart failure patients with oral L-citrulline supplementation. *Cardiol J* 19:612–617.

130. Figueroa, A., Sanchez-Gonzalez, M.A., Perkins-Veazie, P.M., and Arjmandi, B.H. 2011. Effects of watermelon supplementation on aortic blood pressure and wave reflection in individuals with prehypertension: A pilot study. *Am J Hypertens* 24:40–44.

131. Figueroa, A., Sanchez-Gonzalez, M.A., Wong, A., and Arjmandi, B.H. 2012. Watermelon extract supplementation reduces ankle blood pressure and carotid augmentation index in obese adults with prehypertension or hypertension. *Am J Hypertens* 25:640–643.

132. Figueroa, A., Wong, A., Hooshmand, S., and Sanchez-Gonzalez, M.A. 2013. Effects of watermelon supplementation on arterial stiffness and wave reflection amplitude in postmenopausal women. *Menopause* 20:573–577.

133. Aviram, M. and Dornfeld, L. 2001. Pomegranate juice consumption inhibits serum angiotensin converting enzyme activity and reduces systolic blood pressure. *Atherosclerosis* 158:195–198.

134. Aviram, M., Rosenblat, M., Gaitini, D., Nitecki, S., Hoffman, A., Dornfeld, L., Volkova, N., Presser, D., Attias, J., Liker, H. et al. 2004. Pomegranate juice consumption for 3 years by patients with carotid artery stenosis reduces common carotid intima-media thickness, blood pressure and LDL oxidation. *Clin Nutr* 23:423–433.

135. Basu, A. and Penugonda, K. 2009. Pomegranate juice: A heart-healthy fruit juice. *Nutr Rev* 67:49–56.

136. Esmaillzadeh, A., Tahbaz, F., Gaieni, I., Alavi-Majd, H., and Azadbakht, L. 2006. Cholesterol-lowering effect of concentrated pomegranate juice consumption in type II diabetic patients with hyperlipidemia. *Int J Vitam Nutr Res* 76:147–151.

137. Mirmiran, P., Fazeli, M.R., Asghari, G., Shafiee, A., and Azizi, F. 2010. Effect of pomegranate seed oil on hyperlipidaemic subjects: A double-blind placebo-controlled clinical trial. *Br J Nutr* 104:402–406.

138. Sumner, M.D., Elliott-Eller, M., Weidner, G., Daubenmier, J.J., Chew, M.H., Marlin, R., Raisin, C.J., and Ornish, D. 2005. Effects of pomegranate juice consumption on myocardial perfusion in patients with coronary heart disease. *Am J Cardiol* 96:810–814.

139. Arts, I.C., Jacobs, D.R., Jr., Harnack, L.J., Gross, M., and Folsom, A.R. 2001. Dietary catechins in relation to coronary heart disease death among postmenopausal women. *Epidemiology* 12:668–675.

140. Arts, I.C., Hollman, P.C., Feskens, E.J., Bueno de Mesquita, H.B., and Kromhout, D. 2001. Catechin intake might explain the inverse relation between tea consumption and ischemic heart disease: The Zutphen Elderly Study. *Am J Clin Nutr* 74:227–232.

141. Rakici, O., Kiziltepe, U., Coskun, B., Aslamaci, S., and Akar, F. 2005. Effects of resveratrol on vascular tone and endothelial function of human saphenous vein and internal mammary artery. *Int J Cardiol* 105:209–215.

142. Lekakis, J., Rallidis, L.S., Andreadou, I., Vamvakou, G., Kazantzoglou, G., Magiatis, P., Skaltsounis, A.L., and Kremastinos, D.T. 2005. Polyphenolic compounds from red grapes acutely improve endothelial function in patients with coronary heart disease. *Eur J Cardiovasc Prev Rehabil* 12:596–600.

143. Vlachopoulos, C., Aznaouridis, K., Alexopoulos, N., Economou, E., Andreadou, I., and Stefanadis, C. 2005. Effect of dark chocolate on arterial function in healthy individuals. *Am J Hypertens* 18:785–791.

144. Whelan, A.P., Sutherland, W.H., McCormick, M.P., Yeoman, D.J., de Jong, S.A., and Williams, M.J. 2004. Effects of white and red wine on endothelial function in subjects with coronary artery disease. *Intern Med J* 34:224–228.

145. Baba, S., Natsume, M., Yasuda, A., Nakamura, Y., Tamura, T., Osakabe, N., Kanegae, M., and Kondo, K. 2007. Plasma LDL and HDL cholesterol and oxidized LDL concentrations are altered in normo- and hypercholesterolemic humans after intake of different levels of cocoa powder. *J Nutr* 137:1436–1441.

146. Naissides, M., Mamo, J.C., James, A.P., and Pal, S. 2006. The effect of chronic consumption of red wine on cardiovascular disease risk factors in postmenopausal women. *Atherosclerosis* 185:438–445.

147. Covas, M.I., Nyyssonen, K., Poulsen, H.E., Kaikkonen, J., Zunft, H.J., Kiesewetter, H., Gaddi, A., de la Torre, R., Mursu, J., Baumler, H. et al. 2006. The effect of polyphenols in olive oil on heart disease risk factors: A randomized trial. *Ann Intern Med* 145:333–341.

148. Taubert, D., Berkels, R., Roesen, R., and Klaus, W. 2003. Chocolate and blood pressure in elderly individuals with isolated systolic hypertension. *JAMA* 290:1029–1030.

149. Fan, E., Zhang, L., Jiang, S., and Bai, Y. 2008. Beneficial effects of resveratrol on atherosclerosis. *J Med Food* 11:610–614.

150. Tome-Carneiro, J., Gonzalvez, M., Larrosa, M., Garcia-Almagro, F.J., Aviles-Plaza, F., Parra, S., Yanez-Gascon, M.J., Ruiz-Ros, J.A., Garcia-Conesa, M.T., Tomas-Barberan, F.A. et al. 2012. Consumption of a grape extract supplement containing resveratrol decreases oxidized LDL and ApoB in patients undergoing primary prevention of cardiovascular disease: A triple-blind, 6-month follow-up, placebo-controlled, randomized trial. *Mol Nutr Food Res* 56:810–821.

151. Bo, S., Ciccone, G., Castiglione, A., Gambino, R., De Michieli, F., Villois, P., Durazzo, M., Cavallo-Perin, P., and Cassader, M. 2013. Anti-inflammatory and antioxidant effects of resveratrol in healthy smokers a randomized, double-blind, placebo-controlled, cross-over trial. *Curr Med Chem* 20:1323–1331.

152. Tome-Carneiro, J., Gonzalvez, M., Larrosa, M., Yanez-Gascon, M.J., Garcia-Almagro, F.J., Ruiz-Ros, J.A., Tomas-Barberan, F.A., Garcia-Conesa, M.T., and Espin, J.C. 2013. Grape resveratrol increases serum adiponectin and downregulates inflammatory genes in peripheral blood mononuclear cells: A triple-blind, placebo-controlled, one-year clinical trial in patients with stable coronary artery disease. *Cardiovasc Drugs Ther* 27:37–48.

153. Berg, A., Konig, D., Deibert, P., Grathwohl, D., Baumstark, M.W., and Franz, I.W. 2003. Effect of an oat bran enriched diet on the atherogenic lipid profile in patients with an increased coronary heart disease risk. A controlled randomized lifestyle intervention study. *Ann Nutr Metab* 47:306–311.

154. Anderson, J.W., Allgood, L.D., Lawrence, A., Altringer, L.A., Jerdack, G.R., Hengehold, D.A., and Morel, J.G. 2000. Cholesterol-lowering effects of psyllium intake adjunctive to diet therapy in men and women with hypercholesterolemia: Meta-analysis of 8 controlled trials. *Am J Clin Nutr* 71:472–479.

155. Sprecher, D.L., Harris, B.V., Goldberg, A.C., Anderson, E.C., Bayuk, L.M., Russell, B.S., Crone, D.S., Quinn, C., Bateman, J., Kuzmak, B.R. et al. 1993. Efficacy of psyllium in reducing serum cholesterol levels in hypercholesterolemic patients on high- or low-fat diets. *Ann Intern Med* 119:545–554.

156. Keenan, J.M., Pins, J.J., Frazel, C., Moran, A., and Turnquist, L. 2002. Oat ingestion reduces systolic and diastolic blood pressure in patients with mild or borderline hypertension: A pilot trial. *J Fam Pract* 51:369.

157. Pins, J.J., Geleva, D., Keenan, J.M., Frazel, C., O'Connor, P.J., and Cherney, L.M. 2002. Do whole-grain oat cereals reduce the need for antihypertensive medications and improve blood pressure control? *J Fam Pract* 51:353–359.

158. Saltzman, E., Das, S.K., Lichtenstein, A.H., Dallal, G.E., Corrales, A., Schaefer, E.J., Greenberg, A.S., and Roberts, S.B. 2001. An oat-containing hypocaloric diet reduces systolic blood pressure and improves lipid profile beyond effects of weight loss in men and women. *J Nutr* 131:1465–1470.

159. Burdge, G.C., Jones, A.E., and Wootton, S.A. 2002. Eicosapentaenoic and docosapentaenoic acids are the principal products of alpha-linolenic acid metabolism in young men. *Br J Nutr* 88:355–363.

160. Burdge, G. 2004. Alpha-linolenic acid metabolism in men and women: nutritional and biological implications. *Curr Opin Clin Nutr Metab Care* 7:137–144.

161. Burdge, G.C. and Wootton, S.A. 2002. Conversion of alpha-linolenic acid to eicosapentaenoic, docosapentaenoic and docosahexaenoic acids in young women. *Br J Nutr* 88:411–420.

162. Balk, E.M., Lichtenstein, A.H., Chung, M., Kupelnick, B., Chew, P., and Lau, J. 2006. Effects of omega-3 fatty acids on serum markers of cardiovascular disease risk: A systematic review. *Atherosclerosis* 189:19–30.

163. Casula, M., Soranna, D., Catapano, A.L., and Corrao, G. 2013. Long-term effect of high dose omega-3 fatty acid supplementation for secondary prevention of cardiovascular outcomes: A meta-analysis of randomized, placebo controlled trials [corrected]. *Atheroscler Suppl* 14:243–251.

164. Mozaffarian, D., Lemaitre, R.N., King, I.B., Song, X., Huang, H., Sacks, F.M., Rimm, E.B., Wang, M., and Siscovick, D.S. 2013. Plasma phospholipid long-chain omega-3 fatty acids and total and cause-specific mortality in older adults: A cohort study. *Ann Intern Med* 158:515–525.

165. Mozaffarian, D. and Wu, J.H. 2011. Omega-3 fatty acids and cardiovascular disease: Effects on risk factors, molecular pathways, and clinical events. *J Am Coll Cardiol* 58:2047–2067.

166. Park, K. and Mozaffarian, D. 2010. Omega-3 fatty acids, mercury, and selenium in fish and the risk of cardiovascular diseases. *Curr Atheroscler Rep* 12:414–422.

167. Rizos, E.C., Ntzani, E.E., Bika, E., Kostapanos, M.S., and Elisaf, M.S. 2012. Association between omega-3 fatty acid supplementation and risk of major cardiovascular disease events: A systematic review and meta-analysis. *JAMA* 308:1024–1033.

168. Kwak, S.M., Myung, S.K., Lee, Y.J., and Seo, H.G. 2012. Efficacy of omega-3 fatty acid supplements (eicosapentaenoic acid and docosahexaenoic acid) in the secondary prevention of cardiovascular disease: A meta-analysis of randomized, double-blind, placebo-controlled trials. *Arch Intern Med* 172:686–694.

169. 1999. Dietary supplementation with n-3 polyunsaturated fatty acids and vitamin E after myocardial infarction: Results of the GISSI-Prevenzione trial. Gruppo Italiano per lo Studio della Sopravvivenza nell'Infarto miocardico. *Lancet* 354:447–455.

170. Leon, H., Shibata, M.C., Sivakumaran, S., Dorgan, M., Chatterley, T., and Tsuyuki, R.T. 2008. Effect of fish oil on arrhythmias and mortality: Systematic review. *BMJ* 337:A2931.

171. Tavazzi, L., Maggioni, A.P., Marchioli, R., Barlera, S., Franzosi, M.G., Latini, R., Lucci, D., Nicolosi, G.L., Porcu, M., and Tognoni, G. 2008. Effect of n-3 polyunsaturated fatty acids in patients with chronic heart failure (the GISSI-HF trial): A randomised, double-blind, placebo-controlled trial. *Lancet* 372:1223–1230.

172. Lonn, E., Bosch, J., Yusuf, S., Sheridan, P., Pogue, J., Arnold, J.M., Ross, C., Arnold, A., Sleight, P., Probstfield, J. et al. 2005. Effects of long-term vitamin E supplementation on cardiovascular events and cancer: A randomized controlled trial. *JAMA* 293:1338–1347.

173. Roberts, L.J., 2nd, Oates, J.A., Linton, M.F., Fazio, S., Meador, B.P., Gross, M.D., Shyr, Y., and Morrow, J.D. 2007. The relationship between dose of vitamin E and suppression of oxidative stress in humans. *Free Radic Biol Med* 43:1388–1393.

174. Sesso, H.D., Buring, J.E., Christen, W.G., Kurth, T., Belanger, C., MacFadyen, J., Bubes, V., Manson, J.E., Glynn, R.J., and Gaziano, J.M. 2008. Vitamins E and C in the prevention of cardiovascular disease in men: The Physicians' Health Study II randomized controlled trial. *JAMA* 300:2123–2133.

175. Gutierrez, A.D., de Serna, D.G., Robinson, I., and Schade, D.S. 2009. The response of gamma vitamin E to varying dosages of alpha vitamin E plus vitamin C. *Metabolism* 58:469–478.

176. Ye, Z. and Song, H. 2008. Antioxidant vitamins intake and the risk of coronary heart disease: Meta-analysis of cohort studies. *Eur J Cardiovasc Prev Rehabil* 15:26–34.

177. Bazzano, L.A., Reynolds, K., Holder, K.N., and He, J. 2006. Effect of folic acid supplementation on risk of cardiovascular diseases: A meta-analysis of randomized controlled trials. *JAMA* 296:2720–2726.

178. Bleys, J., Miller, E.R., 3rd, Pastor-Barriuso, R., Appel, L.J., and Guallar, E. 2006. Vitamin-mineral supplementation and the progression of atherosclerosis: A meta-analysis of randomized controlled trials. *Am J Clin Nutr* 84:880–887; quiz 954–885.

179. Bonaa, K.H., Njolstad, I., Ueland, P.M., Schirmer, H., Tverdal, A., Steigen, T., Wang, H., Nordrehaug, J.E., Arnesen, E., Rasmussen, K. et al. 2006. Homocysteine lowering and cardiovascular events after acute myocardial infarction. *N Engl J Med* 354:1578–1588.

180. Cavalieri, M., Schmidt, R., Chen, C., Mok, V., de Freitas, G.R., Song, S., Yi, Q., Ropele, S., Grazer, A., Homayoon, N. et al. 2012. B vitamins and magnetic resonance imaging-detected ischemic brain lesions in patients with recent transient ischemic attack or stroke: The VITAmins TO Prevent Stroke (VITATOPS) MRI-substudy. *Stroke* 43:3266–3270.

181. Hankey, G.J., Ford, A.H., Yi, Q., Eikelboom, J.W., Lees, K.R., Chen, C., Xavier, D., Navarro, J.C., Ranawaka, U.K., Uddin, W. et al. 2013. Effect of B vitamins and lowering homocysteine on cognitive impairment in patients with previous stroke or transient ischemic attack: A prespecified secondary analysis of a randomized, placebo-controlled trial and meta-analysis. *Stroke* 44:2232–2239.

182. Lee, M., Markovic, D., and Ovbiagele, B. 2013. Impact and interaction of low estimated GFR and B vitamin therapy on prognosis among ischemic stroke patients: The Vitamin Intervention for Stroke Prevention (VISP) trial. *Am J Kidney Dis* 62:52–57.

183. McNulty, H., Dowey le, R.C., Strain, J.J., Dunne, A., Ward, M., Molloy, A.M., McAnena, L.B., Hughes, J.P., Hannon-Fletcher, M., and Scott, J.M. 2006. Riboflavin lowers homocysteine in individuals homozygous for the MTHFR 677C- > T polymorphism. *Circulation* 113:74–80.

184. Wilson, C.P., McNulty, H., Ward, M., Strain, J.J., Trouton, T.G., Hoeft, B.A., Weber, P., Roos, F.F., Horigan, G., McAnena, L. et al. 2013. Blood pressure in treated hypertensive individuals with the MTHFR 677TT genotype is responsive to intervention with riboflavin: Findings of a targeted randomized trial. *Hypertension* 61:1302–1308.

185. Bradley, R.B. and Oberg, E.B. 2009. Integrative treatments to reduce risk for cardiovascular disease. *Integrative Medicine* 8:7.

186. Pan, J., Lin, M., Kesala, R.L., Van, J., and Charles, M.A. 2002. Niacin treatment of the atherogenic lipid profile and Lp(a) in diabetes. *Diabetes Obes Metab* 4:255–261.

187. Miller, M. 2003. Niacin as a component of combination therapy for dyslipidemia. *Mayo Clin Proc* 78:735–742.

188. Boden, W.E., Probstfield, J.L., Anderson, T., Chaitman, B.R., Desvignes-Nickens, P., Koprowicz, K., McBride, R., Teo, K., and Weintraub, W. 2011. Niacin in patients with low HDL cholesterol levels receiving intensive statin therapy. *N Engl J Med* 365:2255–2267.

189. Mullin, G.E., Greenson, J.K., and Mitchell, M.C. 1989. Fulminant hepatic failure after ingestion of sustained-release nicotinic acid. *Ann Intern Med* 111:253–255.

190. Kendrick, J., Targher, G., Smits, G., and Chonchol, M. 2008. 25-Hydroxyvitamin D deficiency is independently associated with cardiovascular disease in the Third National Health and Nutrition Examination Survey. *Atherosclerosis*.

191. Lee, J.H., O'Keefe, J.H., Bell, D., Hensrud, D.D., and Holick, M.F. 2008. Vitamin D deficiency an important, common, and easily treatable cardiovascular risk factor? *J Am Coll Cardiol* 52:1949–1956.

192. Schleithoff, S.S., Zittermann, A., Tenderich, G., Berthold, H.K., Stehle, P., and Koerfer, R. 2006. Vitamin D supplementation improves cytokine profiles in patients with congestive heart failure: A double-blind, randomized, placebo-controlled trial. *Am J Clin Nutr* 83:754–759.

193. Demir, M., Uyan, U., and Melek, M. 2014. The effects of vitamin D deficiency on atrial fibrillation. *Clin Appl Thromb Hemost* 20:98–103.

194. Perez-Lopez, F.R. 2009. Vitamin D metabolism and cardiovascular risk factors in postmenopausal women. *Maturitas* 62:248–262.

195. Zittermann, A., Frisch, S., Berthold, H.K., Gotting, C., Kuhn, J., Kleesiek, K., Stehle, P., Koertke, H., and Koerfer, R. 2009. Vitamin D supplementation enhances the beneficial effects of weight loss on cardiovascular disease risk markers. *Am J Clin Nutr* 89:1321–1327.

196. Bernini, G., Carrara, D., Bacca, A., Carli, V., Virdis, A., Rugani, I., Duranti, E., Ghiadoni, L., Bernini, M., and Taddei, S. 2013. Effect of acute and chronic vitamin D administration on systemic renin angiotensin system in essential hypertensives and controls. *J Endocrinol Invest* 36:216–220.

197. Forman, J.P., Scott, J.B., Ng, K., Drake, B.F., Suarez, E.G., Hayden, D.L., Bennett, G.G., Chandler, P.D., Hollis, B.W., Emmons, K.M. et al. 2013. Effect of vitamin D supplementation on blood pressure in blacks. *Hypertension* 61:779–785.

198. Margolis, K.L., Ray, R.M., Van Horn, L., Manson, J.E., Allison, M.A., Black, H.R., Beresford, S.A., Connelly, S.A., Curb, J.D., Grimm, R.H., Jr. et al. 2008. Effect of calcium and vitamin D supplementation on blood pressure: The Women's Health Initiative Randomized Trial. *Hypertension* 52:847–855.

199. Larsen, T., Mose, F.H., Bech, J.N., Hansen, A.B., and Pedersen, E.B. 2012. Effect of cholecalciferol supplementation during winter months in patients with hypertension: A randomized, placebo-controlled trial. *Am J Hypertens* 25:1215–1222.

200. Pfeifer, M., Begerow, B., Minne, H.W., Nachtigall, D., and Hansen, C. 2001. Effects of a short-term vitamin D(3) and calcium supplementation on blood pressure and parathyroid hormone levels in elderly women. *J Clin Endocrinol Metab* 86:1633–1637.

201. Traub, M.L., Finnell, J.S., Bhandiwad, A., Oberg, E., Suhaila, L., and Bradley, R. 2014. Impact of vitamin D3 dietary supplement matrix on clinical response. *J Clin Endocrinol Metab*:jc20133162.

202. Michos, E.D. and Melamed, M.L. 2008. Vitamin D and cardiovascular disease risk. *Curr Opin Clin Nutr Metab Care* 11:7–12.

203. Al-Delaimy, W.K., Ferrari, P., Slimani, N., Pala, V., Johansson, I., Nilsson, S., Mattisson, I., Wirfalt, E., Galasso, R., Palli, D. et al. 2005. Plasma carotenoids as biomarkers of intake of fruits and vegetables: Individual-level correlations in the European Prospective Investigation into Cancer and Nutrition (EPIC). *Eur J Clin Nutr* 59:1387–1396.

204. Campbell, D.R., Gross, M.D., Martini, M.C., Grandits, G.A., Slavin, J.L., and Potter, J.D. 1994. Plasma carotenoids as biomarkers of vegetable and fruit intake. *Cancer Epidemiol Biomarkers Prev* 3:493–500.

205. Hozawa, A., Jacobs, D.R., Jr., Steffes, M.W., Gross, M.D., Steffen, L.M., and Lee, D.H. 2007. Relationships of circulating carotenoid concentrations with several markers of inflammation, oxidative stress, and endothelial dysfunction: The Coronary Artery Risk Development in Young Adults (CARDIA)/Young Adult Longitudinal Trends in Antioxidants (YALTA) study. *Clin Chem* 53:447–455.

206. Iribarren, C., Folsom, A.R., Jacobs, D.R., Jr., Gross, M.D., Belcher, J.D., and Eckfeldt, J.H. 1997. Association of serum vitamin levels, LDL susceptibility to oxidation, and autoantibodies against MDA-LDL with carotid atherosclerosis. A case-control study. The ARIC Study Investigators. Atherosclerosis Risk in Communities. *Arterioscler Thromb Vasc Biol* 17:1171–1177.

207. Carroll, Y.L., Corridan, B.M., and Morrissey, P.A. 2000. Lipoprotein carotenoid profiles and the susceptibility of low density lipoprotein to oxidative modification in healthy elderly volunteers. *Eur J Clin Nutr* 54:500–507.

208. Hininger, I.A., Meyer-Wenger, A., Moser, U., Wright, A., Southon, S., Thurnham, D., Chopra, M., Van Den Berg, H., Olmedilla, B., Favier, A.E. et al. 2001. No significant effects of lutein, lycopene or beta-carotene supplementation on biological markers of oxidative stress and LDL oxidizability in healthy adult subjects. *J Am Coll Nutr* 20:232–238.

209. Paterson, E., Gordon, M.H., Niwat, C., George, T.W., Parr, L., Waroonphan, S., and Lovegrove, J.A. 2006. Supplementation with fruit and vegetable soups and beverages increases plasma carotenoid concentrations but does not alter markers of oxidative stress or cardiovascular risk factors. *J Nutr* 136:2849–2855.

210. Kim, J.Y., Paik, J.K., Kim, O.Y., Park, H.W., Lee, J.H., Jang, Y., and Lee, J.H. 2011. Effects of lycopene supplementation on oxidative stress and markers of endothelial function in healthy men. *Atherosclerosis* 215:189–195.

211. McEneny, J., Wade, L., Young, I.S., Masson, L., Duthie, G., McGinty, A., McMaster, C., and Thies, F. 2013. Lycopene intervention reduces inflammation and improves HDL functionality in moderately overweight middle-aged individuals. *J Nutr Biochem* 24:163–168.

212. Silaste, M.L., Alfthan, G., Aro, A., Kesaniemi, Y.A., and Horkko, S. 2007. Tomato juice decreases LDL cholesterol levels and increases LDL resistance to oxidation. *Br J Nutr* 98:1251–1258.

213. Xaplanteris, P., Vlachopoulos, C., Pietri, P., Terentes-Printzios, D., Kardara, D., Alexopoulos, N., Aznaouridis, K., Miliou, A., and Stefanadis, C. 2012. Tomato paste supplementation improves endothelial dynamics and reduces plasma total oxidative status in healthy subjects. *Nutr Res* 32:390–394.

214. Stangl, V., Kuhn, C., Hentschel, S., Jochmann, N., Jacob, C., Bohm, V., Frohlich, K., Muller, L., Gericke, C., and Lorenz, M. 2011. Lack of effects of tomato products on endothelial function in human subjects: Results of a randomised, placebo-controlled cross-over study. *Br J Nutr* 105:263–267.

215. Thies, F., Masson, L.F., Rudd, A., Vaughan, N., Tsang, C., Brittenden, J., Simpson, W.G., Duthie, S., Horgan, G.W., and Duthie, G. 2012. Effect of a tomato-rich diet on markers of cardiovascular disease risk in moderately overweight, disease-free, middle-aged adults: A randomized controlled trial. *Am J Clin Nutr* 95:1013–1022.

216. Zou, Z.Y., Xu, X.R., Lin, X.M., Zhang, H.B., Xiao, X., Ouyang, L., Huang, Y.M., Wang, X., and Liu, Y.Q. 2014. Effects of lutein and lycopene on carotid intima-media thickness in Chinese subjects with subclinical atherosclerosis: A randomised, double-blind, placebo-controlled trial. *Br J Nutr* 111:474–480.

217. Flore, R., Ponziani, F.R., Di Rienzo, T.A., Zocco, M.A., Flex, A., Gerardino, L., Lupascu, A., Santoro, L., Santoliquido, A., Di Stasio, E. et al. 2013. Something more to say about calcium homeostasis: The role of vitamin K2 in vascular calcification and osteoporosis. *Eur Rev Med Pharmacol Sci* 17:2433–2440.

218. Kidd, P.M. 2010. Vitamins D and K as pleiotropic nutrients: Clinical importance to the skeletal and cardiovascular systems and preliminary evidence for synergy. *Altern Med Rev* 15:199–222.

219. McCabe, K.M., Booth, S.L., Fu, X., Shobeiri, N., Pang, J.J., Adams, M.A., and Holden, R.M. 2013. Dietary vitamin K and therapeutic warfarin alter the susceptibility to vascular calcification in experimental chronic kidney disease. *Kidney Int* 83:835–844.

220. Rees, K., Guraewal, S., Wong, Y.L., Majanbu, D.L., Mavrodaris, A., Stranges, S., Kandala, N.B., Clarke, A., and Franco, O.H. 2010. Is vitamin K consumption associated with cardio-metabolic disorders? A systematic review. *Maturitas* 67:121–128.

221. Gast, G.C., de Roos, N.M., Sluijs, I., Bots, M.L., Beulens, J.W., Geleijnse, J.M., Witteman, J.C., Grobbee, D.E., Peeters, P.H., and van der Schouw, Y.T. 2009. A high menaquinone intake reduces the incidence of coronary heart disease. *Nutr Metab Cardiovasc Dis* 19:504–510.

222. Kawashima, H., Nakajima, Y., Matubara, Y., Nakanowatari, J., Fukuta, T., Mizuno, S., Takahashi, S., Tajima, T., and Nakamura, T. 1997. Effects of vitamin K2 (menatetrenone) on atherosclerosis and blood coagulation in hypercholesterolemic rabbits. *Jpn J Pharmacol* 75:135–143.

223. Wallin, R., Schurgers, L., and Wajih, N. 2008. Effects of the blood coagulation vitamin K as an inhibitor of arterial calcification. *Thromb Res* 122:411–417.

224. Hsia, J., Heiss, G., Ren, H., Allison, M., Dolan, N.C., Greenland, P., Heckbert, S.R., Johnson, K.C., Manson, J.E., Sidney, S. et al. 2007. Calcium/vitamin D supplementation and cardiovascular events. *Circulation* 115:846–854.

225. Bolland, M.J., Barber, P.A., Doughty, R.N., Mason, B., Horne, A., Ames, R., Gamble, G.D., Grey, A., and Reid, I.R. 2008. Vascular events in healthy older women receiving calcium supplementation: Randomised controlled trial. *BMJ* 336:262–266.
226. Dickinson, H.O., Nicolson, D.J., Cook, J.V., Campbell, F., Beyer, F.R., Ford, G.A., and Mason, J. 2006. Calcium supplementation for the management of primary hypertension in adults. *Cochrane Database Syst Rev* 3:CD004639.
227. Gums, J.G. 2004. Magnesium in cardiovascular and other disorders. *Am J Health Syst Pharm* 61:1569–1576.
228. Champagne, C.M. 2008. Magnesium in hypertension, cardiovascular disease, metabolic syndrome, and other conditions: A review. *Nutr Clin Pract* 23:142–151.
229. Dickinson, H.O., Nicolson, D.J., Campbell, F., Cook, J.V., Beyer, F.R., Ford, G.A., and Mason, J. 2006. Magnesium supplementation for the management of essential hypertension in adults. *Cochrane Database Syst Rev* 3:CD004640.
230. Jee, S.H., Miller, E.R., 3rd, Guallar, E., Singh, V.K., Appel, L.J., and Klag, M.J. 2002. The effect of magnesium supplementation on blood pressure: A meta-analysis of randomized clinical trials. *Am J Hypertens* 15:691–696.
231. Li, J., Zhang, Q., Zhang, M., and Egger, M. 2007. Intravenous magnesium for acute myocardial infarction. *Cochrane Database Syst Rev*:CD002755.
232. Shechter, M. 2003. Does magnesium have a role in the treatment of patients with coronary artery disease? *Am J Cardiovasc Drugs* 3:231–239.
233. Nakashima, H., Katayama, T., Honda, Y., Suzuki, S., and Yano, K. 2004. Cardioprotective effects of magnesium sulfate in patients undergoing primary coronary angioplasty for acute myocardial infarction. *Circ J* 68:23–28.
234. He, F.J., and MacGregor, G.A. 2003. Potassium: More beneficial effects. *Climacteric* 6(Suppl 3):36–48.
235. Dickinson, H.O., Nicolson, D.J., Campbell, F., Beyer, F.R., and Mason, J. 2006. Potassium supplementation for the management of primary hypertension in adults. *Cochrane Database Syst Rev* 3:CD004641.
236. Zillich, A.J., Garg, J., Basu, S., Bakris, G.L., and Carter, B.L. 2006. Thiazide diuretics, potassium, and the development of diabetes: A quantitative review. *Hypertension* 48:219–224.
237. Hughes, S. and Samman, S. 2006. The effect of zinc supplementation in humans on plasma lipids, antioxidant status and thrombogenesis. *J Am Coll Nutr* 25:285–291.
238. Alsafwah, S., Laguardia, S.P., Arroyo, M., Dockery, B.K., Bhattacharya, S.K., Ahokas, R.A., and Newman, K.P. 2007. Congestive heart failure is a systemic illness: A role for minerals and micronutrients. *Clin Med Res* 5:238–243.
239. Klevay, L.M. 1998. Lack of a recommended dietary allowance for copper may be hazardous to your health. *J Am Coll Nutr* 17:322–326.
240. Prohaska, J.R. 2014. Impact of copper deficiency in humans. *Ann N Y Acad Sci* 1314:1–5.
241. Hoffman, H.N., 2nd, Phyliky, R.L., and Fleming, C.R. 1988. Zinc-induced copper deficiency. *Gastroenterology* 94:508–512.
242. Hummel, M., Standl, E., and Schnell, O. 2007. Chromium in metabolic and cardiovascular disease. *Horm Metab Res* 39:743–751.
243. Lubitz, S.A., Goldbarg, S.H., and Mehta, D. 2008. Sudden cardiac death in infiltrative cardiomyopathies: Sarcoidosis, scleroderma, amyloidosis, hemachromatosis. *Prog Cardiovasc Dis* 51:58–73.
244. Shizukuda, Y., Bolan, C.D., Tripodi, D.J., Yau, Y.Y., Smith, K.P., Sachdev, V., Birdsall, C.W., Sidenko, S., Waclawiw, M.A., Leitman, S.F. et al. 2006. Left ventricular systolic function during stress echocardiography exercise in subjects with asymptomatic hereditary hemochromatosis. *Am J Cardiol* 98:694–698.

245. Elmberg, M., Hultcrantz, R., Simard, J.F., Stal, P., Pehrsson, K., and Askling, J. 2012. Risk of ischaemic heart disease and cardiomyopathy in patients with haemochromatosis and in their first-degree relatives: A nationwide, population-based study. *J Intern Med* 272:45–54.

246. Waalen, J., Felitti, V., Gelbart, T., Ho, N.J., and Beutler, E. 2002. Prevalence of coronary heart disease associated with HFE mutations in adults attending a health appraisal center. *Am J Med* 113:472–479.

247. Zegrean, M. 2009. Association of body iron stores with development of cardiovascular disease in the adult population: A systematic review of the literature. *Can J Cardiovasc Nurs* 19:26–32.

248. Barton, J.C. 2007. Chelation therapy for iron overload. *Curr Gastroenterol Rep* 9:74–82.

249. Houschyar, K.S., Ludtke, R., Dobos, G.J., Kalus, U., Broecker-Preuss, M., Rampp, T., Brinkhaus, B., and Michalsen, A. 2012. Effects of phlebotomy-induced reduction of body iron stores on metabolic syndrome: Results from a randomized clinical trial. *BMC Med* 10:54.

250. Hanaki, Y., Sugiyama, S., Ozawa, T., and Ohno, M. 1991. Ratio of low-density lipoprotein cholesterol to ubiquinone as a coronary risk factor. *N Engl J Med* 325:814–815.

251. Molyneux, S.L., Florkowski, C.M., George, P.M., Pilbrow, A.P., Frampton, C.M., Lever, M., and Richards, A.M. 2008. Coenzyme Q10: An independent predictor of mortality in chronic heart failure. *J Am Coll Cardiol* 52:1435–1441.

252. Keogh, A., Fenton, S., Leslie, C., Aboyoun, C., Macdonald, P., Zhao, Y.C., Bailey, M., and Rosenfeldt, F. 2003. Randomised double-blind, placebo-controlled trial of coenzyme Q, therapy in class II and III systolic heart failure. *Heart Lung Circ* 12:135–141.

253. Cicero, A.F., Derosa, G., Miconi, A., Laghi, L., Nascetti, S., and Gaddi, A. 2005. Possible role of ubiquinone in the treatment of massive hypertriglyceridemia resistant to PUFA and fibrates. *Biomed Pharmacother* 59:312–317.

254. Rosenfeldt, F.L., Haas, S.J., Krum, H., Hadj, A., Ng, K., Leong, J.Y., and Watts, G.F. 2007. Coenzyme Q10 in the treatment of hypertension: A meta-analysis of the clinical trials. *J Hum Hypertens* 21:297–306.

255. Fujioka, T., Sakamoto, Y., and Mimura, G. 1983. Clinical study of cardiac arrhythmias using a 24-hour continuous electrocardiographic recorder (5th report)—Antiarrhythmic action of coenzyme Q10 in diabetics. *Tohoku J Exp Med* 141:453–463.

256. Kamikawa, T., Kobayashi, A., Yamashita, T., Hayashi, H., and Yamazaki, N. 1985. Effects of coenzyme Q10 on exercise tolerance in chronic stable angina pectoris. *Am J Cardiol* 56:247–251.

257. Singh, R.B., Neki, N.S., Kartikey, K., Pella, D., Kumar, A., Niaz, M.A., and Thakur, A.S. 2003. Effect of coenzyme Q10 on risk of atherosclerosis in patients with recent myocardial infarction. *Mol Cell Biochem* 246:75–82.

258. Young, J.M., Florkowski, C.M., Molyneux, S.L., McEwan, R.G., Frampton, C.M., George, P.M., and Scott, R.S. 2007. Effect of coenzyme Q(10) supplementation on simvastatin-induced myalgia. *Am J Cardiol* 100:1400–1403.

259. Langsjoen, P.H., Langsjoen, J.O., Langsjoen, A.M., and Lucas, L.A. 2005. Treatment of statin adverse effects with supplemental coenzyme Q10 and statin drug discontinuation. *Biofactors* 25:147–152.

260. Caso, G., Kelly, P., McNurlan, M.A., and Lawson, W.E. 2007. Effect of coenzyme Q10 on myopathic symptoms in patients treated with statins. *Am J Cardiol* 99:1409–1412.

261. Hidaka, T., Fujii, K., Funahashi, I., Fukutomi, N., and Hosoe, K. 2008. Safety assessment of coenzyme Q10 (CoQ10). *Biofactors* 32:199–208.

262. Tripp, M.E., Katcher, M.L., Peters, H.A., Gilbert, E.F., Arya, S., Hodach, R.J., and Shug, A.L. 1981. Systemic carnitine deficiency presenting as familial endocardial fibroelastosis: A treatable cardiomyopathy. *N Engl J Med* 305:385–390.

263. Malaguarnera, M., Vacante, M., Avitabile, T., Cammalleri, L., and Motta, M. 2009. L-Carnitine supplementation reduces oxidized LDL cholesterol in patients with diabetes. *Am J Clin Nutr* 89:71–76.

264. McMackin, C.J., Widlansky, M.E., Hamburg, N.M., Huang, A.L., Weller, S., Holbrook, M., Gokce, N., Hagen, T.M., Keaney, J.F., Jr., and Vita, J.A. 2007. Effect of combined treatment with alpha-Lipoic acid and acetyl-L-carnitine on vascular function and blood pressure in patients with coronary artery disease. *J Clin Hypertens* (*Greenwich*) 9:249–255.

265. Lango, R., Smolenski, R.T., Narkiewicz, M., Suchorzewska, J., and Lysiak-Szydlowska, W. 2001. Influence of L-carnitine and its derivatives on myocardial metabolism and function in ischemic heart disease and during cardiopulmonary bypass. *Cardiovasc Res* 51:21–29.

266. Singh, R.B. and Aslam, M. 1998. L-carnitine administration in coronary artery disease and cardiomyopathy. *J Assoc Physicians India* 46:801–805.

267. Pauly, D.F. and Pepine, C.J. 2003. The role of carnitine in myocardial dysfunction. *Am J Kidney Dis* 41:S35–43.

268. Witte, K.K., Clark, A.L., and Cleland, J.G. 2001. Chronic heart failure and micronutrients. *J Am Coll Cardiol* 37:1765–1774.

269. Koeth, R.A., Wang, Z., Levison, B.S., Buffa, J.A., Org, E., Sheehy, B.T., Britt, E.B., Fu, X., Wu, Y., Li, L. et al. 2013. Intestinal microbiota metabolism of l-carnitine, a nutrient in red meat, promotes atherosclerosis. *Nat Med* 19(5):576–585.

270. Sinatra, S.T. 2009. Metabolic cardiology: The missing link in cardiovascular disease. *Altern Ther Health Med* 15:48–50.

271. Omran, H., Illien, S., MacCarter, D., St Cyr, J., and Luderitz, B. 2003. D-Ribose improves diastolic function and quality of life in congestive heart failure patients: A prospective feasibility study. *Eur J Heart Fail* 5:615–619.

272. Pliml, W., von Arnim, T., Stablein, A., Hofmann, H., Zimmer, H.G., and Erdmann, E. 1992. Effects of ribose on exercise-induced ischaemia in stable coronary artery disease. *Lancet* 340:507–510.

273. Jabecka, A., Ast, J., Bogdaski, P., Drozdowski, M., Pawlak-Lemaska, K., Cielewicz, A.R., and Pupek-Musialik, D. 2012. Oral L-arginine supplementation in patients with mild arterial hypertension and its effect on plasma level of asymmetric dimethylarginine, L-citruline, L-arginine and antioxidant status. *Eur Rev Med Pharmacol Sci* 16:1665–1674.

274. Bouras, G., Deftereos, S., Tousoulis, D., Giannopoulos, G., Chatzis, G., Tsounis, D., Cleman, M.W., and Stefanadis, C. 2013. Asymmetric Dimethylarginine (ADMA): A promising biomarker for cardiovascular disease? *Curr Top Med Chem* 13:180–200.

275. Lucotti, P., Monti, L., Setola, E., La Canna, G., Castiglioni, A., Rossodivita, A., Pala, M.G., Formica, F., Paolini, G., Catapano, A.L. et al. 2009. Oral L-arginine supplementation improves endothelial function and ameliorates insulin sensitivity and inflammation in cardiopathic nondiabetic patients after an aortocoronary bypass. *Metabolism* 58:1270–1276.

276. Marchesi, S., Lupattelli, G., Siepi, D., Roscini, A.R., Vaudo, G., Sinzinger, H., and Mannarino, E. 2001. Oral L-arginine administration attenuates postprandial endothelial dysfunction in young healthy males. *J Clin Pharm Ther* 26:343–349.

277. Bednarz, B., Jaxa-Chamiec, T., Gebalska, J., Herbaczynska-Cedro, K., and Ceremuzynski, L. 2004. L-arginine supplementation prolongs exercise capacity in congestive heart failure. *Kardiol Pol* 60:348–353.

278. Orozco-Gutierrez, J.J., Castillo-Martinez, L., Orea-Tejeda, A., Vazquez-Diaz, O., Valdespino-Trejo, A., Narvaez-David, R., Keirns-Davis, C., Carrasco-Ortiz, O., Navarro-Navarro, A., and Sanchez-Santillan, R. 2010. Effect of L-arginine or L-citrulline oral supplementation on blood pressure and right ventricular function in heart failure patients with preserved ejection fraction. *Cardiol J* 17:612–618.

279. Ceremuzynski, L., Chamiec, T., and Herbaczynska-Cedro, K. 1997. Effect of supplemental oral L-arginine on exercise capacity in patients with stable angina pectoris. *Am J Cardiol* 80:331–333.

280. Wennmalm, A., Edlund, A., Granstrom, E.F., and Wiklund, O. 1995. Acute supplementation with the nitric oxide precursor L-arginine does not improve cardiovascular performance in patients with hypercholesterolemia. *Atherosclerosis* 118:223–231.

281. Wilson, A.M., Harada, R., Nair, N., Balasubramanian, N., and Cooke, J.P. 2007. L-arginine supplementation in peripheral arterial disease: No benefit and possible harm. *Circulation* 116:188–195.

282. Martina, V., Masha, A., Gigliardi, V.R., Brocato, L., Manzato, E., Berchio, A., Massarenti, P., Settanni, F., Della Casa, L., Bergamini, S. et al. 2008. Long-term N-acetylcysteine and L-arginine administration reduces endothelial activation and systolic blood pressure in hypertensive patients with type 2 diabetes. *Diabetes Care* 31:940–944.

283. Bouckenooghe, T., Remacle, C., and Reusens, B. 2006. Is taurine a functional nutrient? *Curr Opin Clin Nutr Metab Care* 9:728–733.

284. Huxtable, R.J. 1992. Physiological actions of taurine. *Physiol Rev* 72:101–163.

285. Ripps, H. and Shen, W. 2012. Review: Taurine: A "very essential" amino acid. *Mol Vis* 18:2673–2686.

286. Yamori, Y., Liu, L., Ikeda, K., Miura, A., Mizushima, S., Miki, T., and Nara, Y. 2001. Distribution of twenty-four hour urinary taurine excretion and association with ischemic heart disease mortality in 24 populations of 16 countries: Results from the WHO-CARDIAC study. *Hypertens Res* 24:453–457.

287. Yamori, Y., Liu, L., Mizushima, S., Ikeda, K., and Nara, Y. 2006. Male cardiovascular mortality and dietary markers in 25 population samples of 16 countries. *J Hypertens* 24:1499–1505.

288. Yamori, Y., Nara, Y., Mizushima, S., Sawamura, M., and Horie, R. 1994. Nutritional factors for stroke and major cardiovascular diseases: International epidemiological comparison of dietary prevention. *Health Rep* 6:22–27.

289. Zhang, M., Bi, L.F., Fang, J.H., Su, X.L., Da, G.L., Kuwamori, T., and Kagamimori, S. 2004. Beneficial effects of taurine on serum lipids in overweight or obese non-diabetic subjects. *Amino Acids* 26:267–271.

290. Azuma, J., Sawamura, A., Awata, N., Ohta, H., Hamaguchi, T., Harada, H., Takihara, K., Hasegawa, H., Yamagami, T., Ishiyama, T. et al. 1985. Therapeutic effect of taurine in congestive heart failure: A double-blind crossover trial. *Clin Cardiol* 8:276–282.

291. Beyranvand, M.R., Khalafi, M.K., Roshan, V.D., Choobineh, S., Parsa, S.A., and Piranfar, M.A. 2011. Effect of taurine supplementation on exercise capacity of patients with heart failure. *J Cardiol* 57:333–337.

292. Moloney, M.A., Casey, R.G., O'Donnell, D.H., Fitzgerald, P., Thompson, C., and Bouchier-Hayes, D.J. 2010. Two weeks taurine supplementation reverses endothelial dysfunction in young male type 1 diabetics. *Diab Vasc Dis Res* 7:300–310.

293. Jeejeebhoy, F., Keith, M., Freeman, M., Barr, A., McCall, M., Kurian, R., Mazer, D., and Errett, L. 2002. Nutritional supplementation with MyoVive repletes essential cardiac myocyte nutrients and reduces left ventricular size in patients with left ventricular dysfunction. *Am Heart J* 143:1092–1100.

294. Singh, R.B., Kartikey, K., Charu, A.S., Niaz, M.A., and Schaffer, S. 2003. Effect of taurine and coenzyme Q10 in patients with acute myocardial infarction. *Adv Exp Med Biol* 526:41–48.

9 Breast Cancer

Cynthia A. Thomson, PhD, RD
and Deborah Straub, MS, RDN

CONTENTS

INTRODUCTION

Much interest exists about the role nutrition plays in the etiology, treatment, and recurrence of breast cancer. To date, hundreds of studies have been published regarding the role of diet, nutrition, and body weight on breast cancer incidence. Evidence to date provides a rather clear indication that dietary choices, along with physical activity and maintenance of a healthy body weight can significantly reduce breast cancer risk.[1–3]

For women diagnosed with breast cancer, medical nutrition therapy during breast cancer treatment should address not only the usual side effects associated with cancer treatment, but also the symptoms and comorbidity of treatment, including therapies that block endogenous estrogen production. Further, it is estimated that over 80% of breast cancer survivors use complementary and alternative medicine (CAM) including dietary supplementation[4] thus understanding the current state of the evidence in this area is imperative if optimal medical nutrition therapy is to be provided to women with breast cancer.

Finally, the evidence evaluating the role of diet in modifying breast cancer recurrence and/or comorbidity after cancer has grown significantly in recent years. These data suggest modifications in diet (and physical activity) are likely to impact overall health and mortality and provide a viable approach for enhancing well-being after diagnosis and treatment.

BREAST CANCER INCIDENCE AND MORTALITY RATES

Breast cancer is the most common cancer in women. In 2014, it is estimated that 235,670 new cases of invasive breast cancer will be diagnosed.[5] Breast cancer rates had been continuously increasing for more than two decades, but decreased slightly from 2002 to 2003 due to the decline in the use of menopausal hormone therapy (HT) following publication of the results of the Women's Health Initiative (WHI) in 2002, which linked estrogen plus progestin HT use with increased risk of breast cancer and heart disease.[6] Breast cancer rates from 2005 to 2010 remained stable.

An estimated 62,570 new cases of in situ breast cancer are expected to be diagnosed in 2014.[5] While in situ disease is thought to be associated with greater risk for invasive breast cancer, there continues to be some debate in this regard.[7] Of note, no studies have targeted this diagnosis for dietary intervention despite evidence that dietary interventions can modulate early steps in the multistage carcinogenesis process.

Breast cancer is a highly treatable disease. Current estimates suggests that women diagnosed with early-stage disease will have a >95% probability of being alive 10 years following her diagnosis and recurrence rates remain very low.[5,8] Despite a favorable prognosis for early disease, the higher rates of diagnosis make breast cancer the second leading cause of cancer death in women following lung cancer.[8] An estimated 40,430 breast cancer deaths are expected in 2014. Death from breast cancer has steadily declined since 1989—a trend attributable to a combination of early detection and advancements in treatment. Of note, Hispanic and black women are less frequently diagnosed with breast cancer but continue to have poorer overall outcomes after diagnosis.[8]

BREAST ANATOMY AND ESTROGEN METABOLISM

The anatomy of the breast consists of primarily fat, connective tissue, epithelial cells, and glandular tissue arranged into lobules and ducts. The lobules are the milk-producing glands of the breast. Ducts connect the lobules to the nipple. Epithelial cells line the lobules and the ducts. These epithelial cells are the origin of abnormal cell growth and division that leads to a breast cancer diagnosis.

A variety of hormones—including estrogen, progesterone, insulin, and growth factors—contribute to breast tissue development in utero and during puberty, pregnancy, and lactation. After menopause, the glandular tissue atrophies as estrogen and progesterone levels decline. The female hormone estrogen is found in three forms: estradiol, estrone, and estriol. The most potent of these is estradiol. Estrogens circulate in the blood bound to sex-hormone-binding globulin (SHBG). Only unbound estrogens can enter target tissue cells and induce biological activity. Prior to menopause, estrogens are synthesized from cholesterol in the ovaries in response to pituitary hormones. The amount of estrogen produced after menopause, however, is significantly less than the amount produced prior to menopause. After menopause, estrogen is produced primarily by the aromatization of adrenal androstenedione to estrone in the peripheral tissues. Estrogens are also produced by the aromatization of androgens in fat cells, although this source of estrogen is thought to be much lower and may have reduced systemic effects. Estrogen levels are markedly reduced after menopause although the ovaries continue to make small amounts of testosterone, which is converted to estradiol. The metabolism of estrogen takes place predominantly in the liver through Phase I (hydroxylation) and Phase II (methylation, glucuronidation, and sulfation) pathways. Estrogen is excreted in the urine and feces.

Estrogens have a wide range of actions, such that they affect almost all systems of the body in a tissue-specific manner. Estrogens bind with high affinity to estrogen receptors (ER) in target cells. When estrogen is bound to the receptor, it initiates transcription of the estrogen-responsive target gene. Two forms of estrogen receptors are distinguished—alpha and beta—that differ in terms of their tissue distribution, binding affinity, and biological function. Different target cells may respond differently to estrogen depending on the ratio of receptor subtypes. The actions of the selective estrogen receptor modulators (SERMs) known as tamoxifen and raloxifene are examples of this phenomenon. These drugs act as estrogen in some tissue (bone) and block its action in other tissues (breast).

BREAST CANCER SUBTYPES

Breast cancers are primarily carcinomas of the epithelial cells. Breast cancer, historically was classified based only on whether the cancer arose from the epithelial cells of the ducts or the lobules and whether the cells infiltrated through the duct

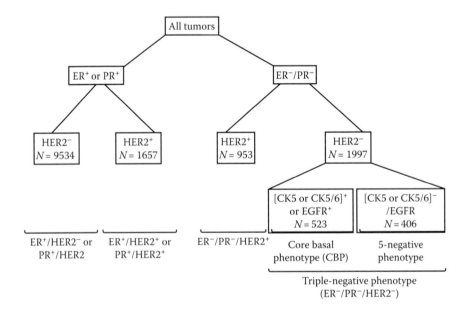

FIGURE 9.1 Breast tumor subtypes defined by the expression of estrogen receptor (ER), progesterone receptor (PR), HER2, cytokeratins 5 or 5/6 (CK5 or CK5/6), and epidermal growth factor receptor (EGFR) in 34 studies participating in the Breast Cancer Association Consortium. The number of case patients for each tumor subtype was pooled across all studies with data on the particular subtype.

or the lobule into the fatty tissue of the breast. More recently, breast tumors have been subtyped based on histological characteristics and molecular profiling as these inform more directly on treatment approaches (Figure 9.1). Luminal A tumors are the most common, accounting for approximately 50% of tumors diagnosed. These are associated with the best prognosis being less aggressive and of lower histological grade; Luminal B have a slightly poorer prognosis than Luminal A tumors. Normal like/unclassified tumors tend to present in younger women and have higher mitotic rates and higher grades resulting in poorer overall prognosis than luminal A and B tumors. ER-alpha negative tumors are associated with an overall poorer prognosis than ER-positive due to the lack of targeted therapy, particularly for women diagnosed with triple negative disease.[9]

Noninvasive breast cancers include ductal carcinoma in situ (DCIS) and lobular carcinoma in situ (LCIS). LCIS is not a true cancer, but it may increase a woman's risk of developing invasive breast cancer in the ipsilateral or in the contralateral breast. Inflammatory breast cancer is a rare but aggressive type of breast cancer; it accounts for 1%–5% of all breast cancer cases. Its symptoms may include redness, swelling, and warmth without a distinct tumor. Other less common ductal breast cancers include medullary, mucinous, papillary, and tubular carcinomas. Paget's disease of the nipple is rare and is responsible for only 1% of all breast cancers.

BREAST CANCER RISK FACTORS

There are several risk factors for breast cancer including age, family history, and prior breast biopsy, especially when atypical hyperplasia is identified. Estrogen exposure is a well-established risk factor for breast cancer given its profound influence on epithelial cell growth.[3] Cumulative, excessive estrogen exposure over the course of a lifetime contributes to breast cancer risk and may be a cause of this disease. Early menarche, late menopause, low parity, or delayed parity all increase a woman's breast cancer risk.[8] Greater estrogen exposure over a women's life course can have direct genotoxic effects by increasing breast cell proliferation and random genetic errors affecting cellular differentiation and gene expression. The mechanisms of carcinogenesis include the metabolism of estrogen to mutagenic, genotoxic metabolites and the stimulation of tissue growth. These processes cause initiation, promotion, and progression of breast cancer.

Risk prediction models can be helpful in assessing a woman's risk for breast cancer. The Breast Cancer Risk Assessment Tool is a computer assessment tool developed by the National Cancer Institute and the National Surgical Adjuvant Breast and Bowel Project (NSABP).[10] It estimates breast cancer risk over the woman's next 5 years and over a lifetime and is based on the Gail model. The risk factors included in this tool are age, age at menarche, age at first live birth, breast cancer among first-degree relatives, and breast biopsies. The Breast Cancer Risk Assessment Tool was developed and validated for primarily non-Hispanic white women in the United States who are age 35 or older. More research is needed to refine and validate this model for other racial and ethnic groups and to develop the recommended individual risk-level standards of care for risk prediction as well as prevention.[11]

Breast density has been strongly associated with breast cancer risk conferring an almost fourfold greater risk for breast cancer as compared to low breast density. Hormonal therapy, particularly estrogen plus progestin, is clearly associated with greater risk for postmenopausal disease based on the large WHI HT trial conducted.[12] Historically, both BMI and adult weight gain have been associated with greater risk for postmenopausal breast cancer but shown to be protective in relation to premenopausal breast cancer.[13] However, more recent evidence suggests this may not hold for young women at greater risk for disease[14] or possibly across race/ethnic groups.[15]

Additionally, radiation exposure to the chest for treatment of childhood or young adulthood cancers has been associated with an increased the risk of breast cancer in adulthood.[16]

GENETIC BREAST CANCER

Genetic breast cancer, in which one dominant cancer gene is passed on to future generations, accounts for only 5%–10% of all breast cancer cases.[8] Most breast cancer cases are sporadic, meaning that there is no family history; indeed, 70%–80% of women who get breast cancer do not have a family history of this disease. A number of genetic mutations have been identified that increase the risk of breast cancer. Notably, mutations in the tumor suppression genes *BRCA1* and *BRCA2* confer up to a 50%–80% lifetime chance of developing breast cancer. *BRCA* mutations are most often found in Jewish women of Ashkenazi (Eastern European) origin, but can appear in any racial or ethnic group.

SCREENING

The goal of screening is to detect breast cancer when it is more likely to be at an early stage, have a better prognosis, and be more successfully treated. Screen-detected breast cancers with or without clinical breast exams are associated with reduced morbidity and mortality. The American Cancer Society has established screening guidelines for breast cancer.[17] Mammography screening is the primary tool for early detection and is recommended annually for women starting at age 40 or 50 years, depending on other risk factors. A 2009 summary statement from the U.S. Preventive Services Taskforce suggested screening could be delayed until age 50 years, depending on risk factors and that insufficient evidence exists for screening beyond age 70 years.[18] More recent analyses suggest that screening after age 75 years results in detection of disease at an earlier stage and thus are likely to be associated with reduced morbidity and mortality even in older women.[19]

DIAGNOSIS

A diagnostic mammogram is performed when a suspicious finding is identified on a screening mammogram. A breast ultrasound (US) and a breast MRI may be performed to obtain additional information. If imaging studies show suspicious findings, a biopsy will be performed. Diagnostic workup and treatment guidelines for breast cancer have been established by the National Comprehensive Cancer Network (NCCN).[20] The guidelines were updated for HER-2 positive metastatic breast cancer in 2013.[21] The workup for invasive cancer includes a history and physical examination, complete blood count, platelets, liver function tests, chest imaging, diagnostic bilateral mammogram, US as necessary, optional breast MRI, and a pathology review, including the determination of tumor estrogen/progesterone receptor status (ER/PR), human epidermal growth factor receptor 2 (HER-2/neu) status, and surgical margins. A bone scan, abdominal computed tomography (CT) scan, or positron emission tomography (PET) scan may also be performed depending on the stage of the cancer and the laboratory findings.

TREATMENT

The treatment of local disease may consist of surgery, radiation therapy (RT), or both. The management of systemic disease, if present, may involve cytotoxic chemotherapy, endocrine therapy, biologic therapies, or combinations of these modalities. Increasingly, neoadjuvant chemotherapy is prescribed prior to surgery. Treatment is determined by numerous factors, including disease stage, tumor histology, clinical and pathologic characteristics of the tumor, axillary node status, tumor hormone receptor status, level of HER-2/neu expression, presence or absence of detectable metastatic disease, comorbid conditions, the patient's age, and menopausal status. Molecular profiling of breast cancers using array technology has confirmed that breast cancer is a heterogeneous group of diseases that are marked by differences in prognosis and response to therapy.[22] Molecular and morphologic predictive models are beginning to influence treatment strategies as well.[23]

STAGING

The American Joint Committee on Cancer's (AJCC) TNM system is used to stage breast cancer. Five stages of breast cancer are distinguished based on the tumor (T) size and spread to the chest wall or skin; the degree of lymph node involvement (N); and metastasis to distant organs (M).[24]

- Stage 0 includes DCIS and LCIS. DCIS is the earliest form of breast cancer, in which the cancer cells are still within the duct and have not invaded the surrounding fatty breast tissue. DCIS is usually treated with lumpectomy, RT, and hormone-modulating medications. LCIS is not considered true breast cancer by most oncologists, but is a marker for increased future risk and is generally treated with Tamoxifen. LCIS may be treated with Tamoxifen in premenopausal women and Raloxifene (Evista) in postmenopausal women.
- Stages I–IV are classified by increasing tumor size, number of positive lymph nodes, and metastases to distant locations. The most common sites for metastatic breast cancer are the bone, liver, brain, or lung.

LOCAL TREATMENT

SURGERY

Breast-conserving lumpectomy and mastectomy are the two types of surgery used to locally remove breast cancer. With lumpectomy, the tumor and healthy tissue surrounding the tumor are removed; the surgical procedure is then usually followed by RT. With mastectomy, the entire breast, including the nipple, is removed. Women may elect to have reconstruction surgery at the same time as mastectomy, after mastectomy, or not at all.

Sentinel node biopsy is the preferred method of determining lymph node involvement. If the sentinel node is positive, an axillary dissection is performed. Complications of surgery vary with the type of surgery performed and the number of lymph nodes removed. Side effects are less common and less severe with sentinel node dissection as compared to full axillary lymph node dissection. Side effects of lymph node dissection may include nerve damage, limitation of arm and shoulder movement, and lymphedema of the arm.

RADIATION THERAPY

Most women treated with breast-conserving surgery will also receive follow-up treatment with RT. RT may also be indicated after mastectomy if the patient has extensive lymph node involvement. External-beam whole-breast radiation therapy with a boost to the tumor bed is the most common form of radiation employed. Brachytherapy or interstitial radiation involving the placement of radioactive seeds may be an option in some cases.

Side effects of radiation to the breast include swelling and heaviness in the breast, sunburn-like skin changes, hair loss in the treated area, and fatigue. Most symptoms occur during the second or third week of treatment and resolve within 2–4 weeks after RT completion. Changes in breast tissue and skin generally resolve in 6–12 months. Long-term risks associated with RT to the breast include rib fractures and secondary cancers caused by the radiation. Women treated with RT to the left breast are more likely than women treated with RT to the right breast to develop cardiac disease, including myocardial infarction and chest pain.[25] Both whole breast RT and targeted RT has been associated with higher cardiovascular mortality after breast cancer.[26]

CHEMOTHERAPY

The decision to initiate adjuvant chemotherapy involves balancing the risk of recurrence from local therapy alone, the degree of benefit from chemotherapy, the toxicity of the therapy, and existing comorbidities. Neoadjuvant chemotherapy may be given to reduce the size of the tumor prior to surgery. Chemotherapy is also used to treat metastatic breast cancer. Multigene testing of the tumor to predict responsiveness to chemotherapy and prognosis is currently available and used as one source of data when clinicians evaluate for individual treatment options.

The side effects of chemotherapy depend on the specific agent used, the dose, and the length of treatment, existing comorbidities, and individual tolerance.

Adjuvant Endocrine Therapy

Adjuvant endocrine therapy is instituted for breast cancers that are estrogen or progesterone receptor-positive (ER-positive and PR-positive).[27] The two SERMs used for treatment of breast cancer, tamoxifen and raloxifene (Evista®), compete with estrogen for receptor sites in target tissues such as the breast. Tamoxifen is used for adjuvant treatment for premenopausal breast cancer. This drug exerts estrogen-like activity on the skeletal and cardiovascular systems, reducing bone loss and improving lipid levels. Side effects of tamoxifen include hot flashes, night sweats, and vaginal dryness. Serious adverse effects include an increased risk of cataracts, endometrial cancer, and pulmonary embolism. The U.S. Food and Drug Administration approved raloxifene for reducing the risk of invasive breast cancer in postmenopausal women with osteoporosis and in postmenopausal women at high risk for invasive breast cancer. The STAR trial that compared Tamoxifen and Raloxifen suggested near equal efficacy supporting a 50% reduction in risk, but with less thrombotic events in the Raloxifen group.[28]

Aromatase inhibitors (AIs) are used to decrease estrogen levels in postmenopausal women through aromatase inhibition. Members of this drug class include anastrozole (Arimidex®), letrozole (Femara®), and exemestane (Aromasin®), all of which are used to treat postmenopausal disease. Nutrition-related side effects of AIs include loss of bone mineral density (BMD). AIs have been associated with abnormal lipid profiles, but these effects vary with agent use and baseline lipid profiles.[29] Because most women presenting with early-stage breast cancer can expect long-term survival, the assessment of cardiovascular adverse effects of AIs is important.

Targeted Therapy

Trastuzumab (Herceptin®) is used to treat HER-2/neu-positive tumors, which tend to be more aggressive. Overexpression of the HER-2/neu protein increases the rate of cell growth and division. Trastuzumab is a recombinant DNA-derived monoclonal antibody that selectively binds to HER-2, thereby inhibiting the proliferation of tumor cells that overexpress HER-2.

Ovarian Ablation

In an effort to decrease estrogen levels, premenopausal women may elect to have an oophorectomy. Side effects of this treatment include early menopause, which may be associated with hot flashes, night sweats, and bone loss.

OTHER PREVENTION THERAPIES

Other therapies are currently being evaluated for potential to further modulate breast cancer risk. These include, but are not limited to retinoids, tyrosine kinase inhibitors, nonsteroidal anti-inflammatory drugs, and metformin.

PROGNOSIS

The most significant prognostic factors predicting future recurrence or death from breast cancer include patient age, stage, comorbidity, tumor size, tumor grade, number of involved axillary lymph nodes, and possibly HER-2/neu level of expression. Algorithms are available that estimate rates of recurrence. A validated computer-based model, Adjuvant! Online, estimates 10-year disease-free and overall survival and is available at http://www.adjuvantonline.com. Evidence from the WHI suggests that premorbid lifestyle (diet, physical activity, weight, and smoking) inform not only in relation to risk for breast cancer, but also prognosis and mortality after breast cancer.[1]

NUTRITION AND LIFESTYLE FACTORS IN THE ETIOLOGY OF BREAST CANCER

Carcinogenesis is a multistage process consisting of several phases including initiation, promotion, and progression (Figure 9.2). Initiation occurs when the cell has been exposed to an agent that results in the first genetic mutation, but by itself initiation is not sufficient for a cancer to develop. Instead, the initiated cell must be activated by a promoting agent that causes cellular proliferation—that is, the process called promotion. Initiated and promoted cells eventually form a tumor mass during the process of progression. At the end of the carcinogenesis process, the cell will have some or all of the characteristics of a cancer cell: growth signal autonomy, insensitivity to antigrowth signals, limitless replicative potential, evasion of apoptosis, sustained angiogenesis, tissue invasion, and metastasis. Diet, including whole foods (vegetables, whole grains, teas, etc.) and bioactive constitutive compounds within foods, can influence cancer development at various stages.

In 2007, a joint panel of the World Cancer Research Fund (WCRF) and American Institute for Cancer Research published its findings on the role of food, nutrition, and physical activity in cancer prevention.[30] These evidence-based reviews are updated periodically on the website at http://www.dietandcancerreport.org/cup/. In their 2010 updated review breast cancer report, the panel members judged the weight of the evidence for the role of nutrition and lifestyle factors in the etiology of breast cancer (http://www.dietandcancerreport.org/cancer_resource_center/downloads/cu/Breast-Cancer-2010-Report). Premenopausal and postmenopausal breast cancers were considered separately in the report. Premenopausal cancers are thought to be mainly genetically driven, with the environment and nutrition playing smaller roles in their genesis. In the genetically associated cancers, a healthy diet along with a physically active lifestyle from an early age may result in the delayed onset of the disease. Diet modulation is most likely to influence postmenopausal disease, which is more prolonged at onset.

PREMENOPAUSAL BREAST CANCER

- *Convincing evidence*: The consumption of alcoholic drinks increases risk; lactation beyond 24 total months decreases risk.
- *Probable evidence*: Adult height and birth weight increases risk.

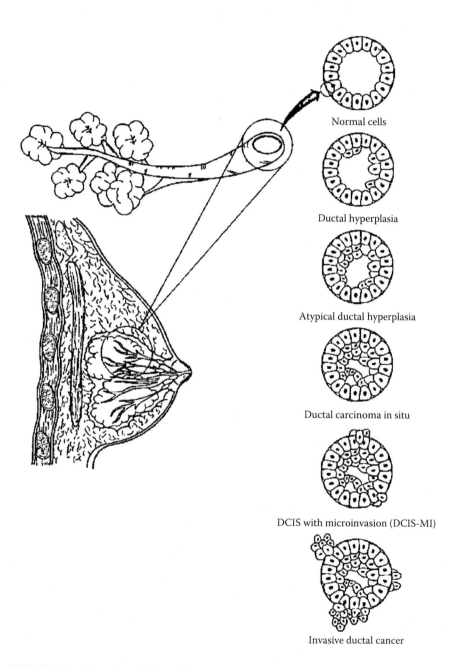

Normal cells

Ductal hyperplasia

Atypical ductal hyperplasia

Ductal carcinoma in situ

DCIS with microinvasion (DCIS-MI)

Invasive ductal cancer

FIGURE 9.2 Illustration of the multistage process of breast carcinogenesis (ductal cancer).

- *Limited suggestive evidence*: Physical activity decreases risk; total fat intake increases risk.
- *No conclusive evidence*: Dietary fiber, fruits and vegetables, meat fish, milk/dairy, total fat, soy, folate, vitamin D, calcium, glycemic index, dietary patterns, adult weight gain, or abdominal fat.

POSTMENOPAUSAL BREAST CANCER

- *Convincing evidence*: Lactation beyond 24 total months decreases risk; consumption of alcoholic beverages, body fatness and obesity, adult height all increase risk.
- *Probable evidence*: Physical activity decreases risk; adult weight gain and abdominal fat increases risk.
- *Limited suggestive evidence*: Total dietary fat increases risk.
- *No conclusive evidence*: Dietary fiber, fruits and vegetables, meat fish, milk/dairy, total fat, soy, folate, vitamin D, calcium, selenium, glycemic index, dietary patterns, energy intake, birth weight.

The panel also found limited evidence and could not draw a conclusion in regard to the risk associated with environmental chemicals. The lack of strong evidence for a relationship between specific dietary constituents and breast cancer may suggests no significant association exists or that no single dietary exposures is likely strong enough to modify cancer risk. Rather a combination of exposures may be responsible for risk modification. Further, challenges related to study designs, including measurement errors in self-reporting intake by study participants likely limits our ability to accurately quantify risk. This was demonstrated in a report from The Women's Health Initiative wherein energy intake by self-report was not associated with greater risk for breast cancer, while energy intake from the more objective measure using doubly-labeled water should a significant increase in breast cancer risk.[31] Additionally, the focus on diet during adult life versus earlier life exposures, particularly during puberty when breast maturation occurs may limit our understanding of the role of diet in modifying risk. Many observational analyses also lack sufficient statistical power (low sample size) to evaluate risk within subgroups of women who are more susceptible to the influence of diet.[32] Further, evidence is mounting that risk may be different dependent on the tumor subtype. As an example, a review of 20 cohort studies showed a reduced risk for triple negative disease in women consuming higher intake of vegetables, but no association overall or for other tumor subtypes.[33]

LACTATION

The evidence that breastfeeding is associated with a decreased risk of breast cancer is mixed.[34,35] In most studies wherein duration of breastfeeding is greater than 24 months total exposure, protection has been reported.[36,37] Specifically, pooled analysis from 47 epidemiological studies showed a decreased risk of 4.3% for each 12 months of breastfeeding.[38] Protection may be conferred by the lower exposure to estrogen during the amenorrhea associated with breastfeeding, increased differentiation of breast cells, exfoliation of breast tissue during lactation, and massive epithelial apoptosis at the end of lactation, which may eliminate cells with potential DNA damage. Little is known about dietary exposures during pregnancy or lactation on future breast cancer risk in the mother or the infant.

WEIGHT, HEIGHT, AND BREAST CANCER

Evidence suggests that adult weight gain may be a risk factor for postmenopausal breast cancer, although recent evidence suggests that risk is only increased after age 69 years and particularly for estrogen and progesterone positive disease.[39] The increased risk of breast cancer after menopause may be due to higher estrogen levels than would normally be present with cessation of menses. In fact, circulating levels of estrogen are twice as high in overweight women as compared to healthy weight controls. The higher estrogen levels are caused by the endogenous production of estrogen by the aromatization of adrenal androgens in the adipose tissue. Overweight women also have lower levels of SHBG as compared to normal weight women, and consequently have more bioavailable estrogen.[40]

Being overweight is also associated with increased levels of insulin and insulin-like growth factor 1 (IGF-1), which produces a hormonal environment that favors breast carcinogenesis.[41,42] Obesity, particularly abdominal obesity, also is associated with increased inflammation. Chronic inflammation may be involved in the initiation and the progression of cancer by damaging DNA, increasing proliferation, inhibiting apoptosis, and increasing angiogenesis.[43]

Epidemiologic data from the Nurses' Health Study found a direct association between weight gain since age 18 and postmenopausal breast cancer risk, especially in women who had never used postmenopausal replacement therapy (PMT).[44] In this prospective cohort, 49,514 women aged 30–55 years who were free of cancer were followed for as long as 26 years. Weight gain of 25 kg or more since age 18 was associated with an increased risk of breast cancer relative risk (RR) equal to 1.45, compared to women who maintained their weight. In women who never took PMT, the RR was 1.98. The data suggest that 15% of breast cancers could be attributed to weight gain of 2 kg or more since age 18 years and that 4.4% could be attributed to weight gain of 2.0 kg or more since menopause. Women who lost 10 kg or more since menopause and kept it off and never used PMT reduced their risk of breast cancer (RR = 0.45) compared to women who maintained their weight. The weaker association of weight gain in women who used PMT may be due to the high levels of circulating exogenous estrogens in these women, unrelated to their weight and adiposity.

The WCRF panel also found convincing evidence that postmenopausal breast cancer risk increases with adult-attained height. Tallness itself is probably not the cause of breast cancer. Rather, height acts as a surrogate for childhood nutritional factors affecting hormonal and metabolic systems that are related to cancer risk, including alterations in levels of growth hormone, insulin-like growth factors, sex hormone-binding proteins, and the age of sexual maturation.

Body Fatness, Greater Weight at Birth, Greater Attained Height, and Premenopausal Risk

In premenopausal women, greater body fatness probably decreases the risk of breast cancer, according to the WCRF panel. The mechanism by which body fatness protects against breast cancer in premenopausal women is still speculative at this time. Proposed mechanisms include irregular menstrual cycles and ovulatory infertility in adulthood, with subsequent alteration in hormone levels. Further, in premenopausal disease, BMI has been shown to be protective; although recent evidence suggests this may only be true in the case of luminal A disease.[45,46]

Premenopausal breast cancer risk is increased with greater weight at birth and greater adult-attained height. The mechanisms are speculative. The factors leading to greater birth weight and attained height may affect the long-term programming of hormonal systems and/or indicate a greater exposure to growth hormones and sex hormones known to promote tumor growth.

Alcohol

Convincing evidence exists that regular alcohol consumption increases the risk of breast cancer although the evidence is stronger for postmenopausal disease.[47] Cumulative exposure, frequency, and quantity all influence risk.[48] Pooled analysis of six prospective studies found a linear increase in breast cancer risk of 9% for each additional 10 g/day of alcohol consumed per day. The specific type of alcohol did not strongly influence risk.[49] In one study, alcohol consumption was associated with ER-positive breast cancer in postmenopausal women but not with ER-negative breast cancer.[50]

Alcohol may affect a number of hormone-dependent pathways by inducing the production of endogenous estrogens, decreasing the metabolic clearance of estradiol, stimulating the proliferation of ER-positive cells, and increasing ER-alpha activity through inactivation of the *BRAC1* gene. Hormone-independent pathways include the induction of carcinogenesis and DNA damage by acetaldehyde (the reactive metabolite of ethanol), lipid peroxidation, and the production of reactive oxygen species. Interestingly, polyphenols in red wine have demonstrated inhibitory activity on the aromatase enzyme associated with estrogen production and as such may not increase breast cancer risk.[51]

Adequate folate status may partially mitigate the increased breast cancer risk associated with moderate alcohol consumption.[47] Folate adequacy should be ensured in women who consume alcohol.

Dietary Fat

The relationship between dietary fat intake and breast cancer risk has been controversial, with mostly observational studies showing inconsistent results. The WCRF panel determined that there is limited evidence suggesting total dietary fat intake is associated with a higher risk of postmenopausal breast cancer, but not premenopausal breast cancer.

The National Institutes of Health/AARP's (NIH-AARP) Diet and Health Study—a prospective study involving 188,736 postmenopausal women—did find a modest increase in the risk of breast cancer in women who were not using menopausal hormone therapy and who had higher total dietary fat intake.[52] Women who consumed 40% of their total calories in the form of fat (90 g/day, highest quintile) had an 11% higher incidence of invasive breast cancer than women who consumed 20% of calories as fat (24.2 g/day, lowest quintile).

In the Women's Health Initiative (WHI)—a randomized, controlled, primary prevention trial involving 48,835 postmenopausal women, ages 50–70—reducing the total fat consumed to 20% of total calories did not result in a statistically significant reduction in invasive breast cancer over an 8.1-year follow-up period.[53] However, those women in the intervention group who consumed the highest percentage of energy in the form of fat at baseline ($\geq$36.8% of calories from fat, $\geq$76 g/day) did see a significant reduction in their risk of invasive breast cancer risk (hazard ratio = 78) when compared to the comparison group. It may be that a subgroup of women with very-high-fat diets would benefit the most from switching to a low-fat dietary pattern.

A review by Sieri et al. suggested risk for ER+/PR+ disease was increased by 20% and 28% in women with higher dietary fat and saturated fat intake, respectively.[54] High saturated fat also was associated with HER2Neu- disease in this same sample of over 337,000 women. Interesting data from the Nurses' health Study has suggested dietary fat is not associated with lethal breast cancers.[55]

If a causal relationship between breast cancer risk and dietary fat does exist, it may reflect any of several mechanisms that affect the initiation and growth of breast cancer that likely vary depending on the specific fatty acids consumed.[56] Among the procarcinogenic mechanisms are increased endogenous production of estrogen with higher-fat diets, modulation of inflammatory response modulation of the immune system, and regulation of gene function.[57]

Red Meat, Processed Meat, and Heterocyclic Amines

Studies of meat consumption, red meat consumption, heterocyclic amines, and breast cancer risk have produced conflicting results. In the UK Women's Cohort Study, which enrolled 35,371 participants, women with the highest total meat consumption (poultry, red meat, and processed meat) had the highest risk of both premenopausal and postmenopausal breast cancer.[58] The effect was larger in postmenopausal women for all types of meat, including red and processed meat.

Evidence from the Nurses' Health Study suggested that for each serving of red meat consumed daily there is an estimated 13% greater risk for breast cancer as compared to no consumption of red meat.[59] Current evidence suggests it is prudent to decrease red meat and processed meat consumption in an effort to reduce overall risk for breast cancer. Further, consideration of alternate protein sources may be protective.[60] A meta-analysis of processed meat intake and breast cancer risk also suggested a significant increase in risk, but associations were weak, accounting for less than a 3% increase in risk with higher intake.[61]

Several mechanisms have been proposed to explain the positive association between meat consumption and breast cancer. In particular, heterocyclic amines, which are produced when meats are charbroiled, fried, or cooked until well done, have been implicated in increasing cancer risk. Heterocyclic amines promote estrogen activity and stimulate ER and PR gene expression in vitro.[62] Processed meats contain nitroso compounds; which are known carcinogens and may also be involved in breast cancer etiology.

Women should be advised to decrease their red and processed meat consumption to an intake below 18 ounces/week, consistent with the AICR/WCRF guidance. Well-done and charbroiled meats should be avoided; roasting, stewing, and slow cooking (Crock-Pot) techniques are the preferred methods of meat preparation.

Diet Patterns, Vegetarian Diets, and Breast Cancer Risk

Several papers have been published in recent years supporting the role of adherence to cancer prevention guidelines for diet and physical activity in relation to breast cancer risk. Generally, risk reduction appears to be between 20% and 30% in terms of lower breast cancer incidence.[63] Further, plant-based diets were associated with a 15% lower breast cancer risk in the California Teachers' cohort, with a particular protective association with ER−/PR− disease.[64]

Intake of a Mediterranean diet pattern may also reduce the risk for breast cancer (particularly for women living in Greece),[65] although not all studies have supported a reduction in risk.[66] A vegetarian diet does not appear to protect against breast cancer. Analysis from the UK Women's cohort showed no protective association with a vegetarian diet, although a diet high in fish was associated with lower postmenopausal disease.[67] Rates of breast cancer remain high among Adventist populations despite their healthy lifestyle, which includes following a lacto-ovo vegetarian diet.[68] However, a diet pattern rich in vegetables and fruit does appear to be associated with lower risk for ER−/PR− disease.[69]

Vegetables and Fruits

Epidemiological studies evaluating the role of fruits and vegetables and breast cancer risk have yielded inconsistent results, including data from the EPIC study.[70] The 2014 WCRF/AICR suggested that "there is no convincing evidence that fruits and vegetables play a role in breast cancer etiology."[71] However, interest exists in specific bioactive compounds found in vegetables and fruit that may confer protection against cancer. According to the WCRF, there is limited, inconclusive evidence that cruciferous vegetables, flavonoids, green tea, and phytoestrogens may play a role in decreasing breast cancer risk.

Cruciferous Vegetables

The cruciferous vegetables of the *Brassica* genus include broccoli, Brussels sprouts, cabbage, collards, cauliflower, kale, kohlrabi, mustard greens, bok choy, Chinese cabbage, turnips, and rutabagas. Cruciferous vegetables are rich in glucosinolates, a group of sulfur-containing compounds. The hydrolysis of glucosinolates by the plant enzyme myrosinase results in biologically active compounds that include indoles.

More than 100 glucosinolates with unique hydrolysis products have been identified in plants. These water-soluble compounds may leach into cooking water; microwaving at high power and steaming and boiling vegetables can also inactivate myrosinase.

Evidence that cruciferous vegetables decrease the risk of breast cancer in population-based studies is limited and inconsistent.[72] The evidence supporting a protective association is more commonly demonstrated among populations residing in areas where cruciferous vegetable intake is generally much higher than the United States as was shown in a recent analysis from Japan wherein intake was associated with a 36% lower risk for premenopausal disease.[73] In addition, genetic polymorphisms may influence the activity of glutathione *S*-transferases (GST) and mediate the effects of cruciferous vegetable intake on cancer risk.[74]

Sulforaphane, indole-3-carbinol (I3C), and diindolylmethane are bioactive constituents of cruciferous vegetables that may offer chemopreventive benefits by shifting the metabolism of 17β-estridiol from 16-α-hydroxyestrone ($16\alpha OHE_1$) to 2-hydroxyestrone ($2OHE_1$). The $16\alpha OHE_1$ metabolite is thought to be genotoxic and tumorigenic, compared to the $2OHE_1$ metabolite. In postmenopausal women, increasing the consumption of cruciferous vegetables significantly increases the urinary ratio of $2OHE_1$ to $16\alpha OHE_1$.[75] However, the relationship between urinary $2OHE_1$:$16\alpha OHE_1$ and breast cancer risk is unclear. Other proposed anticarcinogenic properties of cruciferous vegetables include their ability to induce apoptosis and inhibit angiogenesis.

Flavonoids and Flavonoid-Rich Foods

Flavonoids are a group of more than 5000 polyphenolic compounds that occur naturally in plant foods. Laboratory studies have shown that flavonoids act as anticarcinogens by inhibiting aromatase activity, tumor cell proliferation, and the formation of reactive oxygen species. Epidemiological studies suggest that foods high in specific flavonoids are associated with a decreased risk of breast cancer.[76] Odds ratios (OR) for breast cancer risk were reduced in women with consumption of flavonoids in the highest quintile versus those with consumption in the lowest quintile. The effect was strongest for flavonols (found in onions, cherries, broccoli, tomatoes, tea, red wine, and berries), for which the OR was 0.54; the corresponding ORs were 0.61 for flavones (found in parsley, thyme, and cereal), 0.74 for flavan-3-ols (found in apples, tea, chocolate, red wine, and berries), and 0.69 for lignans (found in flaxseeds, legumes, and whole grains). The data did not support an inverse association between isoflavones (found in soy), anthocyanidins (found in blueberries and raspberries), or flavanones (found in citrus) and breast cancer risk. Importantly, the protective association with flavonoids may be attenuated in women with expression of oxidative stress, carcinogen metabolism and one-carbon metabolism genes that drive risk.[77]

The catechins in tea have also been studied for their potential anticarcinogenic properties. Tea is a popular beverage worldwide, and it has been brewed from the *Camellia sinensis* plant for more than 5000 years. The method used in its processing results in black, green, oolong, or white tea. Black tea is produced by allowing the picked tea leaves to dry indoors, ferment, and oxidize. Green tea is produced by steaming the tea leaves, which inactivates enzymes and preserves the catechin content.

Oolong tea is a partially fermented tea. White tea is the least processed of teas and consequently has even greater antioxidant activity than green tea. White tea is harvested before the leaves are fully opened and the buds are still covered by fine white hair; the leaves are then picked and air-dried. White tea is widely available in the United States but is more expensive than other types of tea.

Population studies suggest that green tea consumption does not decrease the risk of breast cancer.[78,79] Most of these studies have been conducted in Asia; to date, few large-scale epidemiological studies or randomized controlled intervention trials have been carried out in Western populations. Ultimately, the protective effect of green tea may depend on the genotype of an individual. In a population-based, case-controlled study of Asian American women in Los Angeles, a significant inverse relationship was found to exist between tea consumption, breast cancer rate, and polymorphisms in the catechol-*O*-methyltransferase (*COMT*) gene.[80] Women with at least one low-activity *COMT* allele who drank tea had a significantly reduced risk of breast cancer (adjusted OR = 0.48) compared with nontea drinkers. This benefit was observed in drinkers of both green and black teas. However, a similar analysis from Japan considering polymorphisms in COMT showed no protective role from green tea intake.[81]

Phytoestrogens

Phytoestrogens are plant compounds that can bind to ERs. These substances act as SERMs, as they have both estrogenic and antiestrogenic effects, depending on the expression of the ER subtype in the target cell and the amount of endogenous estrogen present. In premenopausal women, phytoestrogens appear to exert antiestrogenic effects; in postmenopausal women, they may exert estrogenic effects and minimize menopausal symptoms. These compounds may influence estrogen metabolism through several mechanisms (1) by promoting C-2 hydroxylation over 16α hydroxylation; (2) by increasing SHBG levels, thereby reducing free estrogens; (3) by inhibiting aromatase activity; and (4) by binding to ERs. The major types of phytoestrogens are isoflavones and lignans.

Isoflavones

Isoflavones are found in soy, legumes, alfalfa, clover, licorice root, and kudzu root. Two isoflavones, genistein and daidzein, are found in soy, for example. The effects of genistein are well documented. The molecular structure of this compound is similar to that of estradiol-17β and binds to both ERα and ERβ, but estrogenic properties have not been demonstrated in human studies.[82] There has been much interest in—and controversy about—the role of soy in breast cancer risk. To date, the data remain inconclusive, but generally refute earlier concerns of proestrogenic effects. A systematic review of studies in Japanese women, women who are known to consume higher intakes of isoflavones throughout life, suggested a modest reduction in breast cancer risk in association with higher lifelong intake of soy foods.[83] Importantly, evidence that earlier life exposure may be important to protective associations has been supported by a primate study in which soy was shown to increase mammary cell differentiation, thus reducing breast cancer risk.[84] Thus, women at risk for breast cancer should not be discouraged from consuming soy, but rather encouraged to consume soy and isoflavones in the form of food (rather than supplements) and to vary soy food sources to optimize the diversity of phytochemical intake.

Lignans

Lignans are compounds found in fiber-rich foods including flaxseed, whole grains, legumes, and vegetables. Flaxseeds are the richest source of lignans (enterodiol and enterolactone) in the diet.

Lignans have been shown to modify estrogen metabolism, stimulate SHBG production in the liver, inhibit aromatase activity in adipose cells, and decrease cellular proliferation in breast cells. In a small, randomized, double-blind, placebo-controlled study of postmenopausal women, supplementation with 25 g of ground flaxseed/day (in the form of a muffin) resulted in increased excretion of the less biologically active estrogen metabolite 2-OHE1; the excretion of 16α-hydroxyestrone did not increase.[85] More trials are needed, but early evidence supports a protective role for dietary lignin intake.[86]

Allium Vegetables

The allium family of vegetables, which includes garlic, onions, and shallots, may have anticarcinogenic properties. Allium vegetables have high concentrations of organosulfur compounds, which may selectively inhibit or induce certain P-450 enzymes; they are also high in antioxidant activity due to their flavonoid content. To date, few data on their role in breast cancer risk have been collected. An Italian case-controlled study failed to find a protective role for garlic and onion consumption and breast cancer risk[87] while the Shanghai Breast Cancer Study suggested a reduction in risk.[88]

Folate

Folate, in the polyglutamate form, occurs naturally in dark-green leafy vegetables, legumes, and fruits. Synthetic folic acid is available in supplements and fortified foods. Several mechanisms have been proposed for the role of folate inadequacy and carcinogenesis. Folate and vitamin B_{12} are coenzymes needed to regenerate methionine from homocysteine. Methionine in the form of S-adenosylmethionine is the principal methyl donor for DNA methylation. Folate inadequacy, in theory, may lead to hypomethylation and, therefore to gene mutation or altered gene expression. Inadequacy of folate may increase cancer risk by the misincorporation of uracil for thymine during DNA synthesis and by impaired DNA repair. Both of these processes can cause DNA strand breaks and chromosome damage.

Epidemiologic evidence supporting an inverse relationship between folate intake and breast cancer risk is inconclusive and generally does not support a protective association.[89] In fact, some studies suggest that high folate intake, above 400 µg/day, may increase breast cancer risk.[90] In the prospective, randomized Prostate, Lung, Colorectal and Ovarian Cancer Screening Trial (PLCO), high folate intake due to supplementation was associated with an increased risk of breast cancer in post-menopausal women.[91] As a methyl donor, folate intake at high levels may promote the growth of an existing cancer or cause epigenetic changes in gene-regulatory mechanisms, leading to gene silencing and cancer development. Ultimately, both deficiency and excess of folate may contribute to breast cancer carcinogenesis.

Vitamin D

Vitamin D is found in fatty fish such as salmon, sardines, mackerel, and tuna as well as mushrooms, egg yolk, and liver. Vitamin D is also found in fortified foods such as milk, orange juice, and breakfast cereals. Multivitamins and some calcium supplements also contain vitamin D. Two forms of supplemental vitamin D are available: vitamin D_3 (also known as cholecalciferol) and vitamin D_2 (also known as ergocalciferol). Cholecalciferol is manufactured through the ultraviolet irradiation of 7-dehydrocholesterol from lanolin; it is the preferred form of supplementation because it has more biological activity. Ergocalciferol is manufactured through the ultraviolet irradiation of ergosterol from yeast, and is less biologically active than cholecalciferol. Humans can produce vitamin D when the skin is exposed to ultraviolet radiation from the sun or from tanning booths.

An estimated 1 billion people worldwide are vitamin D insufficient or deficient. Obese individuals are particularly at risk for vitamin D deficiency. Because vitamin D from the diet or from sunlight is efficiently deposited in the body fat stores, it is not as bioavailable. This process leads to low serum levels in obese persons. Arabic women are also at risk for insufficiency related to cultural practices related to clothing.

Prospective and retrospective studies suggest that serum levels of 25-hydoxy vitamin D less than 20 ng/mL are associated with a 30%–50% increased risk of breast, colon, and prostate cancer and a greater risk of mortality.[92,93] In a 4-year, population-based, double-blind, randomized, placebo-controlled trial involving 1179 women, risk of all cancers—including breast cancer—was reduced in the intervention group receiving 1400–1500 mg of calcium and 1100 IU of vitamin D_3 per day and in the group receiving 1400–1500 mg of supplemental calcium per day.[94] However, the Women's Health Initiative showed no reduction in breast cancer risk[95] nor did a recent review on the topic.[96]

The recommended daily intake of vitamin D developed by the Institute of Medicine is thought by most experts to be inadequate.[92] Most experts agree that without adequate sun exposure, children and adults require approximately 800–1000 IU of vitamin D per day. Supplementation should be in the form of cholecalciferol. Assessment of vitamin D status using serum 25(OH) levels can be helpful in determining individual needs. Optimal vitamin D levels have not been established. Holick has defined vitamin D deficiency measured by 25(OH) vitamin D as less than 20 ng/mL, insufficiency as 21–29 ng/mL, sufficiency as more than 30 ng/mL, and toxicity as more than 150 ng/mL.[92] An optimal range of 40–65 ng/mL has been proposed by other sources.[97]

ENVIRONMENTAL POLLUTANTS

A total of 216 chemicals have been identified in at least one animal study as increasing the incidence of mammary tumors.[98] These substances include industrial chemicals, chlorinated solvents, products of combustion, pesticides, dyes, radiation, drinking water disinfectant by-products, pharmaceuticals and hormones, natural products, and research chemicals. Of these chemicals, 73 are present in consumer products or as contaminants in food, 35 are air pollutants, 25 are associated with occupational exposure, and 29 are produced in the United States in large amounts. Laboratory research indicates that many environmental toxins cause mammary gland tumors in animals by mimicking estrogen or by increasing the susceptibility of the mammary gland to carcinogenesis.

The epidemiologic evidence that environmental pollutants play a role in human breast cancer risk is limited, although support for the relationship is building.[99] Meaningful evidence indicates that polycyclic aromatic hydrocarbons (PAHs) and polychlorinated biphenyls (PCBs) increase the risk of breast cancer in women with certain genetic polymorphisms including *GSTM1*. PHAs include products of combustion from air pollution, tobacco smoke, and cooked food and are prevalent in our environment. PCBs were used in the production of electrical equipment in the past, but were banned in the 1970s. The primary source of PCB exposure is through the consumption of fish from rivers contaminated with the industrial pollutant. PCBs are found in high concentrations in breast milk, and they accumulate in fat. Although breast milk contains PCBs, the American Academy of Pediatrics remains a staunch advocate of breastfeeding infants because of the health, nutritional, immunological, developmental, psychological, social, economic, and environmental benefits associated with this practice.[100]

Bisphenol A has been identified, like diethylstilbestrol, as a synthetic estrogen and is found in polycarbonate plastics, including many packaging materials including plastic water bottles. Exposure has not been directly associated with breast cancer risk, but in theory the mechanistic possibility exists. Certainly evidence to suggest exposure is associated with obesity, diabetes, and insulin production is available.[101] Such metabolic alterations (and diabetes) have been associated with the risk of breast and other cancers,[102] although not consistently.[103] Further research is warranted. Additional epidemiologic research is needed on breast cancer risk and other chemicals that act as endocrine disruptors, including chlorinated solvents, diesel exhaust, dibutyl phthalate, ethylene oxide, perfluorooctanoic acid, and bisphenol A.

NUTRITION CARE DURING AND AFTER CANCER TREATMENT

NUTRITION ASSESSMENT

Evaluation of nutritional status is important during and following treatment. Traditional nutrition assessment includes medical history, diet and weight history, laboratory data, and anthropometric measurements. The Mini Nutritional Assessment (MNA), the scored Patient-Generated Subjective Global Assessment (PG-SGA) and the Malnutrition Screening Tool (MST) are tools that have been studied in the cancer population. Of these tools, the PG-SGA has been validated for use in cancer patients, but is time-consuming and must be administered by a trained individual.[104] The MNA is a simple tool that can be managed by a nontrained person but is validated only for use in the elderly population. The MST has been validated against the SGA resulting in 70.6% sensitivity and 69.5% specificity, below the performance of the SGA; however, it also is less cumbersome to perform.[105]

In a study comparing the two tools in cancer patients, the MNA was found to have high sensitivity but low specificity. It adequately identified patients in need of nutrition intervention but also categorized patients as requiring nutrition intervention when it was not needed.[106] The PG-SGA appears to be more applicable in cancer patients than the MNA, but if staffing and resources are limited, its use may not be realistic. A modification of the MNA could be developed to increase its specificity in the cancer setting.

In clinical practice, many individuals with breast cancer who are treated on an outpatient basis may not require the use of any of these tools. Metastatic breast cancer is more likely to trigger the need for nutrition intervention. Lifestyle and nutrition issues related to survivorship, such as weight gain, exercise, vegetable and fruit intake, and prevention and treatment of the metabolic syndrome—all of which may influence the risk of recurrence—are common nutritional concerns in this population. For this reason, a system for identifying patients and providing education is important. Patients should be asked about the use of CAM, as there is potential for drug–supplement interactions. CAM use has been reported by a significant percentage of breast cancer patients, particularly younger women, and those with higher education.[107]

NUTRITIONAL IMPLICATIONS OF CHEMOTHERAPY

CT side effects affecting nutritional status include nausea and vomiting (N/V), mucositis, altered taste, xerostomia, dysphagia, myelosuppression, fatigue, and diarrhea. Symptoms can be decreased with pharmacologic interventions such as antiemetic, antidiarrheal, and hematopoietic agents, although many patients who are treated with "dose-intensive" regimens experience significant side effects. In premenopausal women treated with CT, infertility and early menopause causing hot flashes and night sweats may occur. These women are also at risk for osteoporosis due to early menopause. Chemotherapeutic agents commonly used to treat breast cancer (summarized in Table 9.1) include cyclophosphamide (Cytoxan®), docetaxel (Taxotere®), doxorubicin (Adriamycin®), epirubicin (Ellence®), 5-fluorouracil(5-FU), methotrexate, and paclitaxel (Taxol®).

Weight Gain Associated with Chemotherapy and Hormonal Therapy

Patients who experience anorexia or N/V often lose weight and should be referred to a registered dietitian nutritionist (RDN) for counseling and advisement to support adequate nutrient intake. In contrast, weight gain during chemotherapy is common in breast cancer patients; the typical increase ranges from 2.5 to 6.2 kg. A study of 98 patients, suggested that about 35% gain weight, 32% lose weight, and the remainder are weight stable during chemotherapy. Weight gain was associated with lower prediagnosis BMI, younger age, and higher hormone dose.[108] In particular, cyclophosphamide, methotrexate, and fluorouracil have been associated with greater weight gain.[109] In the Women's Healthy Eating and Living (WHEL) study, all regimens of chemotherapy were associated with weight gain and only 10% of study participants

TABLE 9.1

Medications Commonly Used in the Treatment of Breast Cancer and Related Nutritional Concerns

Drug (Route of Administration)	Mode of Action	Potential Side Effects/Nutrition Implications
Chemotherapeutic agents		
Cyclophosphamide (Cytoxan®) (intravenous or oral)	Alkylating agent Interferes with RNA transcription, causing growth imbalance and cell death	↑ Uric acid; ↓ platelets, hemoglobin, red blood cells, white blood cells; anorexia, nausea and vomiting, stomatitis, mucositis, abdominal pain, cardiotoxicity in high doses
Docetaxel (Taxotere®) (intravenous)	Inhibits mitosis and leads to cell death	↑ Alkaline phosphatase, alanine aminotransferase, aspartate aminotransferase, and bilirubin; ↓ hemoglobin, platelets, white blood cells; stomatitis, nausea and vomiting, diarrhea, myalgia, arthralgia, nail pigmentation
Doxorubicin (Adriamycin®) (intravenous)	Interferes with DNA-dependent RNA synthesis	↑ Uric acid; ↓ platelets and white blood cells; esophagitis common in patients who have also received radiation; nausea and vomiting, diarrhea, stomatitis, anorexia, cardiotoxicity
Epirubicin (Ellence®) (intravenous)	Inhibits DNA, RNA, and protein synthesis	↓ Hemoglobin, neutrophils, platelets, white blood cells; nausea and vomiting, diarrhea, anorexia, mucositis
5-Fluorouracil (5-FU) (intravenous)	Inhibits DNA and RNA synthesis	↑ Alkaline phosphatase, alanine aminotransferase, aspartate aminotransferase, lactate dehydrogenase, bilirubin; ↓ hemoglobin, platelets, red blood cells, white blood cells, albumin; anorexia, nausea and vomiting, gastrointestinal ulceration; contraindicated in poor nutritional status or following major surgery within previous month
Methotrexate (intravenous)	Antimetabolite Reversibly binds to dihydrofolate reductase, blocking the reduction of folic acid to tetrahydrofolate, a cofactor necessary for purine, protein, and DNA synthesis	↑ Uric acid; ↓ platelets, red blood cells, white blood cells; gingivitis, stomatitis, diarrhea, abdominal distress, anorexia, gastrointestinal ulceration and bleeding, enteritis, nausea and vomiting. May alter results of laboratory assay for folate status. Folic acid derivatives antagonize methotrexate effects and should be avoided. Alcohol may increase hepatotoxicity.
Paclitaxel (Taxol®) (intravenous)	Inhibits normal reorganization of microtubule network needed for mitosis and other vital cellular functions	↑ Alkaline phosphatase, aspartate aminotransferase, triglycerides; ↓ neutrophils, white blood cells, hemoglobin, platelets; nausea and vomiting, diarrhea, mucositis peripheral neuropathy, myalgia, arthralgia

(Continued)

TABLE 9.1 (*Continued*)

Medications Commonly Used in the Treatment of Breast Cancer and Related Nutritional Concerns

Drug (Route of Administration)	Mode of Action	Potential Side Effects/Nutrition Implications
Targeted biologic therapy		
Bevacizumab (Avastin®) (intravenous)	Recombinant humanized monoclonal IgG₁ antibody. Binds and inhibits the biological activity of vascular endothelial growth factor (VEGF) Inhibits angiogenesis	↓ White blood cells; ↑ proteinuria; diarrhea, nausea and vomiting, anorexia, stomatitis, abdominal pain, wound healing complications, gastrointestinal perforations, congestive heart failure, hypertension
Trastuzumab (Herceptin®) (intravenous)	Recombinant DNA-derived monoclonal antibody that selectively binds to HER-2 Inhibits proliferation of cells that overexpress HER-2	↓ Hemoglobin, white blood cells; anorexia, abdominal pain, diarrhea, nausea and vomiting
Hormonal therapy		
Anastrozole (Arimidex®) (oral)	Aromatase inhibitor; aromatase is an enzyme that converts testosterone to estrogen in the peripheral tissue Significantly decreases estrogen levels For use in postmenopausal women with ER/PR-positive tumors	↑ Liver enzymes, hot flashes, bone pain; ↑ risk of osteoporosis Ensure adequate calcium and vitamin D for bone health and encourage weight-bearing exercise.
Exemestane (Aromasin®) (oral)	Aromatase inhibitor Mechanism and indication the same as for Arimidex	↑ Bilirubin, alkaline phosphatase, creatinine, hot flashes; ↑ risk of osteoporosis Ensure adequate calcium and vitamin D for bone health and encourage weight-bearing exercise.
Letrozole (Femara®) (oral)	Aromatase inhibitor Mechanism and indication the same as for Arimidex	↑ Cholesterol, hot flashes; ↑risk for osteoporosis Ensure adequate calcium and vitamin D for bone health and encourage weight-bearing exercise.
Raloxifene	Selective estrogen-receptor modulator (SERM)	Lowers risk by 65%; protective against fracture risk; no increased risk for endometrial cancer.
Tamoxifen (Nolvadex®) (oral)	Selective estrogen-receptor modulator (SERM) For use in premenopausal women or women with DCIS or LCIS	↑ BUN, calcium, T₄, liver enzymes; ↓ white blood cells and platelets; ↑ risk of pulmonary embolism, thromboembolism, endometrial cancer, hot flashes Ensure adequate calcium and vitamin D for bone health and encourage weight-bearing exercise.

Source: Lippincott Williams & Wilkins, *Nursing 2014 Drug Handbook*, 34th edn., Lippincott Williams & Wilkins, Philadelphia, PA, 2014.

returned to their initial weight.[110] Weight stability after breast cancer diagnosis has been associated with lower overall mortality in breast cancer survivors, particularly if correlated with lower comorbid conditions.[111]

Studies to reduce weight gain in breast cancer survivors are limited, but suggest efficacy can be demonstrated.[112] Energy restriction combined with group cooking classes was shown to be effective in one study.[113] Walking interventions also have been associated with less weight gain during therapy.[114] Resistance training, especially that focusing on the lower body, should be encouraged in women undergoing chemotherapy to prevent loss of lean body mass, which leads to a decrease in resting energy expenditure (REE) and subsequent weight gain.

Menopausal Vasomotor Symptoms

The most common complaints in women with ER-positive tumors are the result of early menopause due to chemotherapy-induced ovarian failure, surgical ovarian oblation, or treatment with antiestrogenic drugs including SERMs and AIs.[115] Most women experience vasomotor symptoms, including hot flashes associated with these kinds of treatments.[116] Although hot flashes can affect the quality of life in survivors, they may also be a strong predictor of breast cancer recurrence in women who are treated with tamoxifen.[117] Data from the WHEL study showed that women who reported hot flashes at baseline were less likely after 7.3 years to develop breast cancer recurrence than those who did not report hot flashes at baseline. Hot flashes were a stronger predictor of recurrence than age, hormone receptor status, or the stage of cancer at diagnosis (stage I versus stage II). Additional research is needed to clarify the relationship between hot flashes and recurrence.

Few studies have addressed the management of menopausal symptoms in breast cancer survivors.[118] HRT is contraindicated in breast cancer survivors, especially those with ER-positive tumors. The use of selective serotonin reuptake inhibitors (SSRIs), the selective serotonin and norepinephrine reuptake inhibitor (SSNRI) venlafaxine, and the anticonvulsant gabapentin has been shown to reduce hot flashes, but the long-term safety of these agents is unknown.[119]

Many women are interested in CAM approaches for the alleviation of their menopausal symptoms. The North American Menopause Society (NAMS), in its position paper on the management of hot flashes, suggests lifestyle-related strategies for dealing with mild menopausal symptoms, including keeping the core body temperature cool, using paced respiration, and exercising regularly.[120] NAMS found no benefit with the use of dong quai, evening of primrose oil, ginseng, a Chinese herbal mixture, acupuncture, or magnet therapy. A recent Cochrane review also did not support phytoestrogens for menopausal vasomotor symptom control.[121] Hot flash "triggers" such as alcohol, hot drinks, or spicy foods are also a problem for some, but not all, women. Black cohosh (*Cimicifuga racemosa*) has been approved by the German E Commission for the nonprescription treatment of menopausal symptoms. Black cohosh has a relatively good safety profile. Evidence that supplementation can reduce symptoms is available,[122] but research supporting its use for the treatment of hot flashes in women with breast cancer is inconclusive.[123] This herb is not a phytoestrogen, and its mechanism of action is not clear. Evidence also suggests that weight loss as part of a healthy diet may reduce vasomotor symptoms in postmenopausal women.[124]

Osteoporosis

Breast cancer survivors are at risk for osteoporosis and fractures because of low estrogen levels caused by early menopause as a result of CT or oophorectomy in premenopausal women or the use of AIs in postmenopausal women.[125] Tamoxifen has been shown to preserve bone mineral density (BMD) in the spine and hip in postmenopausal women, although the extent of the protection is not clear—few studies have directly investigated the net BMD increase.[126]

Recommendations for preventing and treating bone loss in breast cancer survivors are similar to those for women without breast cancer. Women are advised to undergo an initial dual-energy x-ray absorptiometry (DEXA) bone scan and then an annual or biennial DEXA to assess BMD.

Recommendations have also been made regarding the use of calcium, vitamin D, and exercise to ward off bone loss. In 2006, for example, NAMS issued a position paper supporting the role of calcium and vitamin D in reducing fractures. It recommends 1200 mg of calcium per day from food and supplements and adequate vitamin D, defined as a serum level of 25 (OH)D of 30 ng/mL (or higher).[127] Yet, a review of the evidence suggests supplementation with vitamin D + calcium is not protective against bone loss in women treated for breast cancer.[128] Women should be advised to engage

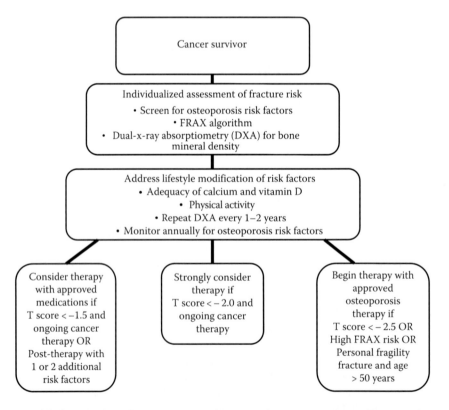

FIGURE 9.3 Algorithm for management of bone loss in cancer survivors. (From Lustberg, M.B. et al., *J. Clin. Oncol.*, 30(30), 3665, 2012.)

in regular weight-bearing and muscle-strengthening exercise to prevent and bone loss and to prevent falls. The use of bisphosphonates in combination with AIs may minimize bone loss.[129] Importantly, all cancer survivors should receive evaluation of bone health and fracture risk at least annually as outlined in Figure 9.3.

Cardiovascular Disease

The risk of cardiovascular disease (CVD) depends on the type of adjuvant systemic therapy received. Radiation to the left chest wall is associated with an increase in the long-term risk of cardiovascular events.[131] Early menopause also increases the long-term risk of CVD because it results in the loss of the protective effects of estrogen. Some concerns have been raised that the reduction of estrogen associated with use of AIs may also increase CVD risk, but studies to date have been inconclusive. For all these reasons, women should follow the standard guidelines for reducing CVD risk, such as maintaining a healthy weight, avoiding smoking, exercising regularly, and controlling blood pressure, blood sugar, and lipids. Congestive heart failure can result from CT consisting of anthracyclines and trastuzumab. Tamoxifen increases the risk of deep venous thrombosis and cerebrovascular disease. Cardiovascular events are associated with poorer survival in women treated with trastuzumab, suggesting this population should receive optimal nutrition therapy to reduce CVD risk.[132]

PREVENTING RECURRENCE

In the United States, the number of breast cancer survivors is estimated to exceed 3 million. Many of these survivors are interested in nutrition and lifestyle interventions beyond conventional treatment to improve their prognosis. Although hundreds of observational studies have focused on the potential links between diet and etiology of breast cancer, the only randomized controlled trial testing the hypothesis that diet can reduce risk was the Women's Health Initiative (results described earlier).[53] Even more alarming is how few studies to date have addressed diet and survival using disease-specific end points.[133] The Women's Intervention Nutrition Study (WINS) and the WHEL study are two randomized trials that focused on lifestyle intervention, including diet and exercise (Table 9.2).[134,135] Both WINS and WHEL enrolled women who had completed primary conventional cancer treatment.

WEIGHT AND RISK OF RECURRENCE AND MORTALITY

Excess adiposity is thought to play a role in reducing overall survival after cancer.[138] However, data specific to breast cancer are less consistent. High body weight prior to diagnosis has been associated with poorer survival in some, but not all association studies.[139,140] Generally, both underweight and morbidly obese women have higher mortality after breast cancer, similar to evidence from studies of nonbreast cancer survivors.[141] Weight gain has also shown inconsistent results in relation to survival. In a study from the pooling project, Caan et al demonstrated weight loss was associated with poorer survival likely related to advanced disease.[111] Concurrently, the same analysis showed a reduced survival among women with comorbid conditions.

TABLE 9.2

Summary of Intervention Trials Evaluating Breast Cancer Recurrence

Name of Study/Year Published/Country	Size of Cohort/Years of Follow-up	Findings
Women's Healthy Eating and Living (WHEL), 2007, United States[136]	1490 women with early-stage breast cancer Mean 6.7 years of follow-up	A combination of consuming five or more servings of vegetables/fruit and accumulating the equivalent of walking 30 min 6 days/week was associated with a significant survival advantage (HR.56). Benefits were observed in both obese and nonobese women.
Women's Intervention Nutrition Study (WINS), 2006, United States[137]	2437 women with early-stage breast cancer 5 years	Reducing dietary fat to 15%–20% of calories was associated with a longer relapse-free survival in women with ER-negative/PR-negative cancers. No benefit was seen in ER-positive/PR positive cancers.

Abrahamson et al., in a large population-based follow-up study, found that breast cancer survival is reduced among younger women aged 20–54 with general or abdominal obesity.[142] Young women who had a BMI of 30 or more or a waist-to-hip ratio (WHR) of 0.80 or more near the time of their diagnosis of breast cancer also had increased mortality. In contrast to these findings, data from the WHEL study revealed that combined healthy lifestyle behaviors, consisting of five servings of vegetables and fruit per day and the equivalent of walking 30 min at a moderate pace 6 days/week, was associated with a 50% reduction in mortality rates in both obese and nonobese women with early-stage breast cancer.[135]

The means by which overweight influences survival include increased endogenous production of estrogen by adipose tissue, decreased levels of SHBG, diagnosis at a later stage, larger tumor size at diagnosis, increased insulin and insulin-like growth factors, and poorer response to treatment.[143] Obesity is also associated with reduced immune function, which could indirectly promote recurrence. Elevated WHR is associated with hyperinsulinemia and insulin resistance independent of BMI and may be a contributing factor in mortality. A higher BMI may also be related to increased mortality as a result of incorrect dosing of chemotherapy incomplete removal of the primary tumor, or difficulty in detecting recurrences in large women.

Importantly, recent evidence suggests the relationship between adiposity and recurrence or survival may be influenced by therapies used to treat the disease. In a recent review, Azrad and Demark-Wahnefried reported that aromatase inhibitor therapy may be less effective in obese as compared to normal weight women.[144]

Finally, efforts to reduce body weight and metabolic abnormalities in women previously treated for breast cancer have been largely effective, suggesting a role for nutrition and activity interventions in this at-risk group.[145,146]

LOW-FAT, HIGH-FIBER, HIGH-VEGETABLE AND FRUIT DIET

A low-fat, high-fiber, high-vegetable and fruit diet does not appear to reduce mortality or recurrence in breast cancer survivors. In the WHEL trial, a diet including five vegetable servings plus 16 ounces of vegetable juice, three fruit servings, 30 g of fiber, and 15%–20% of calories from fat did not reduce mortality from breast cancer, mortality from any cause, or the combined outcome of invasive breast cancer recurrence or new primary breast cancer during the 7.3-year follow-up period in women with early-stage breast cancer (stage I, stage II, or stage IIIa).[134] Women in the control group consumed five servings of vegetables and fruit per day, so it is possible that eating more than five servings of vegetables and fruit per day does not confer additional benefit. This interpretation is supported by evidence that women in WHEL with higher circulating carotenoid concentrations had a survival benefit[147] while those with high C-reactive protein (CRP) did not.[148] Both carotenoids and CRP are biomarkers that are known to be responsive to diet therapy.

DIETARY FAT AND ER-NEGATIVE/PR-NEGATIVE BREAST CANCER RECURRENCE

Dietary fat intake may influence the recurrence or the diagnosis of new breast cancer in women with early-stage breast cancer, according to interim analyses from the Women's Intervention Nutrition Study (WINS).[137] WINS, a randomized, prospective, multicenter trial involving more 2400 participants, showed that a reduction in dietary fat to 15%–20% of total calories was marginally associated with longer relapse-free survival. The benefit was mainly seen in women with ER-negative/PR-negative cancers. Reduced body weight in the intervention group might be responsible for the improvement in relapse-free survival. Although additional research is needed to confirm the relationship between dietary fat and relapse, women with ER-negative/ PR-negative breast cancers should be advised to reduce their dietary fat intake to 20% of calories. The expertise of a registered dietitian–nutritionist should be utilized to help women achieve this goal.

COMBINED HEALTHY LIFESTYLE BEHAVIORS

Healthy lifestyle behaviors, when combined, have been demonstrated to have a beneficial effect on mortality in breast cancer survivors. In an analysis from the Women's Health Initiative, meeting the American Cancer Society's guidelines for cancer prevention reduced cancer-specific mortality by 20%.[1] In addition to evaluating cancer-specific outcomes, several short-term trials have demonstrated positive effects of diet plus physical activity on quality of life, treatment-related symptoms, and function.[149]

Tea

Epidemiologic research in Japan suggests that Asian women who have been treated for stage I or stage II breast cancer and who drink 3–5 cups of green tea per day reduce their risk of recurrence compared to women who drink 0–2 cups of green tea per day (HR stage I = 0.37; HR stage II = 0.80).[150] No benefit was found for stage III and IV breast cancer. Evidence from a large Swedish cohort showed no association between black tea intake and breast cancer survival.[151] Nevertheless, women with early-stage breast cancer may want to consider drinking 3–5 cups of green tea per day, as there is some potential benefit with no known harmful effects.

Vitamin D

Serum vitamin D levels at the time of diagnosis seem to demonstrate a U-shaped association with mortality after breast cancer.[152] In a prospective study involving 512 women with newly diagnosed breast cancer, vitamin D deficiency at the time of breast cancer diagnosis was associated with an increased risk of distant recurrence and death.[153] Vitamin D levels were deficient (<50 nmol/L or <20 ng/mL) in 37.5% of these patients, insufficient (50–72 nmol/L or 20–28.8 ng/mL) in 38.5%, and adequate (>72 nmol/L or 28.8 ng/mL) in 24%. A novel study evaluating the interplay between vitamin D status and response to neoadjuvant chemotherapy showed no survival benefit with vitamin D supplementation.[154]

Epidemiological studies suggest that the season in which diagnosis is made may also affect survival. Diagnosis of breast cancer in the summer is associated with greater survival than diagnosis in the winter. Women of all ages in Norway who were diagnosed in the summer had 25% better survival after standard treatment compared with women who were diagnosed in the winter.[155] Women younger than age 50 had 40% better survival if they were diagnosed in the summer versus the winter. Although no conclusions about the biological mechanism could be made based on this epidemiological study, the authors theorized that women diagnosed in the summer had higher circulating vitamin D levels, which may have modulated cell signaling, induced apoptosis, regulated cell-cycle progression, and reduced angiogenic activity and invasiveness. Similar findings have been reported in the United Kingdom.[156]

Women with a history of breast cancer should have their serum 25(OH) levels measured. Additional research identifying the optimal serum level to prevent recurrence is needed, but the study results suggest that women should take enough vitamin D to maintain an adequate serum level.

Cruciferous Vegetables

The evidence that cruciferous vegetables may reduce recurrence after breast cancer therapy is mixed. In a study of women in the WHEL trial, those on Tamoxifen showed a 35% reduction in recurrence with higher cruciferous vegetable intake.[157] However, a more recent pooled analysis failed to show a significant protective effect.[158] A clinical trial seeking to determine whether cruciferous vegetables are protective against breast cancer recurrence is now under way.[159] In the meantime, it is reasonable to encourage women to increase consumption of cruciferous vegetables because of these foods' proposed anticarcinogenic properties and ability to modulate estrogen metabolites. Currently, there is no evidence to support the use of supplements of I3Cor diindolylmethane, components of cruciferous vegetables, to alter survival.

SUMMARY

The evidence to support diet and lifestyle modification after breast cancer and in the primary prevention of breast cancer is mounting. Table 9.3 summarizes the current

TABLE 9.3
Practical Nutrition Recommendations, Derived from Review of Current Evidence, for Breast Cancer Survivors

1. Engage in the equivalent of brisk walking 6 days/week for ½ h per session.
   - Include resistance training 3 times/week to promote a healthy muscle mass.
2. Eat 3–5 servings of vegetables and 2 servings of fruit per day.
   - Select colorful vegetables including yellow, orange, and deep green vegetables, among others.
   - Select a variety of flavors as well.
3. Achieve and maintain a healthy weight.
   - Consume energy-dense foods sparingly.
   - Stay active, reduce sedentary time.
   - Self-monitor intake, activity, and weight.
4. Limit red or processed meat to less than 18 ounces/week.
   - Select lower fat and plant sources of protein such as eggs, beans, legumes, and fish.
5. Avoid charbroiled and overcooked foods (burnt or charred), including beef, chicken, lamb, pork, or fish.
   - Cook these foods at a temperature below 325°F—the surface temperature at which heterocyclic amines (HCAs) form—whether grilling, pan-frying, or oven-roasting the foods.
   - When grilling, marinating the meat prior to cooking can reduce the formation of HCAs.
   - Avoid cooking over a direct flame, as fat or marinade drippings can cause flare-ups that deposit HCAs and other carcinogens on the surface of food. Flip food once a minute.
   - Microwaving the meat for 1–2 min at a medium setting prior to grilling can inhibit HCAs formation.
   - Use other methods of food preparation such as stewing, poaching, or slow-cooking in a Crock-Pot.
6. Aim for 1000–1500 mg of calcium per day and 800 IU of vitamin D_3 as cholecalciferol.
   - Measure serum 25(OH) vitamin D levels to determine vitamin D sufficiency.
   - Increase vitamin D supplementation as necessary to achieve a sufficient serum level of vitamin D, currently thought to be 30 ng/mL.
   - Optimal serum ranges of vitamin D for the prevention of breast cancer recurrence are not known.
7. Consider regular intake of tea as an alternate to other beverages such as juices, sweetened beverages that provide excess sugar intake with modest bioactive activity.
8. Avoid alcoholic drinks.
   - Even small amounts of alcohol increase breast cancer risk, regardless of the type of alcohol.
   - Red wine may be the best alternative given the aromatase inhibitory effects, but data are limited.
9. For ER-negative/PR-negative breast cancer, dietary fat should be decreased to 15%–20% of total daily calories.
   - Recommend consultation with a registered dietitian nutritionist to achieve this goal.
10. Breast cancer survivors should receive nutritional care from a registered dietitian nutritionist for diet and supplement advice.
    - A registered dietitian nutritionist can help with weight management and the prevention and treatment of the metabolic syndrome.
    - Calcium and vitamin D supplementation is often necessary to meet the recommendations for this nutrient.
    - In general, efforts should be made to obtain nutrients and phytochemicals from food, not from supplements.

(Continued)

TABLE 9.3 (*Continued*)
Practical Nutrition Recommendations, Derived from Review of Current Evidence, for Breast Cancer Survivors

11. Women with ER-positive/PR-positive breast cancers who experience hot flashes due to endocrine therapy or early menopause should avoid taking supplements containing phytoestrogens from soy, lignins, or soy isoflavones.

   • The safety of these supplements has not been established for the management of hot flashes in breast cancer survivors.

   • Lifestyle strategies such as weight loss/control, regular physical activity and avoidance of alcohol may be hot flash triggers in some women.

evidence as practical guidance dietitian–nutritionists can share with their patients/clients. While randomized, controlled clinical trials testing all of these recommendations have not been completed, strong epidemiological evidence combined with the larger body of evidence suggesting health promoting qualities of the selected foods and/or dietary practices supports such guidance for our patients/clients.

FUTURE DIRECTIONS FOR RESEARCH

Nutrition's part in the etiology, treatment, prevention, and recurrence of breast cancer continues to unfold. Although strong evidence is lacking about the relationship between diet and breast cancer, women should continue to embrace healthy eating and lifestyle behaviors for their potential overall health benefits. Additional research is needed about the role of diet during fetal development, infancy, childhood, and adolescence as part of the etiology of breast cancer. Diet during these periods of development may be an important predictor of breast cancer risk, but as yet data are lacking in this area. Areas for additional exploration include how diet influences subgroups of women characterized by certain tumor subtypes and genetic, epigenetic, or hormonal status. Similarly, research is needed on breast cancer risk and chemicals that act as endocrine disruptors. Additionally, studies addressing survivorship and diet are essential, especially those geared toward promotion of healthy eating and physical activity. Dissemination of diet, nutrition, and physical activity guidance for cancer prevention and survival remains limited and efforts to inform and support lifestyle behavior change toward breast cancer risk reduction are needed.

REFERENCES

1. Thomson CA, McCullough ML, Wertheim BC et al. Nutrition and physical activity cancer prevention guidelines, cancer risk, and mortality in the women's health initiative. *Cancer Prevention Research.* January 2014;7(1):42–53.
2. Kushi LH, Doyle C, McCullough M et al. American cancer society guidelines on nutrition and physical activity for cancer prevention reducing the risk of cancer with healthy food choices and physical activity. *CA: A Cancer Journal for Clinicians.* January–February 2012;62(1):30–67.

3. Romaguera D, Vergnaud AC, Peeters PH et al. Is concordance with World Cancer Research Fund/American Institute for Cancer Research guidelines for cancer prevention related to subsequent risk of cancer? Results from the EPIC study. *American Journal of Clinical Nutrition.* July 2012;96(1):150–163.

4. Matsuno RK, Pagano IS, Maskarinec G, Issell BF, Gotay CC. Complementary and alternative medicine use and breast cancer prognosis: A pooled analysis of four population-based studies of breast cancer survivors. *Journal of Women's Health (Larchmt).* 2012;21(12):1252–1258.

5. Siegel R, Ma JM, Zou ZH, Jemal A. Cancer statistics, 2014. *CA: A Cancer Journal for Clinicians.* January 2014;64(1):9–29.

6. Rossouw JE, Anderson GL, Prentice RL et al. Risks and benefits of estrogen plus progestin in healthy postmenopausal women: Principal results From the Women's Health Initiative randomized controlled trial. *JAMA: The Journal of the American Medical Association.* July 17, 2002;288(3):321–333.

7. To T, Wall C, Baines CJ, Miller AB. Is carcinoma in situ a precursor lesion of invasive breast cancer? *International Journal of Cancer.* October 2014;135(7):1646–1652.

8. DeSantis C, Ma J, Bryan L, Jemal A. Breast cancer statistics, 2013. *CA: A Cancer Journal for Clinicians.* 2014;64(1):52–62.

9. Bagaria SP, Ray PS, Sim MS et al. Personalizing breast cancer staging by the inclusion of ER, PR, and HER2. *Jama Surgery.* February 2014;149(2):125–129.

10. NCI. The breast cancer risk assessment tool. http://www.cancer.gov/bcrisktool/. Accessed June 28, 2014.

11. Anderson EE, Hoskins K. Individual breast cancer risk assessment in underserved populations: Integrating empirical bioethics and health disparities research. *Journal of Health Care for the Poor and Underserved.* November 2012;23(4):34–46.

12. Manson JE, Chlebowski RT, Stefanick ML et al. Menopausal hormone therapy and health outcomes during the intervention and extended poststopping phases of the women's health initiative randomized trials. *Obstetrical & Gynecological Survey.* February 2014;69(2):83–85.

13. Huang Z, Hankinson SE, Colditz GA et al. Dual effects of weight and weight gain on breast cancer risk. *JAMA: The Journal of the American Medical Association.* November 5, 1997;278(17):1407–1411.

14. Cecchini RS, Costantino JP, Cauley JA et al. Body mass index and the risk for developing invasive breast cancer among high-risk women in NSABP P-1 and STAR breast cancer prevention trials. *Cancer Prevention Research (Phila).* April 2012;5(4):583–592.

15. Sexton KR, Franzini L, Day RS, Brewster A, Vernon SW, Bondy ML. A review of body size and breast cancer risk in Hispanic and African American women. *Cancer.* December 1, 2011;117(23):5271–5281.

16. Moskowitz CS, Chou JF, Wolden SL et al. Breast cancer after chest radiation therapy for childhood cancer. *Journal of Clinical Oncology.* July 2014;32(21):2217–2223.

17. Smith RA, Manassaram-Baptiste D, Brooks D et al. Cancer screening in the United States, 2014: A review of current American Cancer Society guidelines and current issues in cancer screening. *CA: A Cancer Journal for Clinicians.* 2014;64(1):30–51.

18. Force USPST. Screening for breast cancer. http://www.uspreventiveservicestaskforce. org/uspstf/uspsbrca.htm. Accessed June 28, 2014.

19. Malmgren JA, Parikh J, Atwood MK, Kaplan HG. Improved prognosis of women aged 75 and older with mammography-detected breast cancer. *Radiology.* 2014;5:140209.

20. Network NCC. *NCCN Clinical Practice Guidelines in Oncology: Breast Cancer,* National Comprehensive Cancer Network, 2007.

21. Theriault RL, Carlson RW, Allred C et al. Breast cancer, version 3.2013. *Journal of the National Comprehensive Cancer Network.* 2013;11(7):753–761.

22. Brenton JD, Carey LA, Ahmed AA, Caldas C. Molecular classification and molecular forecasting of breast cancer: Ready for clinical application? *Journal of Clinical Oncology: Official Journal of the American Society of Clinical Oncology.* October 10, 2005;23(29):7350–7360.

23. Daemen A, Griffith OL, Heiser LM et al. Modeling precision treatment of breast cancer. *Genome Biology.* 2013;14(10):R110.

24. Edge SB, Compton CC. The American Joint Committee on Cancer: The 7th edition of the AJCC cancer staging manual and the future of TNM. *Annals of Surgical Oncology.* 2010;17(6):1471–1474.

25. Harris EE, Correa C, Hwang WT et al. Late cardiac mortality and morbidity in early-stage breast cancer patients after breast-conservation treatment. *Journal of Clinical Oncology: Official Journal of the American Society of Clinical Oncology.* September 1, 2006;24(25):4100–4106.

26. Chan EK, Woods R, McBride ML et al. Adjuvant hypofractionated versus conventional whole breast radiation therapy for early-stage breast cancer: Long-term hospital-related morbidity from cardiac causes. *International Journal of Radiation Oncology, Biology, Physics.* 2014;88(4):786–792.

27. Komm BS, Mirkin S. An overview of current and emerging SERMs. *Journal of Steroid Biochemistry and Molecular Biology.* March 22, 2014;143C:207–222.

28. Vogel VG, Costantino JP, Wickerham DL et al. Effects of tamoxifen vs raloxifene on the risk of developing invasive breast cancer and other disease outcomes: The NSABP Study of Tamoxifen and Raloxifene (STAR) P-2 trial. *JAMA: The Journal of the American Medical Association.* June 21, 2006;295(23):2727–2741.

29. Bell LN, Nguyen ATP, Li L et al. Comparison of changes in the lipid profile of postmenopausal women with early stage breast cancer treated with exemestane or letrozole. *The Journal of Clinical Pharmacology.* 2012;52(12):1852–1860.

30. WCRF/AICR. Food, nutrition, physical activity, and the prevention of cancer: A global perspective. 2007; http://www.dietandcancerreport.org/. Accessed May 28, 2014.

31. Prentice RL, Shaw PA, Bingham SA et al. Biomarker-calibrated energy and protein consumption and increased cancer risk among postmenopausal women. *American Journal of Epidemiology.* April 15, 2009;169(8):977–989.

32. Michels KB, Mohllajee AP, Roset-Bahmanyar E, Beehler GP, Moysich KB. Diet and breast cancer: A review of the prospective observational studies. *Cancer.* June 15, 2007;109(12 Suppl):2712–2749.

33. Jung S, Spiegelman D, Baglietto L et al. Fruit and vegetable intake and risk of breast cancer by hormone receptor status. *Journal of the National Cancer Institute.* 2013;105(3):219–236.

34. Phipps AI, Chlebowski RT, Prentice R et al. Reproductive history and oral contraceptive use in relation to risk of triple-negative breast cancer. *Journal of the National Cancer Institute.* 2011;103(6):470–477.

35. Stendell-Hollis NR, Thompson PA, Thomson CA, O'Sullivan MJ, Ray RM, Chlebowski RT. Investigating the association of lactation history and postmenopausal breast cancer risk in the women's health initiative. *Nutrition and Cancer.* 2013;65(7):969–981.

36. Michels KB, Willett WC, Hunter D et al. Prospective assessment of breastfeeding and breast cancer incidence among 89 887 women. *The Lancet.* 1996;347(8999):431–436.

37. London SJ, Colditz GA, Stampfer MJ et al. Lactation and risk of breast cancer in a cohort of US women. *American Journal of Epidemiology.* 1990;132(1):17–26.

38. Collaborative Group on Hormonal Factors in Breast Cancer. Breast cancer and breast-feeding: Collaborative reanalysis of individual data from 47 epidemiological studies in 30 countries, including 50302 women with breast cancer and 96973 women without the disease. *Lancet.* July 20, 2002;360(9328):187–195.

39. Krishnan K, Bassett JK, MacInnis RJ et al. Associations between weight in early adulthood, change in weight, and breast cancer risk in postmenopausal women. *Cancer Epidemiology Biomarkers & Prevention.* 2013;22(8):1409–1416.
40. Zumoff B. Hormonal abnormalities in obesity. *Acta Medica Scandinavica.* 1987;222(S723):153–160.
41. Rose D, Komninou D, Stephenson G. Obesity, adipocytokines, and insulin resistance in breast cancer. *Obesity Reviews.* 2004;5(3):153–165.
42. Renehan AG, Frystyk J, Flyvbjerg A. Obesity and cancer risk: The role of the insulin–IGF axis. *Trends in Endocrinology & Metabolism.* 2006;17(8):328–336.
43. Grivennikov SI, Greten FR, Karin M. Immunity, inflammation, and cancer. *Cell.* 2010;140(6):883–899.
44. Eliassen AH, Colditz GA, Rosner B, Willett WC, Hankinson SE. Adult weight change and risk of postmenopausal breast cancer. *JAMA: The Journal of the American Medical Association.* July 12, 2006;296(2):193–201.
45. Yang XR, Chang-Claude J, Goode EL et al. Associations of breast cancer risk factors with tumor subtypes: A pooled analysis from the Breast Cancer Association Consortium studies. *Journal of the National Cancer Institute.* 2011;103(3):250–263.
46. Sherman ME, Rimm DL, Yang XR et al. Variation in breast cancer hormone receptor and HER2 levels by etiologic factors: A population-based analysis. *International Journal of Cancer.* 2007;121(5):1079–1085.
47. Fagherazzi G, Vilier A, Boutron-Ruault MC, Mesrine S, Clavel-Chapelon F. Alcohol consumption and breast cancer risk subtypes in the E3N-EPIC cohort. *European Journal of Cancer Prevention.* 2014;16:16.
48. Scoccianti C, Lauby-Secretan B, Bello PY, Chajes V, Romieu I. Female breast cancer and alcohol consumption: A review of the literature. *American Journal of Preventive Medicine.* 2014;46(3 Suppl 1):031.
49. Smith-Warner SA, Spiegelman D, Yaun SS et al. Alcohol and breast cancer in women: A pooled analysis of cohort studies. *JAMA: The Journal of the American Medical Association.* February 18 1998;279(7):535–540.
50. Suzuki R, Ye W, Rylander-Rudqvist T, Saji S, Colditz GA, Wolk A. Alcohol and postmenopausal breast cancer risk defined by estrogen and progesterone receptor status: A prospective cohort study. *Journal of National Cancer Institue.* November 2, 2005;97(21):1601–1608.
51. Shufelt C, Merz CN, Yang Y et al. Red versus white wine as a nutritional aromatase inhibitor in premenopausal women: A pilot study. *Journal of Women's Health.* 2012;21(3):281–284.
52. Thiebaut AC, Kipnis V, Chang SC et al. Dietary fat and postmenopausal invasive breast cancer in the National Institutes of Health-AARP Diet and Health Study cohort. *Journal of National Cancer Institute.* March 21, 2007;99(6):451–462.
53. Prentice RL, Caan B, Chlebowski RT et al. Low-fat dietary pattern and risk of invasive breast cancer: The women's health initiative randomized controlled dietary modification trial. *JAMA: The Journal of the American Medical Association.* February 8, 2006;295(6):629–642.
54. Sieri S, Chiodini P, Agnoli C et al. Dietary fat intake and development of specific breast cancer subtypes. *Journal of the National Cancer Institute.* April 2014;106(5):1–6.
55. Boeke CE, Eliassen AH, Chen WY et al. Dietary fat intake in relation to lethal breast cancer in two large prospective cohort studies. *Breast Cancer Research and Treatment.* 2014;146(2):383–392.
56. Abel S, Riedel S, Gelderblom WC. Dietary PUFA and cancer. *Proceedings of the Nutrition Society.* 2014;73(3):361–367.
57. Escrich E, Solanas M, Moral R. Olive oil and other dietary lipids in breast cancer. *Cancer Treatment and Research.* 2014;159:289–309.

58. Taylor EF, Burley VJ, Greenwood DC, Cade JE. Meat consumption and risk of breast cancer in the UK Women's Cohort Study. *British Journal of Cancer.* April 10, 2007;96(7):1139–1146.
59. Wise J. Eating more red meat is linked with raised risk of breast cancer. *BMJ.* 2014;10(348):g3814.
60. Higher red meat intake in young women increases breast cancer risk. *Nursing Standard.* 2014;28(44):16.
61. Alexander DD, Morimoto LM, Mink PJ, Cushing CA. A review and meta-analysis of red and processed meat consumption and breast cancer. *Nutritional Research Review.* 2010;23(2):349–365.
62. Papaioannou MD, Koufaris C, Gooderham NJ. The cooked meat-derived mammary carcinogen 2-amino-1-methyl-6-phenylimidazo[4,5-b]pyridine (PhIP) elicits estrogenic-like microRNA responses in breast cancer cells. *Toxicology Letters.* 2014;229(1):9–16.
63. Catsburg C, Miller AB, Rohan TE. Adherence to cancer prevention guidelines and risk of breast cancer. *International Journal of Cancer.* 2014;10(10):28887.
64. Link LB, Canchola AJ, Bernstein L et al. Dietary patterns and breast cancer risk in the California Teachers Study cohort. *American Journal of Clinical Nutrition.* 2013;98(6):1524–1532.
65. Demetriou CA, Hadjisavvas A, Loizidou MA et al. The mediterranean dietary pattern and breast cancer risk in Greek-Cypriot women: A case-control study. *BMC Cancer.* 2012;12(113):1471–2407.
66. Schwingshackl L, Hoffmann G. Adherence to Mediterranean diet and risk of cancer: A systematic review and meta-analysis of observational studies. *International Journal of Cancer.* 2014;6(10):28824.
67. Cade JE, Taylor EF, Burley VJ, Greenwood DC. Common dietary patterns and risk of breast cancer: Analysis from the United Kingdom Women's Cohort Study. *Nutrition and Cancer.* 2010;62(3):300–306.
68. Willett W. Lessons from dietary studies in Adventists and questions for the future. *American Journal of Clinical Nutrition.* September 2003;78(3 Suppl):539S–543S.
69. Baglietto L, Krishnan K, Severi G et al. Dietary patterns and risk of breast cancer. *British Journal of Cancer.* 2011;104(3):524–531.
70. Bradbury KE, Appleby PN, Key TJ. Fruit, vegetable, and fiber intake in relation to cancer risk: Findings from the European Prospective Investigation into Cancer and Nutrition (EPIC). *American Journal of Clinical Nutrition.* 2014;100(1 Suppl):394S–398S.
71. Norat T, Aune D, Chan D, Romaguera D. Fruits and vegetables: Updating the epidemiologic evidence for the WCRF/AICR lifestyle recommendations for cancer prevention. *Cancer Treatment and Research.* 2014;159:35–50.
72. Higdon JV, Delage B, Williams DE, Dashwood RH. Cruciferous vegetables and human cancer risk: Epidemiologic evidence and mechanistic basis. *Pharmacological Research.* March 2007;55(3):224–236.
73. Suzuki R, Iwasaki M, Hara A et al. Fruit and vegetable intake and breast cancer risk defined by estrogen and progesterone receptor status: The Japan Public Health Center-based Prospective Study. *Cancer Causes Control.* 2013;24(12):2117–2128.
74. Lampe JW, Peterson S. Brassica, biotransformation and cancer risk: Genetic polymorphisms alter the preventive effects of cruciferous vegetables. *Journal of Nutrition.* October 2002;132(10):2991–2994.
75. Fowke JH, Longcope C, Hebert JR. Brassica vegetable consumption shifts estrogen metabolism in healthy postmenopausal women. *Cancer Epidemiol Biomarkers & Prevention.* August 2000;9(8):773–779.
76. Fink BN, Steck SE, Wolff MS et al. Dietary flavonoid intake and breast cancer risk among women on Long Island. *American Journal of Epidemiology.* March 1, 2007;165(5):514–523.

77. Khankari NK, Bradshaw PT, McCullough LE et al. Genetic variation in multiple biologic pathways, flavonoid intake, and breast cancer. *Cancer Causes and Control.* 2014;25(2):215–226.
78. Yuan JM. Cancer prevention by green tea: Evidence from epidemiologic studies. *American Journal of Clinical Nutrition.* 2013;98(6 Suppl):30.
79. Yu F, Jin Z, Jiang H,et al. Tea consumption and the risk of five major cancers: A dose-response meta-analysis of prospective studies. *BMC Cancer.* 2014;14(197):1471–2407.
80. Wu AH, Tseng CC, Van Den Berg D, Yu MC. Tea intake, COMT genotype, and breast cancer in Asian-American women. *Cancer Research.* November 1, 2003;63(21):7526–7529.
81. Iwasaki M, Mizusawa J, Kasuga Y et al. Green tea consumption and breast cancer risk in Japanese women: A case-control study. *Nutrition and Cancer.* 2014;66(1):57–67.
82. Douglas CC, Johnson SA, Arjmandi BH. Soy and its isoflavones: The truth behind the science in breast cancer. *Anticancer Agents in Medicinal Chemistry.* 2013;13(8):1178–1187.
83. Nagata C, Mizoue T, Tanaka K et al. Soy intake and breast cancer risk: An evaluation based on a systematic review of epidemiologic evidence among the Japanese population. *Japan Journal of Clinical Oncology.* 2014;44(3):282–295.
84. Dewi FN, Wood CE, Lees CJ et al. Dietary soy effects on mammary gland development during the pubertal transition in nonhuman primates. *Cancer Prevention Research.* 2013;6(8):832–842.
85. Brooks JD, Ward WE, Lewis JE et al. Supplementation with flaxseed alters estrogen metabolism in postmenopausal women to a greater extent than does supplementation with an equal amount of soy. *American Journal of Clinical Nutrition.* February 2004;79(2):318–325.
86. Mason JK, Thompson LU. Flaxseed and its lignan and oil components: Can they play a role in reducing the risk of and improving the treatment of breast cancer? *Applied Physiology Nutrition and Metabolism.* 2014;39(6):663–678.
87. Galeone C, Pelucchi C, Levi F et al. Onion and garlic use and human cancer. *American Journal of Clinical Nutrition.* November 2006;84(5):1027–1032.
88. Bao PP, Shu XO, Zheng Y et al. Fruit, vegetable, and animal food intake and breast cancer risk by hormone receptor status. *Nutrition and Cancer.* 2012;64(6):806–819.
89. Tio M, Andrici J, Eslick GD. Folate intake and the risk of breast cancer: A systematic review and meta-analysis. *Breast Cancer Research and Treatment.* 2014;145(2): 513–524.
90. Zhang YF, Shi WW, Gao HF, Zhou L, Hou AJ, Zhou YH. Folate intake and the risk of breast cancer: A dose-response meta-analysis of prospective studies. *PLoS One.* 2014;9(6).
91. Stolzenberg-Solomon RZ, Chang SC, Leitzmann MF et al. Folate intake, alcohol use, and postmenopausal breast cancer risk in the prostate, lung, colorectal, and ovarian cancer Sscreening trial. *American Journal of Clinical Nutrition.* April 2006;83(4):895–904.
92. Holick MF. Vitamin D deficiency. *New England Journal of Medicine.* July 19, 2007;357(3):266–281.
93. Feldman D, Krishnan AV, Swami S, Giovannucci E, Feldman BJ. The role of vitamin D in reducing cancer risk and progression. *Nature Reviews Cancer.* 2014;14(5): 342–357.
94. Lappe JM, Travers-Gustafson D, Davies KM, Recker RR, Heaney RP. Vitamin D and calcium supplementation reduces cancer risk: Results of a randomized trial. *American Journal of Clinical Nutrition.* June 2007;85(6):1586–1591.
95. Cauley JA, Chlebowski RT, Wactawski-Wende J et al. Calcium plus vitamin D supplementation and health outcomes five years after active intervention ended: The Women's Health Initiative. *Journal of Womens Health.* 2013;22(11):915–929.

96. Sperati F, Vici P, Maugeri-Sacca M et al. Vitamin D supplementation and breast cancer prevention: A systematic review and meta-analysis of randomized clinical trials. *PLoS One*. 2013;8(7).

97. Vasquez A, Manso G, Cannell J. The clinical importance of vitamin D (cholecalciferol): A paradigm shift with implications for all healthcare providers. *Alternatives Therapies in Health and Medicine*. September–October 2004;10(5):28–36; quiz 37, 94.

98. Rudel RA, Attfield KR, Schifano JN, Brody JG. Chemicals causing mammary gland tumors in animals signal new directions for epidemiology, chemicals testing, and risk assessment for breast cancer prevention. *Cancer*. June 15, 2007;109 (12 Suppl):2635–2666.

99. Brody JG, Moysich KB, Humblet O, Attfield KR, Beehler GP, Rudel RA. Environmental pollutants and breast cancer: Epidemiologic studies. *Cancer*. June 15, 2007;109 (12 Suppl):2667–2711.

100. Gartner LM, Morton J, Lawrence RA et al. Breastfeeding and the use of human milk. *Pediatrics*. February 2005;115(2):496–506.

101. Fenichel P, Chevalier N, Brucker-Davis F. Bisphenol A: An endocrine and metabolic disruptor. *Annales d Endocrinologie*. 2013;74(3):211–220.

102. Xu CX, Zhu HH, Zhu YM. Diabetes and cancer: Associations, mechanisms, and implications for medical practice. *World Journal of Diabetes*. 2014;5(3):372–380.

103. Hernandez AV, Guarnizo M, Miranda Y et al. Association between insulin resistance and breast carcinoma: A systematic review and meta-analysis. *PLoS One*. June 2014;9(6):e99317.

104. Bauer J, Capra S, Ferguson M. Use of the scored Patient-Generated Subjective Global Assessment (PG-SGA) as a nutrition assessment tool in patients with cancer. *European Journal of Clinical Nutrition*. August 2002;56(8):779–785.

105. Abbott J, Teleni L, McKavanagh D, Watson J, McCarthy A, Isenring E. A novel, automated nutrition screening system as a predictor of nutritional risk in an oncology day treatment unit (ODTU). *Supportive Care in Cancer: Official Journal of the Multinational Association of Supportive Care in Cancer*. 2014;22(8):2107–2112.

106. Read JA, Crockett N, Volker DH et al. Nutritional assessment in cancer: Comparing the Mini-Nutritional Assessment (MNA) with the scored Patient-Generated Subjective Global Assessment (PGSGA). *Nutrition and Cancer*. 2005;53(1):51–56.

107. Saghatchian M, Bihan C, Chenailler C, Mazouni C, Dauchy S, Delaloge S. Exploring frontiers: Use of complementary and alternative medicine among patients with early-stage breast cancer. *Breast*. 2014;23(3):279–285.

108. Wang JS, Cai H, Wang CY, Zhang J, Zhang MX. Body weight changes in breast cancer patients following adjuvant chemotherapy and contributing factors. *Molecular and Clinical Oncology*. 2014;2(1):105–110.

109. Liu LN, Wen FH, Miaskowski C et al. Weight change trajectory in women with breast cancer receiving chemotherapy and the effect of different regimens. *Journal of Clinical Nursing*. 2014;7(10):12521.

110. Saquib N, Flatt SW, Natarajan L et al. Weight gain and recovery of pre-cancer weight after breast cancer treatments: Evidence from the women's healthy eating and living (WHEL) study. *Breast Cancer Research and Treatment*. October 2007;105(2):177–186.

111. Caan BJ, Kwan ML, Shu XO et al. Weight change and survival after breast cancer in the after breast cancer pooling project. *Cancer Epidemiol Biomarkers & Prevention*. 2012;21(8):1260–1271.

112. Chaudhry ZW, Brown RV, Fawole OA et al. Comparative effectiveness of strategies to prevent weight gain among women with and at risk for breast cancer: A systematic review. *Springerplus*. June 2013;2(1):277.

113. Villarini A, Pasanisi P, Raimondi M et al. Preventing weight gain during adjuvant chemotherapy for breast cancer: A dietary intervention study. *Breast Cancer Research and Treatment.* 2012;135(2):581–589.

114. Backman M, Wengstrom Y, Johansson B et al. A randomized pilot study with daily walking during adjuvant chemotherapy for patients with breast and colorectal cancer. *Acta Oncology.* 2014;53(4):510–520.

115. Hayes DF. Clinical practice. Follow-up of patients with early breast cancer. *New England Journal of Medicine.* June 14, 2007;356(24):2505–2513.

116. Davis SR, Panjari M, Robinson PJ, Fradkin P, Bell RJ. Menopausal symptoms in breast cancer survivors nearly 6 years after diagnosis. *Menopause.* 2014;10:10.

117. Mortimer JE, Flatt SW, Parker BA et al. Tamoxifen, hot flashes and recurrence in breast cancer. *Breast Cancer Research and Treatment.* April 2008;108(3):421–426.

118. Antoine C, Liebens F, Carly B, Pastijn A, Rozenberg S. Safety of alternative treatments for menopausal symptoms after breast cancer: A qualitative systematic review. *Climacteric.* February 2007;10(1):23–26.

119. Hickey M, Saunders CM, Stuckey BG. Management of menopausal symptoms in patients with breast cancer: An evidence-based approach. *Lancet Oncology.* September 2005;6(9):687–695.

120. North American Menopause Society. Treatment of menopause-associated vasomotor symptoms: Position statement of The North American Menopause Society. *Menopause.* January–February 2004;11(1):11–33.

121. Lethaby A, Marjoribanks J, Kronenberg F, Roberts H, Eden J, Brown J. Phytoestrogens for menopausal vasomotor symptoms. *Cochrane Database Systems Review.* December 2013;10(12):CD001395.

122. Schellenberg R, Saller R, Hess L et al. Dose-dependent effects of the *Cimicifuga racemosa* extract Ze 450 in the treatment of climacteric complaints: A randomized, placebo-controlled study. *Evidence Based Complementary and Alternative Medicine.* 2012;260301(10):23.

123. Walji R, Boon H, Guns E, Oneschuk D, Younus J. Black cohosh (*Cimicifuga racemosa* [L.] Nutt.): Safety and efficacy for cancer patients. *Support Care Cancer.* August 2007;15(8):913–921.

124. Kroenke CH, Caan BJ, Stefanick ML et al. Effects of a dietary intervention and weight change on vasomotor symptoms in the Women's Health Initiative. *Menopause.* 2012;19(9):980–988.

125. Cheung AM, Heisey R, Srighanthan J. Breast cancer and osteoporosis. *Current Opinion in Endocrinology, Diabetes and Obesity.* 2013;20(6):532–538.

126. Ding H, Field TS. Bone health in postmenopausal women with early breast cancer: How protective is tamoxifen? *Cancer Treatment Review.* October 2007;33(6):506–513.

127. North American Menopause Society. The role of calcium in peri- and postmenopausal women: 2006 position statement of the North American Menopause Society. *Menopause.* November–December 2006;13(6):862–877; quiz 878–880.

128. Datta M, Schwartz GG. Calcium and vitamin D supplementation and loss of bone mineral density in women undergoing breast cancer therapy. *Critical Reviews in Oncology Hematology.* 2013;88(3):613–624.

129. Berry J. Are all aromatase inhibitors the same? A review of controlled clinical trials in breast cancer. *Clinical Therapy.* November 2005;27(11):1671–1684.

130. Lustberg MB, Reinbolt RE, Shapiro CL. Bone health in adult cancer survivorship. *Journal of Clinical Oncology: Official Journal of the American Society of Clinical Oncology.* October 20, 2012;30(30):3665–3674.

131. Davis M, Witteles RM. Radiation-induced heart disease: An under-recognized entity? *Current Treatment Options in Cardiovascular Medicine.* 2014;16(6):014–0317.

132. Wang SY, Long JB, Hurria A et al. Cardiovascular events, early discontinuation of trastuzumab, and their impact on survival. *Breast Cancer Research and Treatment.* 2014;146(2):411–419.

133. Kushi LH, Kwan ML, Lee MM, Ambrosone CB. Lifestyle factors and survival in women with breast cancer. *Journal of Nutrition.* January 2007;137(1 Suppl):236S–242S.

134. Pierce JP, Natarajan L, Caan BJ et al. Influence of a diet very high in vegetables, fruit, and fiber and low in fat on prognosis following treatment for breast cancer: The Women's Healthy Eating and Living (WHEL) randomized trial. *JAMA: The Journal of the American Medical Association.* July 18, 2007;298(3):289–298.

135. Rock CL, Flatt SW, Thomson CA et al. Effects of a high-fiber, low-fat diet intervention on serum concentrations of reproductive steroid hormones in women with a history of breast cancer. *Journal of Clinical Oncology.* June 15, 2004;22(12):2379–2387.

136. Pierce JP, Stefanick ML, Flatt SW et al. Greater survival after breast cancer in physically active women with high vegetable-fruit intake regardless of obesity. *Journal of Clinical Oncology.* June 10, 2007;25(17):2345–2351.

137. Chlebowski RT, Blackburn GL, Thomson CA et al. Dietary fat reduction and breast cancer outcome: Interim efficacy results from the Women's Intervention Nutrition Study. *Journal of National Cancer Institute.* December 20, 2006;98(24):1767–1776.

138. Azvolinsky A. Cancer prognosis: Role of BMI and fat tissue. *Journal of National Cancer Institute.* June 6, 2014;106(6):dju177.

139. Ladoire S, Dalban C, Roche H et al. Effect of obesity on disease-free and overall survival in node-positive breast cancer patients in a large French population: A pooled analysis of two randomised trials. *European Journal of Cancer.* 2014;50(3):506–516.

140. Turkoz FP, Solak M, Petekkaya I et al. The prognostic impact of obesity on molecular subtypes of breast cancer in premenopausal women. *Journal of BUON.* 2013;18(2):335–341.

141. Kwan ML, Chen WY, Kroenke CH et al. Pre-diagnosis body mass index and survival after breast cancer in the after breast cancer pooling project. *Breast Cancer Research and Treatment.* 2012;132(2):729–739.

142. Abrahamson PE, Gammon MD, Lund MJ et al. General and abdominal obesity and survival among young women with breast cancer. *Cancer Epidemiology Biomarkers & Prevention.* October 2006;15(10):1871–1877.

143. Can A, Alacacioglu A, Kucukzeybek Y et al. The relationship of insulin resistance and metabolic syndrome with known breast cancer prognostic factors in postmenopausal breast cancer patients. *Journal of BUON.* 2013;18(4):845–850.

144. Azrad M, Demark-Wahnefried W. The association between adiposity and breast cancer recurrence and survival: A review of the recent literature. *Current Nutrition Reports.* 2014;3(1):9–15.

145. Travier N, Fonseca-Nunes A, Javierre C et al. Effect of a diet and physical activity intervention on body weight and nutritional patterns in overweight and obese breast cancer survivors. *Medical Oncology.* 2014;31(1):013–0783.

146. Reeves MM, Terranova CO, Eakin EG, Demark-Wahnefried W. Weight loss intervention trials in women with breast cancer: A systematic review. *Obesity Reviews.* 2014;29(10):12190.

147. Rock CL, Natarajan L, Pu M et al. Longitudinal biological exposure to carotenoids is associated with breast cancer-free survival in the Women's Healthy Eating and Living Study. *Cancer Epidemiology Biomarkers & Prevention.* 2009;18(2):486–494.

148. Villasenor A, Flatt SW, Marinac C, Natarajan L, Pierce JP, Patterson RE. Postdiagnosis C-reactive protein and breast cancer survivorship: Findings from the WHEL study. *Cancer Epidemiology Biomarkers & Prevention.* 2014;23(1):189–199.

149. Ligibel J. Lifestyle factors in cancer survivorship. *Journal of Clinical Oncology.* 2012;30(30):3697–3704.

150. Inoue M, Tajima K, Mizutani M et al. Regular consumption of green tea and the risk of breast cancer recurrence: Follow-up study from the Hospital-Based Epidemiologic Research Program at Aichi Cancer Center (HERPACC), Japan. *Cancer Letters*. June 26, 2001;167(2):175–182.

151. Harris HR, Bergkvist L, Wolk A. Coffee and black tea consumption and breast cancer mortality in a cohort of Swedish women. *British Journal of Cancer*. 2012;107(5):874–878.

152. Huss L, Butt S, Borgquist S, Almquist M, Malm J, Manjer J. Serum levels of vitamin D, parathyroid hormone and calcium in relation to survival following breast cancer. *Cancer Causes Control*. 2014;22:22.

153. Goodwin PJ, Ennis M, Pritchard KI, Hood N. Prognostic effects of 25-hydroxyvitamin D levels in early breast cancer. *Journal of Clinical Oncology*. 2009;27(23):3757–3763.

154. Clark AS, Chen J, Kapoor S et al. Pretreatment vitamin D level and response to neoadjuvant chemotherapy in women with breast cancer on the I-SPY trial (CALGB 150007/150015/ACRIN6657). *Cancer Medicine*. 2014;3(3):693–701.

155. Porojnicu AC, Lagunova Z, Robsahm TE, Berg JP, Dahlback A, Moan J. Changes in risk of death from breast cancer with season and latitude: Sun exposure and breast cancer survival in Norway. *Breast Cancer Research and Treatment*. May 2007;102(3):323–328.

156. Lim HS, Roychoudhuri R, Peto J, Schwartz G, Baade P, Moller H. Cancer survival is dependent on season of diagnosis and sunlight exposure. *International Journal of Cancer*. October 1, 2006;119(7):1530–1536.

157. Thomson CA, Rock CL, Thompson PA et al. Vegetable intake is associated with reduced breast cancer recurrence in tamoxifen users: A secondary analysis from the Women's Healthy Eating and Living Study. *Breast Cancer Research and Treatment*. 2011;125(2):519–527.

158. Nechuta S, Caan BJ, Chen WY et al. Postdiagnosis cruciferous vegetable consumption and breast cancer outcomes: A report from the After Breast Cancer Pooling Project. *Cancer Epidemiology Biomarkers & Prevention*. 2013;22(8):1451–1456.

159. Thomson CA, Rock CL, Caan BJ et al. Increase in cruciferous vegetable intake in women previously treated for breast cancer participating in a dietary intervention trial. *Nutrition and Cancer*. 2007;57(1):11–19.

160. Lippincott Williams & Wilkins. *Nursing 2014 Drug Handbook*, 34th edn., Lippincott Williams & Wilkins, Philadelphia, PA, 2014.

10 Prostate Cancer

Michelle Bratton, RDN, CSO

CONTENTS

INTRODUCTION

The prostate gland is a walnut-shaped gland situated between the bladder and the penis. It is an important part of the male reproductive system in that its primary function is to secrete an alkaline solution that forms part of the seminal fluid. With the exception of skin cancer, prostate cancer is the most common type of cancer diagnosed in American men. Yearly cases total over 220,000 and roughly 27,540 men will die from prostate cancer in 2015 [1]. Prostate cancer is the second leading cause of cancer death in men, following lung cancer. One man in seven will get prostate cancer in his lifetime, and one in thirty-six will die of the disease.

Risk factors include age, with risk increasing considerably after the age of 50 [2]. A family history of prostate cancer increases a man's risk of diagnosis, suggesting an inherited or genetic factor; having a father or brother with prostate cancer more than doubles a man's risk. African-American men have a higher risk of prostate and are more than twice as likely to die of prostate cancer as white men. Finally, country of origin may be a factor. This cancer is most common in North America, northwestern Europe, Australia, and on the Caribbean Islands and less common in Asia, Africa, Central America, and South America. See Table 10.1.

Prostate cancer cases are a heterogenous group. Like many other cancers, it is commonly staged using the TNM (tumor, node, metastasis) system, with tumor representing the extent of the primary tumor or the amount of prostate tissue involved and extension beyond the prostate. Node denotes the degree of regional lymph node involvement, and metastasis is whether or not it has spread to distant parts of the

TABLE 10.1
Risk Factors

- Age
- Family history
- Race
- Ethnicity

body such as the bones. In addition, Gleason score and prostate-specific antigen (PSA) levels are evaluated in a process called stage grouping [1].

Based on data from the Surveillance, Epidemiology, and End Results Program (SEER) for 2004 through 2010, 5-year survival rates for prostate cancer are 98.9% [2]. Most cases of prostate cancer are relatively slow-growing, which means it may take years to detect and even longer to spread beyond the prostate. However, a small percentage of men will be diagnosed with more rapidly growing or aggressive forms of prostate cancer [3]. It is difficult to predict which cancers will grow slowly and which will be more aggressive in nature.

For early-stage disease, or tumors that are confined to the prostate, treatment options most common are surgery (radical prostatectomy), radiation therapy, or active surveillance. The radical prostatectomy is the gold standard of treatment, which all other forms of treatment are compared to. Like any major surgery, there is a risk of infection, bleeding, heart problems, and even death. Removal of the prostate also carries with it the risk of impotence and urinary incontinence [2]. Radiation includes targeting the tumor with external-beam radiation therapy and brachytherapy, the practice of implanting radioactive seeds directly into the tumor [4]. Active surveillance is choosing to delay treatment until it is evident that the cancer may be growing or changing. This is a viable option for men with early-stage disease since the cancer may grow so slowly that it may not cause problems within a man's lifetime. In this way, men are able to avoid treatment costs and complications. Prostate cancer patients are considered to be at low nutrition risk. They infrequently present with nutritional compromise and their treatment causes minimal nutrition-impact symptoms.

Hormonal therapy is used in men with advanced disease and it may also be combined with radiation for high-risk early-stage disease [2]. Since male sex hormones, such as testosterone, can help prostate cancer grow, hormonal therapy works by blocking the effect of these hormones. Hormonal therapy, or androgen deprivation therapy (ADT), leads to several musculoskeletal changes, most of which are undesireable. These include loss of skeletal muscle and strength, osteoporosis, and skeletal fractures [5–9].

Loss of lean body mass has been shown to be 2.4%–2.7%, while increases in percent body fat have been demonstrated at 9.4%–13.8% [9,10]. Smith et al. [10] also noted a modest weight increase of 2.4% after 48 weeks of ADT. Whole body bone mineral density decreased by 2.4% [9]. Several small randomized controlled trials have demonstrated the benefit of an exercise program involving aerobic and resistance components in counteracting some of these deleterious effects [11,12]. Men participating in exercise showed an increase in lean mass compared with usual

---

TABLE 10.2

Maintaining Bone Health in Men on ADT

- Bisphosphonates
- 1000–1500 mg calcium daily
- 400–800 IU vitamin D daily
- Limit caffeine to less than 400 mg/day
- Limit alcohol to less than 2 drinks/day
- Exercise
  - Weight bearing
  - Resistance

---

care controls [11] and gains in body fat mass were also prevented [12]. Both trials found that men in the exercise group had improved muscular strength and reduced fatigue. A systematic review, including one previously cited source [11] and 11 other trials, confirmed the efficacy of exercise in prostate cancer patients, and specifically those on ADT, in improving muscular endurance and strength, as well as reducing fatigue [13]. Current evidence suggests that exercise be considered an important part of the prostate cancer survivorship care plan.

The decrease in bone mineral density can subsequently increase the risk of ADT-related osteoporosis and bone fracture [14]. A systematic review of the literature found that decreased bone mineral density could be addressed with medications (most commonly, bisphosphonates), lifestyle modification, and vitamin/mineral supplementation [15]. In the case of the latter, provision of 1000–1500 mg of calcium per day and 400–800 IU of vitamin D per day was recommended. Lifestyle interventions included limiting caffeine intake to less than 400 mg/day, keeping alcohol consumption to less than 2 drinks/day, and engaging in weight-bearing and resistance exercise. See Table 10.2. Despite the potential for ADT-related bone loss, many physicians do not address this issue with their patients. A retrospective review of 184 medical records of men on ADT showed that only 15% received some type of intervention for the prevention of osteoporosis [16]. Registered dietitians can be excellent resources for these patients. They are trained to be able to consider dietary sources of calcium and vitamin D before recommending supplementation. In this way, excessive calcium intake can be avoided. This is important considering some concern about calcium's role in the promotion of prostate cancer. Davison et al. [17] looked at the impact of a dietitian-led group education session on calcium and vitamin D intake. While intakes did not change significantly, the authors suggested earlier intervention (i.e., closer to the initiation of therapy), and a 6-month follow-up visit. Since men are often on ADT for several years, more frequent follow-up, perhaps incorporated into clinic visits would be more efficacious.

BODY WEIGHT AND EXERCISE

Evidence linking obesity with overall prostate cancer incidence has not been consistent, and in fact, some studies show it may decrease the risk of less-aggressive tumors [18]. However, obesity has been shown to increase the risk of more aggressive prostate cancer [18–20].

Once prostate cancer has been diagnosed, the role of body weight in influencing risk of recurrence and/or progression becomes the focus. Several studies have found no association between obesity and risk of recurrence after prostatectomy [21,22], however, at least two retrospective studies, a prospective study and a meta-analysis, have found an increased risk of biochemical recurrence [23–26]. In one of the trials, the risk elevation seen was at a relatively modest weight gain—men who gained more than 2.2 kg demonstrated twice the recurrence risk [26]. The authors of this trial noted that since obese individuals are more likely to be diagnosed with more aggressive disease, they adjusted for pathologic stage and grade; therefore, they were able to ascertain the independent effects of obesity and weight gain [26]. Similar results have been seen in men treated with radiotherapy; obesity has been associated with higher risk of recurrence and prostate cancer–specific death [27,28]. Data from the National Institutes of Health—AARP Diet and Health Study show that a higher BMI and adult weight gain after age 18 years was associated with an increased risk of dying from prostate cancer [29].

Independent of weight status, physical activity appears to have an inverse association with prostate cancer risk [30]. An exercise benefit has been seen in white men who exercised 9 or more MET (metabolic equivalents) hours per week versus less than 9 MET hours, but not in black men, prompting consideration of a race-specific means by which exercise modifies prostate cancer risk [31]. For those men with a diagnosis of prostate cancer, physical activity, particularly vigorous activity such as biking, swimming, tennis, or jogging, is associated with lower overall mortality and prostate cancer mortality [32].

DIETARY COMPONENTS

SOY

Soy foods, and specifically their isoflavones including genistein and daidzein, are frequently studied for their health benefits including chemoprevention. The liberal use of soy in Asian countries has been postulated as one factor for their lower rates of prostate cancer. This is supported by a meta-analysis of epidemiologic studies, which reported that consumption of soy foods is associated with a reduction in prostate cancer risk in men [33]. An earlier analysis by the same authors quantified similar results, concluding that the consumption of soy foods was related to roughly a 30% reduction in prostate cancer risk [34].

Studies examining the effect of soy protein or isolated isoflavones on PSA levels in prostate cancer patients have shown mixed results. Soy isoflavones did not lead to a decrease in serum PSA levels in any of the eight studies reviewed, however, PSA velocity was decreased in several [35]. Such a decrease, or prolonging PSA doubling time, can be interpreted as a means to delay disease progression and the development of symptoms [35]. The amount of soy isoflavones used in the studies that showed a significant effect of PSA levels was less than or equal to 120 mg/day. As a frame of reference, a serving of soy foods (i.e., 250 mL soy milk, 85 g tofu) contributes approximately 25 mg of isoflavones.

To achieve a consistent intake of 120 mg/day may prove to be a dietary challenge for non-Asians. At least one study has examined the possibility of a soy protein isolate supplement decreasing the rate of prostate cancer recurrence after radical prostatectomy [36]. Men consumed either a daily beverage containing 20 g of soy protein or 20 g of calcium caseinate for a period of 2 years after prostatectomy; soy protein isolate did not reduce biochemical recurrence [36].

VEGETABLES AND FRUITS

A plant-based diet is recommended to reduce cancer risk [37]. Ornish et al. were able to show a decrease in PSA velocity in men who adhered to a low-fat, vegan diet [38].

The experimental arm of the study (n = 44) also included daily soy protein, fish oil supplementation, and stress management, therefore, the benefit seen cannot be attributed solely to the effect of vegetable and fruit consumption.

Looking specifically at the effect of vegetable and fruit intake on the risk of prostate cancer, results have been inconsistent. A meta-analysis of cohort studies failed to find a significant benefit from an increased amount of vegetables and fruits [39]. Data from the Prostate, Lung, Colorectal and Ovarian (PLCO) Cancer Screening Trial did not show any association between vegetable and fruit consumption and overall prostate cancer risk.

However, increasing vegetable intake was associated with a decrease in aggressive disease (in this case defined as Stage III or IV or a Gleason score equal to or greater than 7); and the effect was largely due to intake of cruciferous vegetables, specifically broccoli and cauliflower (i.e., more than 1 serving/week) [40]. This same study found a decreased risk of aggressive disease with increasing spinach consumption, although statistical significance was inconsistent [40]. A meta-analysis also found an inverse relationship between the consumption of cruciferous vegetables and prostate cancer risk [41].

Other specific vegetables may exert an effect on risk; a modest-sized case control study of aggressive prostate cancer found a protective effect from higher consumption of leafy vegetables (spinach, mustard greens, and collards) and high carotenoid vegetables [42].

Garlic has also been identified to possibly decrease the risk of prostate cancer diagnosis [42,43]. In a prospective trial of Iranian men, consuming more than 5.5 g/week (2 cloves) of garlic reduced the risk of prostate cancer diagnosis 42% compared to men eating less than 2.75 g/week [44].

Data analysis from the Cancer of the Prostate Strategic Urologic Research Endeavor (CaPSURE) revealed a reduced risk of prostate cancer progression after diagnosis related to intake of cruciferous vegetables. Men in the fourth quartile (0.92 servings/day) of post-diagnostic intake of cruciferous vegetables had a 59% reduced risk of prostate cancer progression compared to men in the lowest quartile (0.06 servings/day) [45]. No other vegetable or fruit group after diagnosis was statistically significantly associated with risk of prostate cancer progression, although there was a combined benefit seen between walking and total vegetable intake. In men who walked greater than or equal to 7.5 MET hours/week after diagnosis (approximately 150 min/week), total vegetable intake after diagnosis was inversely associated with risk of prostate cancer progression [45]. This finding is similar to that seen in the Women's Healthy Eating and Living trial that followed breast cancer patients after their diagnosis [46]. Women who engaged in physical activity equivalent to walking for 180 min/week and consumed more than five servings of vegetables and fruits daily had a 44% reduced risk of cancer recurrence and mortality. These results suggest a possible synergistic effect of physical activity and plant-based diets.

Tomatoes and tomato products are the predominant source of lycopene, which is a potent phytonutrient. Phytonutrients, bioactive plant-derived compounds, have anticancer activity that targets the processes involved in tumor development [47].

The Health Professionals Follow-up Study follows a prospective cohort of 51,529 male healthcare workers. This study found a statistically significant inverse association between lycopene intake and risk of prostate cancer. High tomato sauce intake was the strongest predictor of lycopene intake; the benefit was seen at a relatively modest level of intake (i.e., one to two servings of tomato sauce per week) [48]. A more recent data analysis from the Health Professionals Follow-up Study found that a higher lycopene intake was inversely associated with total prostate cancer and more strongly with lethal prostate cancer (defined as cancers that caused death or distant metastases) [49].

However, there is conflicting data regarding the efficacy of lycopene and tomato products in reducing risk. Two meta-analyses found only modest effects and at high amounts of tomato intake [50,51].

There is limited data on the use of lycopene supplements in this area, however, a small (n = 26) randomized trial was done on newly diagnosed men awaiting radical prostatectomy. Those receiving a tomato oleoresin extract for 3 weeks prior to surgery versus no supplementation were found to have smaller tumors and less involvement of surgical margins and/or cancer extending beyond the prostate [52]. This was a pilot study and the authors readily acknowledged the need for further trials. The exact mechanism by which lycopene could exert a protective effect is unknown. It has been shown to prevent carcinogenesis by protecting cell DNA [53]. Healthy human subjects with a diet restricted in lycopene or tomato products demonstrate an increase in lipid oxidation [54], and it has been postulated that it may have antioxidant properties similar to that of statins [55]. Finally, it can inhibit proliferation of cancerous cells [56]. Within the larger context of adopting a plant-based diet, it seems prudent for men interested in reducing their risk of prostate cancer or prostate cancer recurrence or progression to increase consumption of tomato and tomato-based products.

Fruit intake has not been associated with the risk of prostate cancer, however, Kirsh et al. [40] identified an increased relative risk from combined fruit juice intake (apple, orange, and other). Pomegranate juice specifically has shown some promise in reducing levels of PSA. The polyphenol content of pomegranate juice, specifically ellagic acid, is thought to be the primary source of protective action. In vitro studies show an inhibition of prostate cancer in several cell lines and studies in mice demonstrated a similar effect [57]. While human trials are small, their results are encouraging. Pantuck et al. [58] were able to demonstrate an increase in PSA doubling time from 15 to 54 months in men who consumed 8 oz of pomegranate juice daily. Consistent use of the juice can be an effective adjunct for men in active surveillance as well as for those with biochemical recurrence after primary treatment. Men often complain about the tart taste of 100% pomegranate juice. The juice is high in sugar (30–32 g/cup) and this can be a concern in men who are diabetic, overweight, or for those who are trying to limit refined carbohydrate intake. In order to derive the therapeutic benefit of pomegranate, individuals often consider pomegranate supplements. There is at least one study that has shown that pomegranate extract, a supplement, can lengthen PSA doubling time, but not to the same degree as shown with juice. Paller et al. reported a difference of 11.9 months at baseline to 18.5 months with use the of POMx supplements [59]. And in men randomized to pomegranate extract (POMx) for 4 weeks prior to radical prostatectomy, no difference was seen in oxidative stress markers [60].

MEAT CONSUMPTION

Research findings on the role of meat in the etiology of prostate cancer have been inconsistent. Any impact on risk could be oversimplified and attributed to the fat content of various types of meat but several other potential carcinogens have been identified [61]. These include (1) zinc, which is needed for testosterone synthesis and may have other significant effects in the prostate gland [62]; (2) displacement of plant foods, and their inherent chemopreventive phytochemicals, by meat in the diet [63]; and (3) compounds formed by high-heat cooking methods, such as heterocyclic amines and polycyclic aromatic hydrocarbons [64].

Analysis of data from the Health Professionals Follow-up Study shows frequent consumers of red meats (i.e., beef, pork, lamb, and processed meat) having a slightly elevated risk of metastatic prostate cancer [65]. This study adjusted for confounding variables including BMI, exercise, and smoking status. It was identified that consumers of red meat were also less likely to have had a PSA test. The lack of PSA testing and a lower likelihood of routine rectal exams also identified might be one reason why cancers would be detected at a later stage. However, in an analysis restricted to those having ever had a PSA test, an even stronger association with red meat intake was seen [65]. After controlling for the effect of saturated fat and alpha-linolenic acid (ASA), a 50% elevation in the risk of metastatic prostate cancer was seen among relatively high consumers of red meat (top versus bottom quintile) [65].

Other studies endorse the association between the consumption of red and processed meat and advanced prostate cancer specifically. John et al. did not find an increased risk of localized prostate cancer; however, weekly consumption of 3 or more servings of red meat or 1.5 or more servings of processed meat was associated with an approximately 50% increased risk of developing advanced prostate cancer [66]. The group also found a similarly increased risk with 1 or more servings of grilled red meat and 1 or more servings of well done red meat. The threshold of processed meat's influence on prostate cancer risk appears to be significantly lower than that for red meat. Men who consumed sausages or bacon once a week or more were significantly more likely to have high-stage prostate cancer compared with nonconsumers [67]. No association was seen between consumption of white meat (chicken and turkey) and prostate cancer incidence [67]. In contrast, a multiethnic cohort study including four racial/ethnic groups did not find any association between meat intake and prostate cancer risk [68]. Fish intake appears to be unrelated to prostate cancer incidence but may reduce prostate cancer-specific mortality [69,70].

DIETARY FAT

There is limited consensus regarding the role of dietary fat in the etiology and progression of prostate cancer and it continues to be an area of active research and debate. There is not much evidence to support a positive association between total dietary fat intake and prostate cancer risk [37,71]. Research has been more focused on types of fat and specific fatty acids. A very large prospective cohort confirmed the lack of association between total fat, poly-unsaturated fat, and total trans-fatty acids and the incidence of total prostate cancer cases as well as any subgroup of cases (TNM classification system) [72]. However, an increased risk of advanced prostate cancer was related to increased intake of saturated fat. Previous studies have demonstrated a link between saturated fat and prostate cancer [73,74]. Dietary recommendations should include a limit on saturated fat intake. There is not a specific amount suggested in the cited studies, but abiding by heart-healthy guidelines of limiting saturated fat to no more than 6% of total calories seems reasonable.

Pelser et al. also identified an increased risk of advanced disease associated with increased intake of ALA [72]. A meta-analysis finding an increased, albeit small, risk of prostate cancer with alpha-linolenic [75] and a similar review finding an inverse association between alpha-linolenic [76] and risk are indicative of the equivocal results related to this topic. As an essential omega-3 fatty acid, ALA is typically regarded as a healthy component of the diet, conferring protection against coronary heart disease [77]. Food sources of ALA are varied, from nuts and flaxseed to red meat, dairy, and soybean oil. Current evidence does not support restriction of ALA from dietary sources.

Another area of debate is the role of omega-3 fatty acids as a contributing factor to prostate cancer. High serum levels of long chain omega-3 polyunsaturated fatty acids have been associated with increased prostate cancer risk overall [78,79]. A review of 12 studies revealed high levels of eicosapentaenoic acid (EPA) and docosahexaenoic acid (DHA) were associated with increased risk of high-grade prostate cancer, while high levels of the less prevalent docosapentaenoic acid (DPA) were linked with reduced total prostate cancer risk [80]. Some laboratory studies showed decreased prostate tumor growth and increased survival in mice fed a diet high in omega-3 fatty acids [81,82]. There is a paucity of research looking at fish oil supplementation and risk of prostate cancer.

Richman et al. sought to examine the association between fat intake and the risk of prostate cancer–related death and all-cause mortality in men with nonmetastatic prostate cancer. They found replacing carbohydrates and animal fat with vegetable fat may reduce the risk of all-cause mortality; however, they could not draw any conclusions on the benefit of vegetable fat intake after diagnosis in reducing prostate cancer–specific mortality [83].

DIETARY SUPPLEMENTS

A high percentage (73%) of men with prostate cancer use dietary supplements, with multivitamins being the most common [84]. It is estimated that over half of men diagnosed with prostate cancer take multivitamins [84]. In spite of their widespread use, multivitamins have not been shown to reduce the risk of prostate cancer and in fact, excessive users of multivitamins (more than seven times per week) may have an increased risk of advanced and fatal prostate cancers [85]. The Physicians' Health Study II reported a modest decrease in the risk of total cancer cases in men on long-term (an average of 11.2 years) multivitamin supplementation; however, it is interesting to note there was no decrease seen in the number of prostate cancer cases diagnosed [86].

Drawing on preclinical and epidemiological evidence supporting a role for selenium and vitamin E in risk reduction for prostate cancer, the Selenium and Vitamin E Cancer Prevention Trial (SELECT) was a large, multi-center trial that sought to identify the effect of supplementation of these two nutrients on the risk of prostate cancer. The study found no benefit from vitamin E and selenium, and study personnel recommended early discontinuation of the supplements [87]. In fact, vitamin E was associated with an increased risk of prostate cancer after extended follow-up [81]. In addition, data analysis found an increased risk, albeit statistically insignificant, of type 2 diabetes mellitus in the selenium group [88]. The Physicians' Health Study II did not find any benefit from vitamin E or vitamin C supplementation in decreasing the risk of prostate cancer [89].

Zyflamend is a unique herbal anti-inflammatory preparation containing 10 different extracts—rosemary, turmeric, ginger, holy basil, green tea, hu zhang, Chinese goldthread, barberry, oregano, and skullcap. Laboratory studies have shown it can inhibit the proliferation of human prostate cancer cells [90–92]. In one case report, a patient with high-grade prostatic intraepithelial neoplasm (HGPIN) was supplemented with Zyflamend for 18 months, at which time he did not show any evidence of PIN or cancer [93]. In a 2009 phase I study, patients (n = 23) with HGPIN took Zyflamend in addition to various other dietary supplements. At the conclusion of the study, 60% of the subjects had only benign tissue at biopsy [94]. Zyflamend was well tolerated and no serious adverse events were noted. This was a small study and the authors acknowledged the need for further trials.

Curcumin, the active ingredient of turmeric, has shown anti-prostate cancers effects in vitro and in vivo (mice) [95]. There is limited data in human subjects regarding the use of turmeric or curcumin in humans. Achieving therapeutic curcumin concentrations similar to that used in cell studies is a challenge and efforts are continuing to improve bioavailability [96].

DAIRY, CALCIUM, AND VITAMIN D

The role of calcium in prostate cancer development and progression has been controversial. A number of cohort studies have revealed a positive association between dairy and calcium intake and prostate cancer [65,67]. However, other similar studies did not find strong support for the hypothesis that calcium and dairy foods increase prostate cancer risk [97,98]. A meta-analysis of prospective studies of dairy product and calcium intake and their impact on prostate cancer concluded that a high intake of dairy and calcium may be associated with an increased risk. The investigators noted the effect was small; total dairy food intake was associated with a 10% increased risk (lowest versus highest) of all prostate cancer cases [99]. Conversely, in a secondary analysis, a small (n = 672) randomized trial of 1200 mg/day of calcium supplementation to prevent recurrence of colorectal adenomas found a statistically nonsignificant decreased risk of prostate cancer [100]. For those men living with a diagnosis of prostate cancer, data from the Health Professionals Follow-Up Study looked at the impact of milk and dairy on disease progression. Among 1202 men diagnosed with prostate cancer, a modest increased risk of biochemical recurrence was seen in men with higher milk consumption [101]. A subsequent study looked at the influence of milk consumption on the risk of metastases and prostate cancer mortality. With the exception of whole milk, there was no association recognized between milk and dairy intake and risk of lethal prostate cancer [102]. There was no association between total high fat dairy and risk of lethal prostate cancer, which led the authors to suggest that some component in whole milk other than saturated fat was contributing to the increased risk.

Several mechanisms have been suggested for dairy foods and calcium to exert an influence on risk. Dairy foods may have an adverse effect by increasing the concentration of insulin growth factor I, which has been associated with an elevated risk of prostate cancer [103]. Suppression of 1,25-dihydroxyvitamin D by high blood calcium levels has been considered as a means by which dairy and calcium could influence risk [97]. However, there has not been consistent evidence on an inverse relationship between vitamin D and the risk of prostate cancer [104,105] making this explanation less viable. Murphy et al. showed that in African-American men undergoing prostate biopsy, vitamin D deficiency (25-OH D < 20 ng/mL) was associated with increased odds of prostate cancer diagnosis. The same study also found that in both European American men and African American men, severe deficiency (25-OH D < 12 ng/mL) was positively associated with higher Gleason grade and tumor stage [106]. In contrast, a recent meta-analysis suggested a positive association between high levels of 25-OH D and increased risk of prostate cancer [107]. Based on their results and earlier studies, the authors recommended cautiousness in interpreting the role of vitamin D in different types of cancer. In spite of the growing popularity of vitamin D and its assumed healthful attributes (nearly 40% of U.S. adults report using vitamin D) [107], supplementation beyond the RDA, in the absence of deficiency or specific cases of increased need, is not indicated.

Overall, the data is mixed regarding dairy products, calcium intake, and risk of prostate cancer. Considering that those trials that did see an increased risk were often limited to higher calcium intakes of 1400–2000 mg/day [67,99], which is below the Dietary Reference Intake of 1000–1200 mg/day for adult men, keeping calcium intake from food and supplements below 1400 mg/day seems prudent.

CARBOHYDRATES

Consumption of refined carbohydrates, including sugar, leads to increased blood levels of glucose, and in turn, higher levels of insulin and insulin-growth factor I.

These hormones have been positively associated with increasing the risk of several cancers, including prostate cancer [108,109]. In vitro studies have shown that both insulin [110] and insulin-like growth factor I [111] can stimulate the growth of prostate cancer cells and epidemiological studies have shown a similar association [112–115]. Human trials have yielded conflicting results. A prospective cohort trial of Swedish men found that a higher intake of refined carbohydrates was associated with an increased risk of prostate cancer, particularly low-risk disease [116]. Examples of refined carbohydrates in this trial were cakes, biscuits, low-fiber cereals, rice, pasta, and sugar-sweetened beverages. A high intake of the latter, representing an intake of close to 300 g of sugar per day, was associated with approximately a 40% increased risk of symptomatic prostate cancer (defined as men who presented with lower urinary tract symptoms or other cancer-related symptoms) [116]. Two case-control studies found a direct relationship between dietary glycemic index and glycemic load and prostate cancer risk [42,117]. Augustin et al. [117] showed a linear relationship between glycemic index and glycemic load and risk even after correcting for confounding variables such as body mass index, physical activity, energy intake, and alcohol consumption, while Hardin et al. found that increased consumption of high glycemic foods, such as bagels, rolls, whole-wheat bread, potato chips, cookies, cakes, and soft drinks, were positively associated with risk of aggressive disease [42]. In contrast, several prospective cohort trials did not show a relationship between glycemic index or glycemic load and prostate cancer risk [118,119].

Several studies have shown an inverse relationship between dietary fiber and prostate cancer incidence [120–122]. There is inconsistency regarding what type of fiber may be most beneficial, however, total fiber and insoluble fiber seems to have more of an impact [120]. Flaxseed is a good source of fiber and has been investigated for its anti-cancer properties. In a mouse model, supplementation with flaxseed was shown to inhibit the growth and development of prostate cancer [123]. A randomized controlled trial was conducted with prostate cancer patients awaiting prostatectomy comparing the effects of a low-fat and/or flaxseed supplemented diet on the biology of the prostate and other biomarkers. Men assigned to the flaxseed arm showed significantly lower proliferation rates although there was no difference in apoptosis and serum end points such as PSA, sex hormone-binding globulin, and insulin-like growth factor-I [124].

SUMMARY

The literature on the role of specific dietary components in influencing risk of prostate cancer diagnosis, recurrence, or progression yields equivocal results. Reviewing this literature for the purpose of formulating dietary recommendations can be frustrating for the nutrition practitioner because of the lack of homogeneous findings. However, small intervention trials, assessing the benefit of an overall plant-based diet, have more consistent results [125–127]. Nguyen et al. were able to show an increased intake of vegetables and whole grains at 3 and 6 months after implementation of a plant-based diet and an accompanying decrease in the rate of rise of PSA [125]. Median vegetable intake increased from 2.8 servings/day at baseline to 5.0 and 4.8 servings/day at 3 and 6 months, respectively. Saxe et al. reported on the rate of PSA rise in this group.

They observed a significant decrease in the rate of PSA rise from prestudy to 0–6 months and 4–10 evaluable subjects experienced an absolute reduction in their PSA levels. The median PSA doubling time went from 11.9 months (prestudy) to 112.3 months (intervention) [126]. The plant-based diet employed was characterized by an increase in whole grains, vegetables, fruits, and legumes and a decrease in meat, dairy, and refined carbohydrates. A review of 8 observational studies and 17 intervention trials found evidence that a shift toward plant foods may serve as an important component of tertiary treatment of prostate cancer [128]. Plant-based diets are similar to the Mediterranean diet; both are characterized by frequent ingestion of vegetarian products (vegetables, fruits, and legumes), a low intake of saturated fat and processed meat, limited milk and dairy products, and an abundance of phytonutrients. Several authors have endorsed a Mediterranean diet as a highly palatable alternative for prostate cancer risk reduction [129,130]. In counseling patients with prostate cancer or those who would like to reduce their risk, there is ample evidence to focus on a plant-based diet, which is also endorsed for overall cancer risk reduction [37], with additional specific recommendations for prostate cancer. See Table 10.3.

TABLE 10.3

Nutrition Recommendations for Prostate Cancer Survivors

- Maintain a healthy weight.
- Engage in regular physical activity.
    - If physical condition allows, choose more vigorous activity (i.e., running, biking, and swimming).
- Include 1 or more servings of whole soy foods daily.
    - 1 serving equals 8 oz of soy milk, 4 oz tofu, ½ cup edamame, ¼ cup soy nuts.
    - Avoid soy supplements.
- Eat 4 or more servings of vegetables daily, including the following:
    - 2–4 servings/week of tomatoes and tomato products.
    - 3–4 servings/week of cruciferous vegetables.
    - Emphasize use of garlic and dark leafy greens.
- Drink 8 oz 100% pomegranate juice daily. Limit other fruit juices.
- Limit red meat consumption to less than 3 servings/week (serving = 3 oz.).
    - Consider adopting one meatless day a weak.
- Avoid processed meats and charred or blackened meats.
- Limit saturated fat to less than 5%–6% of total calories.
    - Avoid alpha-linolenic supplements.
- Limit dairy foods to 2–3 servings/day.
    - Choose low-fat milk and dairy products.
- Keep calcium intake from food sources and supplements <1400 mg/day.
- Choose whole grains over refined carbohydrates.
    - Avoid sugar-sweetened beverages.
    - Incorporate 1–2 tablespoons of ground flaxseed into daily diet.
    - Limit added sugars.

As there continues to be much research in this area, it is incumbent for the nutrition professional to keep abreast of the current literature.

REFERENCES

1. American Cancer Society. *Learn About Cancer: Detailed Guide: Prostate Cancer.* http://www.cancer.org/cancer/prostatecancer/detailedguide/prostate-cancer/index. Accessed April 23, 2015.
2. National Cancer Institute. What you need to know about prostate cancer. http://www.cancer.gov/cancertopics/wyntk/prostate. Accessed July 13, 2014.
3. Prostate Cancer Foundation. Questions about prostate cancer. http://www.pcf.org/site/c.leJRIROrEpH/b.5699537/k.BEF4/Home.htm. Accessed July 13, 2014.
4. Walsh P.C., Worthingon J. 2007. *Dr. Patrick Walsh's Guide to Surviving Prostate Cancer.* New York: Wellness Central.
5. Sharifi N., Gulley J.L., Dahut W.L. 2005. Androgen deprivation therapy for prostate cancer. *JAMA.* 294:238–244.
6. Galvao D.A., Taaffe D.R., Spry N. et al. 2009. Reduced muscle strength and functional performance in men with prostate cancer undergoing androgen suppression: A comprehensive cross-sectional investigation. *Prostate Cancer Prostatic Dis.* 12:198–203.
7. Shahinian V.B., Kuo Y.F., Freeman J.L. et al. 2005. Risk of fracture after androgen deprivation for prostate cancer. *N Engl J Med.* 352:154–164.
8. Spry N.A., Kristjanson L., Hooton B. et al. 2006. Adverse effects to quality of life arising from treatment can recover with intermittent androgen suppression in men with prostate cancer. *Eur J Cancer.* 42:1083–1092.
9. Galvao D.A., Spry N.A., Taaffe D.R. et al. 2008. Changes in muscle, fat and bone mass after 36 weeks of maximal androgen blockade for prostate cancer. *BJU Int.* 102:44–47.
10. Smith M.R., Finkelstein J.S., McGovern F.J. et al. 2002. Changes in body composition during androgen deprivation therapy for prostate cancer. *J Clin Endocrinol Metab.* 87:599–603.
11. Galvao D.A., Taaffe D.R., Spry N.A. et al. 2009. Combined resistance and aerobic exercise program reverses muscle loss in men undergoing androgen suppression therapy for prostate cancer without bone metastases: A randomized controlled trial. *J Clin Oncol.* 28:340–347.
12. Cormie P., Galvao D.A., Spry N.A. et al. 2015. Can supervised exercise prevent treatment toxicity in prostate cancer patients initiating androgen deprivation therapy: A randomized controlled trial. *BJU Int.* 115(2):256–266.
13. Keogh J.W.L., MacLeod R.D. 2012 Body composition, physical fitness, functional performance, quality of life, and fatigue benefits of exercise for prostate cancer patients: A systematic review. *J Pain Symptom Manage.* 43:96–110.
14. Sharifi N., Gulley J.L., Dahut W.L. 2010. An update on androgen deprivation therapy for prostate cancer. *Endocr Relat Cancer.* 17:R305–R315.
15. Millar H., Davison J. 2012. Nutrition education for osteoporosis prevention in men with prostate cancer initiating androgen deprivation therapy. *Clin J Oncol Nurs.* 16(5):497–503.
16. Tanvetyanon T. 2005. Physician practices of bone density testing and drug prescribing to prevent or treat osteoporosis during androgen deprivation therapy. *Cancer.* 103:237–241.
17. Davison B.J., Wiens K., Cushing M. 2012. Promoting calcium and vitamin D intake to reduce the risk of osteoporosis in men on androgen deprivation therapy for recurrent prostate cancer. *Supp Care Cancer.* 20:2287–2294.

18. Rodriguez C., Freedland S.J., Deka A. et al. 2007. Body mass index, weight change, and risk of prostate cancer in the Cancer Prevention Study II Nutrition Cohort. *Cancer Epidemiol Biomarkers Prev.* 16(1):63–69.

19. Allott E.H., Masko E.M., Freedland S.J. 2013. Obesity and prostate cancer: Weighing the evidence. *Eur Urol.* 63(5):800–809.

20. Golabek T., Bukowczan J., Chlosta P. et al. 2014. Obesity and prostate cancer incidence and mortality: A systemic review of prospective cohort studies. *Urol Int.* 92(1):7–14.

21. Tomaszewski J.J., Chen Y.F., Bertolet M. et al. 2013. Obesity is not associated with aggressive pathologic features or biochemical recurrence after radical prostatectomy. *Urology.* 81(5):992–996.

22. Siddiqui S.A., Inman B.A., Sengupta S. et al. 2006. Obesity and survival after radical prostatectomy: A 10-year prospective cohort study. *Cancer.* 107:521–529.

23. Strom S.S., Wang X., Pettaway C.A. et al. 2005. Obesity, weight gain, and risk of biochemical failure among prostate cancer patients following prostatectomy. *Clin Cancer Res.* 11(19):6889–6894.

24. Cao Y., Ma J. 2011. Body mass index, prostate cancer-specific mortality, and biochemical recurrence: A systematic review and meta-analysis. *Cancer Prev Res.* 4(4):486–501.

25. Chalfin H.J., Lee S.B., Jeong B.C. et al. 2014. Obesity and long-term survival after radical prostatectomy. *J Urol.* 192(4):1100–1104.

26. Joshu C.E., Mondul A.M., Menke A. et al. 2011. Weight gain is associated with an increased risk of prostate cancer recurrence after prostatectomy in the PSA era. *Cancer Prev Res.* 4(4):544–551.

27. Strom S.S., Kamat A.M., Gruschkus S.K. et al. 2006. Influence of obesity on biochemical and clinical failure after external-beam radiotherapy for localized prostate cancer. *Cancer.* 107:631–639.

28. Palma D., Pickles T., Tyldesley S. et al. 2007. Obesity as a predictor of biochemical recurrence and survival after radiation therapy for prostate cancer. *BJU Int.* 100:315–319.

29. Wright M.E., Chang S.C., Schatzkin A. et al. 2007 Prospective study of adiposity and weight change in relation to prostate cancer incidence and mortality. *Cancer.* 109(4): 675–684.

30. Liu Y., Hu F., Li D., Wang F. et al. 2011. Does physical activity reduce the risk of prostate cancer? A systematic review and meta-analysis. *Eur Urol.* 60:1029–1044.

31. Singh A.A., Jones L.W., Antonelli J.A. et al. 2013. Association between exercise and primary incidence of prostate cancer: Does race matter? *Cancer.* 119(7):1338–1343.

32. Kenfield S.A., Stampfer M.J., Giovannucci E. et al. 2011. Physical activity and survival after prostate cancer diagnosis in the health professionals follow-up study. *J Clin Oncol.* 29(6):726–732.

33. Yan L., Spitznagel E.L. 2009. Soy consumption and prostate cancer risk in men: A revisit of a meta-analysis. *Am J Clin Nutr.* 89:1155–1163.

34. Yan L., Spitznagel E.L. 2005. Meta-analysis of soy food and risk of prostate cancer in men. *Int J Cancer.* 117:667–669.

35. Messina M., Kucuk O., Lampe J.W. 2006. An overview of the health effects of isoflavones with an emphasis on prostate cancer risk and prostate-specific antigen levels. *J AOAC Int.* 89(4):1121–1134.

36. Bosland M.C., Kato I., Zeleniuch-Jacquotte A. et al. 2013. Effect of soy protein isolate supplementation on biochemical recurrence of prostate cancer after radical prostatectomy a randomized trial. *JAMA.* 310(2):170–178.

37. World Cancer Research Fund/American Institute for Cancer Research. 2007. *Food, Nutrition, Physical Activity, and the Prevention of Cancer: A Global Perspective.* Washington, DC: AICR.

38. Ornish D., Weidner G., Fair W.R. et al. 2005. Intensive lifestyle changes may affect the progression of prostate cancer. *J Urol.* 174(3):1065–1070.

39. Meng H., Hu W., Chen Z. et al. 2014. Fruit and vegetable intake and prostate cancer risk: A meta-analysis. *Asia Pac J Clin Oncol.* 10(2):133–140.

40. Kirsh V.A., Peters U., Mayne S.T. et al. 2007. Prospective study of fruit and vegetable intake and risk of prostate cancer. *J Natl Cancer Inst.* 99:1200–1209.

41. Liu B., Mao Q., Cao M. et al. 2012. Cruciferous vegetables intake and risk of prostate cancer: A meta-analysis. *Int J Urol.* 19(2):134–141.

42. Hardin J., Cheng I., Witte J.S. 2011. Impact of consumption of vegetable, fruit, grain, and high glycemic index foods on aggressive prostate cancer risk. *Nutr Cancer.* 63(6):860–872.

43. Kim J.Y., Kwon O. 2009. Garlic intake and cancer risk: An analysis using the Food and Drug Administration's evidence-based review system for the scientific evaluation of health claims. *Am J Clin Nutr.* 89:257–264.

44. Salem S., Salahi M., Mohseni M. et al. 2011. Major dietary factors and prostate cancer risk: A prospective multicenter case-control study. *Nutr Cancer.* 63(1):21–27.

45. Richman E.L., Carroll P.R., Chan J.M. 2012. Vegetable and fruit intake after diagnosis and risk of prostate cancer progression. *Int J Cancer.* 131:201–210.

46. Pierce J.P., Stefanick M.L., Flatt S.W. et al. 2007. Greater survival after breast cancer in physically active women with high vegetable-fruit intake regardless of obesity. *J Clin Oncol.* 25:2345–2351.

47. Beliveau R., Gingras, D. 2007. *Foods to Fight Cancer.* New York: DK Publishing.

48. Giovannucci E., Rimm E., Liu Y. et al. 2002. A prospective study of tomato products, lycopene, and prostate cancer risk. *J Natl Cancer Inst.* 94(5):391–398.

49. Zu K., Mucci L., Rosner B.A. et al. 2014. Dietary lycopene, angiogenesis, and prostate cancer: A prospective study in the prostate-specific antigen era. *J Natl Cancer Inst.* 106(2):djt430.

50. Etminan M., Takkouche B., Caamano-Isorna F. 2004. The role of tomato products and lycopene in the prevention of prostate cancer: A meta-analysis of observational studies. *Cancer Epidemiol Biomarkers Prev.* 13(3):340–345.

51. Chen J., Song Y., Zhang L. 2013. Lycopene/tomato consumption and the risk of prostate cancer: A systematic review and meta-analysis of prospective studies. *J Nutr Sci Vitaminol.* 59:213–223.

52. Kucuk O., Sarkar F.H., Djuric Z. et al. 2002. Effects of lycopene supplementation in patients with localized prostate cancer. *Exp Biol Med.* 227:881–885.

53. Pool-Zobel B.L., Bub A., Muller H. et al. 1997. Consumption of vegetables reduces genetic damage in humans: First result of a human intervention trial with carotenoid-rich foods. *Carcinogenesis.* 18:1847–1850.

54. Rao A.V., Agarwal S. 1998. Effect of diet and smoking on serum lycopene and lipid peroxidation. *Nutr Res.* 18:713–721.

55. Fuhramn B., Elis A., Aviram M. 1997. Hypocholesterolemic effect of lycopene and beta-carotene is related to suppression of cholesterol synthesis and augmentation of LDL receptor activity in macrophage. *Biochem Biophys Res Commun.* 233:659–662.

56. Matsushima N.R., Shidoji Y., Nishiwaki S. et al. 1995. Suppression by carotenoids of microcystin-induced morphological changes in mouse hepatocytes. *Lipids.* 30:1029–1034.

57. Sartippour M.R., Seeram N.P., Rao J.Y. et al. 2008. Ellagitannin-rich pomegranate extract inhibits angiogenesis in prostate cancer in vitro and in vivo. *Int J Oncol.* 32(2):475–480.

58. Pantuck A.J., Zomorodian M.D., Belldegrun A.S. January 2006. Phase-II study of pomegranate juice for men with prostate cancer and increasing PSA. *Curr Urol Rep.* 7(1): A1.

59. Paller C.J., Ye X., Wozniak P.J. et al. 2013. A randomized phase II study of pomegranate extract for men with rising PSA following initial therapy for localized prostate cancer. *Prostate Cancer Prostatic Dis.* 16(1):50–55.

60. Freedland S.J., Carducci M., Kroeger N. et al. 2013. A double-blind, randomized, neo-adjuvant study of the tissue effects of POMx pills in men with prostate cancer before radical prostatectomy. *Cancer Prev Res (Phila).* 6(10):1120–1127.

61. Kolonel LN. 2001. Fat, meat, and prostate cancer. *Epidemiol Rev.* 23:72–81.

62. Platz E.A., Helzlsouer K.J. 2001. Diet: Selenium, zinc and prostate cancer. *Epidemiol Rev.* 23:93–101.

63. Barnes S. 2001. Diet: Role of phytochemicals in prevention and treatment of prostate cancer. *Epidemiol Rev.* 23:102–105.

64. Norrish A.E., Ferguson L.R., Knize M.G. et al. 1999. Heterocyclic amine content of cooked meat and risk of prostate cancer. *J Natl Cancer Inst.* 91(23):2038–2044.

65. Michaud D.S., Augustsson K., Rimm E.B. et al. 2001 A prospective study on intake of animal products and risk of prostate cancer. *Cancer Causes Control.* 12:557–567.

66. John E.M., Stern M.C., Sinha R. et al. 2011 Meat consumption, cooking practices, meat mutagens, and risk of prostate cancer. *Nutr Cancer.* 63(4):525–537.

67. Rohrmann S., Platz E.A., Kavanaugh C.J. et al. 2007. Meat and dairy consumption and subsequent risk of prostate cancer in a US cohort study. *Cancer Causes Control.* 18:41–50.

68. Park S.Y., Murphy S.P., Wilkens L.R. et al. 2007. Fat and meat intake and prostate cancer risk: The Multiethnic Cohort study. *Int J Cancer.* 121:1339–1345.

69. Chavvarro J.E., Stampfer M.J., Hall M.N. et al. 2008. A 22-y prospective study of fish intake in relation to prostate cancer incidence and mortality1'2'3'. *Am J Clin Nutr.* 88(5):1297–1303.

70. Szymanski K.M., Wheeler D.C., Mucci L.A. 2010. Fish consumption and prostate cancer risk: A review and meta-analysis. *Am J Clin Nutr.* 92:1223–1233.

71. Dennis L.K., Snetselaar L.G., Smith B.J. et al. 2004. Problems with the assessment of dietary fat in prostate cancer studies. *Am J Epidemiol.* 160(5):436–444.

72. Pelser C., Mondul A.M., Hollenbeck A.R. et al. 2013. Dietary fat, fatty acids, and risk of prostate cancer in the NIH-AARP diet and health study. *Cancer Epidemiol Biomarkers Prev.* 22(4):697–707.

73. Whittemore A.S., Kolonel L.N., Wu A.H. et al. 1995. Prostate cancer in relation to diet, physical activity, and body size in blacks, whites and Asians in the United States and Canada. *J Natl Cancer Inst.* 87(9):652–661.

74. Fleshner N., Bagnell P.S., Klotz L. et al. 2004. Dietary fat and prostate cancer. *J Urol.* 171:S19–S24.

75. Simon J.A., Chen Y.H., Bent S. 2009. The relation of alpha-linolenic acid to the risk of prostate cancer: A systematic review and meta-analysis. *Am J Clin Nutr.* 89(5):1558–1564.

76. Carayol M., Grosclaude P., Delpierre C. 2010. Prospective studies of dietary alpha-linolenic acid intake and prostate cancer risk: A meta-analysis. *Cancer Causes Control.* 21(3):347–355.

77. Vedtofte M.S., Jakobsen M.U., Lauritzen L. et al. 2014. Association between the intake of alpha-linolenic acid and the risk or coronary heart disease. *Br J Nutr.* 25:1–9.

78. Brasky T.M., Darke A.K., Song X. et al. 2013. Plasma phospholipid fatty acids and prostate cancer risk in the SELECT trial. *J Natl Cancer Inst.* 105(15):1132–1141.

79. Dahm C.C., Gorst-Rasmussen A., Crowe F.L. et al. 2012 Fatty acid patterns and risk of prostate cancer in a case-control study nested within the European Prospective Investigation into Cancer and Nutrition. *Am J Clin Nutr.* 96:1354–1361.

80. Chua M.E., Sio M.C., Sorongon M.C. et al. 2013 The relevance of serum levels of long chain omega-3 polyunsaturated fatty acids and prostate cancer risk: A meta-analysis. *Can Urol Assoc J.* 7(5–6):e333–e343.

81. Berquin I.M., Min Y., Wu R. et al. 2007. Modulation of prostate cancer genetic risk by omega-3 and omega-6 fatty acids. *J Clin Invest.* 117(7):1866–1875.

82. Kelavkar U.P., Hutzley J., Dhir R. et al. 2006. Prostate tumor growth and recurrence can be modulated by the omega-6:omega-3 ratio in diet:Athymic mouse xenograft model simulating radical prostatectomy. *Neoplasia.* 8(2):112–124.

83. Richman E.L., Kenfield S.A., Chavarro J.E. et al. 2013. Fat intake after diagnosis and risk of lethal prostate cancer and all-cause mortality. *JAMA Intern Med.* 173(14):1318–1326.

84. Wiygul J.B., Evans B.R., Peterson B.L. et al. 2005. Supplement use among men with prostate cancer. *Urology.* 66(1):161–166.

85. Lawson K.A., Wright M.E., Subar A. et al. 2007. Multivitamin use and risk of prostate cacner in the National Institutes of Health-AARP Diet and Health Study. *J Natl Cancer Inst.* 99(10):754–764.

86. Gaziano J.M., Sesso H.D., Christen W.G. et al. 2012. Multivitamins in the prevention of cancer in men The Physicians' Health Study II randomized control trial. *JAMA.* 308(18):1871–1880.

87. Klein E.A., Thompson I.M., Tangen C.M. et al. Vitamin E and the risk of prostate cancer The Selenium and Vitamin E Cancer Prevention Trial (SELECT). *JAMA.* 306(14):1549–1556.

88. Lippman S.M., Klein E.A., Goodman P.J. et al. 2009. Effect of selenium and vitamin E on risk of prostate cancer and other cancers The Selenium and Vitamin E Cancer Prevention Trial (SELECT). *JAMA.* 301(1):39–51.

89. Gaziano J.M., Glynn R.J., Christen W.G. et al. 2009. Vitamins E and C in the prevention of prostate and total cancer in men The Physicians' Health Study II randomized controlled trial. *JAMA.* 301(1):52–62.

90. Yang P., Cartwright C., Chan D. et al. 2007. Zyflamend-mediated inhibition of human prostate cancer PC3 cell proliferation. *Cancer Biol Ther.* 6(2):e1–e9.

91. Bemis D.L., Capodice J.L., Anastasiadis A.G. et al. 2005. Zyflamend, a unique herbal preparation with nonselective OX inhibitory activity, induces apoptosis of prostate cancer cells that lack COX-2 expression. *Nutr Cancer.* 52(2):202–212.

92. Huang E., Chen G., Baek S.J. et al. 2011. Zyflamend reduces the expression of androgen receptor in a model of castrate-resistant prostate cancer. *Nutr Cancer.* 63(8):1287–1296.

93. Rafailov S., Cammack S., Stone B.A. et al. 2007. The role of Zyflamend, and herbal anti-inflammatory, as a potential chemopreventive agent against prostate cancer: A case report. *Integr Cancer Ther.* 6(1):74–76.

94. Capodice J.L., Gorroochurn P., Cammack A.S. et al. 2009. Zyflamend in men with high-grade prostatic intraepithelial neoplasia: Results of a phase I clinical trial. *J Soc Integr Oncol.* 7(2):43–51.

95. Yu X.L., Jing T., Zhao H. et al. 2014. Curcumin inhibits expression of inhibitor of DNA binding 1 in PC3 cells and xenografts. *Asian Pac J Cancer Prev.* 15(3):1465–1470.

96. Klempner S.J., Bubley G. 2012 Complementary and alternative medicines in prostate cancer: From bench to bedside. *Oncologist.* 17(6):830–837.

97. Park Y., Mitrou P.N., Kipnis V. et al. 2007. Calcium, dairy foods, and risk of incident and fatal prostate cancer The NIH-AARP Diet and Health Study. *Am J Epidemiol.* 166(11):1270–1279.

98. Park S., Murphy S.P., Wilkens L.R. et al. 2007. Calcium, vitamin D and dairy product intake and prostate cancer risk The Multiethnic Cohort Study. *Am J Epidemiol.* 166(11):1259–1269.

99. Gao X., LaValley M.P., Tucker K.L. 2005. Prospective studies of dairy product and calcium intakes and prostate cancer risk: A meta-analysis. *J Natl Cancer Inst.* 97(23):1768–1777.

100. Baron J.A., Beach M., Wallace K. et al. 2005. Risk of prostate cancer in a randomized clinical trial of calcium supplementation. *Cancer Epidemiol Biomarkers Prev.* 14:586–589.

101. Chan J.M., Holick C.N., Leitzmann M.F. et al. 2006 Diet after diagnosis and the risk of prostate cancer progression, recurrence, and death (United States). *Cancer Causes Control.* 17:199–208.

102. Pettersson A., Kasperzyk J.L., Kenfield S.A. et al. 2012. Milk and dairy consumption among men with prostate cancer and risk of metastases and prostate cancer death. *Cancer Epidemiol Biomarkers Prev.* 21:428–436.

103. Qin L.Q, He K., Xu J.Y. 2009. Milk consumption and circulating insulin-like growth factor-I level: A systematic literature review. *Int J Food Sci Nutr.* 60(Suppl. 7):330–340.

104. Kristal A.R., Arnold K.B., Neuhouser M.L. et al. 2010. Diet, supplement use, and prostate cancer risk: Results from the Prostate Cancer Prevention Trial. *Am J Epidemiol.* 172:566–577.

105. Ahn J., Peters U., Albanes D. et al. 2008 Serum vitamin D concentration and prostate cancer risk: A nested case-control study. *J Natl Cancer Inst.* 100(11):796–804.

106. Murphy A.B., Nyame Y., Catalona W.J. et al. 2014. Vitamin D deficiency predicts prostate biopsy outcomes. *Clin Cancer Res.* 20(9):2289–2299.

107. Xu Y., Shao X., Yao Y. et al. 2014. Positive association between circulating 25-hydroxyvitamin D levels and prostate cancer risk: New findings from an updated meta-analysis. *J Cancer Res Clin Oncol.* 140(9):1465–1477.

108. Kaaks R. 2004. Nutrition, insulin, IGF-1 metabolism and cancer risk: A summary of epidemiological evidence. *Novartis Found Symp.* 262:247–260.

109. Heald A.H., Cade J.E., Cruickshank J.K. et al. 2003.The influence of dietary intake on the insulin-like growth factor (IGF0 system across three ethnic groups: A population-based study. *Public Health Nutr.* 6(2):175–180.

110. McKeehan W.L., Adams P.S., Rosser M.P. 1984. Direct mitogenic effects of insulin, epidermal growth factor, glucocorticoid, cholera toxin, unknown pituitary factors and possibly prolactin, but not androgen, on normal rat prostate epithelial cells in serum-free, primary cell culture. *Cancer Res.* 44:1998–2010.

111. Iwamura M., Sloss P.M., Casamento J.B. et al. 1993. Insulin-like growth factor I: Action and receptor characterization in human prostate cancer cell lines. *Prostate.* 22:243–252.

112. Chan J.M., Stampfer M.J., Ma J. et al. 2002. Insulin-like growth factor-I (IGF-I) and IGF binding protein-3 as predictors of advanced-stage prostate cancer. *J Natl Cancer Inst.* 94:1099–1106.

113. Hsing A.W., Chua S., Gao Y.T. et al. 2001. Prostate cancer risk and serum levels of insulin and leptin: A population-based study. *J Natl Cancer Inst.* 93:783–789.

114. Chan J.M., Stampfer M.J., Giovannucci E. et al. 1998. Plasma insulin-like growth factor-I and prostate cancer risk: A prospective study. *Science.* 279:563–566.

115. Stattin P., Rinaldi S., Biessy C. et al. 2004. High levels of circulating insulin-like growth factor-I increase prostate cancer risk: A prospective study in a population-based nonscreened cohort. *J Clin Oncol.* 22:3104–3112.

116. Drake I., Sonestedt E., Gullberg B. et al. 2012. Dietary intake of carbohydrates in relation to prostate cancer risk: A prospective study in the Malmo Diet and Cancer cohort 1–3. *Am J Clin Nutr.* 96:1409–1418.

117. Augustin L.S., Galeone C., Dal Maso L. et al. 2004. Glycemic index, glycemic load and risk of prostate cancer. *Int J Cancer.* 112:446–450.

118. Nimptsch K., Kenfield S., Jensen M.K. et al. 2011. Dietary glycemic index, glycemic load, insulin index, fiber and whole-grain intake in relation to risk of prostate cancer. *Cancer Causes Control.* 22:51–61.
119. Shikany J.M., Flood A.P., Kitahara C.M. et al. 2011. Dietary carbohydrate, glycemic index, glycemic load, and risk of prostate cancer in the Prostate, Lung, Colorectal, and Ovarian Cancer Screening Trial (PLCO) cohort. *Cancer Causes Control.* 22:995–1002.
120. Deschasaux M., Pouchieu C., His M. et al. 2014. Dietary total and insoluble fiber intakes are inversely associated with prostate cancer risk. *J Nutr.* 144(4):504–510.
121. Pelucchi C., Talamini R., Galeone C. et al. 2004. Fibre intake and prostate cancer risk. *Int J Cancer.* 109:278–280.
122. Tymchuk C.N., Barnard R.J., Heber D. et al. 2001. Evidence of an inhibitory effect of diet and exercise on prostate cancer cell growth. *J Urol.* 166(3):1185–1189.
123. Lin X., Gingrich J.R., Bao W. et al. 2002. Effect of flaxseed supplementation on prostatic carcinoma in transgenic mice. *Urology.* 60(5):919–924.
124. Demark-Wahnefried W., Polascik T., George S.L. et al. 2008. Flaxseed supplementation (not dietary fat restriction) reduces prostate cancer proliferation rates in men presurgery. *Cancer Epidemiol Biomarkers Prev.* 17(12):3577–3587.
125. Nguyen J.Y., Major J.M., Knott C.J. et al. 2006. Adoption of a plant-based diet by patients with recurrent prostate cancer. *Integr Cancer Ther.* 5(3):214–23.
126. Saxe G.A., Major J.M., Nguyen J.Y. et al. 2006. Potential attenuation of disease progression in recurrent prostate cancer with plant-based diet and stress reduction. *Integr Cancer Ther.* 5(3):206–213.
127. Carmody J., Olendzki B., Reed G. et al. 2008. A dietary intervention for recurrent prostate cancer after definitive primary treatment: Results of a randomized pilot trial. *Urology.* 72(6):1324–1328.
128. Berkow S.E., Barnard N.D., Saxe G.A. et al. 2007. Diet and survival after prostate cancer diagnosis. *Nutr Rev.* 65(9):391–403.
129. Itsiopoulos C., Hodge A., Kaimakamis M. 2009. Can the Mediterranean diet prevent prostate cancer? *Mol Nutr Food Res.* 53(2):227–239.
130. Ferris-Tortajada J., Berbel-Tornero O., Garcia-Castell J. et al. 2012. Dietetic factors associated with prostate cancer: Protective effects of Mediterranean diet. *Actas Urol Esp.* 36(4):239–245.

11 Gastrointestinal Cancer and Complementary Therapies

Lindsay Dowhan, MS, RD, CSO, LD, CNSC
and Monica Habib, MS, RD, LD, CNSC

CONTENTS

INTRODUCTION

Gastrointestinal (GI) cancers are a family of diseases in which malignant cells form in the tissues of the digestive or GI system. This includes esophageal, gastric, and gastrointestinal stromal tumors (GIST), appendix, bile duct, gallbladder, islet cell tumors, pancreatic, liver, small intestine, and colon, rectal, and anal cancers.

Colorectal cancer is the third most common cancer in men and women, with an estimated 105,000 colon cancer and 40,000 rectal cancer cases diagnosed in the United States in the past year. Adding pancreatic cancer (32,000 cases), stomach cancer (22,000 cases), and other cancers of the digestive system, the estimated number of new GI cancer cases totals more than 250,000 annually (National Cancer Institute, 2014). Therefore, GI cancers account for 20% of all newly diagnosed cancers every year (Jemal et al., 2013).

Many cancer survivors are seeking new therapy treatments, in addition to traditional oncological care, in order to help increase the chance of survival and to minimize the risk of disease recurrence. Specifically, patients are turning their attention to more integrative and complementary therapies in their quest for survival.

Of these modalities, some have more evidence supporting their use than others in terms of extent of research in clinically controlled trials.

Upper GI Cancer

Malignancies of the upper GI tract have the worst prognosis of solid tumor malignancies of the entire GI system (Shah and Kurtz, 2010). In the following section, esophageal, stomach, and pancreatic cancers and treatment will be discussed.

Esophageal Cancer

There are two types of esophageal cancer: squamous cell carcinoma and adenocarcinoma. The classification is dependent on the type of cancerous cell growth. Squamous cell carcinoma consists of cancerous cells arising from the squamous cell tissue that line the esophagus. Adenocarcinoma includes cancerous growth from the glandular cells that have replaced squamous cells and tends to be diagnosed more frequently than squamous cell carcinoma, and typically forms in the lower portion of the esophagus near the stomach. Esophageal cancer risk increases with heavy alcohol use, smoking, *Helicobacter pylori* infection, human papillomavirus, esophageal achalasia, consumption of scalding foods and/or fluids, gastroesophageal reflux disease (GERD), and Barrett's esophagus (American Cancer Society, 2013). Risk also tends to be three to four times higher in men than in women with a lifetime risk of 1 in 125 men and 1 in 435 women (American Cancer Society, 2013).

Esophageal cancer presents primarily with dysphagia, but may include increased saliva production, chest pain, hoarseness, chronic cough, hiccups, pneumonia bone pain, and bleeding in the esophagus. Diagnosis is confirmed using barium studies and endoscopy, while endoscopic ultrasound is useful for the determination of size and growth to nearby tissues. Computed tomography (CT) scans, positron emission tomography (PET) scans, bronchoscopy, thoracoscopy, and laparoscopy are used to determine metastasis to surrounding and distant tissues (Mawhinney and Glasgow, 2012).

Traditional treatment options for patients vary depending on the type of cancer and staging based on the American Joint Committee for Cancer staging (Greene et al., 2006) through the determination of the size of the primary tumor, regional lymph node involvement, and the presence of metastasis. Treatment options include chemotherapy, radiation, combination chemotherapy, and radiation and surgery. Each treatment modality poses risks for developing nutrition impact symptoms, ultimately affecting nutrition status. Stent placement, laser therapy, and electrocoagulation are also available; however, these therapies tend to be used more for palliation in esophageal cancer (Mawhinney and Glasgow, 2012).

Nutrition Therapy Recommendations

Adequate nutrition should focus on diet modifications based on recommendations by the American Institute for Cancer Research (see Table 11.1) and arise from consumption of whole foods versus dietary supplementation (WCRF/AICR, 2007). Many nutrition-related side effects exist for patients treated with chemotherapy, radiation, and/or surgery for esophageal cancer. This extensive list includes nausea, vomiting,

TABLE 11.1

American Institute for Cancer Research Diet Recommendations

Maintaining healthy body weight.
- Limit consumption of energy-dense foods.
- Avoid sugary drinks.

Eat mostly foods of plant origin.
- Consume at least 5 servings (14 oz) of variety of nonstarchy fruits and vegetables daily.
- Consume relatively unprocessed grains and legumes at each meal.
- Limit refined starchy foods.

Limit intake of red meat and avoid processed meat.
- Consume less than 18 oz red meat weekly.
- Limit processed meat.
- Limit consumption of animal fats.

Limit alcoholic drinks.

If alcoholic drinks are to be consumed,
- Men should drink no more than 2 drinks daily
- Women should drink no more than 1 drink daily

Limit consumption of salt and avoid moldy grains or legumes.
- Limit salt-preserved, salted, and salty foods.
- Limit consumption of processed foods with added salt.
- Salt intake should be less than 2400 mg daily.
- Minimize exposure to aflatoxins from moldy grains or legumes.

Aim to meet nutritional needs through diet alone.
- Select a wide variety of foods.
- Dietary supplements are not recommended for cancer prevention.

Source: Adapted from WCRF/AICR, *Food, Nutrition, Physical Activity, and the Prevention of Cancer: A Global Perspective,* Washington, DC, AICR, 2007.

anorexia, diarrhea, mucositis, dysphagia, odynophagia, and increased gastric emptying with alterations in digestion and absorption.

Studies completed by Riccardi and Alen (1999) found that 80% of patients show signs of malnutrition at the time of evaluation by a registered dietitian, and that medical nutrition therapy, specifically oral nutrition supplements, enteral nutrition (EN), and parenteral nutrition (PN) have the ability to increase total nutrient intake with the potential to improve and/or prevent malnutrition (Elia et al., 2006). This may help improve nutrition status and weight; and for patients with progressive dysphagia, early intervention with nutrition supplements should be considered.

Following a diet to prevent symptoms of GERD and through maintenance of a healthful body weight with regular physical activity to prevent obesity, thus reducing risk factors for developing GERD and Barrett's esophagus (Fenti et al., 2009) may help prevent occurrence of disease. When portions of the GI tract, specifically the esophagus or stomach, are removed, gastric emptying increases when hyperosmolar chyme is deposited in the small intestine, leading to bloating, abdominal cramping, nausea, and symptoms of dumping. In order to reduce these symptoms, patients should be instructed to follow a low simple sugar, lactose-free diet with emphasis on foods high in soluble fiber and low in fried and greasy foods. Patients should incorporate six small meals daily with beverages sipped between meals (Ukleja, 2006).

Nutrition support has been shown to improve mortality associated with pre-operative nutritional depletion in the malnourished esophageal cancer population (Daly et al., 1982) in which patients had less weight loss and fewer postsurgical complications. EN is commonly used to optimize nutrition status through the use of percutaneous endoscopic gastrostomy (PEG) tube or jejunostomy tube placement postsurgically. Some medical facilities will offer routine placement of feeding tubes for nutrition support prior to initiation of chemotherapy or radiation (Mawhinney and Glasgow, 2012). Beer et al. (2005) had found improved outcomes in patients with upper GI tract cancer who have received EN via PEG at the start of cancer treatment. Debate still exists with the placement of PEG tubes and controversies prevail at different institutions; however, PEG tubes have shown that they are safe and do not compromise the stomach or esophagogastric anastomosis (Margolis et al., 2003). Jejunostomy tubes are used for nutrition support and may prevent potential injury to the stomach. These tubes allow for enteral feeding past the anastomosis, further preventing the interference with postoperative gastric healing (Gupta, 2009).

Locoregional esophageal cancer patients receiving PN have demonstrated tolerance to higher doses of chemotherapy and have surgical outcomes similar to that of patients able to maintain their nutrition status on oral diet alone (Sikora et al., 1998). Preoperative PN to malnourished patients has also been shown to have better outcomes with respect to reduced infection and decreased wound and surgical complications when compared to postoperative PN administration (Daly et al., 1982). PN administration, however, does not improve patient mortality and has the potential to increase infectious complications and impair tumor response to chemotherapy (Koretz et al., 2001). This treatment modality should be reserved for patients who are at risk of increased mortality from starvation than of the disease process itself.

Gastric Cancer

According to predictions from the American Cancer Society (ACS), approximately 21,600 cases of gastric cancer will be diagnosed in 2013 (Seigel et al., 2013) of which the majority of cases (approximately 90%–95%) will consist of adenocarcinoma (Siewert and Sendler, 2001). This type of cancer is typically hereditary and develops from the mucosal cells of the stomach, while other forms include lymphoma, GIST, and carcinoid tumors. Less common forms of gastric cancer include squamous cell carcinoma, small cell carcinoma, and leiomyosarcoma (American Cancer Society, 2013).

Early changes in the mucosa rarely cause symptoms, consequently delaying diagnosis. Early signs of gastric cancer include anorexia, weight loss, abdominal pain or discomfort, sense of fullness, heartburn, nausea and vomiting, and abdominal ascites. Gastric cancer typically affects men more than women, and almost 2/3 of those are 65 years and older (Seigel et al., 2013).

Diagnosis is made through upper endoscopy and biopsy while endoluminal ultrasound determines the depth of cancer growth or metastasis to nearby organs or lymph nodes. Staging and metastasis can be determined using CT scans, CT-guided needle biopsy, MRI, PET scans, and laparoscopy (Siewert and Sendler, 2001).

Lack of refrigeration, presence of *H. pylori* infection, hypochlorhydria and gastritis, history of pernicious anemia, obesity, smoking, and alcohol use have all been shown to increase risk of gastric cancer development. The rate of gastric cancer has declined over the years, possibly due to increased use of refrigeration, increased fruit and vegetable intake (specifically those with high levels of beta carotene and vitamin C), decreased salted and smoked meat consumption, and antibiotic use for the treatment of *H. pylori* (Gonzalez and Agudo, 2012).

Treatment involves the use of chemotherapy, radiation, targeted therapy, and surgery. Classic nutrition-related side effects occurring with chemotherapy and targeted therapy include nausea, vomiting, anorexia, diarrhea, mucositis, and altered taste. Radiation therapy may cause abdominal pain and discomfort, nausea, vomiting, urinary and bladder changes, diarrhea, changes in appetite, anorexia, and fatigue, while surgical therapy may alter digestion and absorption through the removal of portions of the stomach and small intestine. Typical surgical resections include gastroduodenostomy (Bill Roth I), gastrojejunostomy (Bill Roth II), partial gastric resection, and Roux-en-Y (Sah et al., 2009). If surgical reconstruction is planned, surgeons typically do not favor feeding tube placement prior to surgery. Enteral feeding tubes are on average placed during the surgical procedure for postsurgical nutrition support; however, this may be associated with increased postsurgical complications in relation to surgical site infections and increased length of stay (Patel et al., 2013), consequently J tube placement should be considered on an individual basis.

Nutrition Therapy Recommendations

After gastric surgery, patients should follow a low simple sugar diet with six small meals daily and soft, easy-to-digest foods and fluids as tolerated. Patients should include a high-protein food source with each meal, while avoiding high-fat foods and separate fluids from solids at meal times (see Table 11.2 for postsurgical gastric cancer guidelines) (Ukleja, 2006). Patients should be monitored for dumping syndrome and malabsorption of vitamins and minerals. Gastrectomy patients are at increased risk of development of osteoporosis and should have serum 25-hydroxyvitamin D levels monitored. Patients should also increase their calcium intake (up to 1500 mg/day in divided doses) (Bernert et al., 2007) with vitamin D supplementation up to 50,000 IU weekly (Carlin et al., 2009). Malabsorption of iron, folate, and vitamin B12 is common and supplementation may be warranted along with incorporating diet strategies to maximize iron absorption (Bernert et al., 2007; Hyoung-Il et al., 2011).

Pancreatic Cancer

Exocrine tumors are the most common type of pancreatic cancer, with adenocarcinoma ranking among the most difficult cancers to treat coupled with very low 5-year survival rates (O'Reilly, 2009). Endocrine tumors (also called pancreatic neuroendocrine tumors) are less common and make up less than 5% of all pancreatic cancers. These include insulinomas, glucagonomas, gastrinomas, vasoactive intestinal peptideomas, and pancreatic polypeptide-producing tumors (Batcher et al., 2011).

TABLE 11.2

Antidumping Diet Guidelines for Postgastrectomy

General guidelines	• Consume six small meals daily.
	• Eat slowly and chew foods thoroughly.
	• Remain upright for meals and snacks.
Protein	• Consume foods high in protein (meats, poultry, fish, eggs, peanut butter, tofu, cottage cheese, and yogurt).
Fat	• Consume fats in moderation.
	• Butter, mayonnaise, salad dressings used in moderation.
	• May need pancreatic enzyme replacements.
Soluble fiber	• Include apples, oats, beets, carrots, beans, pears, peaches, and Brussels sprouts.
Sweets	• Avoid concentrated sweets/sugars (table sugar, honey, jams/jellies, syrups, candy, etc.).
	• Avoid foods made with sugar alcohols (xylitol, mannitol, sorbitol, etc.).
Beverages	• Drink only 4 oz fluids with meals.
	• Avoid beverages 30 min before meals and 60 min after meals.
	• Avoid caffeinated and carbonated beverages.

Source: Ukleja, A. Dumping syndrome, in: Parrish, C.R. (ed.), *Practical Gastroenterology,* Nutrition Issues in Gastroenterology, Series #35, pp. 32–46, 2006.

Approximately 45,220 people have been diagnosed with pancreatic cancer in the past year, affecting both men and women equally (Seigel et al., 2013). Risk seems to increase with advanced age, smoking, obesity, history of diabetes mellitus, and hereditary pancreatitis; however, contributory factors are not completely understood at present (Li et al., 2004).

Signs and symptoms of exocrine pancreatic cancer include jaundice, abdominal bloating, dyspepsia, back pain, and weight loss (Ghaneh and Neoptolemos, 2012). Symptoms of pancreatic neuroendocrine tumors include abdominal pain, GERD, tachycardia, weight loss, diarrhea and/or steatorrhea, hyper- and hypoglycemia, rash with swelling and blisters (necrolytic migratory erythema), and hypokalemia (National Cancer Institute, 2013).

Some common causes in the development of pancreatic cancer may arise from infection of the stomach with the bacteria *H. pylori* (Xiao et al., 2013), diets high in fat (Theibaut et al., 2009), specifically with consumption of red and processed meats (Larsson and Wolk, 2012), decreased intake of fruits and vegetables (Howe et al., 1990), and heavy alcohol consumption (Lucenteforte et al., 2012). Coffee consumption has historically been associated with increased risk of pancreatic cancer development; however, a meta-analysis completed on 54 human studies completed by Turati et al. (2012) showed no appreciable association.

Diagnosis and staging is made with use of CT scan, CT-guided needle biopsy, somatostatin receptor scintigraphy, and endoscopic ultrasound. MRI and PET scans determine if tumors affect the bile duct, while ERCP and angiography are used to determine if blood flow is affected. They also determine the presence of pancreatic neuroendocrine tumors. Surgical biopsies are obtained through laparoscopy (Michl, 2006).

TABLE 11.3

Signs of Pancreatic Exocrine Insufficiency

- Abdominal cramping
- Steatorrhea (loose, greasy and foul-smelling stools, and stools that have increased volume and are difficult to flush)
- Malnutrition

Source: Adapted from Dominguez-Munoz, J.E., *J. Gastroenterol. Hepatol.*, 2011(Suppl. 2), 12, 2011.

Treatment includes use of chemotherapy, radiation, chemoradiation, targeted therapy (growth factor inhibitors, antiangiogenesis factors), and surgery (NCI accessed 12/2013).

Nutrition Therapy Recommendations

Patients who underwent surgical procedure for treatment historically have been instructed to follow low-fat diets, thus reducing intake and absorption of fat-soluble vitamins. This is no longer the recommendation with the introduction of pancreatic enzyme replacement during meal times to reduce symptoms of steatorrhea. Small, frequent meals are encouraged while avoiding foods and beverages high in sugar. Patients may also be initiated on pancreatic enzyme replacement when symptoms of malabsorption are present (see Table 11.3 for symptoms of malabsorption). In order to provide an additional source of calories, medium-chain triglycerides may be incorporated into the diet for patients with low body weight and weight loss. Supplementation of fat-soluble vitamins may be necessary as close monitoring of vitamin status is essential in the management of this patient population (Dominguez-Munoz, 2011).

EN is common among postoperative patients. One study conducted by Martignoni et al. (2000) demonstrated that patients who did not receive EN after undergoing pancreaticoduodenectomy experienced significantly higher frequency of delayed gastric emptying, longer duration of nasogastric tube decompression and longer hospital stay, when compared with those who did receive EN. Immunonutrition (EN supplemented with arginine, RNA nucleotides, and omega 3 FA) provided to patients undergoing upper and lower GI surgery had significantly reduced overall complications when used pre- and postsurgery, and was also associated with a significantly shorter length of hospital stay (Cerantola et al., 2011). Survivors should focus on obtaining and/or maintaining a healthy body weight as obesity has been linked with pancreatic cancer and decreased survival, specifically prediagnostic weight (Yuan et al., 2013).

COMPLEMENTARY THERAPIES USED IN UPPER GI CANCER

Mind–body medicine includes use of meditation, yoga, tai chi, and music therapy all of which have been shown to improve quality of life (QOL) for cancer survivors (Hilliard, 2003; Mustian et al., 2004; Carlson et al., 2007; Maodel et al., 2007). Some therapies, such as meditation, have demonstrated increased mood, less stress, and improved cortisol levels (Carlson et al., 2007). Hypnosis, another mind–body medicinal technique, has been shown to reduce cancer-related pain (NIH technology assessment panel, 1996), anxiety, anticipatory and postoperative nausea and vomiting (Morrow and Morrell, 1982).

Acupuncture is a therapeutic modality traditionally used in ancient China, now adopted as part of integrative medicine nationally. Evidence shows that acupuncture is a safe method for treating certain ailments, and chemotherapy-induced nausea and vomiting (CINV) is one of them. A review by Naeim et al. (2008) concluded that acupuncture should be incorporated into standard practice for CINV. Acupuncture has demonstrated other benefits as well, including stimulating salivary secretion and flow. This implication is important for patients experiencing radiation-induced xerostomia (Johnstone et al., 2002), typically experienced in head and neck cancer. A randomized controlled trial showed that acupuncture provided concurrently with radiotherapy significantly reduced xerostomia and improved QOL (Zhuang et al., 2013).

In addition to traditional MNT, specific dietary bioactive components are also of interest to cancer survivors. Many studies look at diet manipulation and effects on cancer prevention or mitigation of treatment effects; however, only a few studies show actual benefits. Three studies involving patients with advanced pancreatic and head/neck cancers have demonstrated that diets supplemented with eicosapentaenoic acid and docosahexaenoic acid have improved patients' body weight, provided weight stabilization, gain in lean body mass, and improvements in QOL (Fearon et al., 2003; Dewey et al., 2007; deLuis et al., 2008). High-dose antioxidants, complex botanical agents during chemotherapy and radiation, are not recommended, and patients should discuss with trained professionals prior to their incorporation of treatment due to possible drug supplement interaction and potential for synergistic effects with medication. Data is inconclusive for many of these supplements, and more quality studies need to be performed prior to endorsing such products (Deng et al., 2009).

Two case–control studies have looked at the incidence of garlic consumption and the outcome of esophageal cancer risk; however, both authors concluded there was no correlation between esophageal cancer and garlic consumption (Gao et al., 1994; Hu et al., 1994). Study design is a concern in both cases in which dietary recall was used for information gathering, which may have resulted in recall bias (Hu et al., 1994) and use of general allium consumption versus garlic consumption alone was elucidated, therefore limiting causality (Gao et al., 1994).

Oral mucositis is a common side effect for patients receiving certain chemotherapy drugs. Diet manipulation and guidelines provided by the oncology nutrition practice group have been shown to help improve symptoms of mucositis and several studies that have found a statistically significant benefit for preventing or reducing the severity of mucositis with the use of complementary therapies. Some evidence exists supporting the use of cryotherapy and keratinocyte growth factor for prophylactic treatment of mucositis and sucralfate for the reduction of mucosistic severity. The potential benefits of aloe vera, amifostine, granulocyte-colony stimulating factor, intravenous glutamine, and honey are less clear (Worthington et al., 2011).

Few case-controlled and cohort studies have demonstrated a protective effect on gastric cancer with the consumption of raw and cooked garlic (Buiatti et al., 1989; You et al., 1989; Hansson et al., 1993); however, limitations to the studies include lack of control with other dietary factors and these associations do not include the use of garlic supplements. More definitive research is still needed before conclusions can be made on the inverse relationship between garlic consumption and gastric cancer (Fleischauer and Arab, 2001).

Vegetable intake has been linked to reduced incidence of pancreatic cancer with a strong association with garlic consumption (Chan et al., 2005). A large case-controlled study observed vegetable consumption of residents in the San Francisco Bay area diagnosed with pancreatic cancer and found an inverse relationship with garlic consumption and risk development.

Curcumin (a derivative of the spice turmeric) has been investigated for its purported chemoprotective effect in pancreatic cancer. One study demonstrated that curcumin potentiates the antitumor effect of the chemotherapy drug, gemcitabine, and can enhance this effect and overcome chemoresistance by suppressing genes associated with cell proliferation (Kunnumakkara et al., 2007). Curcumin has been found to be well tolerated in human studies (Kanai et al., 2010) in high doses, and its use may be considered in conjunction with gemcitabine chemotherapy for synergy due to its antitumor effects (Kanai et al., 2010).

LOWER GI CANCER

The lower GI cancers include both small and large intestines, most of which are adenocarcinomas. The next section includes a discussion of the diagnosis, screening, medical and surgical treatment, and complementary therapies for colorectal cancer (CRC).

Colorectal Cancer

According to the National Cancer Institute (NCI) at the National Institutes of Health (NIH), colon and rectal cancer (CRC) forms in the tissues of the colon and or the rectum, most of which are adenocarcinomas, a cancer that begins in the secretory cells (CRC 2013). CRC is the third most commonly diagnosed cancer in males and the second in females and remains the second most common cause of cancer death in the United States (Jemal et al., 2013; National Cancer Institute, 2014) (Table 11.4).

The primary nonmodifiable risk factors include genetic predisposition, family history, age, race, and gender. Familial adenomatous polyposis (FAP) and Lynch syndrome, which are the most common of the familial colon cancers, account for 5% of CRC cases. FAP is caused by a genetic mutation located on chromosome 5, which results in numerous colonic adenomas (Burt et al., 1995). Lynch syndrome, which is also known as hereditary nonpolyposis colorectal cancer, is caused by a defect in the mismatch repair genes (Kempers et al., 2011). Ulcerative colitis, Crohn's disease, acromegaly, renal transplantation, polyps, and abdominal radiation lead to an increased risk of CRC. African Americans have the highest rate of CRC of all ethnic groups. The risk of CRC begins to increase after 40 years of age and rises sharply at

TABLE 11.4

Risk Factors for Colorectal Cancer

Nonmodifiable	Modifiable
Genetic predisposition	Physical inactivity
Family history	Overweight or obese
Age	Diet
Race	Alcohol
Gender	Smoking

Source: Adapted from Smith, R.A. et al., *CA Cancer J. Clin.*,
              51(1), 38, quiz 77–80, January–February 2001.

ages 50–55. Overall, CRC incidence and mortality rates are about 35%–40% higher in men than in women (Smith et al., 2001).

The primary modifiable risk factors include physical inactivity, overweight and obesity, poor diet, and excessive alcohol use and smoking. One of the most consistently seen relationships between colon cancer and behavior is the protective effect of physical activity. The ACS recommends at least 30 min or more on 5 or more days per week as high levels of physical activity decrease risk by as much as 50% (Chan and Giovannucci, 2010). Obesity, specifically abdominal obesity, is associated with a higher risk of colon cancer. Research has shown that increased consumption of red and processed meats and cooking at high temperatures for extended periods of time may increase risk of CRC development (Chan and Giovannucci, 2010). Moderate consumption of alcohol, defined as two to four drinks per day, is associated with a 23% increased risk of CRC compared to consumption of <1 drink/day. (Ferrari et al., 2007). It has been concluded that tobacco is a likely cause of CRC, yet the association is higher for rectal cancer than colon cancer (Secretan et al., 2009).

Once the patient is determined to be at risk, screening should take place. Generally, a flexible sigmoidoscopy, colonoscopy, barium enema, and CT colonography are done to detect adenomatous polyps and cancer. The fecal occult blood test and stool DNA test detect cancer. Those who are at increased risk should begin screening before the age of 50. Colonoscopy is recommended for those who are at high risk (Ransohoff and Lang, 1991).

CRC is often diagnosed after the onset of symptoms as a result of screening. Symptoms usually appear only with more advanced disease. If symptoms are seen, they are generally from growth of the tumor in the lumen of the colon or adjacent structures. Symptoms include change in bowel habits, such as diarrhea, constipation, or narrowing of the stool that lasts for more than a few days, incomplete evacuation, rectal bleeding, dark stools, or blood in the stool, cramping or abdominal pain, weakness and fatigue, or unintentional weight loss (Majumdar et al., 1999). However, many other conditions can cause similar signs or symptoms including other malignancies as well as benign lesions such as hemorrhoids, diverticulitis, infection, or inflammatory bowel disease, therefore a confirmed diagnosis is essential.

Colonoscopy is the most accurate and versatile diagnostic test for CRC since it can localize and biopsy lesions throughout the large bowel, detect synchronous neoplasms, and remove polyps. However, colonoscopy has difficulty detecting flat lesions (Atkin et al., 2013). A flexible sigmoidoscopy is generally not considered to be an adequate diagnostic study for a patient suspected of having CRC unless a palpable mass is felt in the rectum. During the double-contrast barium enema, barium sulfate, a chalky liquid, and air are used to outline the inner part of the colon and rectum to look for abnormal areas on x-rays. If suspicious areas are seen on this test, a colonoscopy will be needed for further explanation (Atkin et al., 2013). A CT colonography provides a computer-simulated endoluminal perspective of the air-filled distended colon. CT colonography has been evaluated in patients with incomplete colonoscopy and as an initial diagnostic test in patients with symptoms suggestive of CRC. CT colonography also has the ability to detect extracolonic lesions, which might explain symptoms and provide information as to the tumor stage (Atkin et al., 2013). A variety of serum markers have been associated with CRC, particularly carcinoembryonic antigen (CEA) (Macdonald, 1999). These markers have a low diagnostic ability to detect primary CRC due to significant overlap with benign disease and low sensitivity for early-stage disease (Macdonald, 1999). In patients receiving chemotherapy for metastatic colon cancer, decreases in CEA levels may be indicative of improvement; however, there is no convincing evidence that CEA monitoring significantly affects either survival or QOL. The overall cost-effectiveness is not clear and convincing definition of the role of postoperative CEA monitoring has yet to be studied (Macdonald, 1999). CEA is used to follow patients during and after treatment to monitor cancer response to treatment or recurrence (Macdonald, 1999).

The type of treatment is dependent upon the extent of the disease and typically includes surgical treatment, chemotherapy, and/or radiation therapy. Surgical resection is the most common modality, with the goal of completely removing the tumor, major vascular pedicles, and the lymphatic drainage of the affected colon. Polyps, both benign or with severe dysplasia or carcinoma, can be managed by endoscopic removal, known as a polypectomy. If the cancer is detected at an early stage (stage I), a local excision is done in which a segment of colon is removed. If the cancer is localized, the tumor is excised along with either side of the colon and nearby lymph nodes (Colon Cancer Treatment, 2013). More advanced stages, such as stage II or III, a partial or total colectomy may be performed along with tissue excision on either side and nearby lymph nodes with an anastomosis, or a diverting stoma is made (Colon Cancer Treatment, 2013). This stoma may be temporary or permanent depending on the location of the cancer. When cancer is advanced, palliative surgery is done simply for the relief of pain and obstructive symptoms or to prevent other local complications (Colon Cancer Treatment, 2013). 5-Fluorouracil or capecitabine are commonly used chemotherapy drugs for stage II CRC (Colon Cancer Treatment, 2013). Oxaliplatin, in combination with 5-fluorouracil/leucovorin (5-FU/LV), is used for adjuvant treatment of stage III colon cancer patients who have undergone complete resection of the primary tumor (National Cancer Institute, 2014).

Neoadjuvant chemotherapy, which is preoperative chemotherapy, is commonly the approach for rectal cancers and is considered in those who have locally advanced colon cancer invading into adjacent organs (Cukier et al., 2012). Adjuvant chemotherapy is indicated in those with stage III cancer to eradicate micometastases that may reduce the likelihood of recurrence. Irinotecan has become a commonly used chemotherapy drug as first-line treatment of metastatic CRC in combination with 5FU/LV (Fuchs et al., 2006). The most common side effects include diarrhea, nausea/vomiting, increased risk of infection, hair thinning or loss, abdominal pain, loss of appetite, and feeling weak (Fuchs et al., 2006).

Adjuvant radiation therapy (postsurgical radiation) is not considered routine care for those with colon cancer; however, chemotherapy in combination with radiation therapy has played a significant role in the management of patients with rectal cancer (Willett et al., 1993).

Nutrition Therapy Recommendations

Diet has the ability to increase and decrease risk for CRC development. Diets high in fat and low in fiber have illustrated associations with increased CRC risk, particularly increased intake of red meats such as beef, pork, or lamb, as well as saturated fats. The heterocyclic amines formed by cooking meat and fish at high temperatures may be a contributor to CRC development (Singh and Fraser, 1998). The excess fat causes more bile acid secretion into the intestine that could change the bacteria in the intestine, possibly leading to cell damage and tumor growth (Reddy et al., 1992). Heme iron commonly found in beef, chicken, turkey, veal, and/or fish is positively correlated to colonic polyps, adenomas, and CRC (Kuhnle and Bingham, 2007).

Diets high in fiber are inversely associated with CRC risk (Jacobs, 1998). The term fiber includes both insoluble and soluble fiber. Ingestion of fiber could modify carcinogenesis in the large bowel by different mechanisms through binding to bile acids, increasing fecal water and possibly diluting carcinogens, and decreasing transit time (Jacobs, 1998). Fiber may act as a substrate for bacterial fermentation with resultant increase in bacterial mass and the production of butyrate (Jacobs, 1998). Butyrate is a short-chain fatty acid (SCFA) that has been shown to have anticarcinogenic effects in vitro and acts as fuel for the colonic epithelium. The proposed mechanism includes the promotion of growth of Lactobacilli, which maintains epithelial health and downregulates the inflammatory response (McGarr et al., 2005). Although many epidemiological studies have examined the relationship between fruit and vegetable intake and the incidence of colon and/or rectal cancer, results from Michels et al. (2000) have found no association.

Alcohol is associated with an increased risk of colonic adenoma as CRC. A meta-analysis of 57 cohort and case–control studies that investigated the association between alcohol consumption and CRC risk showed that people who regularly consumed approximately 3.5 drinks/day had 1.5 times the risk of developing CRC as nondrinkers or occasional drinkers. For every 10 g of alcohol consumed per day, there was a 7% increase in the risk of CRC (Fedirko et al., 2011). The exact mechanism is unknown yet it is proposed that alcohol reduces folate, promotes abnormal DNA methylation, delays DNA repair, and alters the composition of bile salts (Kune and Vitetta, 1992).

As the most common type of surgery for CRC is a colectomy, it is important to note that the colon absorbs water and electrolytes, such as potassium and sodium, to form stool. The colon salvages energy from malabsorbed organic matter through absorption of SCFAs produced in bacterial fermentation (Christl and Scheppach, 1997). Absorption of nutrients in general is not impaired by a colectomy. Therefore, diet after surgery will focus on avoiding diarrhea, dehydration, and gas. Patients are advised to drink plenty of fluids, eat low-fiber, low-fat foods, and avoid heavy, greasy foods, raw fruits and vegetables, strong spices, and caffeine. Liquids should be consumed between meals to avoid dehydration. If patients experience gas and abdominal bloating, then avoidance of carbonated beverages, cruciferous vegetables, beans, eggs, garlic, onions, and foods containing fructose or sorbitol is recommended. Sometimes dairy products may also cause gas, so patients should also try lactose-free items when this occurs.

It is important to note that postsurgical patients may be at risk for obstructions, therefore high residue foods, including nuts, popcorn, seeds, raw fruits and vegetables, and anything with a skin, should be avoided.

Patients need to follow eating patterns that will maintain good health and prevent cancer and other chronic diseases. Although diet has been extensively studied as a risk factor for developing CRC, there are very limited data concerning diet in CRC survivors as related to survival outcomes. The largest prospective study to date includes survivors of stage III colon cancer and demonstrates that a Western dietary pattern is associated with a worse prognosis and decreased overall survival. In contrast, diets characterized by high intakes of fruits and vegetables, poultry, and fish are not significantly associated with cancer recurrence or mortality (Meyerhardt et al., 2007). Emerging data suggest that vitamin D status may influence outcomes in CRC survivors as well, and this is an active area of research as both a secondary preventive and treatment strategy in CRC (Ng et al., 2009).

COMPLIMENTARY THERAPIES USED IN LOWER GI CANCER

Calcium, which is found in dairy products, dark green vegetables, some soy products, fish, nuts, and legumes, is associated with a reduced risk of CRC; however, the results have not always been consistent. The exact mechanism by which calcium may help reduce the risk of CRC is unclear; however, it is known that calcium binds to bile acids and fatty acids in the GI tract to form insoluble calcium soaps. This reduces the ability of the acids to damage cells in the lining of the colon and stimulate cell proliferation. Calcium also may improve signaling within cells and cause cancer cells to differentiate and/or die (Milner et al., 2001). The NCI does not recommend the use of calcium supplements to reduce the risk of CRC.

Vitamin D is found in foods such as fatty fish, fish liver oil, and eggs; however, most dietary vitamin D comes from foods fortified with vitamin D, such as milk, juice, and breakfast cereals. Although many studies provide data to suggest that higher intakes of this vitamin are associated with a reduced risk of CRC, it remains unclear. Vitamin D has been found to slow down or prevent the development of cancer by promoting cellular differentiation, decreasing cancer cell growth, stimulating cell death apoptosis, and reducing tumor blood vessel formation—angiogenesis (Lamprecht and Lipkin, 2001; Ma et al., 2011). In 2005, Gorhem et al. (2005) recommended a daily intake of 1000 IU of vitamin D and a concentration of serum 25-hydroxyvitamin D of

33 ng/mL, which was associated with a 50% lower risk of CRC. NCI does not recommend using vitamin D supplements to reduce the risk of CRC.

A large 1994 study of antioxidant vitamins and cancer conducted by NCI and the National Public Health Institute of Finland found that vitamin E supplements lowered rates of prostate and CRC, especially in persons under 65 years of age (Bostick et al., 1993a,b). This may be due to scavenging free radicals and inhibiting lipid peroxidation, reducing nitrite (a potential carcinogen), and through enhancing immune response (Wu et al., 2002).

Folate, a water-soluble B vitamin and cofactor in 1-carbon transfer, is an important nutritional factor that may modulate the development of CRC (Kim, 2003). Studies show that dietary folate intake and blood folate levels are inversely associated with CRC risk with an approximately 40% reduction (Kim, 2003). Recent studies show that the dose and timing of folate intervention are critical in providing safe and effective chemoprevention (Kim, 2003). High supplemental folate levels and folate intervention after microscopic neoplastic foci promote rather than suppress colorectal carcinogenesis (Giovannucci et al., 1993).

Intake of dietary zinc is associated with a decreased risk of proximal and distal colon cancer (Lee, 2004). It has been shown to have inhibitory effects on proliferation and metabolism of malignant colonocytes (Emil et al., 2008). There has been an inverse association between dietary zinc and rectal cancer in women (Zhang et al., 2011).

Polyphenols found in fruits, vegetables, green tea, coffee, and seeds are known for their antioxidant effects. Polyphenols inhibit cellular proliferation, induce cell cycle arrest, and interact with apoptotic pathways. The polyphenols are divided into five classes: flavonoids, phenolic acids, lignans, stillbenes, and others. Curcumin, a polyphenol found in turmeric, has been shown to reduce the number and size of ileal and cecal adenomas in patients with FAP (Cruz-Correa et al., 2006). Overall, diets high in polyphenols and other phytochemicals such as carotenoids, isothiocyanates, and natural phenols have protective effects against CRC.

Onions, Jerusalem artichokes, garlic, asparagus, and chicory contain oligofructants, which may reduce the number of aberrant crypt foci and influence the activity of natural killer cells (Roller et al., 2004). These are metabolized by colonic microbiota into gases and SCFAs and have been shown to reduce tumorigenesis.

Prebiotics and probiotics have a possible protective role of the gut microbiota in colorectal carcinogenesis (McGarr et al., 2005). The use of probiotic functional foods (beneficial live microorganisms) to modify gut microflora has been suggested in clinical conditions associated with diarrhea, gut–barrier dysfunction, and inflammatory response. There are a vast number of different strains of probiotics; however, much of the clinical research has investigated the species belonging to the family of Lactobacillus and Bifidobacterium for inflammatory bowel disease. Recent studies however illustrate similar results for chemotherapy-induced diarrhea (Bowen et al., 2007). Ohigashi et al. (2013) have demonstrated that patients who underwent CRC surgery had an altered intestinal environment in which levels of SCFA were reduced and pathogenic bacteria were markedly increased. Prebiotics and probiotics have the potential to improve the gut mucosal barrier and help decrease postsurgical infectious complications (Liu et al., 2011).

TABLE 11.5

Cancer of the Colon and Rectum

	Decrease Risk	Increase Risk
Convincing	Physical activity	Red meat
		Processed meat
		Alcoholic drinks (men)
		Body fat
		Abdominal fat
Probable	Food containing dietary fiber	Alcoholic drinks (women)
	Garlic	
	Milk	
	Calcium	
Limited—suggestive	Nonstarchy vegetables	Foods containing iron
	Fruits	Cheese
	Food containing folate	Foods containing animal fats
	Foods containing selenium	Foods containing sugars
	Fish	
	Food containing vitamin D	
	Selenium	
Limited—no conclusion	Cereals (grains); potatoes; poultry; shellfish and other seafood; other dairy products; fatty acid composition; cholesterol; sugar (sucrose); coffee; tea; caffeine; vitamin A; retinol; vitamin C; vitamin E; multivitamins; nondietary sources of calcium; methionine; beta-carotene; alpha-carotene; lycopene	

Source: Adapted from World Cancer Research Fund/American Institute for Cancer Research, Continuous Update Project Report. *Food, Nutrition, Physical Activity, and the Prevention of Colorectal Cancer*, AICR, Washington, DC, 2011.

The World Cancer Research Fund and the American Institute for Cancer Research produced an updated systematic literature review of the evidence on food, nutrition, and physical activity in relation to the prevention of CRC in 2010. Table 11.5 shows the factors that can be found in the report including those that increase and decrease risk of CRC (WCRF/AICR, 2011).

Evidence suggests that glutamine supplementation may decrease the incidence and/or severity of chemotherapy-associated mucositis, diarrhea, neuropathy, and hepatic veno-occlusive disease in the setting of high-dose chemotherapy (Savarese et al., 2003). Vitamin A seems to be very effective in the treatment of radiation-induced anorectal damage as it is known to facilitate wound healing and prevent radiation-induced GI damage (Levitsky et al., 2003).

Studies indicate that ginseng has potential as a chemopreventive agent or adjuvant treatment. Colon cancer has been shown to decrease significantly with ginseng use by inhibition of DNA damage, induction of apoptosis, and inhibition of cell proliferation. It is also becoming increasingly clear that ginseng has potent effects on the inflammatory cascade and may inhibit the inflammation-to-cancer sequence

(Hofseth and Wargovich, 2007). A recent study done by Li et al. (2009), illustrated that panaxadiol, a purified ginseng component, enhances the anticancer effects of 5-FU in human CRC cells.

Physical activity after cancer diagnosis is associated with a reduced risk of cancer recurrence and improved overall mortality among colorectal and prostate cancer survivor groups. At least four large cohort studies have found an inverse association between physical activity after diagnosis and recurrence, CRC-specific mortality, and/or overall mortality, with improvements of up to 50% for each outcome (Meyerhardt et al., 2006). Exercise improves QOL, fatigue, psychosocial distress, depression, and self-esteem.

CONCLUSION

Many cancer survivors are now turning their attention to therapies that will complement their medical treatments in the hopes of survival and improved QOL. A systematic review investigating the use of complementary and alternative therapies in adult populations demonstrated that between 7% and 64% of adults have used these therapies, with the average prevalence totaling 31.4% (Ernst, 1998). Many complementary and alternative therapies have yet to undergo clinical trials, and clinicians involved in the care of these patients need to be attentive and make a conscious effort to understand the science, or lack thereof, behind these alternative approaches in order to provide appropriate guidance relevant to their patients' treatment regimen.

REFERENCES

American Cancer Society. 2013. Esophageal cancer. http://www.cancer.org (accessed December 13, 2013).

Atkin, W. et al. 2013. Computed tomographic colonography versus colonoscopy for investigation of patients with symptoms suggestive of colorectal cancer (SIGGAR): A multicentre randomized trial. *Lancet.* 381:1194–1202.

Batcher, E., Madaj, P., and Gianoukakis, A.G. 2011. Pancreatic neuroendocrine tumors. *Endocr Res.* 36(1):35–43.

Beer, K.T. et al. 2005. Early percutaneous endoscopic gastrostomy insertion maintains nutritional state in patients with aerodigestive tract cancer. *Nutr Cancer.* 52(1):29–34.

Bernert, C.P. et al. 2007. Nutritional deficiency after gastric bypass: Diagnosis, prevention and treatment. *Diabetes Metab.* 33:13–24.

Bostick, M. et al. 1993a. Reduced risk of colon cancer with high intake of vitamin E: The Iowa Women's Health Study. *Cancer Res.* 15:4230–4237.

Bostick, M. et al. 1993b. Relation of calcium, vitamin D, and dairy food intake to incidence of colon cancer among older women. The Iowa Women's Health Study. *Am J Epidemiol.* 137:1302–1317.

Bowen, M. et al. 2007. VSL#3 probiotic treatment reduces chemotherapy-induced diarrhea and weight loss. *Cancer Biol Ther.* 6:1449–1454.

Buaitti, E. et al. 1989. A case–control study of diet and gastric cancer in Italy. *Int J Cancer.* 44:611–616.

Burt, W., DiSario, A., and Cannon-Albright, L. 1995. Genetics of colon cancer: Impact of inheritance on colon cancer risk. *Annu Rev Med.* 46:371–379.

Carlin, A.M. et al. 2009. Treatment of vitamin D depletion after roux-en-y gastric bypass: A randomized prospective clinical trial. *Surg Obes Relat Dis.* 5:444–449.

Carlson, L.E. et al. 2007. One year pre–post intervention follow-up of psychological, immune, endocrine and blood pressure outcomes of mindfulness-based stress reduction (MBSR) in breast and prostate cancer outpatients. *Brain Behav Immun.* 21:1038–1049.

Cerantola, Y. et al. 2011. Immunonutrition in gastrointestinal surgery. *Br J Surg.* 98(1):37–48.

Chan, J.M., Wang, F., and Holly, E.A. 2005. Vegetable and fruit intake and pancreatic cancer in a population-based case–control study in the San Francisco Bay Area. *Cancer Epidemiol Biomarkers Prev.* 14(9):2093–2097.

Chan, T. and Giovannucci, L. 2010. Primary prevention of colorectal cancer. *Gastroenterology.* 138:2029–2043.

Christl, U. and Scheppach, W. 1997. Metabolic consequences of total colectomy. *Scand J Gastroenterol Suppl.* 222:20–24.

Cruz-Correa, M. et al. 2006. Combination treatment with curcumin and quercetin. *Gastroenterol Hepatol.* 4:1035–1038.

Cukier, M. et al. 2012. Neoadjuvant chemoradiotherapy and multivisceral resection for primary locally advanced adherent colon cancer: A single institution experience. *Eur J Surg Oncol.* 38:677–682.

Daly, J.M. et al. 1982. Parenteral nutrition in esophageal cancer patients. *Ann Surg.* 196(2):203–208.

deLuis, D.A. et al. 2008. A randomized clinical trial with two omega 3 fatty acid enhanced oral supplements in head and neck cancer ambulatory patients. *Eur Rev Med Pharmacol Sci.* 12:177–181.

Deng, G.E. et al. 2009. Evidence-based clinical practice guidelines for integrative oncology: Complementary therapies and botanicals. *J Soc Integr Oncol.* 7(3):85–120.

Dewey, A. et al. 2007. Eicosapentaenoic acid for the treatment of cancer cachexia. *Cochrane Database Syst Rev.* 1:CD004597.

Dominguez-Munoz, J.E. 2011. Pancreatic exocrine insufficiency: Diagnosis and treatment. *J Gastroenterol Hepatol.* 26 Suppl 2:12–16.

Elia, M. et al. 2006. Enteral (oral or tube administration) nutritional support and eicosapentaenoic acid in patients with cancer: A systematic review. *Int J Oncol.* 28:5.

Emil, R. et al. 2008. Zinc alters cytoskeletal integrity and migration in colon cancer cells. *Acta Med (Hradec Kralove).* 51:51–57.

Ernst, E. 1998. The prevalence of complementary/Alternative medicine in cancer. *Cancer.* 83:777–782.

Fearon, K.C. et al. 2003. Effect of a protein and energy dense N-3 fatty acid enriched oral supplement on loss of weight and lean tissue in cancer cachexia: A randomised double blind trial. *Gut.* 52:1479–1486.

Fedirko, V. et al. 2011. Alcohol drinking and colorectal cancer risk: An overall and dose-response meta-analysis of published studies. *Ann Oncol.* 22:1958–1972.

Fenti, D. et al. 2009. Body weight, lifestyle, dietary habits and gastroesophageal reflux disease. *World J Gastroenterol.* 15(14):1690–1701.

Ferrari, P. et al. 2007. Lifetime and baseline alcohol intake and risk of colon and rectal cancers in the European prospective investigation into cancer and nutrition (EPIC). *Int J Cancer.* 121:2065–2072.

Fleischhauer, A.T. and Arab, L. 2001. Garlic and cancer: A critical review of the epidemiologic literature. *J Nutr.* 131(3s):1032S–1040S.

Fuchs, C, Mitchell, P., and Hoff, M. 2006. Irinotecan in the treatment of colorectal cancer. *Cancer Treat Rev.* 32:491–503.

Gao, Y.T. et al. 1994. Risk factors for esophageal cancer in Shanghai, China. II. Role of diet and nutrients. *Int J Cancer.* 58:197–202.

Ghaneh, P. and Neoptolemos, J.P. 2012. Pancreatic exocrine tumors, in *Textbook of Clinical Gastroenterology and Hepatology*, 2nd edn. (eds. C.J. Hawkey, J. Bosch, J.E. Richter, G. Garcia-Tsao, and F.K.L. Chan), Wiley-Blackwell, Oxford, U.K.

Giovannucci, E. et al. 1998. Multivitamin use, folate, and colon cancer in women in the Nurses' Health Study. *Ann Intern Med.* 129:517–524.

Gonzalez, C. and Agudo, A. 2012. Carcinogenesis, prevention and early detection of gastric cancer: Where we are and where we should go. *Int J Cancer.* 130(4):745–753.

Gorham, D. et al. 2005. Vitamin D and prevention of colorectal cancer. *J Steroid Biochem Mol Biol.* 97:179–194.

Greene, F.L., Compton, C.C., Fritz, A.G., Shah, J.P., and Winchester, D.P. 2006. The American Joint Committee on Cancer Staging (AJCC) Atlas, in *International Seminars in Surgical Oncology* (ed. G. Singh-Ranger), Springer, Vol. 3, p. 34.

Gupta, V. 2009. Benefits versus risks: A prospective audit. Feeding jejunostomy during esophagectomy. *World J Surg.* 33:1432–1438.

Hansson, L.E. et al. 1993. Diet and risk of gastric cancer: A population-based case–control study in Sweden. *Int J Cancer.* 55:181–189.

Hilliard, R.E. 2003. The effects of music therapy on the quality and length of life of people diagnosed with terminal cancer. *J Music Ther.* 40:113–137.

Hofseth, J. and Wargovich, J. 2007. Inflammation, cancer, and targets of ginseng. *J Nutr.* 137:183S–185S.

Howe, G.R., Jain, M., and Miller, A.B. 1990. Dietary factors and risk of pancreatic cancer: Results of a Canadian population-based case–control study. *Int J Cancer.* 45(4):604.

Hu, J. et al. 1994. Risk factors for oesophageal cancer in northeast China. *Int J Cancer.* 57: 38–46.

Hyoung-Il, K. et al. 2011. Oral vitamin B12 replacement: An effective treatment for vitamin B12 after total gastrectomy in gastric cancer patients. *Ann Surg Oncol.* 18:3711–3717.

Jacobs, R. 1988. Fiber and colon cancer. *Gastroenterol Clin North Am.* 17:747–760.

Jemal, A. et al. 2013. Annual report to the nation on the status of cancer, 1975–2009, featuring the burden and trends in human papillomavirus (HPV)-associated cancers and HPV vaccination coverage levels. *J Natl Cancer Inst.* 105:175.

Johnstone, P.A., Niemtzow, R.C., and Riffenburgh, R.H. 2002. Acupuncture for xerostomia: Clinical update. *Cancer.* 94:1151–1156.

Kanai, M. et al. 2011. A phase I/II study of gemcitabine-based chemotherapy plus curcumin for patients with gemcitabine-resistant pancreatic cancer. *Cancer Chemother Pharmacol.* 68:157–164.

Kempers, J. et al. 2011. Risk of colorectal and endometrial cancers in EPCAM deletion-positive Lynch syndrome: A cohort study. *Lancet Oncol.* 12:49–55.

Kim, I. 2003. Role of folate in colon cancer development and progression. *J Nutr.* 133:3731S–3739S.

Koretz, R.L., Lipman, T.O., and Klein, S. October 2001. American gastroenterological association. AGA technical review on parenteral nutrition. *Gastroenterology.* 121(4):970–1001.

Kuhnle, G. and Bingham, A. 2007. Dietary meat, endogenous nitrosation and colorectal cancer. *Biochem Soc Trans.* 35:1355–1357.

Kune, A. and Vitetta, L. 1992. Alcohol consumption and the etiology of colorectal cancer: A review of the scientific evidence from 1957 to 1991. *Nutr Cancer.* 18:97–111.

Kunnumakkara, A.B. et al. 2007. Curcumin potentiates antitumor activity of gemcitabine in an orthotopic model of pancreatic cancer through suppression of proliferation, angiogenesis, and inhibition of nuclear factor-κB-regulated gene products. *Cancer Res.* 67(8):3853–3861.

Lamprecht, A. and Lipkin, M. 2001. Cellular mechanisms of calcium and vitamin D in the inhibition of colorectal carcinogenesis. *Ann N Y Acad Sci.* 952:73–87.

Larsson, S.C. and Wolk, A. 2012. Red and processed meat consumption and risk of pancreatic cancer: Meta-analysis of prospective studies. *Br J Cancer.* 106(3):603.

Lee, H. 2004. Heme iron, zinc, alcohol consumption, and colon cancer: Iowa Women's Health Study. *J Natl Cancer Inst.* 3:403–407.

Levitsky, J. et al. 2003. Oral vitamin A therapy for a patient with a severely symptomatic postradiation anal ulceration. *Dis Colon Rectum.* 46:679–682.

Li, D. et al. 2004. Pancreatic cancer. *Lancet.* 363(9414):1049–1057.

Li, L. et al. 2009. Panaxadiol, a purified ginseng component, enhances the anti-cancer effects of 5-fluorouracil in human colorectal cancer cells. *Cancer Chemother Pharmacol.* 64:1097–1104.

Liu, Z. et al. 2011. Randomized clinical trial: The effects of perioperative probiotic treatment on barrier function and post-operative infectious complications in colorectal cancer surgery—A double-blind study. *Aliment Pharmacol Ther.* 33:50–63.

Lucenteforte, E. et al. 2012. Alcohol consumption and pancreatic cancer: A pooled analysis in the international pancreatic cancer case–control consortium (PanC4). *Ann Oncol.* 23(2):374.

Ma, Y. et al. 2011. Association between vitamin D and risk of colorectal cancer: A systematic review of prospective studies. *JCO.* 29:3775–3782.

Macdonald, S. 1999. Carcinoembryonic antigen screening: Pros and cons. *Semin Oncol.* 26:556–560.

Majumdar, R., Fletcher, H., and Evans, T. 1999. How does colorectal cancer present? Symptoms, duration and clues to location. *Am J Gastroenterol.* 94:3039–3045.

Margolis, M. et al. 2003. Percutaneous endoscopic gastrostomy tube before multimodality therapy in patients with esophageal cancer. *Ann Thorac Surg.* 76:1694.

Martignoni, M.E. et al. 2000. Enteral nutrition prolongs delayed gastric emptying in patients after Whipple resection. *Am J Surg.* 180(1):18–23.

Mawhinney, M.R. and Glasgow, R.E. 2012. Current treatment options for the management of esophageal cancer. *Cancer Manag Res.* 4:367–377.

McGarr, E., Ridlon, M., and Hylemon, B. 2005. Diet, anaerobic bacterial metabolism, and colon cancer: A review of the literature. *J Clin Gastroenterol.* 39:98–109.

Meyerhardt, A. et al. 2006. Physical activity and survival after colorectal cancer diagnosis. *J Clin Oncol.* 24:3527–3534.

Meyerhardt, A. et al. 2007. Association of dietary patterns with cancer recurrence and survival in patients with stage III colon cancer. *JAMA.* 298:754–764.

Michels, B. et al. 2000. Prospective study of fruit and vegetable consumption and incidence of colon and rectal cancers. *J Natl Cancer Inst.* 92:1740–1752.

Michl, P. 2006. Evidence-based diagnosis and staging of pancreatic cancer. *Best Pract Res Clin Gastroenterol.* 20(2):227–251.

Milner, A. et al. 2001. Molecular targets for nutrients involved with cancer prevention. *Nutr Cancer.* 41:1–16.

Moadel, A.B. et al. 2007. Randomized controlled trial of yoga among a multiethnic sample of breast cancer patients: Effects on quality of life. *J Clin Oncol.* 25:4387–4395.

Morrow, G.R. and Morrell, C. 1982. Behavioral treatment for the anticipatory nausea and vomiting induced by cancer chemotherapy. *N Engl J Med.* 307:1476–1480.

Mustian, K.M. et al. 2004. Health-related quality of life and self-esteem: A randomized trial with breast cancer survivors. *Support Care Cancer.* 12:871–876.

Naeim, A. et al. 2008. Evidence-based recommendations for cancer nausea and vomiting. *J Clin Oncol.* 26:3903–3910.

National Cancer Institute. Colon and Rectal Cancer. http//www.cancer.gov/cancertopics/types/colon-and-recal. Accessed December 11, 2013.

National Cancer Institute. Colon Cancer Treatment. http://www.cancer.gov/cancertopics/pdq/treatment/colon/Patient/page4#Keypoint17. Accessed December 11, 2013.

National Cancer Institute. 2013. Pancreatic neuroendocrine tumors (islet cell tumors) treatment. http://www.cancer.gov (accessed December 12, 2013).

National Cancer Institute. 2014. FDA Approval for Oxaliplatin. http://www.cancer.gov/cancertopics/druginfo/fda-oxaliplatin. Accessed December 11, 2013.

Ng, K. et al. 2009. Prospective study of predictors of vitamin D status and survival in patients with colorectal cancer. *Br J Cancer.* 101:916–923.

NIH Technology. 1996. Assessment panel on integration of behavioral and relaxation approaches into the treatment of chronic pain and insomnia. *JAMA.* 276:313–318.

O'Reilly, E.M. 2009. Pancreatic adenocarcinoma: New strategies for success. *Gastrointest Cancer Res.* 3:S11–S15.

Ohigashi, S. et al. 2013. Significant changes in the intestinal environment after surgery in patients with colorectal cancer. *J Gastrointest Surg.* 17:1657–1664.

Patel, S.H. et al. June 2013. An assessment of feeding jejunostomy tube placement at the time of resection for gastric adenocarcinoma. *J Surg Oncol.* 107(7):728–734.

Ransohoff, F. and Lang, A. 1991. Screening for colorectal cancer. *N Engl J Med.* 325:37–41.

Reddy, S. et al. 1992. Effect of dietary fiber on colonic bacterial enzymes and bile acids in relation to colon cancer. *Gastroenterology.* 102:1475–1482.

Riccardi, D. and Allen, K. 1999. Nutritional management of patient's with esophageal and esophagogastric junction cancer. *Cancer Control.* 6:64.

Roller, M. et al. 2004. Intestinal immunity of rats with colon cancer is modulated by oligo-fructose-enriched inulin combined with *Lactobacillus rhamnosus* and *Bifidobacterium lactis. Br J Nutr.* 92:931–938.

Sah, B.K. et al. 2009. Gastric cancer surgery: Billroth I or Billroth II for distal gastrectomy? *BMC Cancer.* 9:428.

Savarese, M. et al. 2003. Prevention of chemotherapy and radiation toxicity with glutamine. *Cancer Treat Rev.* 29:501–513.

Secretan, B. et al. 2009. A review of human carcinogens—Part E: Tobacco, areca nuts, alcohol, coal, smoke, and salted fish. *Lancet Oncol.* 10:1033–1034.

Shah, M.A. and Kurtz, R.C. 2010. Upper gastrointestinal cancer predisposition syndromes. *Hematol Oncol Clin North Am.* 24(5):815–835.

Siegel, R., Naishadham, D., and Jemal, A. 2013. Cancer statistics. *Cancer J Clin.* 63:11–30.

Siewert, J.R. and Sendler, A. 2001. Preoperative staging for gastric cancer, in *Surgical Treatment: Evidence-Based and Problem-Oriented* (eds. R.G. Holzheimer and J.A. Mannick), Zuckschwerdt, Munich, Germany.

Sikora, S.S. et al. 1998. Role of nutrition support during induction chemoradiation therapy in esophageal cancer. *J Parenter Enteral Nutr.* 22:18.

Singh, N. and Fraser, E. 1998. Dietary risk factors for colon cancer in a low-risk population. *Am J Epidemiol.* 148:761–774.

Smith, R.A. et al. 2001. American Cancer Society guidelines for the early detection of cancer: Update of early detection guidelines for prostate, colorectal, and endometrial cancers. Also: Update 2001—Testing for early lung cancer detection. *CA Cancer J Clin.* 51:38–75.

Thiébaut, A.C. et al. 2009. Dietary fatty acids and pancreatic cancer in the NIH-AARP diet and health study. *J Natl Cancer Inst.* 01(14):1001.

Turati, F. et al. 2012. A meta-analysis of coffee consumption and pancreatic cancer. *Ann Oncol.* 23:311–318.

Ukleja, A. 2006. Dumping Syndrome. In: Nutrition Issues in Gastroenterology, Series #35. Parrish CR, editor. *Practical Gastroenterology*; 32–46.

Willett, G. et al. 1993. Postoperative radiation therapy for high-risk colon carcinoma. *J Clin Oncol.* 11:1112–1117.

World Cancer Research Fund/American Institute for Cancer Research. 2007. *Food, Nutrition, Physical Activity, and Prevention of Cancer: A Global Perspective*, AICR, Washington, DC.

World Cancer Research Fund/American Institute for Cancer Research. 2011. Continuous Update Project Report. *Food, Nutrition, Physical Activity, and the Prevention of Colorectal Cancer*, AICR, Washington, DC. http://www.dietandcancerreport.org/cup/current_progress/colorectal_cancer.php.

Worthington, H.V. et al. 2011. Interventions for preventing oral mucositis for patients with cancer receiving treatment. *Cochrane Database Syst Rev.* Apr 13; (4):CD000978.

Wu, K. et al. 2002. A prospective study on supplemental vitamin E intake and risk of colon cancer in women and men. *Cancer Epidemiol Biomarkers Prev.* 11:1298–1304.

Xiao, M., Wang, Y., and Gao, Y. September 26, 2013. Association between helicobacter pylori infection and pancreatic cancer development: A meta-analysis. *PLoS ONE.* 8(9):e75559.

You, W. et al. 1989. Allium vegetables and reduced risk of stomach cancer. *J Natl Cancer Inst.* 81:162–164.

Yuan, C. et al. 2013. Prediagnostic body mass index and pancreatic cancer survival. *J Clin Oncol.* 31(33):4229–4234.

Zhang, X. et al. 2011. A prospective study of intakes of zinc and heme iron and colorectal cancer risk in men and women. *Cancer Causes Control.* 22:1627–1637.

Zhuang, L. et al. 2013. The preventative and therapeutic effect of acupuncture for radiation-induced xerostomia in patients with head and neck cancer. A systematic review. *Integr Cancer Ther.* 12(3):197–205.

12 Traditional and Nontraditional Treatments for Diabetes

*Patricia G. Davidson, DCN, RDN, CDE, LDN
and Dwight L. Davidson, PhD, MA, LHMC*

CONTENTS

EPIDEMIOLOGY AND PATHOPHYSIOLOGY

The older adult population of the United States has doubled since 1981, and by 2050 is projected to nearly triple. With 29 million people diagnosed with diabetes in the United States in 2012 [1], and an expected additional doubling by the year 2030 [2], it is clear that diabetes has reached the status of an epidemic. The Centers for Disease Control and Prevention (CDC) estimates that there are 79 million people with pre-diabetes (PreDM) and 8.1 million undiagnosed cases of diabetes [1].

Diabetes is classified into two predominant types: type 1 (T1DM) and type 2 (T2DM). A comparison between the characteristics of T1DM and T2DM is illustrated in Table 12.1. T1DM results from the immune system attacking healthy insulin producing beta (β) cells of the pancreas and is a disease of the autoimmune system. This destruction of β cells results in a complete deficiency in insulin production. A virus, such as shingles, or autoimmune diseases, such as hypo/hyperthyroidism, can trigger T1DM. There is also a genetic tendency for T1DM that typically occurs in children. It is increasing in the adult population and is known as latent autoimmune diabetes in adults (LADA), a slow evolving variant of T1DM. Some form of T2DM is found in the majority of older adults. In contrast to T1DM, the etiology of T2DM is hereditary, though triggered by environmental and/or lifestyle factors. Decreased insulin production, insulin resistance, and ultimately insulin deficiency

TABLE 12.1
Comparison of Diabetes Types

Attributes	Type 1	Type 2
Age of onset	Younger onset, with mean age <30	Older onset, with mean age >40, but possible in children
Pathogenesis	Autoimmune	Age <60, primarily hereditary
	Genetic	Age >60, body composition, lifestyle (physical activity, diet, and environment)
Symptoms	Sudden onset	Slow onset
	Very high blood glucose levels	Near normal blood glucose levels with elevated insulin levels
	Normal to thin	Majority overweight or obese
	Symptomatic at onset	Asymptomatic or delayed onset
	Increased urination	Increased urination
	Increased thirst	Increased thirst
	Increased appetite	Increased appetite
	Weakness	Fatigue
	Unintentional, rapid weight loss	Unexplained increase/decrease in weight
	Ketoacidosis, with nausea and vomiting	Proteinuria, without nausea
	Dehydration, with flakey skin and dry mucous membranes	Slow wound healing and repeated fungal and urinary tract infections
Management	Insulin required and DSME/T	DSME/T, including diet and exercise programs, and medications as needed

Source: American Diabetes Association, *Diabetes Care*, 37(1), S81, 2014.

result from a progressive decline in β cell function. Theories of the cause of T2DM include, but are not limited to normal aging body composition changes, increase in visceral adiposity, vitamin D deficiency, and inflammation [3,4].

There is growing evidence supporting the position that genes predispose to the development of T2DM. Over 50 genetic abnormalities have been linked to T2DM, and with the growing number of people included in genetic scans, the number of abnormalities identified is increasing [5]. Various ethnic groups (African Americans, Asians, and Europeans) show significant differences in these gene abnormalities. However, the total aggregate of all of these genetic abnormalities is responsible for <15% predisposition of T2DM [5].

Hyperglycemia is a common diagnostic criterion of diabetes and may originate in one or a combination of the following: an inability to produce any or a sufficient amount of insulin or to utilize insulin properly. There are two key hormones responsible for the regulation of blood glucose, insulin and glucagon. Glucose transport into cells requires the hormone insulin. If there is a drop in the blood glucose level, the body responds by producing glucagon, which stimulates glucose production from the glycogen stores of the liver, known as glycogenolysis, or from noncarbohydrate sources, known as gluconeogenesis. Hyperglycemia (elevated blood glucose levels) from insulin deficiency, poor insulin utilization (insulin resistance), and overproduction of glucose results in a failure of glucose to enter cells, and to accumulate in the blood. Insulin resistance leads to an inability to utilize glucose and concurrent overproduction of insulin, and is known as hyperinsulinemia. This condition can increase glucose levels and worsen insulin resistance. In either case, there is a lack of available insulin to control glucose levels in the blood. With properly functioning glucose metabolism, the body responds to the glucose load of a meal by maintaining blood glucose levels within a certain range and preventing blood glucose level elevations.

There are two hyperglycemic states that occur with the failure of glucose metabolism: continuous or background (basal) and post-meal response (postprandial). When either one of these two conditions exist, hyperglycemia results from either a delayed insulin release, a lack of glucagon suppression, or post-meal insulin hepatic/muscle insulin resistance. In post-prandial hyperglycemia, continued liver glucose production and poor disposal of glucose leads to the body's inability to respond with insulin or to suppress glucagon [6]. In contrast, basal hyperglycemia can be due to inadequate basal insulin levels and/or glycogenolysis or gluconeogenesis, through an overproduction of glucose by the liver in response to poor glucose uptake and fasting blood glucose levels remaining elevated (see Figure 12.1) [6].

CONVENTIONAL AND TRADITIONAL DIABETES MANAGEMENT

The treatment of diabetes involves multiple strategies for managing this complex disease. Medical practitioners in developing countries recognize that T2DM is a multifactorial disease and demands multiple therapeutic approaches [7]. The American Diabetes Standards of Care emphasizes the importance for screening those at risk for diabetes, specifically adults aged 45 years and older, those considered overweight with a BMI ≥ 25 kg/m^2 or at a high risk BMI by ethnicity, plus one or more risk factors, including but not limited to being overweight, family history of diabetes, and/

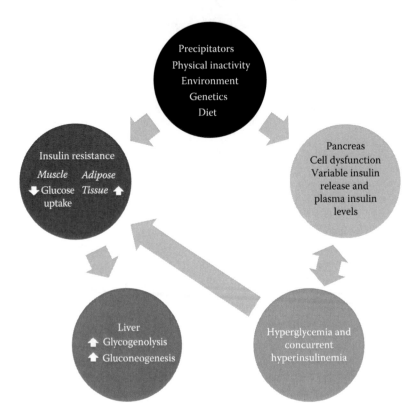

FIGURE 12.1   Relationship between the factors in the development of T2DM.

or ethnicity (African American, Asian American, Native American) [8]. Risk factors that are considered to be modifiable, as lifestyle and dietary factors plan an important role, include being overweight (BMI ≥ 25 kg/m), obesity (BMI ≥ 35), increased waist circumference (>35 in. female and >40 in. males), persons diagnosed with prediabetes, metabolic syndrome (insulin resistance), cardiovascular disease, sleep apnea, or polycystic ovarian syndrome. The guidelines also specify that those at high risk, if the screening test is negative, as well as all adults aged 45 years and older, should be evaluated every 1–3 years, depending on the person's risk factors.

The diagnosis of diabetes is determined either by one or a combination of the following: fasting blood glucose, 2 h 75 g oral glucose tolerance test (OGTT), hemoglobin A1C (A1C) or glycosylated hemoglobin is a test that indicates a person's average glucose level for the previous 90–120 days [8] (Table 12.2 defines the diagnostic criteria for diabetes). If asymptomatic, the test(s) needs to be repeated and confirmed. Research has demonstrated that the A1C best reflects a person's metabolic control and risk for developing complications.

Poor management of diabetes can accelerate natural changes of aging, including bone disease, macro- and micro-vascular changes, dementia, and the development of comorbid conditions, such as heart, cardiovascular, or renal disease (Table 12.3). The diabetes management standards are established primarily with decreasing the risk

TABLE 12.2
Diabetes Diagnostic Criteria

Test[a]	Normal Glucose Tolerance (NGT)	Diabetes ADA
A1C	4.5%–5.7%	≥6.5%
FBG	<100 mg/dL	≥ 126 mg/dL
	(<5.6 mmol/L)	(7.0 mmol/L)
2 h post glucose or glucose challenge (OGTT)—WHO 75 g glucose solution impaired glucose tolerance (IGT)	<140 mg/dL (<7.8 mmol/L)	≥200 mg/dL (11.1 mmol/L)
Symptomatic of hyperglycemia or hyperglycemic crisis	N/A	≥200 mg/dL (11.1 mmol/L)

- All tests should be repeated for confirmation if asymptomatic or if hyperglycemia is absent.
- Repeat test when normal every 1–3 years based on risk factors.

Source: Diabetes Complications, 2014, Retrieved from http://www.diabetes.org/living-with-diabetes/complications/, accessed November 14, 2014.

[a] A1C standardized using the diabetes complication and clinical trial.

for developing comorbid conditions and complications. The diabetes management standards are shown in Table 12.4.

Successful management requires consideration of conventional and complementary/alternative approaches as well as collaboration between a variety of health professionals, including but not limited to physicians, nurses, dietitians, pharmacists, mental health professionals, and the person with diabetes.

It is important to define what is considered to comprise traditional treatment strategies for diabetes self-management. There are three key conventional tenets in the treatment/management of diabetes: diabetes self-management education and support (DSME/S), diet/exercise, and medications. This is considered the traditional approach. However, others consider herbals, mind–body therapies, and other complementary/alternative treatments as traditional and the former method as modern medicine (see Figure 12.2) [9]. This section will discuss each of these as it relates to diabetes management.

CONVENTIONAL MANAGEMENT STRATEGIES

DIABETES SELF-MANAGEMENT EDUCATION AND SUPPORT

At the core for developing any diabetes management plan is the consideration of patient desires and needs, as well as the importance of individualization. Factors that can influence the treatment plan are age, culture, lifestyle (eating patterns/physical activity), schedule (work or school), and social economic determinants.

Diabetes education has as its goal the empowerment of the patient to obtain the knowledge, skills, and confidence to perform self-care behaviors necessary to achieve optimal clinical outcomes and to prevent or delay complications [10].

TABLE 12.3
Chronic and Acute Complications

Complication	Body Changes
Chronic Complications	
Cardiovascular and vascular damage	Elevated blood lipids, blood pressure, stroke, heart attack and heart failure, peripheral vascular disease and poor wound healing, foot infections and deformities
Mental health	Depression and diabetes distress
Nerve damage	Neuropathy—damage to nerves throughout the body
	Can lead to numbness; foot deformities; burning and tingling sensation hands, feet, and legs; decreased sensitivity to extreme temperatures; decreased recognition of symptoms of hypoglycemia
Eye/ears	Retinopathy and other visual changes
	Damage blood vessels of the retina can lead to impaired vision, blindness, higher risk for cataracts and glaucoma
	Hearing problems associated with neuropathy and vascular disease
Kidney disease	Nephropathy—changes in the small and large blood vessels decreasing kidney filtration rates and kidney insufficiency and failure
Stomach and digestion	Gastroparesis—poor stomach emptying or rapid emptying causing blood glucose variability
Dental	Periodontal disease, tooth loss, gum disease causing changes in appetite, taste, and textures of foods consumed
Acute Complications	
Ketoacidosis	Occurs in those with T1DM primarily
	High risk during an infection or trauma and caused by hyperglycemia, insulin deficiency, and rapid fat metabolism
Hyperosmolar hyperglycemic nonketotic syndrome (HHNS)	Occurs in those with T2DM primarily, elderly. Can be caused by an acute infection, medications (i.e., glucocorticoids); peritoneal dialysis; renal failure
Hypoglycemia	T1DM or T2DM—if taking insulin and possibly oral hypoglycemic agents

Source: Diabetes Complications, http://www.diabetes.org/living-with-diabetes/complications/ (accessed November 14, 2014), 2014.

There is also a supportive component that assists people with diabetes to establish and implement a plan of action for behavior change and continued care [10,11].

According to the CDC, great strides have been made over the past few decades in the management and quality of care of diabetes. Despite these changes, limited advances have been made to achieve the metabolic control goals for diabetes management, including blood glucose, blood pressure, and lipid levels [12]. Approximately 35% of the people with diabetes still have abnormal lipid levels and/or poor control of their blood pressure and glucose levels [12]. The findings of these studies emphasize the continuing need for efforts to identify all barriers to achieving optimal diabetes management.

TABLE 12.4
Diabetes Management Standards

Clinical Parameter	Non-Diabetes Normal Range	Diabetes Standard
Glycemic targets—modified based on age, risk of hypoglycemia, or complications		
A1C	4.0%–6.0%	<7.0% (higher based on age or risk of hypoglycemia)
Fasting blood glucose	70–99 mg/dL	70–130 mg/dL
Postprandial blood glucose	140–199 mg/dL	<180 mg/dL
Lipid targets—modified based on age, risk of complications, and co-morbid conditions		
LDL-C	65–180 mg/dL	<100 mg/dL
HDL-C	30–70 mg/dL	Men > 40 mg/dL Women > 50 mg/dL
Triglycerides	65–180 mg/dL	<150 mg/dL
Blood pressure target—modified based on age, risk of complications, and co-morbid conditions		
	120/80 mmHg	130/80 mmHg

Source: American Diabetes Association, *Diabetes Care*, 37(1), S14, 2014.

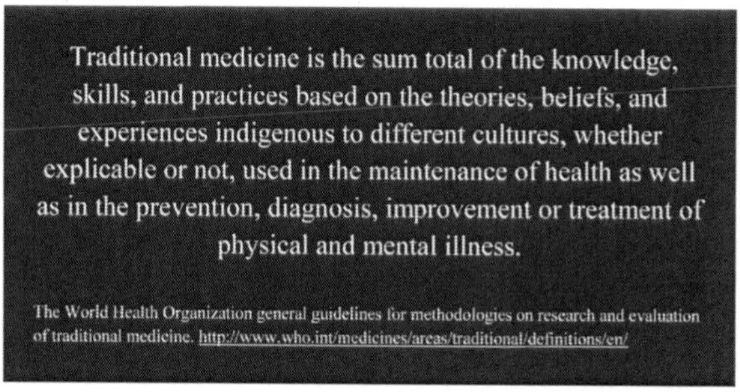

Traditional medicine is the sum total of the knowledge, skills, and practices based on the theories, beliefs, and experiences indigenous to different cultures, whether explicable or not, used in the maintenance of health as well as in the prevention, diagnosis, improvement or treatment of physical and mental illness.

The World Health Organization general guidelines for methodologies on research and evaluation of traditional medicine. http://www.who.int/medicines/areas/traditional/definitions/en/

FIGURE 12.2 World Health Organization (WHO) traditional medicine definition.

Diabetes self-management education (DSME) plays a pivotal role in successful diabetes care and management [13–16]. Two large hallmark studies in the area of diabetes management, along with smaller clinical trials, emphasize the role of education and promoting diabetes self-management in adults [17–20]. Diabetes self-management is the conventional, multidisciplinary approach that encourages the development of self-management skills in the patient [21–23].

There are two main methods for monitoring glucose control: self-monitoring blood glucose (SMBG) and the A1C. SMBG is a monitoring activity performed by those with diabetes for obtaining a blood glucose level at a single point in time with a finger stick using a lancet, test strip, and blood glucose meter. It is considered a foundation for evaluating a person's on going progress and response to their treatment plan and changes. SMBG supports patient involvement in self-care, and in turn develops a symbiotic relationship between the health team and the patient. SMBG data is typically used to detect or confirm variations in blood glucose levels and to take corrective action. Clinicians perform a retrospective analysis of SMBG data, typically communicated by the patient's logbook or diary. It is recommended that for those taking insulin multiple times per day or on an insulin pump, perform this test at least prior to each meal or snack, exercise, and bedtime [8]. For those with less stringent treatment regimens, the frequency for testing should be driven by the person's treatment goals [8]. Similarly, A1C testing should be based on a patient's treatment goals and individualized. It should be measured a minimum of twice a year for those patients meeting their treatment goals and considered in good metabolic control, with a value greater than 6.5 and less than or equal to 7.0%, and every 3 months if not meeting metabolic treatment goals or when changes have been made to the management plan.

There are many barriers that can inhibit self-management, including the patient's knowledge base, personal beliefs, medication regimens, and lifestyle [10]. If self-management is to be effective, it must include the ability to self-monitor and to influence the cognitive, behavioral, and emotional responses required to maintain a palatable quality of life. Therefore, self-management requires more than just adherence to treatment guidelines. It must incorporate the psychosocial factors associated with living with a chronic disease [24]. While integrating these psychosocial factors, three key components of traditional diabetes management are necessary: nutrition (including diet and weight management), physical activity, and medication (if needed) [9].

NUTRITION AND LIFESTYLE

Nutrition plays an important part in the management of diabetes [25,26]. An individualized nutrition plan must take into account comorbid conditions, energy needs based on the individual lifestyle, and the person's base belief structure. A thorough nutrition assessment (including food, nutrition, and client histories), anthropometric measures, and all appropriate clinical lab work will assist in the structuring and individualization of the diabetes management plan.

DIET

Two prominent, national organizations, the American Diabetes Association (ADA) and the Academy of Nutrition and Dietetics (The Academy), advise that in the care of adults with diabetes, evidence-based nutritional guidelines individualized to the patient/client (Medical Nutrition Therapy) be utilized [8,25,27]. An individualized eating plan, promoting optimal metabolic control (hemoglobin A1C [A1C], serum lipids, and blood pressure), an ideal/healthy body weight, and delaying/preventing complications is the goal of the dietary intervention [25,27].

The dietary intervention is shaped by the patient's diabetes type and comorbid conditions. Evidence-based research analysis by the Academy and the ADA advocates the use of specific dietary patterns, such as a Mediterranean diet, dietary approaches to stop hypertension (DASH), and a low-fat or low-carbohydrate diet [25,27]. Clinical studies have demonstrated that a Mediterranean diet is effective in the reduction of insulin resistance and inflammation, resulting in significant weight loss and reduction in the progression to T2DM and related comorbidities. The Mediterranean diet emphasizes fruits and vegetables, nuts, olive oil, legumes, and whole grains. Increasing intake of seafood, lean meats, and low-fat milk products as sources of protein is encouraged, as is moderate amounts of wine with meals. Following this type of diet also increases the intake of fiber. The ADA daily recommendation of 25–35 g of dietary fiber, either as a supplement or in foods, has been shown to improve glycemic control [8,27,28]. Food sources of fiber include chickpeas, beans, peas, lentils, grains, fruits, and vegetables.

Though the Mediterranean style of eating is relatively high in total fat as a percentage of total calories (30%–40%), it is higher in the beneficial monounsaturated fatty acids (MUFA), and higher in omega-3 polyunsaturated fatty acids (PUFA) compared to omega-6 PUFAs, and lower in saturated fatty acids (SFA) [29–32]. Researchers of the Mediterranean diet surmised that altering the macronutrient composition, substituting unsaturated fat for a portion of the carbohydrate, and increasing the omega-3 fatty acids from fish reduces insulin resistance [30,31,33–35].

STRATEGIES FOR MEAL PLANNING

The focus for most meal planning strategies is on the macronutrient carbohydrate, as they exhibit the most impact on blood glucose levels. The exchange system of meal planning strategy is the most complex, categorizing foods based on its macronutrient composition in one serving. It includes the major food groups: carbohydrates (starches, fruits, milk, and sweets), meat or meat substitutes, non-starchy vegetables, and fats. This method allows for flexibility in food choices, as foods within a group can be replaced or traded for another in that food group. For example, a 1 oz slice of bread has the same carbohydrate content as 1/3 cup of rice or pasta. The main feature of the exchanges is portion sizes. By using portions, a structured but individualized meal plan can be developed for maintaining a carbohydrate, macronutrient, and energy-consistent meal plan.

Consuming carbohydrates higher in fiber in combinations with lower glycemic index (GI) and glycemic load (GL) have been shown in some studies to be beneficial in controlling insulin levels, postprandial blood glucose levels, and reduced occurrence of cardiovascular complications as well as other associated co-morbid conditions of diabetes in interventional and observational research [28,36–39]. In addition, this dietary pattern may improve the utilization of insulin and glucose while preserving pancreatic function. In theory, following a lower GI/GL-type diet, there is greater stability in glucose levels by consuming a better quality of carbohydrates [25,27,37]. Based on the research, the 2014 ADA Clinical Practice Recommendations promote combining a carbohydrate-consistent diet with consuming lower GI-type foods as an effective dietary strategy [8]. Foods such as brown rice, barley, sweet potatoes, legumes, and whole wheat bread are considered to be low/intermediate GI foods, compared to high GI foods such as white bread, puffed rice, white potatoes, instant oatmeal, and thin pasta. When using the GI method, ADA recommends selecting lower/intermediate GI foods or to minimize the GL (useable carbohydrate = GI × grams of carbohydrate) by combining foods of lower GI with higher GI. This type of diet has been shown to stabilize blood glucose levels and significantly improve A1C and other metabolic parameters, such as blood pressure and blood lipids [36,38].

Carbohydrate counting, another method for meal planning, focuses only on maintaining a consistent amount of this macronutrient throughout the day by meals and snacks. The guidelines stress carbohydrate counting should be considered as a foundational dietary strategy for maintaining glycemic control [8,27]. According to the Academy of Nutrition and Dietetics, evidence-based guidelines for persons with type 1 or type 2 diabetes taking multiple insulin injections or who are on an insulin pump, carbohydrate intake should be matched with insulin needs. This is accomplished by using carbohydrate counting and established, individualized carbohydrate-to-insulin ratios [25]. Even though there is clear evidence that maintaining a consistent carbohydrate intake is beneficial, the ideal amount of carbohydrate as a percentage of the total calories is inconclusive. Therefore, it is recommended that "experience-based estimation" and carbohydrate counting are two good methods to use when establishing the ideal carbohydrate content of a person's diet [27]. Maintaining a carbohydrate-consistent diet has shown improvement in blood glucose stability and plays an important role in regulating post-meal blood glucose excursions, as carbohydrate quality and amount are the best predictors of changes in blood glucose levels [35,36,40].

Weight Loss and Obesity

Obesity due to the causal relationship to insulin resistance and decreasing beta-cell function is a major risk factor in T2DM and the comorbid conditions that often proceed the development of diabetes [5]. Even though research indicates that weight loss can delay disease progression and decrease treatment costs, the strong pathological link between obesity and diabetes makes weight loss difficult [5,41,42]. Weight loss through dietary modification has shown to improve the key metabolic alterations in diabetes: beta cell function and insulin resistance [43,44]. For those with a BMI greater than 40 kg/m^2 thus requiring extreme weight loss, bariatric surgery significantly improved all the key metabolic parameters [25,45,46]. There is immediate remission and glucose homeostasis of T2DM following bariatric surgery, which seems to be related to metabolic and gut hormonal changes [47]. The changes that occur appear to be associated to both weight loss improving insulin sensitivity and beta cell function, as well as the surgical anatomical alteration leading to improved hormonal response to eating. Observational research indicates that the duration of diabetes, glycemic control prior to surgery, and severity of diabetes influence remission rates. Those experiencing diabetes for 5 years or less and A1C levels between 6.5% and 7.9% had higher remission rates, 96% and 77%, respectively, than those with longer duration and poor glycemic control [48,49]. Similarly, the recurrence rate is associated with the severity and duration of diabetes.

According to the Academy, the primary focus of dietary intervention should be on methods to improve blood glucose levels, as the research is inconsistent on the effects of sustained weight loss interventions of greater than or equal to 1 year on overall glycemic control, A1C. The research is not clear as to whether weight loss alone improves glucose levels or results from a combination including lifestyle changes and physical activity. Studies have demonstrated that a moderate weight loss of even 7% improves blood glucose levels and the body's ability to use insulin [8,25,27].

The 2014 ADA Clinical Recommendations encourage that continuous monitoring and lifestyle interventions, including diet and physical activity, are needed to ascertain the long-term effects of weight loss and maintenance of the clinical outcomes [25,27]. Knowing that weight loss is often maximized in the early stages of diabetes, intensive programs and long-term follow-up is required for assessing factors that may impede weight loss and maintenance, including socioeconomic conditions, medication regimens, and hormonal changes occurring with disease progression and the body's compensation to weight loss that promote adiposity and insulin resistance [50]. Research shows that behaviors can improve success with weight maintenance following weight loss. These include consuming breakfast, regular physical activity, weighing weekly, portion control, and consuming nutrient dense, low-calorie foods [51,52].

PHYSICAL ACTIVITY

Physical activity (PA), such as moderate walking, cycling, or structured group activities, in combination with diet and medication are recognized as foundation to diabetes management and lead to improved metabolic control, quality of life, and physical fitness [4,53–55]. The research clearly shows improvements in glycemic control with increased PA and/or implementation of an exercise routine as part of the therapeutic regimen in diabetes self-management [55–57]. In those with T2DM, moderate to light physical activity improves insulin sensitivity, enhances mobility, metabolic control, and reduces abdominal visceral body fat but has no effect on β cell function [58]. The type of exercise did not significantly influence the improvements in glucose control (A1C) as the changes were similar between those performing aerobic exercise or resistance training, emphasizing the importance of increasing PA in general, not the type of exercise [56–58]. In contrast, a study by Sigal et al. found that a combination of both resistance and aerobic exercise led to significantly better outcomes than a single method alone [59]. ADA Clinical Recommendations supports PA for all adults but stresses that before exercising a physical assessment be conducted by a medical professional to ascertain the level of fitness and to minimize risks [8]. If there are no contraindications, it is recommended combining resistance training, a minimum of two times per week, with moderate aerobic activity a minimum of 3 days/week, equaling at least 150 min total aerobic activity per week [4,8,60]. Encouraging the maintenance and incorporation of exercise, as part of the care plan, is a role of the diabetes care team. Behavior modification strategies assist diabetic patients to maintain or increase PA. Research confirms this recommendation and the clinical benefits of behavioral methods in promoting PA and exercise [61].

MEDICATION MANAGEMENT

An important tenet in diabetes management is a patient-centered approach to making diet, lifestyle, and medication choices. If diet and physical activity or other chosen treatment strategies do not achieve optimal glycemic control, then oral hypoglycemic medications should be considered. In the selection of the type of medication, the team should consider the desires of the patient, effects on weight

TABLE 12.5
Diabetes Medications

Medication	Class	Action	Risks
Glyburide Amaryl Glucotrol	Sulfonylurea	Improves basal insulin by stimulating pancreatic β-cells and insulin secretion	Hypoglycemia (low blood glucose). Hyperinsulinemia and weight gain. Sensitivity to the sun. Drug–herbal interactions, e.g., bitter melon and fenugreek.
Prandin Starlix	Meglitinide	Improves post-meal insulin by stimulating pancreatic β-cells and insulin secretion in response to glycemic load of the meal	Low risk of hypoglycemia, increased if taken with medication or herbals that act as insulin mimetics. Drug–herbal interactions, e.g., ginger extract, gower plant, ginseng, cinnamon. Drug to drug interaction, e.g., sulfonylurea.
Glucophage	Biguanide	Decreases insulin resistance and hepatic glucose production Preserves β-cell function	May cause digestive changes, e.g., gas, bloating, diarrhea, nausea. Caution use in certain populations, e.g., heart failure, renal or hepatic failure. Drug to herbal interactions, e.g., *Galena officinalis* (high in guanidine).
Actos/ Avandia	Thiazolidinediones	Improves insulin sensitivity of muscle and liver cells	Weight gain and edema. Caution use with certain populations, e.g., heart failure, liver or renal impairment. Monitor liver and renal function.
Januvia Onglyza Tradjenta	DPP4-inhibitor	Increases release of insulin; decreases release of glucagon; decreases stomach emptying; leads to weight loss and increased satiety	Caution use with certain populations, e.g., heart failure, renal impairment. Monitor renal function. Dose based on renal function. Drug to herbal interactions, e.g., ginseng, legume extracts.
Precose	α-Glucosidase inhibitor	Alters the absorption and utilization of glucose in the gut; creates a sensation of fullness or satiety	May cause digestive changes, e.g., cramping and gas. Potential drug–herbal interaction: mulberry.

(Continued)

TABLE 12.5 (*Continued*)
Diabetes Medications

Medication	Class	Action	Risks
Amylin Symlin	Injectable amylin analogs	Improves gut hormone action leading to decreased glucose production and delayed stomach emptying, decreased appetite, decreases glucagon, and timely insulin release	Caution use in certain populations, e.g., history of pancreatitis, multiple endocrine neoplasia syndrome type 2, gastroparesis Drug–drug interactions, e.g., sulfonylureas and meglitinide. May cause gastrointestinal changes, e.g., nausea. Risk of hypoglycemia with other anti-hyperglycemic drugs or herbals.
Invokana	Canagliflozin	Improves kidney reabsorption of glucose	Urinary tract infections. Caution use in certain populations, e.g., elderly, pregnant and nursing mothers, or those with renal/liver impairment. Drug to drug or herbal interactions, e.g., digoxin.

management, cost, other treatment modalities, comorbid conditions, and the patient's management goals [8].

In Table 12.5, a list of common medications used in the treatment of T2DM is provided, including their actions and side effects. Metformin causes digestive changes, including decreased gastrointestinal motility, bacteria overgrowth, and a decrease of the intrinsic factor–B12 complex, leading to poor absorption and deficiency of B12, an increase in megaloblastic anemia, and neuropathy [62,63]. It is recommended that those taking biguanides (Metformin) long-term have their B12 status monitored, with supplementation considered, if needed. Insulin is also used in the treatment of both types of diabetes, but it is essential in T1DM. For those with T2DM, insulin may be added to the treatment regimen when oral hypoglycemic agents and lifestyle changes do not maintain blood glucose levels within the patient's targeted goals or insulin may be needed in the newly diagnosed T2DM patient who is markedly symptomatic or has elevated blood glucose levels [8].

Diabetes management is goal oriented and should be individualized [10,11]. Though decisions regarding alternative methods are patient-driven, incorporating a team approach is fundamental to the treatment of diabetes. Continuous assessment of a person's lifestyle habits and behavior modification are important in the treatment and management of diabetes and have been shown to improve clinical outcomes [8,10,11].

"TRADITIONAL" AND ALTERNATIVE TREATMENT STRATEGIES

Integrative medicine, the blending of traditional and alternative treatment strategies, is applicable in the management of a complex chronic disease, such as diabetes. In combining conventional and alternative therapies, we emphasize the natural, less invasive evidence-based options. Healthcare professionals and patients need to know which integrative strategies have evidence to support their use in conjunction with pharmaceutical management of T2DM [64]. In this chapter, we have focused on those supplements that have been studied in use with humans with DM. While there are a variety of animal studies on other supplements, the absence of evidence-based, human randomized clinical trials (RCTs) were used by the authors as a criteria for exclusion.

According to 2003–2006 National Health and Nutrition Examination Study data, approximately 50% of all Americans use supplements [65]. Studies are unclear on exactly how people use supplements, that is, the specifics of dosing, which products and/or botanical parts are used, who is using them, and for what reasons. The products used most often by patients with diabetes include cinnamon, coenzyme Q10 (CoQ10), hibiscus, magnesium, chromium, mulberry, ginseng, vinegar, and probiotics [66].

Since the 2002 National Health Interview Survey, which indicated that 22% of patients with diabetes used herbal products, use has been reported as high as 67% [65]. The reason(s) for patients with diabetes choosing supplements is not clear; increasing costs of medication and/or provider visits are possible explanations. Other possibilities are beliefs/fears of adverse effects associated with medications, inability of conventional treatments to completely manage the disease, the belief that supplements are without risk, and the recommendations of peers and/or family members [66].

In contrast, a study of Latino/Hispanic immigrants found that some choose to incorporate the use of supplements and herbal remedies because herbals are not only effective for treating diabetes, but in their belief system offer a cure [67]. They have had no education or counsel concerning the risks for herb–herb or herb–drug interactions, overmedication, environmental contamination of the herb, possible allergic reactions or toxicities, and the exacerbation of illness. In this study of Latinos/Hispanics, 69% reported incorporating herbal treatments for self-care of diabetes. Most commonly used were prickly pear cactus, aloe vera, celery, cinnamon, and chayote. Three-fourths of those reported concurrent use of a herbal with prescribed medications but failed to report their herbal use to their healthcare providers [67].

An important finding was that the dosage is a matter of self-determination, without consideration for the other medications included in the treatment regimen, with 68% taking oral hypoglycemic agents, 26.7% taking insulin, 52% taking lipid-lowering medications (like statins), and 63% taking anti-hypertensive medications [67]. In this study, 69.3% (n = 52) reported using one or more of 49 herbals, from 1 to 9 simultaneously, with individualized dosing and frequency. Of a variety of reasons stated for using herbals, no respondents reported their use due to the cost of diabetes medication or lack of health insurance. More trusted the combination of herbals and prescribed medications than prescribed medications alone [67]. Only a few reported trusting herbals alone.

Clinicians must recognize that these "natural" products have active chemical constituents and are the source of many of the conventional medications of similar pharmacologic activity [57,59]. An example is the diabetes medication Metformin, which was derived from the plant *Galega officinalis* that is high in guanidine, an anti-hyperglycemic agent [68]. Due to its potency in its natural form, the synthetic form was developed. Adverse effects and drug interactions are very real possibilities when using supplements. Supplements continue to be used even without strong evidence of their efficacy for human use. For example, fenugreek, bitter melon, and prickly pear are consumed as part of the diet or in a supplement form. It is important to ask patients what supplements they are consuming and what they hope to achieve with their use, for example, a desire to lower their A1C level, blood pressure, or cholesterol level. Clinicians should also encourage patients to continue their conventional medications and monitor for potential interactions.

HERBALS AND SUPPLEMENTS

Before the development and use of insulin and oral hypoglycemic agents (OHAs), diabetes was treated with plant extracts or plant preparations [7]. World Health Organization (WHO) recommendations state that hypoglycemic agents of plant origin used in traditional medicine are important in diabetes management [9]. Herbal drugs with antidiabetic activity can be classified in the following manner, by their mode of action [7]:

First group—Insulin mimetics, for example, *Momordica charantia*, extracted from the bitter gourd produces hypoglycemic effects with the polypeptide isolated from its seeds and tissues.

Second group—Acts on the β cells to increase insulin production, for example, *Allium cepa*, an onion extract, and *Pterocarpus marsupium*, extracted from aloe tree and bark. Double-blind trials by the Indian Council Medical Research have shown *P. marsupium* as effective as Tolbutamide (a first-generation sulfonylurea).

Third group—Act by enhancing glucose utilization, for example, *Zingiber officinale* from ginger, *Cyamopsis tetragonolobus* from the gower plant, and *Grewia asiatica* from the phalsa plant. By increasing the viscosity of gastrointestinal contents, the seeds of the gower plant slow down gastric emptying and glucose uptake by the cells.

Fourth group—Act by miscellaneous mechanisms, these include the legumes *Euphorbia prostrata*, *Fumaria parvia*, *Panax ginseng*, and *Phyllanthus emblica*, which may increase the fiber content of the diet and thus the rate of absorption of glucose.

HERBAL AND MINERAL SUPPLEMENTS

CINNAMON

Of over 400 supplements that have been used for treating diabetes, only cinnamon has evidence from several RCTs for improving glucose utilization, postprandial blood glucose levels, insulin sensitivity, and glucose uptake [69–71]. A 2011 meta-analysis [72] found that cinnamon supplementation resulted in significant improvement in fasting blood glucose (FBG). Cinnamon (*Cinnamomum cassia*) is the most commonly used natural treatment for diabetes and hyperlipidemia and probably has more benefits than drawbacks. Studies have shown it to be less effective in T1DM and slightly, but significantly, effective in T2DM [66]. A 2013 Cochrane systematic review on the use of cinnamon concluded it could be beneficial as an adjunct therapy, as the results showed the use of *C. cassia* taken from 4 to 16 weeks significantly improved A1C and/or serum insulin levels over the placebo groups. More research is needed as to the efficacy of different types of cinnamon, their preparation, and forms of administration [73] though there is insufficient evidence to support the recommendation of cinnamon as a treatment of diabetes [8].

MULBERRY

Mulberry (*Morus alba*) leaf tea and extract have been widely used in Asia for the treatment of diabetes. It significantly decreased fasting glucose levels (from 153 to 110 mg/dL), low-density lipoprotein (LDL) cholesterol, and triglyceride levels, and significantly increased high-density lipoprotein cholesterol (HDL) levels [66,74]. The overall benefits may be the result of diminished or delayed carbohydrate absorption [75,76]. The suggested mechanism for the blood glucose lowering effect of the mulberry leaf extract is digestion and utilization of carbohydrates, whose absorption is inhibited by limiting α glucosidase activity [76]. In addition to the effects on post-meal blood glucose levels, mulberry leaf extracts enhance weight loss and satiety [77].

GINSENG

The most studied medicinal plant for its hypoglycemic activities is Ginseng, which decreases blood glucose by affecting various pathways [75]. Geographical source, method of processing, dosage/concentration, and type of diabetes impact its efficacy and potency. *P. ginseng* (Chinese or Korean ginseng) is highest in therapeutic potency, *Panax quinquefolius* (American ginseng) is of medium potency, and *Panax japonicus* (Japanese ginseng) is of the lowest potency. *P. ginseng* is the most commonly used in treating DM. A systematic review of RCTs for the use of red ginseng in T2DM management indicated limited effectiveness of this type of ginseng on blood glucose levels as compared to placebo [78]. To date the research is inconclusive to the exact mechanism, but American ginseng seems to stimulate insulin release in response to a meal or glucose load [79]. It is speculated that some of the effects of ginseng on blood glucose control is related to improving both mood and the psychophysical state of the person with diabetes, leading to increased physical activity and ability to perform self-management [80].

Ginseng is not without side effects, which can include severe headache, insomnia, diarrhea, vaginal bleeding, and pain in the breast. There have even been reports of Stevens–Johnson syndrome, a rare, serious, and sometimes fatal disorder of the skin and mucous membranes [75]. The safe, recommended dosage is 1–3 g of ginseng root or 200–600 mg of ginseng extract [81].

CHROMIUM

Two factors have led clinicians and researchers to evaluate the role of chromium (Cr) and Cr supplementation. First, its role is a necessary cofactor for glucose metabolism and insulin regulation, and second, altered Cr metabolism is linked to increased excretion and low blood levels in those with diabetes. Though present in many foods, including grains, broccoli, spinach, carrots, and potatoes, food processing may eliminate the availability of absorbable Cr and increase the need to supplement the diets of those with diabetes. A large clinical trial conducted by Anderson et al. [82] using Cr picolinate led to a 2% decrease in A1C, but later was found to have methodological concerns and was conducted with those with Cr deficiency. Later studies, as demonstrated in a meta-analysis, found limited effects of Cr supplementation on glucose control and insulin activity or were inconclusive [83]. A review by Landman et al. [84] confirmed the previous systematic review that Cr supplementation is not recommended for persons with diabetes especially T2DM. Reasons cited for this recommendation were study design, type of chromium, level of diabetes control, and consideration for pre-existing chromium deficiency.

MAGNESIUM

In the early to mid-1970s, an association between magnesium (Mg) deficiency and blood glucose dysregulation was verified in humans. Mg deficiency is associated with decreased absorption or increased elimination of Mg, as well as the development of insulin resistance in people with T2DM [85]. Mg plays an integral role in glucose metabolism serving as an enzyme cofactor in several glucose metabolic pathways and is involved in insulin secretion, binding, and activity. Rich sources of magnesium are whole grains, leafy green vegetables, legumes, and nuts.

Many patients with diabetes consume insufficient amounts of Mg-containing foods and have been shown to have low Mg concentrations in the blood plasma [86]. A meta-analysis of randomized controlled trials evaluating Mg supplements showed a significant decrease in fasting glucose levels of 10 mg/dL but a nonsignificant decrease in A1C [87]. Based on the research, there is consensus that recommending supplementation of Mg for those with diabetes (T2DM) or at risk for developing DM is beneficial. Supplementation with Mg in those at risk for diabetes improved insulin release by the β cells and insulin utilization [88]. Although Mg supplementation is beneficial as either adjunct therapy for those with diabetes or used as a preventive measure, the exact form or supplementation and amount have not been determined. It is important before supplementing to evaluate renal function, as the kidney plays a central role in magnesium homeostasis and renal insufficiency and can lead to the toxicity of this nutrient. There is limited evidence supporting routine supplementation of magnesium, also of chromium, vitamin D, and other micronutrients [8]. Before it can be recommended as an adjunct therapy for glucose management, clinical evaluation is needed [8].

ALPHA LIPOIC ACID

Alpha lipoic acid (ALA) is an antioxidant made by the body and is also found in very small amounts in foods. Due to its antioxidant properties, research has focused on its use in the treatment or prevention of inflammatory-type diseases, such as diabetes, as well as the associated complications, as in retinopathy and neuropathy. ALA supplementation of 300 mg/day showed promising results in preventing vision loss in those with T1DM and T2DM, as documented in a RCT. Participants in all groups showed either visual acuity stability or improvement and decreased progression of retinopathy [89].

ALA is widely used in Europe in the treatment of diabetic neuropathy. Small studies have found that ALA may improve insulin sensitivity and reduce oxidative stress in patients with diabetes [90–93]. Some studies showed that after a brief supplementation of ALA, there was a statistically significant decrease in FBG and postprandial glucose [90]. In addition, ALA has shown promising results in the prevention of cardiovascular complications and vascular dysfunction [94].

PROBIOTICS

Due to the relationship between gut flora, systematic inflammation, and the immune system, research has focused on the benefits of probiotics, either by supplements or food source, in the prevention and treatment of diabetes [95]. WHO defines probiotics as "microorganisms ... able to confer defined health benefits on the host" [96]. Probiotic supplementation appears to play a role in enhancing cholesterol metabolism, decreasing inflammation, and improving insulin resistance, as well as managing weight [95]. Research has demonstrated a difference in the gut flora of obese as compared to lean people. Dietary factors, by introducing multiple types of probiotics or supplements containing a variety of bacterium species, can improve or alter the gut flora, weight loss, and weight maintenance [97–99].

The flora in the gut of the healthy, normal weight person includes a combination of *Bacteroidetes*, *Firmicutes*, and *Actinobacteria* [95]. In both T2DM and obesity, there is a higher proportion of *Bacteroidetes*, which is a bacteria that contains lipopolysaccharides and precipitates or functions in the development of insulin resistance in the obese and T2DM [100]. Type 2 diabetes patients have significantly reduced populations of *Firmicutes* and a higher proportion of *Bacteroidetes*. This alteration has a direct correlation with increased plasma glucose levels [100].

Interest in the role of probiotics in the prevention of gestational diabetes (GDM) has prompted research that has shown probiotics to be a cost-effective approach in the prevention of GDM. Further, it has demonstrated gut flora composition correlates with insulin resistance and the incidence of GDM. A study by Luoto et al. demonstrated a significant decrease in the occurrence of GDM in normal-weight pregnant women provided with dietary intervention by probiotics [101]. Research shows that the gut flora of normal weight and overweight pregnant women differ, and that not only did the overweight women have higher levels of *Bacteroidetes*, but correlated higher levels of this bacteria with excessive weight gain [102]. Probiotics have shown to influence the gut bacteria and that changing the composition of gut flora can reduce inflammation, decrease insulin resistance, and effect blood glucose levels. Supplementation amounts have not been determined; however, probiotic food products, such as yogurt, and other fermented foods, including kefir, kimchi, kombucha, miso, and sauerkraut, may be beneficial.

MIND–BODY STRATEGIES

Adherence to a treatment regimen is critical in any chronic disease. High adherence levels to the treatment of diabetes have been observed to encourage near normal development and lifespan in T1DM children. However, such a life long commitment to a treatment regimen that focuses heavily on self-management is difficult for the patient, and by extension the family. External influences endanger adherence, not only in children with DM but in adults as well [103]. Adherence has been defined by WHO as "the extent to which a person's behavior—taking medication, following a diet and/or executing lifestyle changes—corresponds with agreed recommendations from a health care provider" [104]. Patients with depression and DM have less adherence to treatments, poorer glycemic control, higher A1C levels [105], higher rates of hospital admissions, and increased diabetic complications [106]. Mind–body strategies represent one of the most widely used alternatives to or adjuncts with anti-depressive medications [64].

In the 2007 National Health Interview Survey (NHIS), it was estimated that in the previous 12 months, nearly one in five adults in the United States used at least one mind–body technique [107]. Techniques or modalities cited in the report included biofeedback and yoga as the most studied mind–body interventions for the management of DM.

BIOFEEDBACK

In a small RCT of patients with T2DM that compared biofeedback-assisted relaxation training with diabetes education alone, the biofeedback group had significant improvement in HbAlc (decreased from 7.4% to 6.8%), meeting the standard for metabolic control, as well as in average blood glucose levels. The biofeedback sessions were weekly, 45 min in duration, for a period of 10 weeks [108]. Volitional warming with biofeedback has been associated with more rapid healing of diabetic ulcers, increased circulation with improvement or elimination of intermittent claudication pain, and improved functional status in patients with T2DM [109].

YOGA

Patients with T2DM were shown to benefit in two systematic reviews from yoga techniques. These studies concluded that yoga training could lead to lower blood sugar, LDL-C and triglyceride levels, decreased body weight and waist-to-hip ratio, improved AlC, and higher HDL-C [110,111]. It also appears yoga has beneficial effects in patients with T2DM on heart rate and blood pressure, oxidative stress, and pulmonary function. With these various physiometric improvements, there is a reduction in medication needed for metabolic control [102].

MEDITATION

A study that compared transcendental meditation (TM) practitioners with a control group found that the regular practice of TM is associated with a reduction of catecholamine (a stress hormone connected to alterations in blood glucose) levels [112]. Another study focused on the relationship between diabetes and depression found persuasive and convincing evidence of an association between hypothalamic-pituitary-adrenal (HPA) axis hyperactivity and mental stress [113]. This hyperactivity and long-term dysregulation of the HPA axis can result in several abnormalities that enhance the vulnerability to depression [114]. These findings by Dusek suggest that reducing stress levels through meditation might lead to improved glycemic control as decreased catecholamine levels affect glucose transport and insulin resistance. Similar to TM, stress management consists of progressive muscle relaxation, deep breathing, and mental imagery. Research comparing diabetes education alone with education plus stress management found at 1 year that AlC levels decreased by 0.5 in the combined group [115].

SUMMARY AND CONCLUSION

The decision to use complementary or alternative (CAM) treatments for diabetes remains largely the domain of the person with diabetes. They may make that decision without the benefit of the information in this chapter and without the knowledge or participation of the members of the diabetes care/education team. It is imperative that healthcare professionals acquire a thorough, working foundation of all evidence-based CAM treatments related to diabetes, whether supplements and/or mind–body methodologies. Research shows that a significant portion of patients, including those with established diabetic treatment plans, will use one or more of these modalities [65]. We must ensure that their decision is an informed one.

REFERENCES

1. Centers for Disease Control and Prevention. National Fact Sheet: General Information and National Estimates of Diabetes in the United States, 2011. Altanta, GA: U.S. Department of Health and Human Services Centers for Disease Control and Prevention, 2011. http://www.cdc.gov/diabetes/pubs/factsheet11/fastfacts.htm (accessed July 2, 2014).
2. Boyle, J.P., T.J. Thompson, L.E. Barker et al. 2010. Projection of the year 2050 burden of diabetes in the US adult population: Dynamic modeling of incidence, mortality, and prediabetes prevalence. *Popul Health Metr* 22(8):29–40.
3. Gambert, S.R. and S. Pinkstaff. 2006. Emerging epidemic: Diabetes in the older adults: Demographic, economic, impact and pathophysiology. *Diabetes Spectr* 19(6):221–228.
4. Kirkman, M., V.J. Briscoe, N. Clark et al. 2012. Diabetes and the older adult: Consensus Report. *J Am Ger Soc* 60(12):242–256.

5. Lebovitz, H.E. 2012. Type 2 diabetes: The evolution of a disease. *Br J Diabetes Vasc Dis* 12:290–298.
6. Aronoff, S., K. Berkowitz, B. Shreiner, and L. Want. 2004. Glucose metabolism and regulation: Beyond insulin and glucagon. *Diabetes Spectr* 7(3):183–190.
7. Jayakumar, R.V. 2010. Herbal medicines for type-2 diabetes. *Int J Diab Dev Ctries* 30(3):111–112.
8. American Diabetes Association. 2014. Standards of medical care in diabetes. *Diabetes Care* 37(1):S14–S80.
9. The World Health Organization. 2000. General guidelines for methodologies on research and evaluation of traditional medicine. http://www.who.int/medicines/areas/traditional/definitions/en/ (accessed July 3, 2014).
10. Haas, L., M. Maryniuk, J. Beck et al. 2014. On behalf of the national 2012 standards revision task force. Standards for diabetes self-management education and support. *Diabetes Care* 37(1):S144–S153.
11. Funnell, M.M., T.L. Brown, B.P. Childs et al. 2010. National standards for diabetes self-management and education. *Diabetes Care* 33(1):S89–S96.
12. Centers for Disease Control. 2011. National diabetes fact sheet, risk factors for complications. http://apps.nccd.cdc.gov/DDTSTRS/default.aspx (accessed May 12, 2014).
13. Funnell, M.M., R.M. Anderson, A. Austin, and S.J. Gilespie. 2007. AADE position statement: Individualization of diabetes self-management education. *Diabetes Educator* 33:45–49.
14. Norris, S.L., M.M. Engelgau, and K.M.V. Narayan. 2001. Effectiveness of self-management training in type 2 diabetes: A systematic review of randomized control trials. *Diabetes Care* 24:561–587.
15. Mensing, C., J. Boucher, M. Cypress et al. 2004. National standards for diabetes self-management education. *Diabetes Care* 27(1):S143–S150.
16. Mulcahy, K., M. Maryniuk, M. Peeples et al. 2003. Diabetes self-management education core outcomes measures: Technical review. *Diabetes Educator* 29(5):768–816.
17. The Diabetes Control and Complications Trial Research Group. 1993. The effect of intensive treatment of diabetes on the development and progression of long-term complications in insulin-dependent diabetes mellitus. *N Engl J Med* 329:977–986.
18. United Kingdom Prospective Diabetes Study (UKPDS) Group. 1998. Effect of intensive blood-glucose control with metformin on complications in overweight patients with type 2 diabetes (UKPDS 34). *Lancet* 352:854–865.
19. United Kingdom Prospective Diabetes Study (UKPDS) Group. 1998. Intensive blood-glucose control with sulphonylureas or insulin compared with conventional treatment and risk of complications in patients with type 2 diabetes (UKPDS 33). *Lancet* 352:837–853.
20. United Kingdom Prospective Diabetes Study (UKPDS) Group. 1990. UK Prospective Diabetes Study: Response of fasting plasma glucose to diet therapy in newly presenting type II diabetic patients. *Metabolism* 39:905–912.
21. Peterson, K.A., D.M. Radosevich, P.J. O'Connor et al. 2008. Improving diabetes care in practice. Findings from the TRANSLATE trial. *Diabetes Care* 31: 2238–2243.
22. Zgibor, J.C., H. Rao, J. Wesche-Thobaben et al. 2004. Improving the quality of diabetes care in primary care practice. *J Health Qual* 26(4):14–21.
23. Bodenheimer, T., E.H. Wagner, and K. Gumbach. 2002. Improving primary care for patients with chronic illness. *JAMA* 288(14):1775–1779.
24. Hicks, D. 2010. Self-management skills for people with type 2 diabetes. *Nursg Standard* 25(6):48–56.
25. ADA Evidence Analysis Library. 2008. Diabetes type 1 and 2 evidence-based nutrition practice guideline for adults. http://andevidencelibrary.com (accessed July 3, 2014).

26. Miller, C.K.E.L., I. Edwards, and G. Kissling. 2002. Nutrition education improves metabolic outcomes among older adults with diabetes mellitus: Results from a randomized control trial. *Prev Med* 34:252–259.

27. Evert, A.B., J.L. Boucher, M. Cypress et al. 2014. Nutrition therapy recommendations for the management of adults with diabetes. *Diabetes Care* 37:S120–S143.

28. Riccardi, G., A.A. Rivellese, and R. Giacco. 2008. Role of glycemic index and glycemic load in the healthy state, in pre-diabetes and in diabetes. *Am J Clin Nutr* 87:269–274.

29. Orchard, T.J., M. Temprosa, R. Goldberg et al. 2005. The effect of metformin and intensive lifestyle intervention on the metabolic syndrome: Diabetes Prevention Program randomized trial. *Ann Intern Med* 142(8):611–619.

30. Shai, I., D. Schwarzfuchs, Y. Henkin et al. 2008. Weight loss with a low-carbohydrate, Mediterranean, or low-fat diet. *N Engl J Med* 359:229–241.

31. Sofi, F., R. Abbate, G.F. Gensini, and A. Casini. 2010. Accruing evidence on benefits of adherence to the Mediterranean diet on health: An updated systematic review and meta-analysis. *Am J Clin Nutr* 92(5):1189–1196.

32. Hoffman, R. and M. Gerber. 2013. Evaluating and adapting the Mediterranean diet for non-Mediterranean populations: A critical appraisal. *Nutr Rev* 71(9):573–584.

33. Esposito, K., R. Marfella, M. Ciotola et al. 2004. Effect of a Mediterranean-style diet on endothelial dysfunction and markers of vascular inflammation in the metabolic syndrome: A randomized trial. *JAMA* 292(12):1440–1446.

34. InterAct Consortium. 2011. Mediterranean diet and type 2 diabetes risk in the European prospective investigation into cancer and nutrition (EPIC) study. The InterAct project. *Diabetes Care* 34:1913–1918.

35. Kastorini, C.M. and D.B. Panagiotakos. 2009. Dietary patterns and prevention of type 2 diabetes: From research to clinical practice: A systematic review. *Curr Diabetes Rev* 5(4):221–227.

36. Thomas, D.E. 2010. The use of low-glycaemic index diets in diabetes control. *Br J Nutr* 104(6):797–802.

37. Burani, J. and P.J. Longo. 2006. Low-glycemic index carbohydrates. An effective behavioral change for glycemic control and weight management in patients with type 1 and type 2 diabetes. *Diabetes Educator* 32(1):78–88.

38. Barclay, A.W., P. Petocz, J. McMillian-Price et al. 2008. Glycemic index, glycemic load, and chronic disease risk- a meta-analysis of observational studies. *Am J Clin Nutr* 87:627–63.

39. Brand-Miller, J., S. Hayne, P. Petocz, and S. Colagiur. 2003. Low–glycemic index diets in the management of diabetes: A meta-analysis of randomized controlled trials. *Diabetes Care* 26:2261–2267.

40. Thomas, D. and E.J. Elliott. 2009. Low glycaemic index, or low glycaemic load, diets for diabetes mellitus. *Cochrane Database Syst Rev* 1:CD006296.

41. Davis, W.A., D.G. Bruce, and T.M. Davis. 2011. Economic impact of moderate weight loss in patients with type 2 diabetes: The Fremantle diabetes study. *Diabet Med* 28:1131–1135.

42. Kyrou, I. and S. Kumar. 2010. Weight management in overweight and obese patients with type 2 diabetes mellitus. *Br J Diabetes Vasc Dis* 10(6):274–283.

43. Utzschneider, K.M., D.B. Carr, S.M. Barsness et al. 2004. Diet induced weight loss is associated with an improvement in beta-cell function in older men. *J Clin Endocrinol Metab* 89(6):2704–2710.

44. Barina-Mitchell, E., L. Kuller, K. Sutton-Tyrrell et al. 2006. Effect of weight loss and nutritional intervention on arterial stiffness in type 2 diabetes. *Diabetes Care* 29:2218–2222.

45. Pinkney, J. 2010. Bariatric surgery for diabetes: Gastric banding is simple and safe. *Br J Diabetes Vasc Dis* 10:139–42.

46. Buchwald, H., R. Estok, K. Fahrbach et al. 2009. Weight and type 2 diabetes after bariatric surgery: Systematic review and meta-analysis. *Am J Med* 122:248–256.
47. Sala, P.C., R.S. Torrinhas, D. Giannella-Netos, and D. Linetzky. 2014. Relationship between gut hormones and glucose homeostasis after bariatric surgery. *Diabetol Metab Syndrome* 6:87–102.
48. Hall, T.C., M.G. Pellen, P.C. Sedman, and P.K. Jain. 2010. Preoperative factors predicting remission of type 2 diabetes mellitus after Roux-en-Y gastric bypass surgery for obesity. *Obes Surg* 20:1245–1250.
49. Sala, P.C., R.S. Torrinhas, S.B. Heymsfield, and D.L. Waitzberg. 2012. Type 2 diabetes mellitus: A possible surgically reversible intestinal dysfunction. *Obes Surg* 22:167–176.
50. Look AHEAD Research Group. 2013. Cardiovascular effects of intensive lifestyle intervention in type 2 diabetes. *N Engl J Med* 369:145–154.
51. Raynor, H.A., R.W. Jeffery, A.M. Ruggiero et al.; Look AHEAD (Action for Health in Diabetes) Research Group. 2008. Weight loss strategies associated with BMI in overweight adults with type 2 diabetes at entry into The Look AHEAD (Action for Health in Diabetes) trial. *Diabetes Care* 31:299–1304.
52. Wheeler, M.L., S.A. Dunbar, L.M. Jaacks et al. 2012. Macronutrients, food groups, and eating patterns in the management of diabetes: A systematic review of the literature, 2010. *Diabetes Care* 35:434–445.
53. Jakicic, J.M., S.A. Jaramillo, A. Balasubramanyam et al. 2009. Look AHEAD Study Group. Effect of a lifestyle intervention on change in cardiorespiratory fitness in adults with type 2 diabetes: Results from the Look AHEAD Study. *Int J Obes* 233:305–316.
54. Praet, S.F.E. and L.J.C. van Loon. 2009. Exercise therapy in type 2 diabetes. *Acta Diabetol* 46:263–278.
55. Zanuso, S., A. Jimenez, G. Pugliese, G. Corigliano, and S. Balducci. 2010. Exercise for the management of type 2 diabetes: A review of the evidence. *Acta Diabetol* 47:15–22.
56. Thomas, D.E., E.J. Elliott, and G.A. Naughton. 2006. Exercise for type 2 diabetes mellitus. *Cochrane Database Syst Rev* 3:CD002968.
57. Umpierre, D., P.A.B. Ribeiro, C.K. Kramer et al. 2011. Physical activity advice only or structured exercise training and association with HbA1c levels in type 2 diabetes: A systematic review and meta-analysis. *JAMA* 305:1790–1799.
58. Bacchi, E., C. Negri, M. Zanolin et al. 2012. Metabolic effects of aerobic training and resistance training in type 2 diabetic subjects: A randomized controlled trial the RAED2 study. *Diabetes Care* 35:676–682.
59. Sigal, R.J., G.P. Kenny, N.G. Boulé et al. 2007. Effects of aerobic training, resistance training, or both on glycemic control in type 2 diabetes: A randomized trial. *Ann Intern Med* 147:357–369.
60. Sigal, R.J., G.P. Kenny, D.H. Wasserman, C. Castaneda-Sceppa, and R.D. White. 2006. Physical activity/exercise and type 2 diabetes: A consensus statement from the American Diabetes Association. *Diabetes Care* 29:1433–1438.
61. Avery, L., D. Flynn, A. van Wersch et al. 2012. Changing physical activity behavior in type II diabetes. *Diabetes Care* 35:2681–2689.
62. Reinstatler, L., Y. Ping-Qi, R.S. Williamson et al. 2012. Association of biochemical B12 deficiency with metformin therapy and vitamin B12 supplements. *Diabetes Care* 35(2): 327–333.
63. Liu, Q., S. Li, H. Quan, and J. Li. 2014. Vitamin B12 status in metformin treated patients: Systematic review. *PLoS ONE* 9(6):e100379.
64. Redtner, J., E. Longmier, and P. Wedel. 2013. Targeting diabetes: The benefits of an integrative approach. *J Fam Prac* 62(7) 337–344.
65. Bailey, R.L., J. Gahache, C.V. Lentino et al. 2011. Dietary supplement use in the United States, 2003–2006. *J Nutr* 141(2):261–266.

66. Shane-McWhorter, L. July 2012. Dietary supplements and probiotics for diabetes. *AJN* 112(7):47–53.
67. Amirehsani, K.A. and D.C. Wallace. 2013. Tés, licuados, and cápsulas: Herbal self-care remedies of Latino/Hispanic immigrants for type 2 diabetes. *Diabetes Educator* 39:828–840.
68. Modak, M., P. Dixit, J. Londhe et al. 2007. Indian herbs and herbal drugs used in the treatment of diabetes. *J Clin Biochem Nutr* 40:163–173.
69. Crawford, P. 2009. Effectiveness of cinnamon for lowering hemoglobin A1C in patients with type 2 diabetes: A randomized, controlled trial. *J Am Board Fam Med* 22:507–512.
70. Akilen, R., A. Tsiami, D. Devendra, and N. Robinson. 2010. Glycated haemoglobin and blood pressure-lowering effect of cinnamon in multi-ethnic type 2 diabetic patients in the UK: A randomized, placebo-controlled, double-blind clinical trial. *Diabet Med* 27(10):1159–1167.
71. Hlebowicz, J., A. Hlebowicz, S. Lindstedt et al. 2009. Effects of 1 and 3 g cinnamon on gastric emptying, satiety, and postprandial blood glucose, insulin, glucose-dependent insulinotropic polypeptide, glucagon-like peptide 1, and ghrelin concentrations in healthy subjects. *Am J Clin Nutr* 89(3):815–821.
72. Davis, P.A. and W. Yokoyama. 2011. Cinnamon intake lowers fasting blood glucose: Meta-analysis. *J Med Food* 14:884–689.
73. Leach, M.J. and S. Kumar. 2012. Cinnamon for diabetes mellitus. *Cochrane Database Syst Rev* 9:Art. No.:CD007170.
74. Mudra, M., N. Ercan-Fang, L. Zhong, J. Furne, and M. Levitt. 2007. Influence of mulberry leaf extract on the blood glucose and breath hydrogen response to ingestion of 75 g sucrose by type 2 diabetic and control subjects. *Diabetes Care* 30(5):1272–1274.
75. Prabhakar, P.K. and M. Doble. 2011. Mechanism of action of natural products used in the treatment of diabetes mellitus. *Chin J Integr Med* 17(8):563–574.
76. Banu, S., N.R. Jabir, N.C. Manjunath. 2014. Reduction of post-prandial hyperglycemia by mulberry tea in type-2 diabetes patients. *Saudi J Bio Sci* 22(1):32–36.
77. Blaak, E.E., J.M. Antoine, D. Benton et al. 2012. Impact of postprandial glycaemia on health and prevention of disease. *Obes Rev* 13:923–984.
78. Kim, S., B.C. Shin, M.S. Lee, H. Lee, and E. Ernst. 2011. Red ginseng for type 2 diabetes mellitus: A systematic review of randomized controlled trials. *Chin J Integr Med* 17(12):937–944.
79. Mucalo I., D. Rahelic, E. Jovanovski et al. 2012. Effect of American ginseng (*Panax quinquefolius* L.) on glycemic control in type 2 diabetes. *Coll Antropol* 36(4):1435–1440.
80. Geng J., J. Dong, H. Ni et al. 2010. Ginseng for cognition. *Cochrane Database Syst Rev* (12):CD007769.
81. Vuksan V., J.L. Sievenpiper, V.Y. Koo et al. 2000. American ginseng (*Panax quinquefolius* L.) reduces postprandial glycemia in nondiabetic subjects and subjects with type 2 diabetes mellitus. *Arch Intern Med* 160:1009–1013.
82. Anderson R.A., N. Cheng, N.A. Bryden et al. 1997. Elevated intakes of supplemental chromium improve glucose and insulin variables in individuals with type 2 diabetes. *Diabetes* 46: 1786–1791.
83. Balk, E.M., A. Tatsioni, A.H. Lichtenstein, J. Lau, and A.G. Pittas. 2007. Effect of chromium supplementation on glucose metabolism and lipids: A systematic review of randomized controlled trials. *Diabetes Care* 30:2154–2163.
84. Landman, G.W.D., H.J.G. Bilo, S.T. Houweling, and N. Kleefstra. 2014. Chromium does not belong in the diabetes treatment arsenal: Current evidence and future perspectives. *World J Diabetes* 5(2):160–164.
85. Pham, P.C.T., P.M.T. Pham, S.V. Pham, J.M. Miller, and P.T.T. Pham. 2007. Hypomagnesemia in patients with type 2 diabetes. *Clin J Am Soc Nephr* 2(2):366–373.

86. Lopez-Ridaura, R., W.C. Willett, E.B. Rimm, S. Liu et al. 2004. Magnesium intake and risk of type 2 diabetes in men and women. *Diabetes Care* 27:270–271.

87. Song, Y., K. He, E.B. Levitan, J.E. Manson, and S. Liu. 2006. Effects of oral magnesium supplementation on glycaemic control in type 2 diabetes: A meta-analysis of randomized double-blind controlled trials. *Diabetes Med* 23(10):1050–1056.

88. Guerrero-Romero, F. and M. Rodríguez-Morán. 2011. Magnesium improves the beta-cell function to compensate variation of insulin sensitivity: Double-blind, randomized clinical trial. *Eur J Clin Invest* 41(4):405–410.

89. Gębka, A., E. Serkie-Minuth, and D. Raczyńska. 2014. Effect of the administration of alpha-lipoic acid on contrast sensitivity in patients with type 1 and type 2 diabetes. *Med Inflam*. 2014:Article ID 131538.

90. Singh, U. and I. Jialal. 2008. Alpha-lipoic acid supplementation and diabetes. *Nutr Rev* 66(11):646.

91. Ziegler, D., H. Schatz, F. Conrad et al. 1997. Effects of treatment with the antioxidant α-lipoic acid on cardiac autonomic neuropathy in NIDDM patients: A 4-month randomized controlled multicenter trial (DEKAN Study). *Diabetes Care* 20(3):369–373.

92. Mijnhout, G., B.J. Kollen, A. Alkhalaf, N. Kleefstra, and H.J.G. Bilo. 2012. Alpha lipoic acid for symptomatic peripheral neuropathy in patients with diabetes: A meta-analysis of randomized controlled trials. *Int J Endocrinol* 2012:456279. Published online January 26, 2012.

93. Ziegler, D., A. Ametov, A. Barinov et al. 2006. Oral treatment with α-lipoic acid improves symptomatic diabetic polyneuropathy. The SYDNEY 2 trial. *Diabetes Care* 29(11):2365–2370.

94. Heinisch, B.B., M. Francesconi, F. Mittermayer et al. 2010. Alpha-lipoic acid improves vascular endothelial function in patients with type 2 diabetes: A placebo-controlled randomized trial. *Eur J Clin Invest* 40(2):148.

95. Barrett, H.L., L.K. Callaway, and M.D. Nitert. 2012. Probiotics: A potential role in the prevention of gestational diabetes? *Acta Diabetol* 49(1):S1–S13.

96. Food and Agriculture Organization/World Health Organization (FAO/WHO). 2001. Health and nutritional properties of probiotics in food including powder milk with live lactic acid bacteria, Report of a Joint FAO/WHO Expert Consultation on Evaluation of Health and Nutritional Properties of Probiotics in Food including Powder Milk with Live Lactic Acid Bacteria, Cordoba, AR. http://www.who.int/foodsafety/publications/fs_management/en/probiotics.pdf.

97. Harte, A.L., M.C. Varma, G. Tripathi et al. 2012. High fat intake leads to acute postprandial exposure to circulating endotoxin in type 2 diabetic subjects. *Diabetes Care* 35:375–382.

98. Chapman, C.M., G.R. Gibson, and I. Rowland. 2011. Health benefits of probiotics: Are mixtures more effective than single strains? *Eur J Nutr* 50:1–17.

99. Hildebrandt, M.A., C. Hoffmann, S.A. Sherrill-Mix et al. 2009. High-fat diet determines the composition of the murine gut microbiome independently of obesity. *Gastroenterology* 137:1716–1724.

100. Giongo, A., K.A. Gano, D.B. Crabb et al. 2011. Toward defining the autoimmune microbiome for type 1 diabetes. *ISME J* 5:82–91.

101. Luoto, R., K. Laitinen, M. Nermes, and E. Isolauri. 2010. Impact of maternal probiotic-supplemented dietary counselling on pregnancy outcome and prenatal and postnatal growth: A double-blind, placebo-controlled study. *Br J Nutr* 103(12):1792–1799.

102. Collado, M.C., E. Isolauri, K. Laitinen, and S. Salminen. 2008. Distinct composition of gut microbiota during pregnancy in overweight and normal-weight women. *Am J Clin Nutr* 88(4):894–899.

103. Kongkaew, C., K. Jampachaisri, C.A. Chaturongkul, and C.N. Scholfield. 2014. Depression and adherence to treatment in diabetic children and adolescents: A systematic review and meta-analysis of observational studies. *Eur J Ped* 173(2):203–212.

104. Yach, D.X. 2003. Adherence to long-term therapies—Evidence for action. World Health Organization. http://whqlibdoc.who.int/publications/2003/9241545992.pdf (accessed July 3, 2014).

105. Johnson, B., C. Eiser, V. Young, S. Brierley, and S. Heller. 2013. Prevalence of depression among young people with type 1 diabetes: A systematic review. *Diabetic Med* 30:199–208.

106. Fogel, N.R. and J. Weissberg-Benchell. 2010. Preventing poor psychological and health outcomes in pediatric type 1 diabetes. *Curr Diab Rep* 10:436–443.

107. Bames, P.M., B. Bloom, and R.L. Nahin. 2008. Complementary and alternative medicine use among adults and children: United States, 2007. *Natl Health Stat Rep* 12:1–23.

108. McGinnis, R.A., A. McGrady, S.A. Cox et al. 2005. Biofeedback-assisted relaxation in type 2 diabetes. *Diabetes Care* 28:2145–2149.

109. Galper, D.I., A.G. Taylor, and D.J. Cox. 2003. Current status of mind-body interventions for vascular complications of diabetes. *Fam Commun Health* 26:34–40.

110. Alexander, G.K., A.G. Taylor, K.E. Innes et al. 2008. Contextualizing the effects of yoga therapy on diabetes management. *Fam Commun Health* 31:228–239.

111. Innes, K.E. and H.K. Vincent. 2007. The influence of yoga-based programs on risk profiles in adults with type 2 diabetes mellitus: A systematic review. *Evidence Based Complement Alternat Med* 4:469–486.

112. Infante, J.R., M. Torres-Avisbal, P. Pinei et al. 2001. Catecholamine levels in practitioners of the transcendental meditation technique. *Physiol Behav* 72:141–146.

113. Dusek, J.A. and H. Benson. 2009. Mind-body medicine: A model of the comparative clinical impact of the acute stress and relaxation responses. *Minn Med* 92:47–50.

114. Masi, G. and P. Brovedani. 2011. The hippocampus, neurotrophic factors and depression: Possible implications for the pharmacotherapy of depression. *CNS Drugs* 25:913–931.

115. Surwit, R.S., M.A.L. Van Tilburg, N. Zucker et al. 2002. Stress management improves long-term glycemic control in type 2 diabetes. *Diabetes Care* 25:30–34.

116. American Diabetes Association. 2014. Diagnosis and classification of diabetes mellitus. *Diabetes Care* 37(1):S81–S90.

117. Diabetes Complications. 2014. Retrieved from http://www.diabetes.org/living-with-diabetes/complications/ (accessed November 14, 2014).

13 Obesity

Sherif El Behiry, MD, Laura E. Matarese,
PhD, RND, LDN, FADA, CNSC, FASPEN,
FAND and Hossam M. Kandil, MD, PhD

CONTENTS

INTRODUCTION

The two major causes of death in middle- and high-income countries worldwide are ischemic heart disease and cerebrovascular diseases. Obesity is a risk factor for each of these diseases as well as many other health problems [1]. Numerous factors play a role in the development of obesity, including diet, lifestyle, medications, endocrine disorders, and genetic predisposition. Recently, gut microorganisms residing in the intestine have been shown to play an important role in metabolic disorders such as obesity [2]. Weight loss can be induced through dietary modification, increased physical activity, and behavior changes. In some cases, prescription medications or weight loss surgery may be indicated [3]. This chapter will focus on the prevalence and distribution of obesity worldwide, the mechanisms of its development, and the available treatment interventions.

EPIDEMIOLOGY OF OBESITY

Obese individuals have an excessive amount of body fat; however, the exact meaning of excess has not been defined [4]. Consequently, obesity has been defined as a body mass index (BMI) of >30 kg/m^2. A BMI of 30 represents an excess of body weight of approximately 30 lb (14 kg) for any given height [5]. The use of BMI to classify people as obese may result in false positives in those individuals who have a higher percentage of muscle and lower percentage of fat; the rate of false positives is 9.9% of nonobese men and 1.8% of nonobese women [6]. Women are less likely to be inaccurately classified as obese on the basis of BMI because they are less likely to have a heavy musculature. Based on these findings, it was concluded that the ability of BMI in particular, and weight–height indices in general, to identify obesity using direct measures of fatness is *suboptimal* [6]. Moreover, the inferiority of BMI at predicting health outcomes relative to more accurate measures of fatness led a 2005 editorial in the British medical journal *The Lancet* to conclude "…current practice with body-mass index as the measure of obesity is obsolete, and results in considerable underestimation of the grave consequences of the overweight epidemic" [7].

In children and teens, the BMI number is plotted on the Centers for Disease Control and Prevention BMI-for-age growth charts (for either girls or boys) to obtain a percentile ranking. Percentiles are the most commonly used indicator to assess the size and growth patterns of individual children in the United States. The percentile indicates the relative position of the child's BMI number among children of the same sex and age. The growth charts show the weight status categories used with children and teens (underweight, healthy weight, overweight, and obese) [8]. BMI-for-age weight status categories and the corresponding percentiles are shown in Table 13.1.

In 2008, more than 1.4 billion adults were overweight and more than half a billion were obese worldwide. At least 2.8 million people each year die as a result of being overweight or obese. The prevalence of obesity has nearly doubled between 1980 and 2008. Once associated with high-income countries, obesity is now prevalent also in low- and middle-income countries [9]. It is often difficult to compare the prevalence of obesity between countries due to inconsistencies in the classification used for obesity [9].

TABLE 13.1
Percentile Range according to Weight among Children and Adolescents

Weight Status Category	Percentile Range
Underweight	Less than the 5th percentile
Healthy weight	5th percentile to less than the 85th percentile
Overweight	85th to less than the 95th percentile
Obese	Equal to or greater than the 95th percentile

Source: Mei, Z. et al., *Am. J. Clin. Nutr.*, 75, 978, 2002.

The prevalence of overweight and obesity was highest in the World Health Organization (WHO) regions of the Americas (62% for overweight in both sexes, and 26% for obesity). In the WHO region for South East Asia, overweight was 14% in both sexes and 3% for obesity. In the WHO regions for Europe, Eastern Mediterranean, and the Americas, over 50% of women were overweight. For all three of these regions, roughly half of overweight women are obese (23% in Europe, 24% in the Eastern Mediterranean, 29% in the Americas). In all WHO regions, women were more likely to be obese than men. In the WHO regions for Africa, Eastern Mediterranean, and South East Asia, women had roughly double the obesity prevalence of men [10]. The latest survey conducted in the United States during 2009–2010 revealed that more than one-third of the population was overweight or obese [11].

With soaring obesity rates, the United States had been regarded as the fattest country in the Organization for Economic Co-operation and Development. Recently, Mexico became the number one country with the highest level of obesity. New projections for 2010–2020 indicate that overweight and obesity rates are expected to grow by 8% during that period. There are also ethnic and cultural differences. Obesity rates are 17% higher in African American women and 6% higher in Mexican American women than in non-Hispanic white women [12]. Overweight and obesity have dramatically increased among children, and almost one-third of children and adolescents in the United States are either overweight or obese [13]. The prevalence of overweight and obesity among children is summarized in Table 13.2.

Interestingly, obesity is also more prevalent among low-income populations. For example, 14.9% of low-income preschool-aged children were obese in 2010, as compared with 12.1% in this age group in the general population [14]. Among the low-income children, 2.1% had extreme obesity (BMI ≥120% of the 95th percentile). The prevalence of obesity among the low-income preschool-aged population increased from 1998 to 2003, but plateaued between 2003 and 2010 [15]. Children and adolescents who are obese are likely to be obese as adults [16,17] and are therefore more at risk for adult health problems such as heart disease, type 2 diabetes, stroke, several types of cancer, and osteoarthritis [18].

Childhood obesity is more common among American Indian, non-Hispanic blacks, and Mexican Americans than in non-Hispanic whites [13,19,20]. Having an obese parent increases the risk of obesity by two- to threefold.

TABLE 13.2
Obesity Prevalence among Children and Adolescents

	Preschool Children (2–5 Years)	School-Aged Children (6–11 Years)	Adolescents (12–19 Years)
Overweight or obese (BMI ≥ 85th percentile)	26.7%	12.1%	9.7%
Obese (BMI ≥ 95th percentile)	32.6%	18.0%	13.0%
Severe obesity (BMI ≥ 97th percentile)	33.6%	18.4%	13.0%

PATHOGENESIS

How Do We Get Fat?

Obesity results from a greater consumption of energy than is needed. As this energy is stored, fat cells enlarge [21]. Hypertrophy (increase in the cell size) occurs prior to hyperplasia (increase in the cell number) to meet the need for additional fat storage capacity in the progression of obesity [22]. Cell size distribution can be used to estimate total cell number within a fat pad from its mass. Furthermore, it is believed that some specific metabolic properties, for example, insulin resistance [23] and adipokine (hormones released by fat cells) secretion [24], depend on the precise cell size distribution rather than the mean cell size. Obesity is a complex multifactorial chronic disease developing from interactive influences of numerous factors—social, behavioral, physiological, metabolic, cellular, hormonal, and molecular.

Social and Behavioral Influences

Pervasive series of social and economic changes that have occurred in the United States during the past several decades have resulted in what is termed a toxic environment [25]. These changes include the increased portion sizes and the *supersizing* of commercially available foods, the proliferation of fast-food restaurants, the reduced cost of fast-food products, the increasing access to energy-dense foods in schools, the increased use of labor-saving devices that reduce physical activity, and reduced opportunities for physical activity in schools, at safe playgrounds, and neighborhoods [26,27]. Although strong causal inferences cannot be easily made from these observational trends, it is thought that these changes in the environment are largely responsible for the increase in obesity prevalence.

Several studies have documented that the lower the socioeconomic status (SES), the greater the occurrence of obesity [28]. A National Longitudinal Survey of Youth found that children from lower SES families were more likely to have been overweight during the prior year than children from higher SES families. Regardless of the ethnicity and other demographic variables, there is a negative association between obesity, SES, household income and parental education [29].

The link between low SES and obesity could be influenced by many factors such as limited access to resources, poor knowledge of nutrition and health, increased exposure to fast-food outlets, and limited physical activity due to deprived or unsafe neighborhoods [30]. It may also be influenced by differential costs of more expensive, healthy, nutrient-dense foods such as fruits and vegetables versus energy-dense, less nutritious foods [31]. For this reason, the availability of fruits and vegetables was shown to be greater among families from high compared to low SES strata [32].

Another behavioral habit that can influence obesity is a phenomenon called *social facilitation* in which energy intake at meals is increased when eating in the presence of other people [33]. It has been shown that overweight and normal-weight subjects consumed more when eating in groups of four or five persons compared to eating alone [34]. The mechanism underlying social facilitation of eating has been termed *time-extension* and has received the most empirical support as the presence of people at a meal serves to lengthen eating time, which, in turn, promotes further energy intake [33]. Ingestion rate, satiation, and meal size are influenced by the *bite size*.

Decreasing the bite size of test foods was associated with a lower ingestion rate for the whole meal. Interestingly, this decrease in the rate of eating was offset by an increase in meal duration such that overall meal sizes did not differ across conditions. This result was found true for both lean and obese individuals. It is generally advisable to monitor the bite size in addition to the meal duration during meal consumption [35,36].

Screen time, including television, computers, tablets, video game, and other electronic devices, plays an important role in weight gain. The mechanisms for this association are multifold including increase in sedentary behavior, which in turn displaces time spent in physical activity. It also provides a setting during which food can be consumed, in particular energy-dense snack foods, especially with the increased exposure to food advertising [36,37]. The patient should therefore be instructed on a technique of mindful eating. Clearly, obesity is a multifactorial and complex disorder that has significant implications for affected subjects and the health-care services required to deal with the consequences of this disorder. Physiologically, energy homeostasis involves the interplay of various secreted signals from the periphery. Obesity results in excessive adiposity, which over time leads to an imbalance in adiposity signals to the brain and in turn may contribute to pathways involved in the development of associated comorbidities.

Hormonal Causes

Multiple hormones are involved in the regulation and pathophysiology of energy metabolism, including gut-related hormones (insulin and glucagon), adipokines, and others. Several hormones are involved in regulating appetite. Ghrelin, a circulating peptide hormone, is derived from the stomach. It plays an important role in regulating energy balance and food intake and stimulating adipogenesis and weight gain [38]. Peripheral ghrelin administration reliably induces the sensation of hunger and increases food intake in lean and obese as well as in healthy and malnourished individuals [39].

Another hormone, which plays a role in the delay of gastric emptying and reduction of gastric secretion, is peptide YY (PYY). PYY is released after meal ingestion and signals to the hypothalamus. It is found throughout the intestine at progressively higher levels distally, with the highest levels in the colon and the rectum. It is secreted by the L cells of the distal small bowel and colon. Administration of PYY before meals results in decreased food consumption [40]. Cholecystokinin (CCK), which is produced in the gallbladder, pancreas, and stomach, and concentrated in the small intestine, also controls gastric emptying and gut motility. CCK acts centrally by increasing satiety and decreasing appetite [41]. Glucagon-like peptide-1 enhances satiety and reduces food intake when administered intravenously to humans [42]. It is a potent regulator of food intake in humans.

Fat cells (adipocytes) produce several hormones, collectively referred to as adipokines. The key secretory products are tumor necrosis factor-alpha (TNF-α), interleukin-6 (IL-6), leptin, resistin, and adiponectin. Elevated levels of pro-inflammatory metabolites such as TNF-α and IL-6 are observed in obese subjects and have been linked to insulin resistance and inhibition of insulin receptor signal transduction in hepatocytes and increasing circulating free fatty acids from adipose tissue.

TABLE 13.3

Summary of Hormones Influencing the Obesity Pathogenesis

Hormone	Origin	Contributing to Obesity
Ghrelin	Stomach	Adipogenesis, weight gain, and regulation of energy balance
PYY	Intestines	Decrease food consumption
CCK	Pancreas and gallbladder	Increase satiety, slow down gastric emptying
Glucagon-like peptide-1	Intestinal L-cells	Enhance satiety and reduce food intake
Proinflammatory mediators	Immune cells	Increase serum glucose and fatty acids
Leptin	Fat cells	Inhibit the appetite
Adiponectin	Adipose tissue	Reduce the metabolism

Leptin is a protein hormone that plays a key role in regulating energy intake and expenditure, including appetite and hunger, metabolism, and behavior. It is transported across the blood–brain barrier and binds to specific receptors on appetite-modulating neurons and the hypothalamus resulting in an inhibition of appetite. Furthermore, leptin deficiency reduces energy expenditure [43]. Adiponectin is an adipokine derived from plasma protein. It is insulin sensitizing, anti-inflammatory, and antiatherogenic [44]. The origin and effects of hormones are summarized in Table 13.3.

Genetic Causes

Genetic influences are difficult to elucidate, and identification of the genes is not easily achieved in familial or pedigree studies [45]. There is no one diet prescription that can be used universally for all individuals. Different people will respond to different diet prescriptions based on their individual metabolic makeup, comorbid factors, and lifestyle behaviors. At least 24 genetic mutations have been shown to play a role in obesity development. The inheritance of 9 of these disorders is autosomal dominant, 10 are autosomal recessive, and 5 are X-linked [46]. There is approximately 1.5-fold increase in the risk of obesity with the inherited risk genotype of fat mass and obesity-associated gene (FTO), which was seen in both children and adults. This gene variant may account for 22% of common obesity [47]. Many other genes can contribute to the development of obesity including mutations in prohormone convertase 1/3 gene (PC1/3) and the gene for peroxisome-proliferator-activated receptor (PPAR) gamma 2 [48,49]. Inactivating mutations of the gene encoding PPARγ are associated with insulin resistance, type 2 diabetes, and hypertension, whereas a rare gain of function mutation causes extreme obesity [50].

Prenatal and Postnatal Influences

During pregnancy, a mother's body weight may influence body size, shape, and later body composition of her infant. High pre-pregnancy BMI and excessive gestational weight gain are risk factors for childhood obesity. In addition, maternal smoking or diabetes increases the risk of obesity in the offspring [51]. The amount of weight a woman gains during pregnancy may be a potentially important modifiable risk factor that influences the growth and health of the fetus as well as outcomes later during

TABLE 13.4
Recommended Gestational Weight according to BMI

BMI Category (kg/m²)	Recommended Gestational Weight Gain in kg
<19.8	12.5–18
19.8–26.0	11.5–16
>26.0–29.0	7–11.5
>29.0	≥6.8

childhood and adulthood [52]. The recommended maternal gestational weight gain based on prepregnancy BMI, as defined by the Institute of Medicine, is summarized in Table 13.4.

After delivery, breast-feeding, when compared to formula feeding, may be associated with a lower risk of overweight and obesity. As an example, feeding infants solely with breast milk during the first 3 or more months of life reduces the risk of being overweight in childhood [53]. The predictive value of childhood obesity varies with the age at onset of obesity and the family history. It has been found that obese children under 3 years of age were at low risk of becoming obese adults unless one or both parents were obese. On the other hand, obesity among older children was an increasingly important predictor of adult obesity, regardless of parents' weights. For both obese and nonobese children less than 10 years of age, having an obese parent more than doubled the risk of obesity as an adult [54]. Between the age of 5 and 7, the BMI may begin to increase, which is referred to as adiposity rebound [55]. Earlier onset of rebound and body weight over 95th percentile in childhood increase the chance of obesity in adulthood by two- or threefold [55,56].

ROLE OF GUT MICROBIOTA IN OBESITY

There is great interest in the mechanistic links between gut microbes and specific conditions associated with obesity [57]. Microbiota is a collection of microorganisms including bacteria, archaea, viruses, and some unicellular eukaryotes associated with every multicellular organism on earth. There are approximately 10^{14} microorganisms, which reside in various parts of the body including the surface of skin and in the gastrointestinal (GI), genitourinary, and respiratory tracts. The GI tract has the largest pool of microorganisms in humans. The chemical environment and habitable microorganisms differ tremendously in each section of the GI tract. In the colon, up to 10^{12} microorganisms are reported, and this is by far the highest density found in humans [58–60]. Most of the bacterial taxa present in the GI tract have not yet been successfully cultured, identified, or otherwise characterized [61]. Normally, the majority of bacteria in the GI tract are beneficial or harmless to the host health, while only a minority represents potentially harmful bacteria. The GI microbiota is a complex system that has a major influence on human health. It is known to contribute to, for example, the maturation of the gut, nutrition of the host, resistance to pathogens, and the maintenance of host health [62].

Gut physiology and function are altered during the aging process [63], which is often accompanied by an increased incidence of GI infections. While they can be explained by changes in environmental circumstances, and altered dietary and physiological factors, bacterial community shifts in the gut can also have great effects on host physiology and metabolism [64]. The colonic microflora of infants is generally viewed as being adult-like after the age of 2 years, although facultative anaerobes in these children have been reported to be higher than in adults [65]. Indeed, it is likely that the intestinal microflora does not completely resemble that of adults until much later in childhood. Once the climax gut microflora has become established, the major bacterial groups in the feces of adults remain relatively constant over time [66]. There are reports, however, that elderly subjects harbor fewer bifidobacteria and higher levels of fungi and enterobacteria with reduced biodiversity of the gut microbiome when compared with younger adults, and it seems, therefore, that the gut microbiota continues to evolve throughout the life span of the host [67]. The extremes of life have reduced biodiversity of the gut microbiota, which correlate with suboptimal immunity.

Obesity and type 2 diabetes are associated with altered communities of gut microbiota, inflammation, and gut barrier disintegration. However, intestinal microbial composition and the mechanisms of interaction with the host that affect gut barrier function during obesity and type 2 diabetes have not been clearly defined [68].

Microbiota can influence host adiposity by energy extraction from the diet, with variable efficiency depending on community composition or by influencing metabolism throughout the body [69,70]. Gut microbiota increase serum levels of glucose and short-chain fatty acids, which induce triglyceride production in the liver, and are associated with greater adiposity and reduced glucose tolerance [70]. Mice raised in aseptic isolators are significantly leaner than conventionally raised mice despite their considerably greater food intake. Additionally, they are resistant to diet-induced obesity and insulin resistance [70]. Prevotellaceae, a subgroup of Bacteroidetes, are significantly enriched in obesity, again raising the potentially important issue of gut microbiota as a confounding factor [71].

The vast majority of microorganisms belong to the family of Firmicutes, Bacteroidetes, Actinobacteria, and Proteobacteria, with relatively lower numbers belonging to Fusobacteria, Verrucomicrobia, and TM7 [60,72]. Interestingly, Firmicutes were found to be dominant in lean and obese individuals and decreased in three patients undergoing Roux-en-Y gastric bypass surgery [73]. Occupation can also affect the gut bacteria in humans, for example, those who had regular contact with livestock, such as farmers and their wives, had bacterial communities dominated by special type of bacteria that is also abundant in the gut microbiota of cattle and sheep [74]. Overweight pregnant patients (week 24) have reduced numbers of Bacteroidetes, whereas increased numbers of certain Firmicutes (e.g., *Staphylococcus*) or Proteobacteria (e.g., Enterobacteriaceae such as *Escherichia coli*) were detected [75].

The intestinal microbiota, as a whole, provides metabolic functions, which improve the ability to extract and store energy from the diet and play a role in body weight gain and thus the obesity. Imbalances in the gut microbiota and increases in plasma lipopolysaccharide may also act as inflammatory factors related to the development of atherosclerosis, insulin resistance, and body weight gain.

Recently, a mucin-degrading bacterium, *Akkermansia muciniphila*, which resides in the mucous layer, has been isolated. The presence of this bacterium inversely correlates with body weight [76]. However, the precise physiological roles played by this bacterium during obesity and metabolic disorders are unknown. The multitude of these bacteria decreased in obese and type 2 diabetic, and a prebiotic feeding normalizes this multitude in intestine, which correlated with an improved metabolic profile. In addition, it has been demonstrated that treatment with these bacteria reverses high-fat-diet-induced metabolic disorders, including fat-mass gain, metabolic endotoxemia, adipose tissue inflammation, and insulin resistance. Furthermore, administration of *A. muciniphila* increased the intestinal levels of endocannabinoids that control inflammation, the gut barrier, and gut peptide secretion. However, viable *A. muciniphila* is required to achieve these effects because treatment with heat-killed cells did not improve the metabolic profile or the mucous layer thickness [76]. The intricate mechanisms of bacterial regulation of the cross talk between the host and gut microbiota are still currently under investigation.

In contrast, specific probiotics, prebiotics, and related metabolites might exert beneficial effects on lipid and glucose metabolism, the production of satiety peptides, and the inflammatory tone related to obesity and associated metabolic disorders. Better knowledge of these mechanisms may contribute to our understanding of how environmental factors influence obesity and associated diseases, providing new opportunities to design improved dietary intervention strategies to manage these disorders [68].

DIETARY SUPPLEMENTS

The Dietary Supplement Health and Education Act defined dietary supplements as a product containing one or more of the following: a vitamin, mineral, amino acid, herb, other botanical, concentrate, metabolite, constituent, or extract; furthermore, it placed dietary supplements in a distinct category from drugs. Labels of dietary supplements are required to state the following: "this product is not intended to diagnose, treat, cure, or prevent any disease." However, product labels are allowed to make health claims, such as *promotes prostate health* or *supports the circulatory system*. Dietary supplements are not required to demonstrate efficacy, safety, or quality of a product prior to marketing. Supplement manufacturers are also not obligated to report postmarketing adverse events to the FDA. However, the new good manufacturing practices require dietary supplements to be properly labeled, free of adulterants, and manufactured according to specified standards for personnel and equipment [77,78]. The use of dietary supplements is common in industrialized countries. More than 50 individual dietary supplements and 125 proprietary products are listed in the Natural Medicines Comprehensive Database as commonly being used for weight loss [79].

Commonly used dietary supplements for weight loss are listed in Table 13.5 according to their mechanism of action. Approximately one half of the most commonly used individual supplements in weight loss products have not been studied in randomized controlled trials (RCTs) in humans. Criteria adapted from a recent

TABLE 13.5

Common Dietary Supplements Used for Weight Loss

Mechanism of Action	Supplements
Increase energy expenditure	Guarana—caffeine
	Country mallow—yerba maté
Modulate carbohydrate metabolism	Chromium—ginseng
Increase fat oxidation or reduce fat synthesis	L-Carnitine—hydroxycitric acid
	Green tea—vitamin B_5
	Licorice—conjugated linoleic acid
	Pyruvate
Increase satiety	Guar gum—glucomannan
	Psyllium
Block dietary fat absorption	Chitosan
Increase water elimination	Dandelion—cascara
Enhance mood	St. John's wort
Miscellaneous or unspecified	Laminaria—spirulina (blue-green algae)
	Guggul—apple cider vinegar

review [80] can be used to develop clinical recommendations for each supplement. If there is strong evidence for a product's quality, safety, and efficacy, it may be reasonable to recommend that product and closely monitor the patient. In contrast, it would be appropriate to discourage use of products when there is strong evidence for lack of quality, safety, or efficacy. For example, use of products that contain ephedra should be actively discouraged because of serious safety concerns. Chitosan appears to be ineffective for weight loss and should also be discouraged. Table 13.6 summarizes the evidence for quality, safety, and efficacy for each supplement discussed and provides a suggested clinical stance [80,81–93].

WEIGHT LOSS DIETS AND COMMERCIAL PROGRAMS

"I am on a diet" is commonly stated when starting to follow a program to induce weight loss. *Diet* is a word commonly used in weight reduction programs. Hundreds of weight loss diets have been proposed in the lay literature and media. Few of them have achieved a consensus approval of inducing or maintaining weight loss. Adding, eliminating, or substituting one or more of food groups or recommending consumption of one type of food in excess determines the basic concept of this dietary program. There is no doubt that prescribing a diet modification program is an essential way to reduce weight, but the pathogenesis of obesity is multifactorial, complicated, and includes other factors in addition to diet. Therefore, there is no one diet prescription that can be used universally for all individuals. Different people will respond to different diet prescriptions based on their individual metabolic makeup, comorbid factors, and lifestyle behaviors.

TABLE 13.6
Evidence of Quality, Safety, and Efficacy of Commonly Used Dietary Supplements

Supplement	Product Quality	Product Safety	Product Efficacy	Clinical Stance[a]
Chromium	Present	Uncertain	Uncertain	Caution and monitor
Ginseng	Uncertain	Uncertain	Uncertain	Caution and monitor
L-Carnitine	Present	Present	Uncertain	Caution and monitor
Hydroxycitric acid	Uncertain	Uncertain	Uncertain	Caution and monitor
Green tea	Uncertain	Present	Uncertain	Caution and monitor
Vitamin B_5	Present	Present	Uncertain	Caution and monitor
Licorice	Uncertain	Uncertain	Uncertain	Caution and monitor
Guar gum	Uncertain	Present	Absent	Discourage
Chitosan	Uncertain	Present	Absent	Discourage
Dandelion	Uncertain	Uncertain	Uncertain	Caution and monitor
St. John's wort	Uncertain	Uncertain	Uncertain	Caution and monitor
Laminaria	Uncertain	Uncertain	Uncertain	Caution and monitor
Spirulina	Uncertain	Uncertain	Absent	Discourage
Apple cider vinegar	Uncertain	Uncertain	Uncertain	Caution and monitor
Cascara	Present	Uncertain	Uncertain	Caution and monitor

Sources: Shekelle, P.G. et al., *JAMA*, 289, 1537, 2003; Althuis, M.D. et al., *Am. J. Clin. Nutr.*, 76, 148, 2002; Vincent, J.B., *Sports Med.*, 33, 213, 2003; Sotaniemi, E.A. et al., *Diabetes Care*, 18, 1373, 1995; Mattes, R.D. and Bormann, L., *Physiol. Behav.*, 71, 87, 2000; Heymsfield, S.B. et al., *JAMA*, 280, 1596, 1998; Dulloo, A.G. et al., *Am. J. Clin. Nutr.*, 70, 1040, 1999; Armanini, D. et al., *J. Endocrinol. Invest.*, 26, 646, 2003; Ernst, E. and Pittler, M.H., *Perfusion*, 11, 461, 1998; Pittler, M.H. et al., *Eur. J. Clin. Nutr.*, 53, 379, 1999; Wuolijoki, E. et al., *Methods Find. Exp. Clin. Pharmacol.*, 21, 357, 1999; Ho, S.C. et al., *Singapore Med. J.*, 42, 6, 2001; Food and Drug Administration, FDA Consumer, 3, 1981; Weiger, W.A. et al., *Ann. Intern. Med.*, 137, 889, 2002.

[a] If there is strong evidence for the presence of quality, safety, and efficacy, then the suggested clinical stance is to recommend. If there is strong evidence for the absence of quality, safety, or efficacy, then the suggested clinical stance is to discourage. If the evidence does not meet the criteria for recommend or discourage (i.e., evidence for quality, safety, or efficacy is uncertain with no strong evidence for absence of quality, safety, or efficacy), then the suggested clinical stance is to provide caution and monitor [101].

The optimal management of overweight and obesity requires a combination of diet, exercise, and behavioral modification. In addition, some patients eventually require pharmacologic therapy and, if there is an inadequate response, then bariatric surgery. Before starting any treatment program, the risk of overweight to the subject should be evaluated. Selection of treatment can then be made using a risk–benefit assessment. The choice of therapy is dependent on several factors including the degree of overweight or obesity and patient preference.

Goals should be clear before discussing a dietary weight loss program with an individual patient. The first goal for any overweight individual is to prevent further weight gain and keep body weight stable (within 5 lb of its current level). An initial weight loss goal of 5%–7% of body weight is realistic for most individuals. Most patients have unrealistic weight loss goal as 30% or more below current weight [94]. Five percent weight loss or more has been shown to reduce risk factors for cardiovascular disease, such as dyslipidemia, hypertension, and diabetes mellitus [95]. For example, reduction of progression rate from impaired glucose tolerance to frank diabetes by 58% occurs with a weight loss of 7% [96]. It should be clear that loss of 5% of initial body weight and maintenance of this loss is a good medical result, even if the subject does not reach his or her desired body weight.

Despite the complicated mechanism of obesity development, the rate of weight loss is directly related to the difference between the subject's energy intake and energy requirements. Reducing caloric intake below expenditure results in a predictable initial rate of weight loss that is related to the energy deficit. However, prediction of weight loss for an individual subject can be difficult because of marked variability in initial body composition, adherence, and energy expenditure [97]. Prediction of weight loss is difficult due to the fact that food records are often inaccurate as most of the normal-weight people underreport what they eat by 10%–30%, while overweight people underreport by 30% or more [98]. In addition, energy requirements are influenced by many factors as gender, age, and genetic factors. For example, men generally lose more weight than women of similar height and weight when they comply with any given diet modification plan due to the higher lean body mass, lower percent body fat, and therefore higher energy expenditure. Older subjects of either sex have lower energy expenditure and therefore lose weight more slowly than younger subjects; metabolic rate declines by approximately 2%/decade (about 100 kcal/decade) [99].

Approximately 22 kcal/kg is required to maintain a kilogram of body weight in a normal adult [100]. Thus, the expected or calculated energy expenditure for a woman weighing 100 kg is approximately 2200 kcal/day. With a variability of ±20%, the range of energy needs may be as high as 2620 kcal/day or as low as 1860 kcal/day. An average deficit of 500 kcal/day should result in an initial weight loss of approximately 0.5 kg/week (1 lb/week). However, after 3–6 months of weight loss, energy expenditure adaptations occur, which slow down body weight response to a given change in energy intake, thereby diminishing ongoing weight loss [100].

There are several methods of formally estimating energy expenditure. If possible, direct measurement is the best. The WHO method allows a direct estimate of resting metabolic rate (RMR) and calculation of daily energy requirement. The low activity level (1.3 × RMR) includes subjects who lead a sedentary life. The high activity level (1.7 × RMR) applies to those in jobs requiring manual labor or patients with regular daily physical exercise programs [101].

Weight loss maintenance is also difficult because of changes in the hormone signals that regulate appetite. Hormonal adaptations favoring weight gain persist for at least 1 year after diet-induced weight loss [102]. The general unanimity is that excess intake of calories from any source, associated with a sedentary lifestyle, causes weight gain and obesity. The goal of weight management program, therefore, is to decrease energy intake and maintain active lifestyle in addition to behavior modification. Conventional weight loss diets are defined as those below energy requirements but above 800 kcal/day [103]. These diets fall into the following groups:

1. Balanced low-calorie diets/portion-controlled diets
2. Low-fat diets
3. Low-carbohydrate diets
4. Mediterranean diet
5. Fad diets (diets involving unusual combinations of foods or eating sequences)

HIGH-PROTEIN, LOW-CARBOHYDRATE DIET PROGRAMS

Proponents of low-carbohydrate diets have argued that the increasing obesity epidemic may be in part due to low-fat, high-carbohydrate diets. But this may be dependent upon the type of carbohydrates that are consumed, such as energy-dense snacks and sugar or high-fructose containing beverages.

The carbohydrate content of the diet is an important determinant of short-term (less than 2 weeks) weight loss. Low (60–130 g of carbohydrates) and very-low-carbohydrate diets (0 to <60 g) have been popular for many years [103]. Restriction of carbohydrates leads to glycogen mobilization, and if carbohydrate intake is less than 50 g/day, ketosis will develop. Initial rapid weight loss occurs, primarily due to fluid loss rather than fat loss. The rationale for a carbohydrate restriction is that, in response to lower glucose availability, there will be reduced insulin concentrations, which in turn will shift metabolism from lipogenesis to lipolysis. The exact carbohydrate level required to produce this metabolic shift is thought to be between 20 and 50 g/day in the initial phases of the diet in comparison to the carbohydrate content of the typical Western diet, which often exceeds 300 g/day [104].

Low- and very-low-carbohydrate diets are more effective for short-term weight loss than low-fat diets, although probably not for long-term weight loss. The difference in weight loss at 6 months, favoring the low-carbohydrate over low-fat diet, is not sustained at 12 months [105]. However, a recent randomized trial demonstrated that the low-carbohydrate diet was more effective for weight loss and cardiovascular risk factor reduction than the low-fat diet [106].

ATKINS DIET

Phase 1: This is a 2-week induction phase in which the consumption of calories from carbohydrates is limited to 20 g each day. Carbohydrate sources are mainly from vegetables.

Phase 2: Other carbohydrate sources are added as fiber-rich foods, at an increased rate of 25 g during the first week of this phase. Carbohydrate intake is gradually increased in 5 g increments each week until the weight loss stops. At that point, 5 g of carbs is taken from the daily intake until weight loss begins again.

Phase 3: This is the premaintenance phase in which the patient has achieved the goal weight. The carbohydrate intake is increased by 10 g each week until the weight loss is very gradual. Carbohydrate is added until weight loss stops.

Phase 4: This is the lifetime maintenance phase in which a wider range of carbohydrate sources are included while carefully monitoring body weight [107–109].

Dukan Diet

Dukan diet is another example of a low-carbohydratem high-protein diet, which proposes an eating plan including 100 foods, of which 72 are from animal sources and 28 come from plants. The amounts are unrestricted as long as consumption is limited to those 100 foods. Exercise is encouraged throughout all of the four phases.

Phase 1: The aim of phase 1 is rapid weight loss of 3–4 kg (4.4–6.6 lb) within 10 days. The plan begins with unlimited amounts of low-fat protein in the form of beef, fish, chicken, eggs, soy, and cottage cheese. The only carbohydrate allowed in this phase is oat bran, which is believed to be less carbohydrate rich and suppresses hunger because it grows to up to 20 times its size in the stomach. However, the carbohydrate content of the dairy products is never addressed. Thus, it is possible to consume enough carbohydrate from cottage cheese to prevent conversion to ketosis.

Phase 2: Vegetables are added by 28 specific kinds. Fruit is not allowed. This phase aims to achieve the target bodyweight more gradually. Although based on specific personal conditions, the vegetables can be consumed in unlimited amounts as long as they are not starchy.

The plan alternates between lean protein and vegetables. Thus, one day, the individual eats just lean protein, and the next day lean proteins combined with unlimited low-starch vegetables. This alternation persists throughout this stage.

Phase 3: This phase aims to sustain the achieved weight loss by consuming unlimited quantities of protein and vegetables daily, as well as one piece of low-sugar fruit (e.g., strawberry, watermelon, peach), one portion of cheese, and two slices of whole-grain bread. One or two servings of a starchy food is allowed, and one or two open meals are permitted each week. In an open meal, people can eat whatever they want. This type of approach can easily convert the metabolism from lipolysis to lipogenesis if enough carbohydrate is consumed.

Phase 4: This phase focuses on long-term simple rules such as including one all-protein day each week, as in phase 1. Three tablespoons of oat bran should be consumed each day, and exercise is increased to 20 min of walking each day [110].

South Beach Diet

The South Beach Diet is sometimes called a modified low-carbohydrate diet because it is lower in carbohydrates and higher in protein and healthy fats than is a typical eating plan. But it is not a strict low-carbohydrate diet [111]. The South Beach Diet has three phases:

Phase 1: This 2-week phase is designed to eliminate food cravings and jump-start weight loss. Almost all carbohydrates are cut out from the diet, particularly starches and sugars, including pasta, rice, bread, and fruit. There are no fruit juices or alcohol allowed. It focuses on eating lean protein, such as seafood, skinless poultry, lean beef, and soy products. Also high-fiber vegetables, low-fat dairy, and foods with healthy unsaturated fats, including avocadoes, nuts, and seeds can be eaten.

Phase 2: This is a long-term weight loss phase. Some of the previously banned foods, such as whole-grain breads, whole-wheat pasta, brown rice, fruits, and more vegetables are reintroduced. This phase continues until the goal weight is reached [112,113].

Phase 3: This is a maintenance phase, which is based on continuation of the diet and lifestyle principles learned in the two previous phases. Most foods can be consumed, including occasional indulgences [114,115].

COMMERCIAL PROGRAMS (MEDIFAST, WEIGHT WATCHERS)

There are several commercial programs, which vary in effectiveness, and the ability to provide, follow, and maintain good nutrition and safety. Weight Watchers is one of the most recognized and oldest commercial weight loss programs.

The overall program is based on calorie reduction. A point system is applied for foods, which are categorized, based on their calorie, fat, and fiber content. One of the advantages of Weight Watchers is the flexibility in food choices as long as the individual stays within the desired points. The disadvantage to this, however, is that one could easily consume all the prescribed points as a slice of chocolate cake or a candy bar. Because of this, Weight Watchers changed the point system in 2013.

The new program encourages people to use the points wisely by eating foods rich in protein and fiber, which have a high satiety value and help to lose weight in a healthier and more nutritious way. Exercise is encouraged, and group support is provided at local meetings and via the Internet to provide behavioral modification techniques as well as emotional support.

In a 2-year randomized trial study conducted by Heshka et al. [116], participants in Weight Watchers lost 4.3 kg in 1 year as compared to 1.3 kg in the group who received two 20 min counseling sessions and provision of self-help resources. Additionally, those in the Weight Watchers group maintained a weight loss of 2.9 kg (vs. 0.2 kg) after 2 years. The Lighten Up RCT compared a range of 12-week commercial and National Health Service (NHS) weight reduction programs with traditional self-help programs [117]. The NHS programs consisted of a group weight loss program and two primary care programs—one led by a nurse and one led by a pharmacist. The participants in the self-help group were provided with 12 vouchers to a local fitness center. At 12 weeks, all programs achieved significant weight loss range 1.37 (NHS) to 4.43 kg (Weight Watchers), and all except NHS programs resulted in significant weight loss at 1 year. At 1 year, only the Weight Watchers group had significantly greater weight loss than did the self-help group (2.5 kg greater loss). Other several follow-up studies by the NHS demonstrated that referrals from primary care practitioners into a pragmatically delivered weight management program led to a clinically significant loss with Weight Watchers demonstrating the greatest weight loss for the least cost [118,119].

The Medifast brand has been available for a number of decades and, at one time, was available only via physicians. Medifast offers meal replacement products, generally formulated to be low calorie and low fat, with optimum levels of vitamins. The formula will generally take users into a mild state of ketosis.

The most popular plan is called 5 and 1. This plan (800–1000 calories daily) comprises five meal replacements and one *real* meal containing a lean protein and vegetables and salad. Medifast claims a weight loss of 2–5 lb/week. Most of these meals are low glycemic, low fat, and gluten free. During the first phase of the Medifast diet, dairy, fruits, and starch products are not allowed. Dieters will be asked to avoid high-sugar, greasy, and fried foods even during the maintenance phase. Dieters must drink approximately 64 oz of noncaloric drinks every day. Good choices would be water, tea, coffee, and sugar-free drinks like diet sodas. Caffeinated drinks, however, should be limited to a maximum of three servings per day since the low-calorie Medifast diet may make people more sensitive to the side effects of caffeine.

The total carbohydrate intake per day must be limited to around 80–85 g until the transition phase wherein they are brought back into your diet gradually. The Medifast diet suggests celery stalks, dill pickles, and sugar-free popsicles, gelatin, and gum as snacks.

The next phase is the transition phase, which aims to increase the calorie intake and gradually reintroduces the body to the foods that it had to abstain from (i.e., starches, dairy, and fruits) during the first phase. The length of the transition period is connected to how much losing weight is required. For instance, losing 100 lb would require a 12-week transition period, while losing less than 50 lb would necessitate only 8 weeks. The last part of the Medifast diet is maintenance in which a balanced diet is required, and a list of ideal foods to eat is given to the dieter in order to maintain body weight [119].

CONCLUSION

Obesity is a serious and highly prevalent disease associated with increased morbidity and mortality. The pathogenesis of obesity is multifactorial including diet, lifestyle, medications, endocrine disorders, genetic predisposition, and cardinal role of gut microorganisms. Primary treatment should be directed at achieving and maintaining desirable body weight. Body weight can be reduced with a number of scientifically based weight loss diets if implemented correctly and with adequate compliance.

The weight loss diet should be individualized for each patient based on BMI, metabolic risk factors, lifestyle, cultural, religious, and food preferences. A strong educational component is essential to include not only the mechanics of the diet, but also portion control, eating in restaurants, and how to change behaviors for lifelong health.

It is important to help the patient find a balance between food and physical activity for overall well-being and fitness. The use of behavior modification will aid in compliance.

REFERENCES

1. World Health Organization. who.int/mediacentre/factsheets/fs310/en/ (Accessed October 16, 2013).
2. Million M, Lagier JC, Yahav D et al. Gut bacterial microbiota and obesity. *Clin Microbiol Infect.* April 2013; 19(4):305–313.
3. Fitch A, Everling L, Fox C et al. Prevention and management of obesity for adults. Institute for Clinical Systems Improvement (ICSI), Bloomington, MN, May 2013, 99p.
4. Defining overweight and obesity. Centers for Disease Control & Prevention. http://www.cdc.gov/obesity/adult/defining.html (Accessed April 24, 2015).
5. NIH-NHLBI, Obesity Initiative Task Force. Clinical guidelines on the identification, evaluation, and treatment of overweight in adults—The evidence report. *Obes Res.* 1998; i6:1–209.
6. Smalley KJ, Knerr AN, Kendrick ZV et al. Reassessment of body mass indices. *Am J Clin Nutr.* 1990; 52:405–408.
7. Kragelund C and Omland T. A farewell to body-mass index? *Lancet.* 2005; 366:1589–1591.
8. Mei Z, Grummer-Strawn LM, Pietrobelli A et al. Validity of body mass index compared with other body-composition screening indexes for the assessment of body fatness in children and adolescents. *Am J Clin Nutr.* 2002; 75:978–985.
9. WHO. 2014. 10 facts about obesity. http://who.int/features/factfiles/obesity/en/ (Accessed May 21, 2014).
10. WHO, 2014. Global Health Observatory. Obesity, situation and trend. http://who.int/gho/ncd/risk_factors/obesity_text/en/index.html (Accessed May 21, 2014).
11. Centers for Disease Control and Prevention. Summary health statistics for U.S. adults: National Health Interview Survey, 2010. Hyattsville, MD: National Center for Health Statistics. Vital and Health Statistics 10(252); 2012. Available online: http://www.cdc.gov/nchs/data/series/sr_10/sr10_252.pdf.
12. Flegal KM, Carroll MD, Kit BK et al. 2012. Prevalence of obesity and trends in the distribution of body mass index among US adults, 1999–2010. *JAMA.* 2012; 307(5):491–497.
13. Ogden CL, Carroll MD, Kit BK et al. Prevalence of obesity and trends in body mass index among US children and adolescents, 1999–2010. *JAMA.* 2012; 307(5):483.
14. Eagle TF, Sheetz A, Gurm R et al. Understanding childhood obesity in America: Linkages between household income, community resources, and children's behaviors. *Am Heart J.* 2012; 163(5): 836.
15. Pan L, Blanck HM, Sherry B et al. Trends in the prevalence of extreme obesity among US preschool-aged children living in low-income families, 1998–2010. *JAMA.* December 2012; 308(24):2563–2565.
16. Freedman DS, Kettel L, Serdula MK et al. The relation of childhood BMI to adult adiposity: The Bogalusa Heart Study. *Pediatrics.* 2005; 115:22–27.
17. Guo SS and Chumlea WC. Tracking of body mass index in children in relation to overweight in adulthood. *Am J Clin Nutr.* 1999; 70:S145–S148.
18. Berenson GS, Srinivasan SR, Bao W, et al. Association between multiple cardiovascular risk factors and atherosclerosis in children and young adults. The Bogalusa Heart Study. *N Engl J Med.* Jun 4 1998; 338(23):1650–1656.

19. Dietz WH and Robinson TN. Clinical practice. Overweight children and adolescents. *N Engl J Med.* 2005; 352(20):2100.

20. Anderson SE and Whitaker RC. Prevalence of obesity among US preschool children in different racial and ethnic groups. *Arch Pediatr Adolesc Med.* 2009; 163(4):344.

21. Bray GA. Etiology and pathogenesis of obesity. *Clin Cornerstone.* 1999; 2(3):1–15.

22. Faust IM, Johnson PR, Stern JS et al. Diet-induced adipocyte number increase in adult rats: A new model of obesity. *Am J Physiol.* 1978; 235:279–286.

23. McLaughlin T, Sherman A, Tsao P et al. Enhanced proportion of small adipose cells in insulin-resistant vs. insulin-sensitive obese individuals implicates impaired adipogenesis. *Diabetologia.* 2007; 50:1707–1715.

24. Skurk T, Alberti-Huber C, Herder C et al. Relationship between adipocyte size and adipokine expression and secretion. *J Clin Endocrinol Metab.* 2007; 92:1023–1033.

25. Jacobson MF and Brownell KD. Small taxes on soft drinks and snack foods to promote health. *Am J Public Health.* 2000; 90(6):854–857.

26. French SA, story M, Neumark-Sztainer D et al. Fast food restaurant use among adolescents: Associations with nutrient intake, food choices and behavioral and psychosocial variables. *Int J Obes Relat Metab Disord.* 2001; 25(12):1823–1833.

27. Crawford DA, Jeffery RW, French SA et al. Television viewing, physical inactivity and obesity. *Int J Obes Relat Metab Disord.* 1999; 23(4):437–440.

28. Jeffery RW, Forester AR, Folsom RV et al. The relationship between social status and body mass index in the Minnesota Heart Health Program. *Int J Obes.* 1989; 13(1):59–67.

29. Goodman E. The role of socioeconomic status gradients in explaining differences in U.S. adolescents' health. *Am J Public Health.* 1999; 89(10):1522–1528.

30. Boslaugh SE, Douglas A, Ross C et al. Perceptions of neighborhood environment for physical activity: Is it "who you are" or "where you live"? *J Urban Health.* 2004; 81(4):671–681.

31. Drewnowski A, Wall M, Perry C et al. Obesity and the food environment: Dietary energy density and diet costs. *Am J Prev Med.* 2004; 27(3 Suppl.):154–162.

32. Neumark-Sztainer D, Wall M, Perry C et al. correlates of fruit and vegetable intake among adolescents. Findings from Project EAT. *Prev Med.* 2003; 37(3):198–208.

33. Herman CP, Roth DA, Polivy J et al. Effects of the presence of others on food intake: A normative interpretation. *Psychol Bull.* 2003; 129(6):873–886.

34. Edelman B, Engell D, Bronstein P et al. Environmental effects on the intake of overweight and normal-weight men. *Appetite.* 1986; 7(1):71–83.

35. Spiegel TA, Kaplan JM, Tomassinin A et al. Bite size, ingestion rate, and meal size in lean and obese women. *Appetite.* 1993; 21(2):131–45.

36. Francis LA, Lee Y, Birch LL et al. Parental weight status and girls' television viewing, snacking, and body mass indexes. *Obes Res.* 2003; 11(1):143–151.

37. Henderson VR and Kelly B. Food advertising in the age of obesity: Content analysis of food advertising on general market and African American television. *J Nutr Educ Behav.* 2005; 37(4):191–196.

38. Tschop M, Weyer C, Tataranni PA et al. Circulating ghrelin levels are decreased in human obesity. *Diabetes.* 2001; 50:707–709.

39. Wren AM, Seal LJ, Cohen MA et al. Ghrelin enhances appetite and increase food intake in humans. *J Clin Endocrinol Metab.* 2001; 86:5992.

40. Degen L, Oesch S, Casanova M et al. Effect of peptide YY3–36 on food intake in humans. *Gastroenterology.* 2005; 129:1430–1436.

41. Cohen MA, Ellis SM, Le Roux CW et al. Oxyntomodulin suppresses appetite and reduces food intake in humans. *J Clin Endocrinol Metab.* 2003; 88:4696–4701.

42. Flint A, Raben A, Astrup A et al. Glucagon-like peptide 1 promotes satiety and suppresses energy intake in humans. *J Clin Invest.* 1998; 101:515–520.

43. Mizuno TM, Kelley KA, Pasinetti GM et al. Transgenic neuronal expression of proopiomelanocortin attenuates hyperphagic response to fasting and reverses metabolic impairments in leptin-deficient obese mice. *Diabetes.* 2003; 52:2675–2683.
44. Matsuzawa Y, Funahashi T, Kihara S et al. Review Adiponectin and metabolic syndrome. *Arterioscler Thromb Vasc Biol.* January 2004; 24(1):29–33.
45. Bouchard C, Perusse L, Leblanc C et al. Inheritance of the amount and distribution of human body fat. *Int J Obes.* 1988; 12:205–215.
46. Rankinen T, Pérusse L, Weisnagel SJ et al. The human obesity gene map: The 2001 update. *Obes Res.* 2002; 10(3):196.
47. Dina C, Meyre D, Gallina S et al. Variation in FTO contributes to childhood obesity and severe adult obesity. *Nat Genet.* 2007; 39(6):724.
48. Meyre D, Delplanque J, Chèvre JC et al. Genome-wide association study for early-onset and morbid adult obesity identifies three new risk loci in European populations. *Nat Genet.* 2009; 41(2):157.
49. Han JC, Liu QR, Jones M. Brain-derived neurotrophic factor and obesity in the WAGR syndrome. *N Engl J Med.* 2008; 359(9):918.
50. Francesco S and Alan R. The role of peroxisome proliferator-activated receptor gamma in Diabetes and Obesity. *Shuldiner* 2002; 2(2):179–185.
51. Power C and Jefferis BJ. Environment and subsequent obesity: A study of maternal smoking. *Int J Epidemiol.* 2002; 31(2):413.
52. Gillman MW, Rifas-Shiman S, Berkey CS et al. Maternal gestational diabetes, birth weight, and adolescent obesity. *Pediatrics* 2003; 111:e221–e226.
53. Hediger ML, Overpeck MD, Kuczmarski RJ et al. Association between infant breastfeeding and overweight in young children. *JAMA.* 2001; 285(19):2453.
54. Whitaker RC, Wright JA, Pepe MS et al. Predicting obesity in young adulthood from childhood and parental obesity. *N Engl J Med.* 1997; 337(13):869.
55. Siervogel RM, Roche AF, Guo SM et al. Patterns of change in weight/stature2 from 2 to 18 years: Findings from long-term serial data for children in the Fels longitudinal growth study. *Int J Obes.* 1991; 15(7):479.
56. Whitaker RC, Pepe MS, Wright JA et al. Early adiposity rebound and the risk of adult obesity. *Pediatrics.* 1998; 101(3):E5.
57. Reinhardt C, Reigstad CS, and Bäckhed F. Intestinal microbiota during infancy and its implications for obesity. *J Pediatr Gastroenterol Nutr.* 2009; 48:249–256.
58. Suau A, Bonnet R, Sutren M et al. Direct analysis of genes encoding 16S rRNA from complex communities reveals many novel molecular species within the human gut. *Appl Environ Microbiol.* 1999; 65(11):4799–4807.
59. Savage DC. Microbial ecology of the gastrointestinal tract. *Annu Rev Microbiol.* 1977; 31:107–133.
60. Andersson A, Lindberg M, Jakobsson H et al. Comparative analysis of human gut microbiota by barcoded pyrosequencing. *PLoS ONE* 2008; 3(7): Article ID e2836.
61. Hayashi H, Sakamoto M, and Benno Y. Phylogenetic analysis of the human gut microbiota using 16S rDNA clone libraries and strictly anaerobic culture-based methods. *Microbiol Immunol.* 2002; 46(8):535–548.
62. Stecher B and Hardt WD. The role of microbiota in infectious disease. *Trends Microbiol.* 2008; 16(3):107–114.
63. Lovat LB. Age related changes in gut physiology and nutritional status. *Gut.* 1996; 38:306–309.
64. Phillips SF, Pemberton JH, Shorter RG, Macfarlane GT, and Cummings JH. The colonic flora, fermentation and large bowel digestive function. In *The Large Intestine: Physiology, Pathophysiology and Disease,* (eds.) Phillips SF, Pemberton JH, Shorter RG (Raven Press, New York), 1991, pp. 51–92.

65. Stark PL and Lee A. The microbial ecology of the large bowel of breast-fed and formula-fed infants during the first year of life. *J Med Microbiol.* 1982; 15:189–203.

66. Hentges DJ, Finegold SM, Sutter VL et al. Normal indigenous intestinal flora. In *Human Intestinal Microflora in Health and Disease*, (ed.) Hentges DJ (Academic Press, New York), 1983, pp. 3–31.

67. Gorbach SL, Nahas L, Lerner PI et al. Effects of diet, age, and periodic sampling on numbers of faecal microorganisms in man. *Gastroenterology* 1967; 53:845–855.

68. Everard A, Belzer C, Geurts L et al. Cross-talk between *Akkermansia muciniphila* and intestinal epithelium controls diet-induced obesity. *Proc Natl Acad Sci USA.* 2013; 110(22):9066–9071.

69. Bäckhed F, Manchester J, Semenkovich C et al. Mechanisms underlying the resistance to diet-induced obesity in germ-free mice. *Proc Natl Acad Sci USA.* 2007; 104:979–984.

70. Bäckhed F, Ding H, Wang T et al. The gut microbiota as an environmental factor that regulates fat storage. *Proc Natl Acad Sci USA.* 2004; 101:15718–15723.

71. Ley RE, Turnbaugh PJ, Klein S et al. Microbial ecology: Human gut microbes associated with obesity. *Nature.* 2006; 444(7122):1022–1023.

72. Hattori M and Taylor TD. The human intestinal microbiome: A new frontier of human biology. *DNA Res.* 2009; 16(1):1–12.

73. Zhang H, DiBaise JK, Zuccoto A et al. Human gut microbiota in obesity and after gastric bypass. *Proc Natl Acad Sci USA.* 2009; 106(7):2365–2370.

74. Margaret L, Brandi L, and Zhenqiu L. Analysis of the gut microbiota in the old order amish and its relation to the metabolic syndrome. *PLoS ONE.* 2012; 7(8):e43052.

75. Santacruz A, Collado M, Garcia L et al. Gut microbiota composition is associated with body weight, weight gain and biochemical parameters in pregnant women. *Br J Nutr.* 2010; 104(1):83–92.

76. Sanzy Y, Santacruz A, Gauffin P. Gut microbiota in obesity and metabolic disorders. *Proceedings of the Nutrition Society,* August 2010; 69(3):434–441.

77. Goldman P. Herbal medicines today and the roots of modern pharmacology. *Ann Intern Med.* 2001; 135(8 Pt 1):594.

78. FDA. 2007. Issues dietary supplements final rule. Available at: www.fda.gov/bbs/topics/NEWS/2007/NEW01657.html (Accessed on March 18, 2008).

79. Therapeutic Research Faculty. 2002. Natural medicines comprehensive database. Available at: http://www.naturaldatabase.com (Accessed online August 18, 2004).

80. Weiger WA, Smith M, Boon H et al. Advising patients who seek complementary and alternative medical therapies for cancer. *Ann Intern Med.* 2002; 137:889–903.

81. Shekelle PG, Hardy ML, Morton SC et al. Efficacy and safety of ephedra and ephedrine for weight loss and athletic performance: A meta-analysis. *JAMA.* 2003; 289:1537–1545.

82. Althuis MD, Jordan NE, Ludington EA et al. Glucose and insulin responses to dietary chromium supplements: A meta-analysis. *Am J Clin Nutr.* 2002; 76:148–155.

83. Vincent JB. The potential value and toxicity of chromium picolinate as a nutritional supplement, weight loss agent and muscle development agent. *Sports Med.* 2003; 33:213–230.

84. Sotaniemi EA, Haapakoski E, Rautio A. Ginseng therapy in non-insulin-dependent diabetic patients. *Diabetes Care.* 1995; 18:1373–1375.

85. Mattes RD and Bormann L. Effects of (−)-hydroxycitric acid on appetitive variables. *Physiol Behav.* 2000; 71:87–94.

86. Heymsfield SB, Allison DB, Vasselli JR et al. Cambogia (hydroxycitric acid) as a potential antiobesity agent: A randomized controlled trial. *JAMA.* 1998; 280:1596–1600.

87. Dulloo AG, Duret C, Rohrer D et al. Efficacy of a green tea extract rich in catechin polyphenols and caffeine in increasing 24-h energy expenditure and fat oxidation in humans. *Am J Clin Nutr.* 1999; 70:1040–1045.

88. Armanini D, De Palo CB, Mattarello MJ et al. Effect of licorice on the reduction of body fat mass in healthy subjects. *J Endocrinol Invest.* 2003; 26:646–650.

89. Ernst E and Pittler MH. Chitosan as a treatment for body weight reduction? A meta-analysis. *Perfusion.* 1998; 11:461–465.

90. Pittler MH, Abbot NC, Harkness EF et al. Double blind trial of chitosan for body weight reduction. *Eur J Clin Nutr.* 1999; 53:379–381.

91. Wuolijoki E, Hirvela T, and Ylitalo P. Decrease in serum LDL cholesterol with micro-crystalline chitosan. *Methods Find Exp Clin Pharmacol.* 1999; 21:357–361.

92. Ho SC, Tai ES, Eng PH et al. In the absence of dietary surveillance, chitosan does not reduce plasma lipids or obesity in hypercholesterolaemic obese Asian subjects. *Singapore Med J.* 2001; 42:6–10.

93. Food and Drug Administration. FDA Consumer. SMG 2180.1, transmittal Number 81–87, 1981:3.

94. Foster GD, Wadden TA, Vogt RA et al. What is a reasonable weight loss? Patients' expectations and evaluations of obesity treatment outcomes. *J Consult Clin Psychol.* 1997; 65(1):79.

95. Douketis JD, Macie C, Thabane L et al. Systematic review of long-term weight loss studies in obese adults: Clinical significance and applicability to clinical practice. *Int J Obes (Lond).* 2005; 29(10):1153.

96. Knowler WC, Barrett E, Fowler SE et al. Reduction in the incidence of type 2 diabetes with lifestyle intervention or metformin. *N Engl J Med.* 2002; 346(6):393.

97. Heymsfield SB, Harp JB, Reitman ML et al. Why do obese patients not lose more weight when treated with low-calorie diets? A mechanistic perspective. *Am J Clin Nutr.* 2007; 85(2):346.

98. Trabulsi J and Schoeller DA, Evaluation of dietary assessment instruments against doubly labeled water, a biomarker of habitual energy intake. *Am J Physiol Endocrinol Metab.* 2001; 281(5):E891.

99. Roberts SB and Rosenberg I. Nutrition and aging: Changes in the regulation of energy metabolism with aging. *Physiol Rev.* 2006; 86(2):651.

100. Hall KD, Sacks G, Chandramohan D et al. Quantification of the effect of energy imbalance on bodyweight. *Lancet.* August 2011; 378(9793):826–837.

101. Lin PH, Proschan MA, Bray GA et al. Estimation of energy requirements in a controlled feeding trial. *Am J Clin Nutr.* 2003; 77(3):639.

102. Sumithran P, Prendergast LA, Delbridge E et al. Long-term persistence of hormonal adaptations to weight loss. *N Engl J Med.* October 2011; 365(17):1597–1604.

103. Freedman MR, King J, Kennedy E. Popular diets: A scientific review. *Obes Res.* 2001; 9(Suppl 1):1S.

104. Dietary Reference Intakes (DRIs). 2001. Energy, Carbohydrate, Fiber, Fat, Fatty Acids, Cholesterol, Protein, and Amino Acids (Macronutrients). Institute of Medicine. http://www.nap.edu/openbook.php?isbn = 0309085373 (Accessed May 1, 2009).

105. Howard BV, Manson JE, Stefanick ML et al. Low-fat dietary pattern and weight change over 7 years: The Women's Health Initiative Dietary Modification Trial. *JAMA.* 2006; 295(1):39.

106. Lydia A, Tian Hu, Kristi R et Al. Effects of low-carbohydrate and low-fat diets: A randomized trial. *Ann Intern Med.* 2014; 161(5):309–318.

107. Atkins RC. *Dr. Atkins' New Diet Revolution.* New York: Avon Books; 2002.

108. Astrup A, Meinert T, Harper A. Atkins and other low-carbohydrate diets: Hoax or an effective tool for weight loss? *Lancet.* 2004; 364:897.

109. Atkins RC. *Atkins for Life.* New York: St. Martin's Press; 2003.

110. WebMD. http://www.m.webmd.com/diet/dukan-diet (Accessed April 25, 2015).

111. Goff SL, Foody JM, Inzucchi S et al. Nutrition and weight loss information in a popular diet book: Is it fact, fiction, or something in between? *J General Internal Med.* 2006; 21:769.

112. Rutten LF, Yaroch A, Colon-Ramos U et al. Awareness, use, and perceptions of low-carbohydrate diets. *Prevent Chronic Dis.* 2008; 5(4):A130.

113. Last AR and Wilson SA. Low-carbohydrate diets. *Am Family Phys.* 2006; 73:1942.
114. South Beach Diet recipes. 2009. South beach diet online. http://www.southbeachdiet.com/sbd/publicsite/south-beach-diet-recipes.aspx (Accessed on March 22, 2011).
115. Agatston AS. *The South Beach Diet: The Delicious, Doctor-Designed, Foolproof Plan for Fast and Healthy Weight Loss.* Emmaus, PA: Rodale; 2003.
116. Heshka S, Anderson JW, Atkinson RL et al. Weight loss with self-help compared with a structured commercial program: A randomized trial. *JAMA.* 2003; 289(14):1792.
117. Jolly K, Lewis A, Beach J et al. Comparison of range of commercial or primary care led weight reduction programmes with minimal intervention control for weight loss in obesity: Lighten up randomised controlled trial. *BMJ.* 2011; 343:d6500.
118. Ahern AL, Olson AD, Aston LM et al. Weight Watchers on prescription: An observational study of weight change among adults referred to Weight Watchers by the NHS. *BMC Public Health.* 2011; 11:434.
119. Dixon KJL, Shcherba S, Kipping RR. Weight loss from three commercial providers of NHS primary care slimming on referral in North Somerset: Service evaluation. *J Public Health.* 2012; 34(4):555–561.

14 Nutritional Management of Upper Gastrointestinal Disorders

Francis Okeke, MD, MPH
and Bani Chander Roland, MD

CONTENTS

INTRODUCTION

Over the past decade, the increasing importance of nutritional supplements as items of medicinal value has gained increasing recognition. The critical need for optimizing nutrition, as a means to rapid recovery from acute illness and convalescent periods after prolonged illness, has recently carved a niche within the medical field. This came about when the government and insurance providers began to recognize the value of nutritional status to the comprehensive evaluation and approach to disease treatment and subsequently began reimbursing medical practitioners for demonstrating that this aspect of patient care was addressed in both the inpatient and outpatient clinical settings.

In this chapter, we will review some of the common upper gastrointestinal (GI) disorders, including gastroesophageal reflux disease (GERD), eosinophilic esophagitis (EoE), gastroparesis, celiac disease (CD), and irritable bowel syndrome (IBS), with a look at the definition, etiology, pathophysiology, diagnosis, and management of each disorder. The majority of our focus will be on the nutritional management aspects of these disorders.

GASTROESOPHAGEAL REFLUX DISEASE

INTRODUCTION

Gastroesophageal reflux is thought to be a physiological phenomenon that occurs in individuals of all ages. Physiological gastroesophageal reflux simply involves the retrograde transition of gastric or duodenal contents into the esophagus (typically the lower third of the esophagus). GERD, on the other hand, is defined as symptoms or complications resulting from the reflux of gastric contents into the esophagus or beyond, into the oral cavity (including larynx) or lung [1]. It can be further classified as the presence of symptoms without erosions on endoscopic examination (nonerosive disease or NERD) or GERD symptoms with erosions present (ERD) [1].

Symptoms of GERD can be divided into typical esophageal, atypical, and extra-esophageal, and are listed in Table 14.1.

TABLE 14.1
Symptoms of GERD

GERD Symptoms		
Esophageal Symptoms	**Atypical Symptoms**	**Extraesophageal Symptoms**
Heartburn	Dyspepsia	Noncardiac chest pain
Regurgitation	Epigastric pain	Cough
Dysphagia	Nausea	Dental erosions
	Bloating	Erosions of dental enamel
	Belching	Sinusitis
		Chronic laryngitis
		Globus
		Voice disturbances—hoarseness
		Otitis media

TABLE 14.2
Factors That Contribute to GERD

Gastric	**Esophageal**	**Others**
Large meals	Esophageal dysmotility	Decreased salivation
Delayed gastric emptying	LES dysfunction—TLESR, hypotensive LES	Duodenal dysmotility
Pyloric dysfunction	Impaired mucosal resistance	Connective tissue disorders (scleroderma)
H. pylori	Increased esophageal acid exposure	Lying down
		Increased
		Obesity
		Pregnancy
		Hypothyroidism (leads to LES dysfunction)
		Medications

PATHOPHYSIOLOGY

The pathophysiology of GERD is in simple terms exposure of the esophagus and other extraesophageal structures to gastric and duodenal contents, in the presence of conditions that promote this. Some physiological measures are in place to help decrease these reflux episodes and include the lower esophageal sphincter (LES), crural diaphragm, and remaining supine after meals. Certain conditions tend to favor this recurrent and prolonged exposure to gastric and duodenal contents; these conditions are listed in Table 14.2.

DIAGNOSIS

The diagnosis of GERD involves evaluation of clinical symptoms, use of endoscopic findings, coupled with gastric and esophageal biopsies, and histopathologic findings.

TABLE 14.3
Establishing the Diagnosis of GERD

Recommendations

1. A presumptive diagnosis of GERD can be established in the setting of typical symptoms of heartburn and regurgitation. Empiric medical therapy with a PPI is recommended in this setting. (Strong recommendation, moderate level of evidence)

2. Patients suspected to have noncardiac chest pain due to GERD should have diagnostic evaluation before institution of therapy. (Conditional recommendation, moderate level of evidence) A cardiac cause should be excluded in patients with chest pain before the commencement of a gastrointestinal evaluation. (Strong recommendation, low level of evidence)

3. Barium radiographs should not be performed to diagnose GERD. (Strong recommendation, high level of evidence)

4. Upper endoscopy is not required in the presence of typical GERD symptoms. Endoscopy is recommended in the presence of alarm symptoms and for screening of patients at high risk for complications. Repeat endoscopy is not indicated in patients without Barrett' s esophagus in the absence of new symptoms. (Strong recommendation, moderate level of evidence)

5. Routine biopsies from the distal esophagus are not recommended specifically to diagnose GERD. (Strong recommendation, moderate level of evidence)

6. Esophageal manometry is recommended for preoperative evaluation, but has no role in the diagnosis of GERD. (Strong recommendation, low level of evidence)

7. Ambulatory esophageal reflux monitoring is indicated before consideration of endoscopic or surgical therapy in patients with NERD, as part of the evaluation of patients refractory to PPI therapy and in situations when the diagnosis of GERD is in question. (Strong recommendation, low level evidence.) Ambulatory reflux monitoring is the only test that can assess reflux symptom association. (Strong recommendation, low level of evidence)

8. Ambulatory reflux monitoring is not required in the presence of short- or long-segment Barrett's esophagus to establish a diagnosis of GERD. (Strong recommendation, moderate level of evidence)

9. Screening for *Helicobacter pylori* infection is not recommended in GERD. Eradication of *H. pylori* infection is not routinely required as part of antireflux therapy. (Strong recommendation, low level of evidence)

Source: Katz, P.O. et al., *Am. J. Gastroenterol.*, 108(3), 308, 2013.

Other objective diagnostic modalities include ambulatory pH monitoring (24 h pH impedance monitoring and BRAVO capsule for 48–96 h pH monitoring). In certain cases, a modified barium swallow and esophageal manometry can also be helpful. Finally, one of the most useful diagnostic methods is a proton-pump inhibitor (PPI) trial. Katz et al. [1] in their 2013 guidelines on the diagnosis of GERD summarized the current recommendations that are adapted in Table 14.3.

MANAGEMENT

Current recommendations favor the use of PPIs empirically as part of the initial approach and management of those patients who present with classic symptoms of GERD (e.g., heartburn and regurgitation).

A main component of the initial management recommendations for GERD is dietary and lifestyle modifications including

- Avoidance of ingestion of large or heavy meals, instead replacing with smaller and more frequent meals
- Avoidance of eating at least 2–3 h prior to bed
- Avoidance of items that decrease LES pressure including caffeinated beverages, alcohol, chocolate, citrus-based foods, tomato-based foods, spicy foods, heavily processed foods, garlic, onions, peppermint, fried/fatty foods
- Avoidance of medications that may trigger or aggravate GERD (e.g., nitrates, theophylline, alpha-adrenergic blockers, beta-adrenergic agonists, NSAIDs, anticholinergics, benzodiazepines, tricyclic antidepressants, bisphosphonates)
- Elevate the head of the bed (use of multiple pillows to try to achieve this is not advised since this tends to aggravate the problem by increasing the pressure on the lower sternum and causing reflux of gastric contents, one can use cinder blocks, or wooden-shaped blocks)
- Weight loss, if obese
- Avoid tight-fitting clothes around the abdomen or chest area
- Avoidance of nicotine

Some nutritional supplements that have preliminarily been recommended for use in the management of GERD include the following:

- Acupuncture [2,3].
- Almonds.
- Apples.
- Apple cider vinegar—has been used over decades as an old household remedy for GERD symptoms, typically taken as 1–2 tablespoons diluted in a glass of water during acute symptoms.
- Chamomile tea.
- Deglycyrrhizinated licorice (DGL) [4], slippery elm, and marshmallow are herbs that soothe irritated tissues (aka demulcents).
- D-Limonene—often times used as a fragrance and flavoring agent in body products and is found in citrus oils [5]. The purported mechanism of action is by improving gastric emptying and GI motility.
- Ginger—used in multiple different formulations and one of the common methods is ginger ale, ginger candy/mints.
- Gingko biloba [4].
- Glutamine—not been studied extensively, but has been suggested at a dose of 1,000–10,000 mg/day, for 1–2 months to help alleviate symptoms of GERD [4]. The pathogenesis of NERD is partly from defective barrier function of the esophageal lining, permitting luminal refluxed hydrogen ions to irritate submucosal nerves. Glutamine helps facilitate healing of small intestine lining cells, but it is unclear whether its effect upon GERD is from the normalization of esophageal permeability.

- Green tea polyphenols [4].
- Iberogast: this herbal remedy contains nine different herbs (angelica, caraway, clown's mustard plant, German chamomile, greater celandine, lemon balm, licorice, milk thistle, and peppermint), and it is still not clear which of the herbs helps with heartburn [6].
- Lonicerae (Chinese Honeysuckle flower, jin yin jua)—no human studies to date, but animal study was promising.
- Low carbohydrate diet [2,7–9].
- Melatonin [2,10,11].
- Milk: prior to the advent of acid-suppressive therapy such as H_2 blockers (ranitidine, cimetidine) or PPIs, people ingested milk to treat their symptoms, which was thought to act as a natural antacid to palliate symptoms of GERD. However, as with peptic ulcers, the calcium in milk actually increases gastric acid secretion, and whole milk fat may decrease LES pressure and theoretically worsen GERD.
- Okra extracts have been used to help with symptoms of GERD; however, some of the formulations have alginate as an ingredient, and this anionic polysaccharide when it binds with water forms a viscous gum, which has been used in some antacid formulations to help with symptoms of GERD.
- Prebiotics [4].
- Probiotics [4].
- Raft-forming agents (natural substances like alginate, pectin, and carbenoxolone—which is a synthetic derivative of glycyrrhizin) are so called as they form a viscous gel when they interact with gastric acid and coat the top of the gastric content protecting the gastroesophageal junction and the lower esophagus from refluxate [12–15].
- Spearmint/peppermint oil [16,17].
- Zinc L carnosine is a supplement that theoretically facilitates healing of the lining of the hyperpermeable esophageal mucosa in GERD [95,96].

ESOPHAGEAL EOSINOPHILIA AND EOSINOPHILIC ESOPHAGITIS

INTRODUCTION

In 1993, Attwood et al. described the histological and phenotypic features of EoE [18]. Later on in 2007, the consensus recommendations/guidelines on the management of EoE were published [19]; these were subsequently revised in 2011 [20] and also in 2013 [21] with the availability of new information about the disease process. Since the first publication on EoE in 1993, the number of publications on EoE has increased dramatically, and with this increased awareness of the disease, the prevalence has steadily increased, as more gastroenterologists, allergists, and immunologists diagnose patients with the disorder.

Esophageal eosinophilia (EE) is the finding of an abnormal increase in eosinophils in the squamous epithelium of the esophagus in patients without any clinical symptoms of EoE. Conditions that are associated with EE include achalasia; CD; Crohn's disease; connective tissue disease; drug hypersensitivity response; EoE; eosinophilic gastroenteritis and other eosinophilic GI diseases (EGID); GERD; graft vs. host disease; hypereosinophilic syndrome (HES); pemphigoid vegetans; PPIs; vasculitis, and should be looked for if EE is found on histology.

In the 2011 guidelines, EoE was defined as a chronic, immune/antigen-mediated esophageal disease characterized clinically by symptoms related to esophageal dysfunction and histologically by eosinophil-predominant inflammation [20]. In the 2013 guidelines, EoE was defined as a primary clinicopathologic disorder of the esophagus, characterized by esophageal and/or upper GI tract symptoms in association with esophageal mucosal biopsy specimens containing ≥15 intraepithelial eosinophil's/HPF in one or more biopsy specimens and absence of pathologic GERD as evidenced by a normal pH monitoring study of the distal esophagus or lack of response to high-dose PPI medication [21].

PPI-responsive EE is described as patients with both clinical and histologic features of EoE; however, they respond histologically to PPI treatment unlike in EoE [21,22].

EoE is a condition that has been observed in both children and adults, and as with most other diseases, presentation differences have been documented for both groups. Children typically present with the findings listed in Table 14.4, and adults more often present with the symptoms listed in Table 14.5.

TABLE 14.4
Presenting Symptoms of EoE in Children

Feeding refusal
GERD symptoms: heartburn, regurgitation
Dysphagia
Food impaction
Failure to thrive
Emesis
Chest pain
Abdominal pain
Diarrhea

TABLE 14.5
Presenting Symptoms of EoE in Adults

Intermittent dysphagia
Food impaction
GERD like symptoms—heartburn, regurgitation
Chest pain
Abdominal pain
Diarrhea
Weight loss

PATHOPHYSIOLOGY

The pathophysiology of EoE is not fully understood, but both genetic and environmental factors have been implicated. The underlying immune response has been linked to adaptive T-cell immunity driven mostly by type 2 T helper cells [23], involving interleukin (IL) 13, 15, and 5 expressions [24–26].

A significant number of patients with EoE report a history of atopy/allergies and peripheral eosinophilia [27–29]. This association of atopy and allergies with EoE has led to the hypothesis that recruitment of eosinophils in the esophagus may be an immune response to environmental antigens in individuals that are genetically susceptible or predisposed. This theory has been supported by a few observations including feeding children with EoE an elemental diet has led to the resolution of both histologic findings and clinical symptoms [30], and fewer cases are seen in the winter months when it is assumed that outdoor allergens are greatly reduced [31].

The evidence of familial clustering supports a genetic basis for EoE, and this is further supported with the identification of a possible susceptibility locus on chromosome 5q22 [32]. A positive family history of EoE has also been observed in some patients. Some genetic defects have additionally been identified that may predispose to EoE, including a defect in filaggrin, a barrier-protective molecule, typically found in the skin [33] and in thymic stromal lymphopoietin, a cytokine involved in Th 2 cell determination [32].

DIAGNOSIS

The diagnosis of EoE requires both the clinical symptoms and histological presence of eosinophils >15/hpf following a trial of acid-suppressive therapy. The suggested diagnostic approach is detailed in the 2013 AGA guidelines, on diagnosis and management of EoE [21].

Some endoscopic features of the esophageal mucosa have been described in patients with EoE; these are not pathognomonic for EoE because they have also been seen in other conditions, and a meta-analysis in 2012 showed that endoscopic findings had a low sensitivity ranging from 15% to 48% for diagnosing EoE, but a high specificity ranging from 90% to 95%. The endoscopic findings include the following:

- Fixed esophageal rings (sometimes called corrugated rings or trachealization), transient esophageal rings (sometimes called feline folds or felinization, or stacked circular rings) 44%
- Whitish exudates/papules (representing eosinophil microabscesses) 27%
- Longitudinal/linear furrows 48%
- Attenuation of the subepithelial vascular pattern 41%
- Edema
- Diffuse esophageal narrowing
- Narrow-caliber/small-caliber esophagus 9%

- Esophageal lacerations induced by passage of the endoscope (a sign of mucosal fragility when severe, the esophagus has been described as crepe paper)
- Strictures

Other diagnostic modalities that have been implemented include the following:

- Esophageal pH monitoring (and pH impedance, where available) is a useful diagnostic test to evaluate for GERD in patients with EE [20].
- Radiographic studies—barium studies may show mucosal abnormalities associated with EoE, but as noted in the endoscopic findings are nonspecific and will still require histologic diagnosis via mucosal biopsies.
- Endoscopic ultrasonography role in EoE Dx or management?
- Impedance planimetry (EndoFlip)—an imaging technique that displays the distensibility of hollow viscera and has been applied to the esophagus to characterize the biomechanical properties of the esophagogastric junction, the esophageal body, and the pharyngoesophageal sphincter [34].
- Esophageal manometry—EoE has been associated with esophageal dysmotility including panesophageal pressurization [35] and esophageal dysmotility of uncertain clinical significance [36]. These findings, however, are not pathognomonic for EoE.

MANAGEMENT

EoE can be effectively managed by a variety of approaches including, more prominently, dietary/nutritional, pharmacologic, and endoscopic approaches. There are currently no clear guidelines outlining an evidence-based treatment approach to EoE, and most treatment approaches at the present time are based on clinician experience, a handful of case reports, and smaller controlled trials.

Dietary/Nutritional

The primary goal of the dietary approach in the management of EoE is to decrease the exposure to food allergens, which are thought to be the primary triggers for the immune reaction that leads to recruitment of eosinophils. The role of food allergens as triggers for EoE was corroborated after studies were conducted showing that feeding children having EoE with an elemental diet (made up of amino acids, e.g., vivonex, thereby eliminating exposure to any food allergens) led to the resolution of EE [30].

Three primary approaches are currently recognized for the initiation of a dietary avoidance of food allergen triggers in patients with EoE:

- *Elemental diet*—this approach uses an elemental diet that basically consists of amino acids leading to the elimination of any potential food allergens entirely as macronutrients are predigested. This approach usually works in children, but is difficult to adhere to in adults and can sometimes be very expensive if not covered by insurance.

- *Directed elimination diet/testing-based elimination diet*—with this approach, patients with EoE typically undergo skin prick testing and atopy patch testing looking for any IgE-mediated food allergies. Any foods that test positive are removed from the diet; cow milk is removed empirically since it has a poor negative predictive value on testing.
- *Empiric elimination diet/six food elimination diet*—involves empirically avoiding foods that have a high prevalence of leading to immediate hypersensitivity in a population (IgE-mediated food reactions). The six foods that have been studied include milk, egg, soy, wheat, peanuts/tree nuts, and fish/shellfish.

The choice of an approach is often driven by multiple factors including efficacy of diet, cost, ease of compliance, convenience, as well as physician and patient preference. It often makes sense to include the family/spouse in the diet plan if the patient lives with other family members, as this has been shown to help maintain adherence. Studies have shown varying degrees of nonadherence to diet in EoE patients placed on an elimination diet, with one study reporting that up to 33% of patients are noncompliant [37].

GASTROPARESIS

INTRODUCTION

The normal motor function of the GI tract has been identified as a complex series of events requiring coordination of the autonomic nervous system (both sympathetic and parasympathetic nervous systems), the enteric nervous system (neurons and pacemaker cells—known as the interstitial cells of Cajal (ICC), found within the stomach, intestine, and smooth muscle cells of the GI tract), and finally the smooth muscle cells of the GI tract (with excitable membranes that contain specific receptors that bind to amines, peptides, and other transmitters that are propagated via neurocrine, endocrine, or paracrine routes) [38]. Any disruptions within this complex series of events are usually associated with some dysfunction of the motor function of the GI tract.

Gastroparesis is a syndrome of objectively delayed gastric emptying in the absence of a mechanical obstruction along with associated symptoms of nausea, emesis, early satiety, bloating, and upper abdominal pain [38]. The inherent problems associated with gastroparesis are myriad and lead not only to decreased productivity, but also to a host of psychosocial problems.

The etiology of gastroparesis has been associated with a few conditions, but overall the most common causes include idiopathic, diabetic, postsurgical, and postinfectious [39].

1. *Idiopathic*—this has been estimated to be the etiology of approximately one half of the patients with delayed gastric emptying [39].
2. *Iatrogenic/postsurgical*—this mechanism is thought to involve inadvertent or intended damage to the vagus nerve during thoracic or upper abdominal surgery.

3. *Diabetes mellitus (DM)*—has been recognized as the systemic illness associated with gastric dysfunction more often than any other. Multiple mechanisms have been proposed as the possible etiologies of the gastric dysfunction associated with DM, and these are discussed in detail in the next section on pathophysiology.

4. *Postinfectious*—a postinfectious *nerve-stunning* effect has been ascribed to the dysmotility that ensues following an infection of the GI tract. This effect usually is thought to be self-limiting after a few years.

5. *Neurologic disorders*—certain neurologic disorders may lead to either damage of the vagus nerve, the autonomic nervous system, the enteric nervous system, and/or the myenteric plexus including multiple sclerosis, cerebrovascular accident of the brainstem, amyloid neuropathy, diabetic neuropathy, primary dysautonomias, AIDS neuropathy, and parkinsonism. Some medications used to treat neurologic disorders are associated with gastric dysfunction, including dopaminergics and anticholinergics.

6. *Medications*—some medications are well known to cause delay in gastric emptying and also total gut dysfunction with the commonest culprit being narcotic medications. Other medications that have been implicated in delayed gastric emptying include alpha 2 adrenergic agonists, amylin analogues, calcium channel blockers, cyclosporine, dopamine agonists, glucagon-like peptide (GLP)-1 agonists, muscarinic cholinergic receptor antagonists, octreotide, phenothiazines.

7. *Connective tissue disorders*—connective tissue disorders and infiltrative disorders have been associated with gastroparesis, and often, other areas of the GI tract are involved.

PATHOPHYSIOLOGY

The pathophysiology of gastroparesis may be explained based on the differing etiologies, as it appears that each etiology has a separate or multiple mechanisms leading to the gastric dysfunction and subsequently the symptoms associated with the syndrome. Additional theories suggest that different areas of the stomach (e.g., antral, fundic, cardia) can be affected differently by a variety of diseases.

Common etiologies of gastroparesis include the following:

1. *Idiopathic*—the pathophysiological mechanism underlying idiopathic gastroparesis is still poorly understood, but one postulated mechanism has been a possible autoimmune GI dysmotility [40], which may be idiopathic or occur in association with a remote neoplasm (most commonly small cell lung cancer).

2. *Postsurgical/iatrogenic*—damage to the vagus nerve usually leads to a dysfunction in the accommodation response of the stomach and also the phasic contractility of the stomach is lost [41].

3. *DM*—multiple mechanisms have been proposed on the pathogenesis of gastroparesis in diabetics; some are clearly understood and have been studied

extensively, while others are still hypotheses that need further research. Some of the mechanisms that have been proposed include the following:

a. *Hyperglycemia*—elevated serum glucose levels have been implicated in gastric emptying dysfunction. This has been postulated to occur via reduction in the levels of gastric inhibitory peptide and GLP-1 [42], reduction in the postprandial antral contractile activity [43], antroduodenal incoordination [44], and pyloric spasm, which has been shown to rarely exist alone, but is typically associated with hypomotility of the antrum of the stomach [45].

b. *Autonomic dysfunction*—involving damage to the intrinsic nervous system—the ICC, nitrergic neurons—the pacemaker system of the GI tract. Due to a decreased production of stem cell factor by smooth muscles, which has been identified as an important ICC survival factor [46–50].

c. *Oxidative stress*—has also been implicated as a possible mechanism for the gastric dysfunction seen in diabetes. This is thought to be due to failure of the usual upregulation of the enzyme macrophage heme oxygenase-1 seen in diabetics [51].

DIAGNOSIS

A scintigraphic gastric emptying scan after a solid meal showing delay in emptying is usually the gold standard for the diagnosis of gastroparesis. Evaluation of patients suspected to have gastroparesis should be systematic, and mechanical obstruction should be ruled out. Table 14.6 adapted from the AGA technical review [52] on the diagnosis and treatment of gastroparesis summarizes this.

MANAGEMENT

As with most obscure diseases, the management of gastroparesis is still very difficult.

The only currently FDA approved medication for this condition is metoclopramide (despite its inherent black box warning for irreversible tardive dyskinesia)—which naturally espouses hesitation among providers to prescribe it and additionally lends to poor patient compliance given the known significant associated risks.

Other medications that are often used off-label in the management of gastroparesis include the following:

1. *Promotility agents*—domperidone, erythromycin
2. *Increase antral accommodation*—Buspar
3. *Antinausea and antiemetic agents*—Zofran, Compazine, Phenergan
4. *Other drugs*—Mirtazapine, tricyclic medications, selective serotonin reuptake inhibitors, cannabis, and its derivatives such as marinol

Most times, the initial management approach usually aims to palliate some of the symptoms, which are mostly diet related; therefore, the usual approach is to adopt a *gastroparesis diet* as described in detail later—which for the most part is interpreted very differently by different individuals. Regardless, to date, there has not been a single study evaluating the efficacy of an appropriate diet in these patients.

TABLE 14.6

Evaluation of Patients Suspected to Have Gastroparesis

STEP I: Initial investigation
- Targeted history and physical
- Laboratory tests
  - Complete blood count
  - Complete metabolic profile
  - Amylase if abdominal pain is a significant symptom
  - Lipase
  - Pregnancy test if appropriate
- Abdominal obstruction series if vomiting or pain is acute

STEP II: Evaluate for organic disorders
- Upper endoscopy to evaluate for mechanical obstruction or mucosal lesions (alternative: barium upper gastrointestinal series, often with small bowel follow-through)
- Biliary ultrasound if abdominal pain is a significant symptom

STEP III: Evaluate for delayed gastric emptying
- Solid-phase gastric emptying test
- Screen for secondary causes of gastroparesis—thyroid function test, rheumatologic serologies (ANA, Scl 70, dsDNA, etc.), glycosylated hemoglobin

STEP IV: Treatment trial with a prokinetic agent and or antiemetic agent

STEP V: If no clinical response consider further investigations
- Electrogastrogram (EGG)
- Antroduodenal manometry
- Small bowel evaluation with enteroclysis or small bowel follow-through
- Further laboratory tests if indicated—ANNA, tissue transglutaminase antibody
- Lactulose hydrogen breath test if bloating is a significant symptom

Source: Parkman, H.P. et al., *Gastroenterology*, 127(5), 1592, 2004.

The current understanding of a gastroparesis diet is one with low fat and residue, and more liquid items. The rationale for this is that since the stomach has a difficult time handling digestion of many solid food items (particularly fat and fiber), low residue items are usually better tolerated. Most patients with gastroparesis usually have preserved management of liquid content by the stomach. In this respect, patients are then advised to try to blenderize most of their intake if possible. One of the most important aspects of dietary change is to try to eat smaller-sized more frequent meals throughout the day. Randomized controlled trials are needed looking at the efficacy of different diets on symptom palliation.

When oral intake is inadequate and cannot be tolerated, enteral feeding can be attempted with placement of a jejunal feeding tube. Some studies have shown that in some patients with gastroparesis, a feeding jejunostomy is associated with favorable outcomes (decreased hospitalizations, maintaining nutrition, and improvement in symptoms) [52,53]. But in some patients, this can be difficult if there is concomitant small bowel dysmotility associated with gastroparesis, which is frequently seen in collagen vascular disease. Some providers will insert a trial nasojejunal tube for a few weeks to assess for tolerance to jejunal feeding. Some other tests that have been suggested to evaluate small intestinal transit, but are done mostly for academic and research purposes, include antroduodenojejunal manometry, wireless motility capsule, and small intestinal transit scintigraphy before placement of the jejunal feeding tube [38].

If enteral feeding is not tolerated and patient is unable to maintain their weight and nutritional status, then central parenteral nutrition can be initiated.

Other nutritional remedies that have been used in the management of gastroparesis include the following:

1. *Ginger formulations*—these usually help with nausea in some patients and have evidence to improve gastroparesis when using 1500 mg daily in divided doses [54].
2. *Peppermint formulations*—also known to help with nausea and has also been reported to accelerate the early phase of gastric emptying, increase the relaxation time of the pylorus, and decrease the resting pressure of the LES [17].
3. *Iberogast (STW 5)*—this is a combination of nine herbs, which have different effects on the stomach including inhibitory effects on the proximal stomach and increased motility of the distal stomach [55]. Large prospective studies are needed to determine any therapeutic benefits of Iberogast in patients with gastroparesis.
4. *Melatonin*—close to 500× more melatonin is synthesized in the GI tract than in the pineal gland [56]. Studies of the effects of melatonin on the GI tract have included its effect on GERD symptoms [2,10,11], and colonic transit times [57], but large-scale prospective studies are needed to look at these effects in patients with gastroparesis.
5. *Cinnamon*—in one study was shown to delay gastric emptying if taken in doses of up to 6 g or higher, but was also shown to reduce the postprandial glucose response [58].
6. *Tangweikang (TWK)*—this traditional Chinese herb showed promise in a study investigating its effects on diabetic gastroparesis and was significant in symptom improvement clinically, increasing gastric emptying rate, shortening gastric emptying time, enhancing GI kinetics, and also postprandial glucose control.

CELIAC DISEASE

INTRODUCTION

CD is a chronic, immune-based reaction to dietary gluten (storage protein in wheat, barley, and rye) that primarily affects the small intestine in those with a genetic predisposition and resolves with exclusion of gluten from the diet [59].

Non-celiac gluten sensitivity is thought to be a state of heightened immunological responsiveness to ingested gluten in genetically susceptible individuals [60,61]. CD is thought to occur primarily in Caucasians of Northern European ancestry.

TABLE 14.7
Classification of CD

1. *Classic CD*—which is defined as CD with the following features: villous atrophy, malabsorption symptoms (steatorrhea, weight loss, and other signs of nutrient or vitamin deficiency), and resolution of the mucosal injury following withdrawal of gluten-containing foods. Most patients with classic disease usually have antibodies against gliadin (especially tissue transglutaminase).
2. *Atypical CD*—patients classified as atypical CD usually have minor GI symptoms, but present with other systemic involvement including anemia, enamel defects, arthritis, osteoporosis, abnormal liver transaminases, neurologic symptoms, and infertility, and they all have severe mucosal disease and positive antibodies.
3. *Asymptomatic/Silent CD*—as the name implies, patients in this category are usually asymptomatic or have smoldering nonspecific symptoms like malaise and fatigue. They are usually diagnosed incidentally, and most have the typical architectural remodeling of the intestinal mucosa seen in CD.
4. *Latent CD*—patients in this classification have had normal jejunal mucosa and minor symptoms/no symptoms at some time point while they were on a normal, gluten-containing diet [85]. Two variants of latent CD have been described in the literature:
   a. History of CD in the past, but patient had full recovery with gluten-free diet and remained so even after reintroduction of a normal diet.
   b. Normal mucosa noted at an earlier time while on a normal diet but CD developed later.

The classification of CD is shown in Table 14.7.

The symptoms associated with CD are myriad, and if a clinician is not highly suspicious, the diagnosis is often overlooked. In the past, celiac was classically regarded as a disease of infants who presented with failure to thrive and symptoms of malabsorption. CD has recently been associated with later presentations in life from age 10 to 40 years, thought to be in part due to the longer breast-feeding periods, increased use of formula feeding, and later introduction of gluten in many infants' diet and possibly an association with Cesarean section [62]. Symptoms that have been associated with CD are listed in Table 14.8.

Certain diseases/conditions have been shown to be associated with CD, and the presence of these conditions should raise the suspicion for underlying CD and should also be excluded in patients with previously diagnosed CD. They are listed in Table 14.9.

PATHOPHYSIOLOGY

CD is an autoimmune disorder, as evidenced by the recognition of antibodies to self (autoantibodies—tissue transglutaminase, an enzyme that is involved in the disease pathogenesis). Some of the pathophysiological mechanisms underlying CD are discussed in Table 14.10.

DIAGNOSIS

Diagnostic testing, when performed, should be done with the patient on a gluten diet. This has become somewhat more of a diagnostic challenge as most patients now

TABLE 14.8
Signs and Symptoms of CD

Gastrointestinal

Classic signs/symptoms: diarrhea (stools are usually bulky, foul smelling, and float), flatulence, malabsorption, and its consequences (growth failure in children, weight loss, anemia, neurologic dysfunction from vitamin B deficiencies, osteopenia from vitamin D and calcium deficiencies).

Atypical symptoms: in more recent times, patients have been presenting with atypical symptoms and on occasion asymptomatic—one study found a 38% pooled prevalence of CD patients presenting with IBS-like symptoms [86].

Non-gastrointestinal

1. *Neuropsychiatric*: headache, peripheral neuropathy, ataxia, depression, dysthymia, anxiety, seizures
2. *Musculoskeletal*: osteoarthritis, metabolic bone disease (osteopenia, osteoporosis)
3. *Hematologic*: Iron-deficiency anemia, hyposplenism
4. *Renal*: IgA deposition in the glomerulus
5. *Pulmonary*: Idiopathic pulmonary hemosiderosis (also known as Lane-Hamilton syndrome) has been described to coexist with celiac disease

Oncologic

Multiple studies have been done looking at the mortality and cancer risk in patients with celiac disease and a small absolute increase in the overall mortality of patients with celiac disease when compared to the general population. The strongest cancer link has been linked with lymphoma (non-Hodgkin's lymphoma) and other GI cancers.

TABLE 14.9
Conditions Associated with CD

Dermatitis herpetiformis

Down's syndrome

Selective IgA deficiency

Autoimmune conditions

Type 1 diabetes mellitus

Polyglandular autoimmune syndrome type III (immune-mediated diabetes combined with autoimmune thyroiditis)

Thyroid disease

Liver disease (chronic low-grade elevations in serum aminotransferases; primary biliary cirrhosis

Eosinophilic esophagitis

Inflammatory bowel disease: ulcerative colitis > Crohn's

Gastroesophageal reflux disease (GERD)

Reproductive and menstrual issues

Cardiovascular: myocarditis, cardiomyopathy, ischemic heart disease

Atrophic glossitis

Pancreatitis

TABLE 14.10

Pathophysiological Mechanisms of CD

1. *Genetic Factors*

   There is a close association of CD with HLA-DQ2 and DQ8 gene loci, with an estimated 36% contribution rate to the development of the disease among siblings [87]. Some non-HLA locus genes that increase the risk for developing CD have also been identified [88,89].

2. *Gliadin Reactive T Cells*

   Tissue transglutaminase is an intracellular enzyme released by inflammatory and endothelial cells and fibroblasts in response to mechanical irritation. It has also been found to be able to deamidate glutamine residues in gluten to glutamic acid, which leads to negatively charged gluten peptides, which then increases its ability to bind to HLA-DQ2 and DQ8, potentiating their T-cell-stimulating capacity [90,91].

3. Innate Immunity

   It has been suggested that an innate immune response to wheat proteins is also involved in the pathogenesis of CD and might even be necessary to trigger the gliadin-specific (adaptive) T-cell response in genetically predisposed individuals described earlier [92].

4. Autoantibodies

   Antigliadin antibodies—it has been suggested that antigliadin antibodies are not essential for the pathogenesis of CD [93].

   Endomysial antibodies—while these are rarely found in the absence of CD and have been implicated in the pathogenesis of the disease.

   Tissue transglutaminase antibodies—which target the antigen within the endomysium, have also been implicated to have some pathogenetic import.

   Other antibodies—patients with CD have been found to have antibodies to other food proteins—including beta-lactoglobulin, ovalbumin, and casein [94].

have a heightened awareness of the disease (with the age of the Internet) and end up simply taking themselves off gluten and if they feel better stay that way. Since no single test can definitely diagnose CD in every individual with the disease, it makes it more important to be aware of the clinical features associated with the disease and have a high index of suspicion.

The AGA position paper on CD [63] suggests serologic testing as the initial diagnostic approach in detecting CD. Two tests, the IgA antiendomysial antibody (EMA) and the IgA tissue transglutaminase antibody (tTGA), are proposed as the initial tests of choice in the primary care setting, with evidence indicating that addition of IgG antigliadin antibody and IgA antigliadin antibody (which are tests that predate the first two tests) is no longer necessary.

Depending on the results of serologic testing, and the degree of suspicion for the presence of CD, other diagnostic testing may be employed including the following:

1. Positive serology: proceed to treatment
2. Negative serology + elevated suspicion:
    a. Presence of documented IgA deficiency—can do IgG EMA or IgG tTGA
    b. Serum levels of IgA

3. Negative serology + high suspicion:
   a. Disease associated HLA alleles—if present can proceed to upper endoscopy and biopsies

It is also reasonable to proceed directly to an upper endoscopy, with small intestinal biopsies, particularly if the patient presents with symptoms that warrants this diagnostic test.

The gold standard for establishing a diagnosis of CD remains distal duodenal/jejunal biopsies that demonstrate the characteristic histologic changes in the intestinal mucosa including the following—range from partial to total villous atrophy, crypt lengthening with an increase in lamina propria, and intraepithelial lymphocytes.

Because several patients with CD have CD-associated alleles (DQ2: 95% of patients, DQ8: 3%–5% of patients), the absence of both of these alleles is often considered sufficient to definitively deem that a patient does not have CD as it has a close-to-99% negative predictive value [63].

MANAGEMENT

CD is the one disease with a clearly known food allergen trigger, and treatment with the resolution of most symptoms comes about with strict avoidance of the allergen. That said, the mainstay in the treatment of CD is the maintenance of a strict gluten-free diet (GFD).

The patient should be managed along six identified elements that make up the term *CELIAC*, as follows:

1. Consult with a dietitian (especially one versed in CD).
2. Education (about CD, consequences of poor compliance).
3. Lifelong maintenance of a GFD.
4. Identify nutritional deficiencies and treat as necessary.
5. Access to support (family, friends, support/advocacy groups).
6. Continuous/constant follow-up by a multidisciplinary team.

Although most patients with CD will respond to a GFD, some patients despite strict GFD and adherence to the diet still have persistent symptoms, with or without serologic and histologic changes, and these patients are termed nonresponders. They have been placed into certain categories, including the following:

1. Poor compliance or inadvertent gluten ingestion (for these patients, further consultation with a dietitian might help increase compliance)
2. Clinical/histologic features that overlap with CD but are caused by other disorders (other disease conditions associated with villous atrophy should be ruled out in these patients)
3. Concurrent disorders (should be sought out and treated if found including lactose intolerance, IBS, small intestinal bacterial overgrowth (SIBO), pancreatic insufficiency, and microscopic colitis)
4. Refractory sprue (trial of immunosuppression)
5. Ulcerative jejunitis or intestinal lymphoma

IRRITABLE BOWEL SYNDROME

INTRODUCTION

IBS is one of the most common GI disorders in the United States and is highly prevalent in young adults, particularly in women [64]. It also remains one of the common causes of work absenteeism. IBS remains a diagnosis of exclusion in patients who present with typical symptoms of this disorder and also after excluding organic conditions such as CD, inflammatory bowel disease, infections, and microscopic colitis. At present, there are a few known effective therapies for this syndrome, given that the pathophysiology of the disorder remains elusive.

PATHOPHYSIOLOGY

Although the pathophysiology of this disorder remains uncertain, the role of altered GI motility, visceral hypersensitivity, food sensitivity, alterations in intestinal permeability, dysbiosis, and an altered brain–gut axis have all been implicated in IBS.

Intestinal Dysmotility

Altered GI motility and intestinal spasm are among the commonly implicated mechanisms in IBS. Intestinal transit time appears to be delayed in patients with constipation and increases in patients with diarrhea. Preliminary data have suggested that these alterations may be related to serotonin signaling.

Visceral Hypersensitivity/Hyperalgesia

Patients with IBS typically have an enhanced pain perception to rapid stimuli but not to a gradual stimulus. A plausible mechanism for this may be oversensitization of afferent pathways in the dorsal horns. Preliminary data have also suggested that receptor hypersensitivity of the gut wall plays some role in these patients. In fact, prior studies have demonstrated that intrarectal balloon distention at lower volumes elicits pain in IBS subjects as compared to healthy controls [65]. Interestingly, patients with IBS often complain of abdominal fullness (bloating); however, nearly all of these patients have been found to have normal amounts of gas production as compared to healthy, non-IBS patients [66].

Altered Brain–Gut Axis

Altered CNS perception of visceral events is demonstrated in the pathophysiology of IBS, but the reason for this significant difference is yet unknown. Anxiety and stress initiate these symptoms in these patients. Autonomic dysfunction may also play a significant role in the pathophysiology.

Intestinal Inflammation and Permeability

Patients with predominance of diarrhea, may be postinfectious, have some markers and particular immune cell alterations. The terminal ileum, jejunum, and colon of IBS patients show higher number of mucosal and submucosal mast cells [67,68].

These activated mast cells in colon have correlation with the pain symptoms in IBS patients. Lymphocytes are also increased in small gut and colon in these patients [69]. As these cells release stimulatory substances such as histamine and nitric oxide, this in turn presumably causes impairment in visceral sensations and intestinal motility. Elevated levels of cytokines have also been observed in these patients [70].

Altered Gut Microbiota

It has been hypothesized that an alteration in colonic gut flora leads to overproduction of intestinal gas and results in a change in stool consistency. There has been a well-known association between IBS and SIBO as several studies not only show a markedly increased SIBO prevalence in the IBS population, but also demonstrate an improvement in IBS symptoms following treatment with rifaximin and normalization of breath hydrogen levels [71,72]. Other studies have reported a deficiency in bifidobacteria as one of the most consistent findings in IBS. Probiotics using different strains have been reported to be beneficial in several meta-analyses in the IBS population [73].

Postinfectious

There appears to be an increased risk of IBS development following an acute GI illness [74,75]. (The severity and duration of the infection appears to directly increase the risk of developing IBS.)

Food Sensitivity

Prior studies have also implicated a relationship and overlap between IBS and CD [74,75]. Additionally, even among patients with IBS who test negative for CD (based on histopathology along with serologic and genetic testing), some have been found to have an increase in IgG antibody titers to gluten and to other food antigens [13,14]. FODMAPs (fermentable oligo-, di-, monosaccharides, and polyols) induce symptoms in several IBS patients, which is thought to be in part due to fermentation in the small intestinal and colon. This leads to increased gas production and impaired intestinal permeability. FODMAPs are discussed in more detail in the following later.

Diagnosis

The diagnosis of IBS is largely based on a detailed medical history and clinical symptoms. The physical exam is often unremarkable and of little help in the majority of cases. Common tests that should be done prior to establishing a diagnosis of IBS include celiac testing, hydrogen breath testing for SIBO, stool studies for infectious causes included to evaluate for ova and parasites, complete blood count, comprehensive metabolic panel, and thyroid function testing. Further investigation should of course be done in those patients with any alarm symptoms including weight loss and/or rectal bleeding.

In an attempt to standardize the diagnosis of the condition, diagnostic criteria were developed for IBS. The two most commonly quoted criteria are the Manning and the ROME Criteria.

1. *Manning criteria*—developed in 1978, after Manning and colleagues formulated a symptom complex suggestive of IBS [76].
2. *Rome criteria*—this consensus guideline was published in 1992 (and revised in 2005) in an effort to standardize clinical research protocols involving IBS patients [77]. IBS was defined as a syndrome associated with recurrent abdominal pain or discomfort associated with altered defecation [77]. Some symptoms that are not part of the Rome III criteria, but support a diagnosis of IBS include abnormal stool frequency (<3 bowel movements/ week or >3 bowel movements/day), abnormal stool form, straining during defecation, fecal urgency, sensation of incomplete evacuation, mucus in stool, and bloating.

MANAGEMENT

There have been various approaches implemented in the management of IBS, but all of these approaches mainly target alleviating symptoms, but fail to address the underlying pathophysiological defect of the disorder. Current management approaches include establishment of a close physician–patient relationship, antispasmodics (e.g., dicyclomine and hyoscyamine), laxatives and stool-bulking agents (in IBS-D or IBS-M), probiotics, antidepressants, and dietary management.

Dietary Management

Dietary management remains a mainstay of therapy in IBS. In fact, a careful survey of daily meals often illustrates patterns of symptoms related to specific foods. Dietary management is focused in large part on eliminating foods that may cause increased gas production, leading to abdominal distention and bloating, particularly in those who are hypersensitive. Commonly implicated foods that produce symptoms in IBS include dairy products, caffeine, carbonated beverages, fatty foods, alcohol, and foods high in gluten and FODMAPs. At present, there is no substantial evidence, however, to recommend routine food allergy testing in patients with IBS.

Low-FODMAP Diet

A trial of a low-FODMAP diet may be successful in reducing symptoms in patients with IBS. FODMAPs, a group of short-chain carbohydrates, are poorly absorbed in the small intestine and undergo rapid fermentation in the gut, leading to increased gas production and intestinal distention. FODMAP restriction appears to result in significant improvement in certain patients with IBS, specifically the diarrhea-predominant subtype [78]. In one study, FODMAPs were eliminated from the diet for up to 8 weeks and then successfully reintroduced gradually with foods with highly fermentable carbohydrates to determine the tolerance of each individual food item [79]. Many experts would recommend that all patients with IBS undergo formal dietary counseling to provide FODMAP education and additionally to ensure that individuals do not become undernourished on this diet [80,81].

Exclusion of Additional Foods That Are Gas Producing

Patients with IBS appear to be more sensitive to gas-producing foods as compared to the general population and may be related to visceral hypersensitivity. Therefore, it is recommended that they avoid foods that increase gas production and flatulence such as onions, prunes, bagels, pretzels, beans, and Brussels sprouts.

Gluten Avoidance

Gluten avoidance should be recommended only in those patients who have persistent symptoms of bloating and flatulence despite a trial of a low-FODMAP diet and avoidance of typical gas-producing food. At present, there is limited scientific evidence to support the use of a GFD in patients with IBS without CD.

Lactose Avoidance

In patients with persistent symptoms despite a trial of the earlier diets, empiric trial of a lactose-free diet is recommended. Despite this, improvement of symptoms may occur even in those patients who do not have a clear evidence of lactose maldigestion [82].

Fiber

Psyllium supplementation may be trialed in patients with constipation-predominant IBS. Given the potential to precipitate symptoms such as abdominal bloating and flatulence, a low dose should be trialed (one half tablespoon daily) and gradually uptitrated. To date, there is little evidence to support the use of fiber to improve symptoms in patients with IBS. In one large systematic review looking at 12 studies, no benefit was found as compared to placebo in patients with IBS for improving abdominal pain or global symptom scores [83]. However, in a subsequent meta-analysis that looked at the same trials but instead used a combined end point for abdominal pain and global IBS symptoms found that psyllium was associated in a small improvement in symptoms as compared to placebo (number needed to treat = 6) [84].

REFERENCES

1. Katz, P.O., L.B. Gerson, and M.F. Vela, Guidelines for the diagnosis and management of gastroesophageal reflux disease. *Am J Gastroenterol*, 2013, 108(3): 308–328; quiz 329.
2. Patrick, L., Gastroesophageal reflux disease (GERD): A review of conventional and alternative treatments. *Altern Med Rev*, 2011, 16(2): 116–133.
3. Dickman, R. et al., Clinical trial: Acupuncture vs. doubling the proton pump inhibitor dose in refractory heartburn. *Aliment Pharmacol Ther*, 2007, 26(10): 1333–1344.
4. Wright, E.M. and M. Hyman. Gastroesophageal reflux disease. In: *Advancing Medicine with Food and Nutrients*, Kohlstadt I (ed.). Boca Raton, FL, CRC Press/Taylor & Francis, pp. 203–228.
5. Wilkins, J.S. Jr., Method for treating gastrointestinal disorders. US Patent. USA 2002. Patent Version Number 6,420,435.
6. Melzer, J. et al., Meta-analysis: Phytotherapy of functional dyspepsia with the herbal drug preparation STW 5 (Iberogast). *Aliment Pharmacol Ther*, 2004, 20(11–12): 1279–1287.
7. Yancy, W.S. Jr., D. Provenzale, and E.C. Westman, Improvement of gastroesophageal reflux disease after initiation of a low-carbohydrate diet: Five brief case reports. *Altern Ther Health Med*, 2001, 7(6): 120, 116–119.

8. Yudkin, J., E. Evans, and M.G. Smith, The low-carbohydrate diet in the treatment of chronic dyspepsia. *Proc Nutr Soc*, 1972, 31(1): 12a.
9. Austin, G.L. et al., A very low-carbohydrate diet improves gastroesophageal reflux and its symptoms. *Dig Dis Sci*, 2006, 51(8): 1307–1312.
10. Lahiri, S. et al., Melatonin protects against experimental reflux esophagitis. *J Pineal Res*, 2009, 46(2): 207–213.
11. Pereira Rde, S., Regression of gastroesophageal reflux disease symptoms using dietary supplementation with melatonin, vitamins and aminoacids: Comparison with omeprazole. *J Pineal Res*, 2006, 41(3): 195–200.
12. Waterhouse, E.T., C. Washington, and N. Washington, An investigation into the efficacy of the pectin based anti-reflux formulation-Aflurax. *Int J Pharm*, 2000, 209(1–2): 79–85.
13. Amdrup, E. and B.M. Jakobsen, Reflux esophagitis treated with Gaviscon. *Acta Chir Scand Suppl*, 1969, 396: 16–17.
14. Chatfield, S., A comparison of the efficacy of the alginate preparation, Gaviscon Advance, with placebo in the treatment of gastro-oesophageal reflux disease. *Curr Med Res Opin*, 1999, 15(3): 152–159.
15. Thomas, E. et al., Randomised clinical trial: Relief of upper gastrointestinal symptoms by an acid pocket-targeting alginate-antacid (Gaviscon Double Action)—A double-blind, placebo-controlled, pilot study in gastro-oesophageal reflux disease. *Aliment Pharmacol Ther*, 2014, 39(6): 595–602.
16. Bulat, R. et al., Lack of effect of spearmint on lower oesophageal sphincter function and acid reflux in healthy volunteers. *Aliment Pharmacol Ther*, 1999, 13(6): 805–812.
17. Inamori, M. et al., Early effects of peppermint oil on gastric emptying: A crossover study using a continuous real-time 13C breath test (BreathID system). *J Gastroenterol*, 2007, 42(7): 539–542.
18. Attwood, S.E. et al., Esophageal eosinophilia with dysphagia. A distinct clinicopathologic syndrome. *Digest Dis Sci*, 1993, 38(1): 109–116.
19. Furuta, G.T. et al., Eosinophilic esophagitis in children and adults: A systematic review and consensus recommendations for diagnosis and treatment. *Gastroenterology*, 2007, 133(4): 1342–1363.
20. Liacouras, C.A. et al., Eosinophilic esophagitis: Updated consensus recommendations for children and adults. *J Allergy Clin Immunol*, 2011, 128(1): 3–20.e6; quiz 21–2.
21. Dellon, E.S. et al., ACG clinical guideline: Evidenced based approach to the diagnosis and management of esophageal eosinophilia and eosinophilic esophagitis (EoE). *Am J Gastroenterol*, 2013, 108(5): 679–692; quiz 693.
22. van Rhijn, B.D., P.W. Weijenborg, J. Verheij, M.A. van den Bergh Weerman, C. Verseijden, R.M. van den Wijngaard, et al. Proton pump inhibitors partially restore mucosal integrity in patients with proton pump inhibitor-responsive esophageal eosinophilia but not eosinophilic esophagitis. *Clin Gastroenterol Hepatol*. 2014, 12(11): 1815–1823.
23. Straumann, A. et al., Idiopathic eosinophilic esophagitis is associated with a T(H)2-type allergic inflammatory response. *J Allergy Clin Immunol*, 2001, 108(6): 954–961.
24. Rothenberg, M.E., Biology and treatment of eosinophilic esophagitis. *Gastroenterology*, 2009, 137(4): 1238–1249.
25. Zuo, L. et al., IL-13 induces esophageal remodeling and gene expression by an eosinophil-independent, IL-13R alpha 2-inhibited pathway. *J Immunol* (Baltimore, MD.: 1950), 2010, 185(1): 660–669.
26. Zhu, X. et al., Interleukin-15 expression is increased in human eosinophilic esophagitis and mediates pathogenesis in mice. *Gastroenterology*, 2010, 139(1): 182–193.e7.
27. Dobbins, J.W., D.G. Sheahan, and J. Behar, Eosinophilic gastroenteritis with esophageal involvement. *Gastroenterology*, 1977, 72(6): 1312–1316.
28. Roy-Ghanta, S., D.F. Larosa, and D.A. Katzka, Atopic characteristics of adult patients with eosinophilic esophagitis. *Clin Gastroenterol Hepatol*, 2008, 6(5): 531–535.

29. Khan, S. et al., Eosinophilic esophagitis: Strictures, impactions, dysphagia. *Digest Dis Sci*, 2003, 48(1): 22–29.

30. Kelly, K.J. et al., Eosinophilic esophagitis attributed to gastroesophageal reflux: Improvement with an amino acid-based formula. *Gastroenterology*, 1995, 109(5): 1503–1512.

31. Wang, F.Y., S.K. Gupta, and J.F. Fitzgerald, Is there a seasonal variation in the incidence or intensity of allergic eosinophilic esophagitis in newly diagnosed children? *J Clin Gastroenterol*, 2007, 41(5): 451–453.

32. Rothenberg, M.E. et al., Common variants at 5q22 associate with pediatric eosinophilic esophagitis. *Nat Gen*, 2010, 42(4): 289–291.

33. Blanchard, C. et al., Coordinate interaction between IL-13 and epithelial differentiation cluster genes in eosinophilic esophagitis. *J Immunol* (Baltimore, MD.: 1950), 2010, 184(7): 4033–4041.

34. Lenglinger, J., Impedance planimetry, in *Dysphagia*, O. Ekberg (ed.). Springer-Verlag, Berlin, Germany, 2012, pp. 329–337.

35. Martín Martín, L. et al., Esophageal motor abnormalities in eosinophilic esophagitis identified by high-resolution manometry. *J Gastroenterol Hepatol*, 2011, 26(9): 1447–1450.

36. Moawad, F.J. et al., Esophageal motor disorders in adults with eosinophilic esophagitis. *Digest Dis Sci*, 2011, 56(5): 1427–1431.

37. Henry, M.L. et al., Factors contributing to adherence to dietary treatment of eosinophilic gastrointestinal diseases. *J Pediatr Gastroenterol Nutr*, 2012, 54(3): 430–432.

38. Camilleri, M. et al., Clinical guideline: Management of gastroparesis. *Am J Gastroenterol*, 2013, 108(1): 18–37; quiz 38.

39. Soykan, I. et al., Demography, clinical characteristics, psychological and abuse profiles, treatment, and long-term follow-up of patients with gastroparesis. *Digest Dis Sci*, 1998, 43(11): 2398–2404.

40. Dhamija, R. et al., Serologic profiles aiding the diagnosis of autoimmune gastrointestinal dysmotility. *Clin Gastroenterol Hepatol*, 2008, 6(9): 988–992.

41. Azpiroz, F. and J.R. Malagelada, Gastric tone measured by an electronic barostat in health and postsurgical gastroparesis. *Gastroenterology*, 1987, 92(4): 934–943.

42. Vollmer, K. et al., Hyperglycemia acutely lowers the postprandial excursions of glucagon-like Peptide-1 and gastric inhibitory polypeptide in humans. *J Clin Endocrinol Metabol*, 2009, 94(4): 1379–1385.

43. Samsom, M. et al., Gastrointestinal motor mechanisms in hyperglycaemia induced delayed gastric emptying in type I diabetes mellitus. *Gut*, 1997, 40(5): 641–646.

44. Camilleri, M., M.L. Brown, and J.R. Malagelada, Relationship between impaired gastric emptying and abnormal gastrointestinal motility. *Gastroenterology*, 1986, 91(1): 94–99.

45. Mearin, F., M. Camilleri, and J.R. Malagelada, Pyloric dysfunction in diabetics with recurrent nausea and vomiting. *Gastroenterology*, 1986, 90(6): 1919–1925.

46. Zarate, N. et al., Severe idiopathic gastroparesis due to neuronal and interstitial cells of Cajal degeneration: Pathological findings and management. *Gut*, 2003, 52(7): 966–970.

47. Forster, J. et al., Absence of the interstitial cells of Cajal in patients with gastroparesis and correlation with clinical findings. *J Gastrointest Surg*, 2005, 9(1): 102–108.

48. Iwasaki, H. et al., A deficiency of gastric interstitial cells of Cajal accompanied by decreased expression of neuronal nitric oxide synthase and substance P in patients with type 2 diabetes mellitus. *J Gastroenterol*, 2006, 41(11): 1076–1087.

49. Battaglia, E. et al., Loss of interstitial cells of Cajal network in severe idiopathic gastroparesis. *World J Gastroenterol*, 2006, 12(38): 6172–6177.

50. Farrugia, G., Interstitial cells of Cajal in health and disease. *Neurogastroenterol Motil*, 2008, 20(Suppl. 1): 54–63.

51. Choi, K.M. et al., Heme oxygenase-1 protects interstitial cells of Cajal from oxidative stress and reverses diabetic gastroparesis. *Gastroenterology*, 2008, 135(6): 2055–2064, 2064.e1–e2.
52. Parkman, H.P., W.L. Hasler, and R.S. Fisher, American Gastroenterological Association technical review on the diagnosis and treatment of gastroparesis. *Gastroenterology*, 2004, 127(5): 1592–1622.
53. Fontana, R.J. and J.L. Barnett, Jejunostomy tube placement in refractory diabetic gastroparesis: A retrospective review. *Am J Gastroenterol*, 1996, 91(10): 2174–2178.
54. Wu, K.L. et al., Effects of ginger on gastric emptying and motility in healthy humans. *Eur J Gastroenterol Hepatol*, 2008, 20(5): 436–440.
55. Schemann, M. et al., Region-specific effects of STW 5 (Iberogast) and its components in gastric fundus, corpus and antrum. *Phytomedicine*, 2006, 13(Suppl. 5): 90–99.
56. Bubenik, G.A. et al., Melatonin concentrations in the luminal fluid, mucosa, and muscularis of the bovine and porcine gastrointestinal tract. *J Pineal Res*, 1999, 26(1): 56–63.
57. Lu, W.Z. et al., The effects of melatonin on colonic transit time in normal controls and IBS patients. *Dig Dis Sci*, 2009, 54(5): 1087–1093.
58. Hlebowicz, J. et al., Effect of cinnamon on postprandial blood glucose, gastric emptying, and satiety in healthy subjects. *Am J Clin Nutr*, 2007, 85(6): 1552–1556.
59. Rubio-Tapia, A. et al., ACG clinical guidelines: Diagnosis and management of celiac disease. *Am J Gastroenterol*, 2013, 108(5): 656–676; quiz 677.
60. Biesiekierski, J.R. et al., Gluten causes gastrointestinal symptoms in subjects without celiac disease: A double-blind randomized placebo-controlled trial. *Am J Gastroenterol*, 2011, 106(3): 508–514; quiz 515.
61. O'Bryan, T., R. Ford, and C. Kupper, Celaic disease and non-celiac gluten sensitivity, in Kohlstadt, I. (ed.), *Advancing Medicine with Food and Nutrients*. CRC Press Taylor & Francis Group, Boca Raton, FL, 2013, pp. 305–329.
62. Schuppan, D. and W. Dieterich, Pathogenesis, epidemiology and clinical manifestations of celiac disease in adults, UptoDate. 2014.
63. Rostom, A., J.A. Murray, and M.F. Kagnoff, AGA Institute Medical Position Statement on the Diagnosis and Management of Celiac Disease. *Gastroenterology*, 2006, 131(6): 1977–1980.
64. Brandt, L.J. et al., An evidence-based position statement on the management of irritable bowel syndrome. *Am J Gastroenterol*, 2009, 104(Suppl. 1): S1–S35.
65. Whitehead, W.E. et al., Tolerance for rectosigmoid distention in irritable bowel syndrome. *Gastroenterology*, 1990, 98(5 Pt 1): 1187–1192.
66. Lasser, R.B., J.H. Bond, and M.D. Levitt, *The role of intestinal gas in functional abdominal pain. N Engl J Med*, 1975, 293(11): 524–526.
67. Guilarte, M. et al., Diarrhoea-predominant IBS patients show mast cell activation and hyperplasia in the jejunum. *Gut*, 2007, 56(2): 203–209.
68. Barbara, G. et al., Activated mast cells in proximity to colonic nerves correlate with abdominal pain in irritable bowel syndrome. *Gastroenterology*, 2004, 126(3): 693–702.
69. Chadwick, V.S. et al., Activation of the mucosal immune system in irritable bowel syndrome. *Gastroenterology*, 2002, 122(7): 1778–1783.
70. Dinan, T.G. et al., Hypothalamic-pituitary-gut axis dysregulation in irritable bowel syndrome: Plasma cytokines as a potential biomarker? *Gastroenterology*, 2006, 130(2): 304–311.
71. Pimentel, M., E.J. Chow, and H.C. Lin, Eradication of small intestinal bacterial overgrowth reduces symptoms of irritable bowel syndrome. *Am J Gastroenterol*, 2000, 95(12): 3503–3506.
72. Lupascu, A. et al., Hydrogen glucose breath test to detect small intestinal bacterial overgrowth: A prevalence case-control study in irritable bowel syndrome. *Aliment Pharmacol Ther*, 2005, 22(11–12): 1157–1160.

73. Ford, A.C. et al., Efficacy of prebiotics, probiotics, and synbiotics in irritable bowel syndrome and chronic idiopathic constipation: Systematic review and meta-analysis. *Am J Gastroenterol*, 2014, 109(10): 1547–1561.

74. Wang, L.H., X.C. Fang, and G.Z. Pan, Bacillary dysentery as a causative factor of irritable bowel syndrome and its pathogenesis. *Gut*, 2004, 53(8): 1096–1101.

75. Halvorson, H.A., C.D. Schlett, and M.S. Riddle, Postinfectious irritable bowel syndrome—A meta-analysis. *Am J Gastroenterol*, 2006, 101(8): 1894–1899; quiz 1942.

76. Manning, A.P. et al., Towards positive diagnosis of the irritable bowel. *Br Med J*, 1978, 2(6138): 653–654.

77. Longstreth, G.F. et al., Functional bowel disorders. *Gastroenterology*, 2006, 130(5): 1480–1491.

78. Austin, G.L. et al., A very low-carbohydrate diet improves symptoms and quality of life in diarrhea-predominant irritable bowel syndrome. *Clin Gastroenterol Hepatol*, 2009, 7(6): 706–708.e1.

79. McKenzie, Y.A. et al., British Dietetic Association evidence-based guidelines for the dietary management of irritable bowel syndrome in adults. *J Hum Nutr Diet*, 2012, 25(3): 260–274.

80. Magge, S. and A. Lembo, Low-FODMAP diet for treatment of irritable bowel syndrome. *Gastroenterol Hepatol* (NY), 2012, 8(11): 739–745.

81. Halmos, E.P. et al., A diet low in FODMAPs reduces symptoms of irritable bowel syndrome. *Gastroenterology*, 2014, 146(1): 67–75.e5.

82. Yang, J. et al., Prevalence and presentation of lactose intolerance and effects on dairy product intake in healthy subjects and patients with irritable bowel syndrome. *Clin Gastroenterol Hepatol*, 2013, 11(3): 262–268.e1.

83. Ruepert, L. et al., Bulking agents, antispasmodics and antidepressants for the treatment of irritable bowel syndrome. *Cochrane Database Syst Rev*, 2011, (8): Cd003460.

84. Ford, A.C. and N.J. Talley, Irritable bowel syndrome. *BMJ*, 2012, 345: e5836.

85. Troncone, R. et al., Latent and potential coeliac disease. *Acta Paediatr Suppl*, 1996, 412: 10–14.

86. Sainsbury, A., D.S. Sanders, and A.C. Ford, Prevalence of irritable bowel syndrome-type symptoms in patients with celiac disease: A meta-analysis. *Clin Gastroenterol Hepatol*, 2013, 11(4): 359–65.e1.

87. Petronzelli, F. et al., Genetic contribution of the HLA region to the familial clustering of coeliac disease. *Ann Hum Genet*, 1997, 61(Pt 4): 307–317.

88. Romanos, J. et al., Analysis of HLA and non-HLA alleles can identify individuals at high risk for celiac disease. *Gastroenterology*, 2009, 137(3): 834–840, 840.e1–e3.

89. Trynka, G. et al., Coeliac disease-associated risk variants in TNFAIP3 and REL implicate altered NF-kappaB signalling. *Gut*, 2009, 58(8): 1078–1083.

90. Molberg, O. et al., Tissue transglutaminase selectively modifies gliadin peptides that are recognized by gut-derived T cells in celiac disease. *Nat Med*, 1998, 4(6): 713–717.

91. van de Wal, Y. et al., Selective deamidation by tissue transglutaminase strongly enhances gliadin-specific T cell reactivity. *J Immunol*, 1998, 161(4): 1585–1588.

92. Maiuri, L. et al., Association between innate response to gliadin and activation of pathogenic T cells in coeliac disease. *Lancet*, 2003, 362(9377): 30–37.

93. Maki, M. The humoral immune system in coeliac disease. *Baillieres Clin Gastroenterol*, 1995, 9(2): 231–249.

94. Hvatum, M., H. Scott, and P. Brandtzaeg, Serum IgG subclass antibodies to a variety of food antigens in patients with coeliac disease. *Gut*, 1992, 33(5): 632–638.

95. Mahmood, A., A. Fitzgerald, and Marchbank, T. et al. *Gut*. 2007, 56(2): 168–175.

96. Matsukura, T. and H. Tanaka, *Biochemistry (Mosc)*. 2000, 65(7): 817–823.

15 Inflammatory Bowel Disease

Alyssa Parian, MD

CONTENTS

INTRODUCTION

Inflammatory bowel diseases (IBDs) including ulcerative colitis (UC) and Crohn's disease (CD) are relapsing, remitting chronic inflammatory diseases. UC is characterized by inflammation limited to the colonic mucosa, whereas CD can affect the entire GI tract from mouth to anus and produce transmural inflammation. Despite an unknown pathogenesis of IBD, there is some evidence that diet and nutrition may play a role. There has been increasing interest in diet therapy, nutritional therapy, and vitamin supplementation as *alternative* treatments to integrate into the care plan for IBD patients.

This chapter will review alternative treatments for IBD, including diets aimed at reducing gut inflammation, probiotics to alter the gut microbiome, nutritional therapies shown to improve inflammation, and herbal therapies. Additionally, common vitamin and mineral deficiencies in IBD patients will be discussed.

EPIDEMIOLOGY

The incidence of IBD is increasing worldwide. The prevalence of UC in the United States is estimated to be 230 per 100,000 people, and the prevalence of CD is estimated to be about 201 per 100,000 people [1]. Within the United States, the incidence has been stable over the past 20 years, but rates within Asia and South America are increasing. The Ashkenazi Jewish population has the highest incidence of IBD. There are two peaks of initial IBD presentation, the first between ages 15 and 40 and the second between ages 50 and 80 [2]. CD has a slight female predominance, and UC a slight male predominance [3,4]. IBD appears to be more prevalent in urban areas compared to rural areas and more common in higher socioeconomic classes than lower socioeconomic classes.

PATHOPHYSIOLOGY OF INFLAMMATORY BOWEL DISEASE

The exact etiology of IBD has yet to be identified, but it has been proposed that genetically susceptible individuals develop the disease when there is an exaggerated immune response to an environmental trigger in the gut microbiota. The exact triggers have yet to be identified. Several studies have suggested that diet may be a risk factor in the development of IBD. High intake of refined sugar, total fat, and complex carbohydrates have been associated with an increased risk of IBD, whereas a diet high in fiber and omega-3 fatty acids is negatively associated with CD [5–9].

An alteration in the gut microbiome is also believed to play a role in the pathogenesis of IBD. Infections and antibiotics interfere with the normal microbiota and are possible triggers for IBD. Acute gastroenteritis, *Salmonella*, and *Campylobacter* are associated with an increased risk of developing IBD [10,11]. IBD patients are more likely to have taken antibiotics in the 2 years leading up to their diagnosis than controls [12].

An aberrant mucosal immune system has also been implicated in the pathogenesis of IBD. Abnormalities in the mucosal epithelium and increased gut permeability in the setting of altered microbiota may invoke inflammation within the intestines [13].

This chapter will review alternative treatments for IBD, including diets aimed at reducing gut inflammation, probiotics to alter the microbiome, nutritional therapies shown to improve inflammation, and herbal therapies. Additionally, common vitamin and mineral deficiencies in IBD patients will be discussed.

DIET THERAPY IN IBD

Diet may play an important role in the development and treatment of IBD. Diet patterns have been shown to affect the composition of the microbiome and the permeability of the intestines [14]. The rates of IBD have seemingly increased with the spread of the Western diet. Diets high in animal fats, refined carbohydrates, and sugars, and low in fiber may lead to the formation of IBD, although the retrospective studies demonstrating this are difficult to interpret as environmental factors cannot be controlled [15]. Meats and other high-protein foods produce hydrogen sulfide in the gut, which has been shown to induce inflammation, and sulfites in the colon worsen endoscopic activity of UC [16]. A separate observational study found that higher intake of meat, eggs, protein (excluding fish), and alcohol was associated with an increased number of UC flares [17]. High-fiber diet in the NHANES study was found to be associated with a lower risk of CD, but not UC [9].

The role of dietary therapy for the treatment or improvement of IBD is a common question practitioners are asked. The Internet is filled with blogs and websites claiming to have the dietary cure for IBD. Unfortunately, the majority of these diets have not been studied in a randomized, controlled fashion making the data difficult to interpret. The following are the most common diets for the treatment of IBD, with supporting data.

ENTERAL (ELEMENTAL, SEMI-ELEMENTAL, AND POLYMERIC) FORMULAS

Elemental and polymeric formulas have shown promising results especially in the pediatric population. Despite positive results, these diets are unpalatable and expensive, frequently requiring nasogastric tube delivery, and are difficult to maintain for long-term treatment. Polymeric feeds taste better and are less expensive than elemental feeds, and a systematic review found polymeric feeds equivalent in efficacy to elemental feeds. A polymeric formula was compared to steroids in a study of 40 children with active CD. Both therapies improved the serum inflammatory markers and increased the body mass index, but only the polymeric formula was found to improve both endoscopic and histologic scores of the small bowel and colon [18]. Fell et al. studied the effects of an oral elemental diet on CD patients and observed mucosal healing as well as a decrease in mucosal proinflammatory cytokines [19]. Beattie et al. found not only a decrease in inflammatory markers with a polymeric diet, but also an increase in insulin-like growth factor 1 and insulin-like growth factor binding protein 3. Insulin-like growth factor plays a pivotal role in healthy cell growth and development [20]. Several other studies have observed similar results suggesting that elemental and polymeric enteral feedings have anti-inflammatory properties [21–23].

In children with CD, the response rate to an enteral diet is greater than 80%. Even when only half of the calories were obtained from an elemental diet, the flare rate was decreased by half [24].

Enteric nutrition has been shown to be effective for both small and large bowel inflammation [19,25,26]. Of note, enteral nutrition has not shown efficacy in UC, despite its effectiveness in Crohn's colitis [27]. The anti-inflammatory mechanism of enteral feeding has yet to be fully elucidated. Ensuring appropriate essential nutrients and vitamins, decreasing the fat content, altering the microbiota, and improving the immune status are all plausible theories, but no evidence currently exists to support them [28].

ELIMINATION DIETS

Elimination diets are commonly recommended for a plethora of GI conditions including IBD. The idea is to eliminate foods that can cause hypersensitivity in the gut for 2–4 weeks and then reintroduce foods one by one while maintaining a food dairy. On review of the food diary, one can determine which foods the patient is sensitive to and permanently eliminate these from the diet. Almost 50% of CD patients report at least one food sensitivity. This is thought to be due to a compromised mucosal barrier in IBD patients, which increases their rate of food intolerances [29]. The most common food allergens are milk, egg, peanuts, tree nuts, fish, shellfish, soy, and wheat. At times, skin testing is performed to determine food allergies although this is notoriously unreliable. There have been multiple studies evaluating the elimination diet especially in CD patients, with the majority showing beneficial effects with reduced symptoms and less relapses [30–34].

One study eliminated foods based on food-triggered elevated serum IgG4 levels. The most common foods eliminated were beef and eggs. There was no control group, but the 29 patients on this exclusion diet had a significant decrease in symptoms and a decrease in the erythrocyte sedimentation rate [35]. A small study by Chiba gave 22 postoperative patients a semi-vegetarian diet vs. an omnivorous diet in the hospital with the option to continue the diet upon discharge. A greater portion of patients on the semi-vegetarian diet maintained a clinical remission compared to the omnivorous diet (94% vs. 33%) [36].

SPECIFIC CARBOHYDRATE DIET

The specific carbohydrate diet (SCD) was first introduced as a treatment for celiac disease in 1924. Elaine Gottschall, in her book titled *Breaking the Vicous Cycle*, describes the cure of her daughter's UC with the SCD and greatly popularized this diet. There are minor variations within different publications on the SCD, but the concept is that disaccharide and polysaccharide carbohydrates are difficult to absorb in the human gut. Therefore, these carbohydrates are broken down by intestinal bacteria and result in dysbiosis with bacterial and yeast overgrowth. This microbial overgrowth is theorized to lead to a breakdown in gut barrier function and chronic intestinal inflammation. The diet must be strictly followed as any exposure to these carbohydrates will flare the inflammatory process and lead to further intestinal damage. The diet allows all fruits, most vegetables, meat, nuts, and honey (raw honey preferred), and prohibits potatoes, yams, legumes, processed meats, grains, milk, beer, chocolate, corn syrup, sugar, and margarine.

A small study of seven pediatric CD patients on an SCD was retrospectively evaluated. The average amount of time the diet was followed was 14.6 months. All symptoms were noted to resolve and the albumin levels, inflammatory markers, hematocrit, and stool calprotectin either significantly improved or returned to normal [37]. A prospective trial was undertaken to evaluate the efficacy of SCD in pediatric CD patients for which nine patients completed the initial 12-week study. After 12 weeks, the Harvey Bradshaw index and pediatric CD activity index significantly decreased. Four of the nine patients achieved mucosal healing, with another four showing improved disease activity as measured by capsule endoscopy [38]. There was a single case report of two adult patients with IBD who had clinical and endoscopic remission after 1–2 years of the SCD [39]. The rest of the reports are all anecdotal and without a control group. Larger randomized studies are needed to confirm the efficacy of this diet.

Low-FODMAP Diet

The concept of the low-FODMAP diet is similar to the SCD in that it limits carbohydrates that are difficult to digest and absorb that can lead to small intestine bacterial overgrowth. Bacterial overgrowth has been shown in animal models to increase intestinal permeability, which is believed to be one part of the pathogenesis of CD and other autoimmune conditions [40]. The biggest difference between the two diets is the limits on fruits and vegetables in the FODMAP diet, which prohibits apples, apricots, cherries, pears, watermelon, Brussels sprouts, cabbage, legumes, onions, and artichokes. Milk products are also recommended to be avoided as are all sweeteners and honey with a suggestion of using maple syrup for sweetening. The FODMAP diet has been shown to be effective in treating irritable bowel syndrome and functional abdominal pain [41].

Gearry et al. evaluated the FODMAP diet in 72 IBD patients (52 CD, 20 UC) and found an improvement in abdominal pain, bloating, flatus, and diarrhea in patients who were compliant with the diet. No endoscopic endpoints were evaluated, so it is unclear if the symptomatic improvement resulted from a treatment of concomitant irritable bowel syndrome symptoms rather than the inflammatory disease [42]. A pilot study investigated eight UC patients with a history of colectomy with either an ileal pouch formation or an ileorectal anastomosis. The FODMAP diet decreased the median number of stools from eight to four in the patients without pouchitis, but did not help in patients with pouchitis. The authors concluded that a low-FODMAP diet may help decrease the number of bowel movements in colectomy patients without pouchitis [43].

Paleolithic Diet

The theory behind the Paleo diet is that our gastrointestinal system is not equipped to handle the fiber-depleted refined sugars and complex carbohydrates that the

Westernized diet has introduced. It encourages us to return to a diet eaten by our ancestors hundreds of years ago when many of these modern-day diseases did not exist. There are several variations among this diet as well, but the overall concept is to eat lean nondomesticated (game) meats, unlimited fruits and vegetables, legumes, and nuts. The Paleo diet suggests avoiding domesticated meats that have been raised on a grain-based diet due to an increased *inflammatory* fat content of the meat. The goal is to decrease the amount of n-6 polyunsaturated fatty acids (PUFAs) in which the modern diet is very high. The Paleo diet also recommends avoiding cereal grains, all dairy, soda, beer, fruit juice, and refined sugars. There are no studies evaluating the efficacy of the Paleo diet and therefore has to be taken with caution.

GENERAL IBD DIET RECOMMENDATIONS

Overall, data on the efficacy of any particular diet for IBD are scarce. Although patients desire a natural diet approach for relief of their symptoms, caution has to be taken to not eliminate too many essential vitamins and minerals from the diet as IBD patients are already at risk for nutritional deficiencies. The SCD and Paleo diet especially can lead to vitamin D deficiency, which is critical in IBD patients and discussed in detail later [44]. There is general agreement that high-fat and fried foods can cause or exacerbate IBD and should be minimized if not eliminated. Dietary fiber, fruits, and vegetables seem to shift the gut microbiota to a highly diverse, more favorable, and less inflammatory bacterial species. High-fibrous foods are not recommended in Crohn's patients with stricturing disease as this can precipitate a bowel obstruction. Artificial sweeteners containing sugar alcohols such as sorbitol commonly cause diarrhea even in the general population and can worsen diarrheal symptoms in IBD patients. Lactose intolerance is common among IBD patients especially CD, and dairy may cause bloating, abdominal discomfort, and diarrhea. If that is the case, dairy should be eliminated, but care should be taken to check vitamin D levels and supplement with calcium and vitamin D. Caffeine and alcohol are two other common triggers for abdominal discomfort and diarrhea and may best be avoided in IBD patients. The best recommendation may be for patients to keep a food dairy and track their symptoms to find out which foods trigger their symptoms as each patient seems to have individual food sensitivities. Based on the food and symptom diary, personal recommendations can be made for each patient [44].

PREBIOTICS AND PROBIOTICS IN INFLAMMATORY BOWEL DISEASE

There have been significant data implicating an inappropriate inflammatory response to commensal intestinal bacteria as part of the pathogenesis in IBD. The microbiota of IBD patients has been proven to be different from the microbiota of healthy patients. Therefore, it makes sense that alteration of the intestinal microbiota back to *normal flora* could provide a viable treatment option. This may be possible with prebiotics and probiotics.

PREBIOTICS

Prebiotics are nondigestible fibrous products that selectively promote the growth or activity of beneficial bacteria and fungi, which improve the well-being of the host [45]. The majority of prebiotics are not digestible by the human gastrointestinal tract, but instead act as nutrients for commensal (good) bacteria especially in the distal small bowel and colon. Examples of prebiotics include fructo-oligosaccharides (FOS), inulin, galacto-oligosaccharides (GOS), soybean oligosaccharides, and complex polysaccharides. Inulin and oligofructoses increase the population of lactobacilli and bifidobacteria, which are thought be anti-inflammatory bacteria. As opposed to *Escherichia coli*, *Enterobacter aerogenes*, *Klebsiella pneumonia*, *Streptococcus viridans*, *Bacteroides fragilis*, *Bacteroides uniformis*, and *Clostridium ramosum* have been shown to invoke inflammatory reactions, infiltration of monocytes, and accumulation of collagen.

The majority of the studies are small without controls groups and focus on UC patients, not CD patients. The prebiotic *P. ovata* was studied and found to improve symptoms of UC and increase the concentration of fecal butyrate, although the significant side effects of constipation and flatulence required cessation of therapy in many patients [46,47]. Inulin was able to decrease the fecal calprotectin levels in UC patients, in a small trial [48]. FOS studies for active CD had mixed results with a significant drop-out rate making the results difficult to interpret [49,50]. Germinated barley foodstuff decreased the UC clinical activity score in active UC [51] and also maintained remission [52] compared to placebo without any adverse events reported. A summary of the majority of prebiotic trials is listed in Table 15.1. There is a paucity of high-quality trials investigating the use of prebiotics for the treatment of IBD, and further studies are needed on this topic.

PROBIOTICS

Probiotics are defined by the World Health Organization as "live micro-organisms which, when administered in adequate amounts, confer a health benefit on the host." To be considered a probiotic, specific criteria must be met [53]. First, probiotics must be alive when administered and therefore be able to survive processing, storage, and transition through the foregut. Second, probiotics must have human controlled studies evaluating the health benefits to the host. Third, each probiotic should be defined by genus, species, and strain levels. Last and most important, probiotics should be safe for their intended use.

When prebiotics and probiotics are combined into one, it is called synbiotic. Probiotics work through several different mechanisms in the treatment of IBD. Many probiotic strains have anti-inflammatory properties due to a decrease in pro-inflammatory cytokine secretion and an increase in anti-inflammatory cytokines. Probiotics induce regulatory T-cells, which balances immune and inflammatory responses. Prebiotics and probiotics can increase the production of short-chain fatty acids (SCFAs), which is known to lower the pH of the colon and inhibit the growth of pathogenic bacteria. Probiotics have also been found to decrease intestinal permeability and improve the gut barrier function [54]. As one may expect, each probiotic strain has a different effect on the gastrointestinal system.

TABLE 15.1
Prebiotics for Treatment of IBD

Prebiotic Name	Author (Year)	No. of Patients	Comparison	Outcomes	Side Effects
Plantago ovata	Fernandez-Banares (1999)	105 UC	*P. ovata* ± mesalamine 1500 mg/day	Equal to mesalamine, increased fecal butyrate	Constipation, flatulence
P. ovata	Hallert (1991)	29 UC	*P. ovata* vs. placebo	Improved symptom scores, less flares	N/A
Inulin	Casellas (2007)	19 UC	Inulin vs. placebo	Decreased calprotectin, improved symptom scores	None
Inulin	Welters (2002)	20 pouchitis	Inulin vs. placebo	Decreased pouch inflammation, increased fecal butyrate, decreased *B. fragilis*	None
Inulin	Furrie (2005)	18 UC	Inulin + *B. longum* probiotic vs. placebo	Improved sigmoid scores, decreased inflammatory cytokines	None
Inulin	Joosstens (2012) and De Preter (2013)	67 CD	Inulin vs. placebo	Improved symptoms, decreased *Ruminococcus gnavus*; increased *B. longum* increased butyrate	Abdominal complaints
Fructo-oligosaccharides (FOS)	Lindsay (2006)	10 CD	FOS open trial	Improved Harvey Bradshaw Index, increased bifidobacteria	None
Fructo-oligosaccharides (FOS)	Benjamin (2011)	103 CD	FOS vs. placebo	No difference	Abdominal pain, flatulence, borborygmi
Germinated barley	Kanauchi (2002)	18 UC	Barley + std therapy vs. std therapy alone	Improved clinical scores, increased bifidobacterium and *Eubacterium limosum*	None
Germinated barley	Kanauchi (2003)	21 UC	Barley open label	Improved symptoms, decreased bleeding, decreased nocturnal diarrhea	None
Germinated barley	Hanai (2004)	59 UC	Barley + std therapy vs. std therapy alone	Improved symptom scores, decreased flares	None

Probiotics in UC

Multiple probiotics have been studied for the induction and maintenance of remission in UC. VSL#3 is one of the newer studied probiotics, which contains three genera of bacteria: *Lactobacilli* (*L. casei*, *L. plantarum*, *L. acidophilus*, *L. delbrueckii*), *Bifidobacteria* (*B. longum*, *B. breve*, *B. infantis*), and *Streptococcus* (*S. salivarius*). The VSL#3 trials for UC are listed in Table 15.2. All trials did show some mild-to-modest benefit although most of the studies were quite small. Importantly, there were no adverse events related to VSL#3 in any studies. A meta-analysis by Jonkers et al. [55] showed VSL#3-induced remission in active UC 70% more frequently than placebo.

BIO-THREE is an additional probiotic that contains three genera of *good* bacteria. In a study of 20 patients for the treatment of refractory mild-to-moderate distal UC, remission was seen in 45% of patients, although there was no comparison placebo group. Stool analysis found an increase in the levels of *Bifidobacteria* after BIO-THREE use [56]. No adverse effects were reported, and the authors concluded that BIO-THREE improved clinical symptoms, is safe, and is efficacious for the treatment of UC [56].

Another commonly studied probiotic for the treatment of UC is *E. coli* Nissle 1917. The majority of studies found *E. coli* Nissle 1917 to be at least as efficacious as mesalamine therapy in both induction and maintenance of remission, although low doses of mesalamines were used in the comparison group [57–59]. *E. coli* Nissle 1917 enemas were found to be effective in inducing remission of distal acute UC [60].

Bifidobacteria-fermented milk (BFM) contains *Bifidobacterium breve*, *B. bifidum*, and *Lactobacillus acidophilus*, and has been shown to be effective in treating active UC in a small randomized placebo-controlled trial of 20 patients. BFM was found

---

TABLE 15.2
VSL#3 for Ulcerative Colitis

Author	Year	No. of Patients on VSL#3	Comparison Group	Outcomes
Tursi [46]	2004	30 adults	VSL#3/balsalazide vs. balsalazine vs. mesalazine	Faster and more frequent remission
Bibiloni [47]	2005	32 adults	None	53% remission induced
Huynh [48]	2009	18 children	None	56% remission induced
Sood [49]	2009	77 adults	Placebo	Improved UCDAI, higher remission rate
Miele [50]	2009	14 adults	Placebo	Induced and maintained remission
Tursi [51]	2010	65 adults	Placebo	Improved UCDAI, decreased rectal bleeding

These are studies evaluating VSL#3 for the induction and/or maintenance of remission in ulcerative colitis. Only statistically significant outcomes are reported.

to increase the stool concentration of butyrate and SCFAs [61]. Another trial showed BFM maintains remission and can prevent flares [62].

Multiple other probiotics have been studied in small trials with mixed results [63–67]. Meta-analyses have been hard to perform on probiotic trials due to the large variation in methodology, dosage, probiotic strain, and measured outcomes. One meta-analysis by Sang et al. [68] demonstrated the remission rate for probiotics compared to non-probiotics trended toward significance—1.35 (95% CI 0.98–1.85), and the remission rate for probiotics compared to placebo was significant—2.00 (95% CI 1.35–2.96).

Probiotics in Pouchitis

In severe UC refractory to medication, a colectomy may be performed, and an ileo-anal pouch or reservoir created to maintain continence and avoid an ostomy bag. Up to 50% of patients with an ileoanal pouch suffer from at least one episode of pouchitis or inflammation of the pouch. The exact etiology is unknown, although it is thought to be due to dysbiosis and is frequently treated with antibiotics with some success and frequent recurrence [55,69].

Lactobacillus GG did not improve active pouchitis symptoms or inflammation despite a proven change in the microbiome [70]. Most impressive are the data on VSL#3 preventing recurrence of pouchitis. In a randomized, placebo-controlled trial, VSL#3 had a 15% relapse rate of pouchitis compared to 100% relapse rate with placebo after 9 months of follow-up [71]. Gionchetti et al. then studied VSL#3 as a primary prevention of pouchitis in patients within the first year after pouch formation. Only 10% of VSL#3-treated patients developed pouchitis compared to 40% in the placebo group [72]. The clinical guidelines for the management of pouchitis from 2009 suggests VSL#3 be used in patients with recurrent pouchitis, but it is not recommended currently for the treatment of acute pouchitis [73].

Probiotics in Crohn's Disease

Probiotics have also been studied, albeit less so, for the induction and maintenance of remission in CD with disappointing results. The data on the use of probiotics for the treatment of *active* CD are conflicting [74,75]. Two recent studies investigating syn-biotics had positive results [76,77] both with >50% response rates. Steed et al. [77] found a reduction in TNF-α as well as an increase in *Bifidobacteria*. A small study found some promising evidence that *Saccharomyces boulardii* when combined with regular medical maintenance therapy may be helpful in maintaining remission in CD [78]. On the other hand, two Cochrane reviews found no evidence that probiotics decrease relapse rates [79] or prevent postoperative recurrences [80]. Two meta-analyses also concluded that probiotics were not effective in maintaining remission [81,82]. The small size of the studies, the heterogeneous methodology, and the varied measured outcomes may be to blame for the negative meta-analyses and Cochrane review. Larger trials are needed to better evaluate probiotics in the treatment of CD.

In summary, there is a paucity of research on the efficacy of prebiotics and pro-biotics for the treatment of UC and CD. Concurrent medications, diet variability, and heterogeneous methodologies all contribute to lack of good data in this field. The only current approved indication for probiotic use is VSL#3 for the prevention of recurrent pouchitis. Probiotic use appears promising for mild-to-moderate active UC, albeit more studies are needed. Larger, randomized placebo-controlled trials are needed to further elucidate the role prebiotics and probiotics may have in the treatment of IBD.

FATTY ACIDS IN IBD

Essential fatty acids (EFAs) cannot be endogenously produced and need to be obtained from the diet. EFAs consist of two families: omega-3 and omega-6 PUFAs. Linoleic acid is the parent compound to omega-6 fatty acids, whereas α-linolenic acid is the parent compound to omega-3. Omega-6 fatty acids are found in red meat, corn, soybean, and safflower oils, and omega-3 fatty acids are found in flaxseed, canola, walnuts, and oils from deep-sea fish. The two omega-3 EFAs are eicosapentaenoic acid (EPA) and docosahexaenoic acid (DHA). Omega-3 fatty acids have been shown to have beneficial health effects, whereas omega-6 fatty acids are thought to contribute to certain inflammatory diseases. These two EFAs compete for the same rate-limiting enzyme, so a diet high in omega-6 fatty acids is associated with a pro-thrombotic and inflammatory state. The dietary ratio of omega-6 to omega-3 fatty acids should be less than 4:1, although a *Westernized diet* typically has ratios >10:1, which may explain the increased incidence of IBD as more countries are adopting this Western diet.

Omega-3 EFAs have been shown to inhibit cyclooxygenase and 5-lipoxygenase pathways, which are the essential inflammatory pathways. Omega-3 EFAs also decrease proinflammatory cytokines anti-TNF-α, IL-1β, and NFκB. A diet with increased omega-3 PUFA can improve immune cell function [83,84]. A mouse model demonstrated that omega-3 PUFA decreased colitis by decreasing proinflammatory cytokine synthesis, improving the epithelial barrier function and improved mucosal healing [85].

Fish oil is a valuable source of omega-3 because humans do not readily transform α-linolenic acid to EPA and DHA, which are the main precursors for desirable eicosanoids. Fish oil affects the gut immune system by suppressing T-cell signaling, inhibiting proinflammatory cytokine synthesis, reducing inflammatory cell recruitment, and enhancing epithelial barrier function. Fish oil consumption has been correlated with a decreased risk of the development of colitis as well as a treatment to reduce colitis activity. There have been several conflicting studies on the effects of omega-3 PUFA as a treatment modality for both UC and CD. Overall, there seems to be at least a mild benefit to fish oil to decrease inflammation in IBD patients [86].

SCFAs have also been studied in the pathogenesis and treatment of IBD. SCFAs such as pyruvic, acetic, and butyric acids are monocarboxylic hydrocarbons produced in the colon from fermentation of nonabsorbed carbohydrates. Butyrate is a major source of energy for colonocytes and has shown promise as an anti-inflammatory agent that can be used as a treatment for IBD. Studies have found that IBD patients have a lower concentration of butyric acid and higher concentration of lactic acid and pyruvic acid compared to controls [87]. It is thought that butyrate can decrease the synthesis of inflammatory cytokines through the inactivation of NFκB pathway [88] as well as promote sodium absorption within the colon, therefore, decreasing diarrhea. A number of human studies are investigating the role of butyrate enemas for the treatment of distal UC with improvement seen in stool frequency, volume of blood in the stool, clinical symptoms, and endoscopic healing [89–93]. Other studies on butyrate for the treatment of UC have been negative [93,94]. The amount, duration, and type of enemas varied without studies, and larger, randomized, placebo-controlled trials are needed to determine the role of SCFA for the treatment of IBD inflammation.

HERBAL THERAPIES IN IBD

CURCUMIN

Turmeric, traditionally found in curry dishes, contains a biologically active component known as curcumin. Curcumin is a naturally occurring substance from the plant *Curcuma longa*. Curcumin appears to have anti-inflammatory properties mediated through the inhibition of NFκB, which decreases the production of proinflammatory cytokines [95]. It is also reported to suppress the immune system by inhibiting IL-2 synthesis and TNF-α. Impressively, it has been shown to decrease polyp growth in familial polyposis [96,97]. Topical and oral formulations of curcumin have proven to have an excellent safety profile and are well tolerated [98,99]. Initial studies in mice and rats found curcumin both prevented and treated chemically induced colitis [100–102].

In the first open-label human study, 10 IBD patients (5 UC, 5 CD) received oral curcumin. All of the UC patients and four of five CD improved both symptomatically and serologically. Four of the patients were even able to decrease or eliminate their other colitis medications [103]. A larger, randomized, double-blind, placebo-controlled trial of 89 patients with quiescent UC on baseline mesalamine therapy was performed by Hanai et al. in 2006. One gram of curcumin twice a day compared to placebo for 6 months resulted in symptomatic and endoscopic improvement plus a decrease in the number of flares [104]. A trial of curcumin enemas was performed in patients with distal UC compared to placebo although the drop-out rate of both arms was quite high leaving the intention-to-treat analysis insignificant. The per-protocol analysis was significant in terms of symptomatic and endoscopic improvement [105]. Curcumin definitely appears to have promise in the treatment of UC and even possibly CD; however, larger studies with longer follow-up times are needed. Due to its known chemopreventive activity against colon cancer, curcumin may be an ideal therapy for IBD patients who are at an increased risk of colorectal cancer.

BOSWELLIA

Boswellia serrata is a plant native to India, which has been used for hundreds of years as a herbal remedy for inflammatory conditions. *B. serrata* is a leukotriene inhibitor leading to a blunted release of pro-inflammatory cytokines explaining its anti-inflammatory effects [106]. Gupta et al. demonstrated an improvement in 70% of UC patients treated with *B. serrata*, which was equally as effective as sulfasalazine therapy [107]. Gerhardt et al. found that *B. serrata* was equivalent to mesalamine in the treatment of CD [108]. A double-blind randomized controlled trial of 108 patients confirmed the safety and patient tolerability of *B. serrata*, although it was not efficacious in maintaining remission in CD patients after 52 weeks of therapy [109]. Another study demonstrated a possible improvement of collagenous colitis treated with *B. serrata*, although due to a high drop-out rate, only the per-protocol analysis was statistically significant.

Aloe Vera

Aloe vera is an antioxidant with possible anti-inflammatory properties. Aloe vera was observed to decrease reactive oxygen metabolite production in a dose-dependent manner in in vitro studies. A decreased production of prostaglandin E_2 and IL-8 was also observed without any effect on thromboxane B_2 during in vitro studies of human colorectal mucosa [110]. There have been anecdotal patient reports of improved colitis with aloe vera therapy. A randomized, double-blind placebo-controlled trial found aloe vera gel superior to placebo in achieving clinical and histological improvement in moderately active UC patients [111]. Aloe vera was well tolerated with minimal insignificant side effects.

Wheatgrass Juice

Wheatgrass juice (*triticum aestivum*) has antioxidant properties [112] and has been used for the treatment of thalassemias and intestinal diseases for some time now. The main component of wheatgrass is pigenin, which has been shown to block production of proinflammatory cytokines IL-1β, IL-8, and TNF through inactivation of NFκB [113]. A randomized, double-blind, placebo-controlled trial was performed to determine the efficacy of wheatgrass for the treatment of active distal UC. Twenty-three patients were treated for 1 month with either 100 mL of wheatgrass juice or placebo. Treatment with wheatgrass juice was associated with reduction in overall disease activity and degree of rectal bleeding. There was some mild nausea reported with wheatgrass intake. The authors concluded that wheatgrass juice is safe and effective in the treatment of active distal UC [114].

VITAMIN AND MINERAL DEFICIENCIES AND SUPPLEMENTATION IN IBD

Vitamin D

Vitamin D plays a key role in the regulation of cell growth as well as the adaptive and innate immune system. Vitamin D deficiency has been linked to multiple inflammatory conditions. Supplementation of vitamin D has been shown to induce cathelicidin, which activates the innate immune system against microbes such as mycobacterium [115–117]. T helper cells and T regulatory cells of the adaptive immune system are also modulated by vitamin D [115,116,118]. Dysregulated autophagy (degradation of dysfunctional cells or cellular components required for the health of the host) has been shown to be important in the pathogenesis of CD, and vitamin D is thought to be a regulator of autophagy [119,120]. Low levels of vitamin D are associated with anergy, while vitamin D supplement restores immunoreactivity [121]. Supplementation with vitamin D has been used in the treatment of tuberculosis (TB) [122–124] and to decrease the rate of TB conversion [125,126]. In a cellular model, vitamin D has been shown to decrease monocyte production of IL-6 and TNF-α [127].

The main source of vitamin D is from endogenous production in the skin secondary to UVB exposure from the sun. Dietary products high in vitamin D include fattier fishes (e.g., tuna, mackerel, salmon), cod-liver oil, beef liver, egg yolks, and fortified milk or orange juice [128]. The metabolism of both endogenously produced and diet-consumed vitamin D is shown in Figure 15.1. Normal vitamin D levels are serum 25(OH)D 30 ng/mL or higher. Vitamin D deficiency is classified as serum 25(OH)D levels <20 ng/mL. A level between 20 and 29 ng/mL is considered vitamin D insufficiency [128].

As shown in Figure 15.1, the conversion of vitamin D to its active form requires multiple steps and organ systems to be functioning appropriately. Therefore, vitamin D deficiency in IBD patients can be the result of a number of different mechanisms including lack of sunlight exposure, inadequate dietary intake, poor absorption through the GI tract, impaired conversion to active vitamin D, increased metabolic requirement for vitamin D, and an increased excretion of vitamin D [128,129]. Vitamin D is absorbed in the proximal small bowel, and inflammation in the upper GI tract of Crohn's patients can inhibit absorption [130]. Additionally, patients who have had an ileal small bowel resection (common in CD) are at increased risk for vitamin D deficiency. This is due to decreased bile acid resorption in the ileum and therefore decreased bile acid recycling into the small bowel, which is essential for vitamin D absorption [131,132].

Higher levels of vitamin D have been associated with a decreased risk of developing IBD. On the other hand, the incidence of IBD is more common in northern parts of the world with less exposure to sunlight. IBD flares are more common during low sunlight months of the year [133–135]. Vitamin D deficiency has been reported in IBD patients in varying degrees [136–143]. Severe IBD tends to be associated with low levels of vitamin D. A Canadian population cohort demonstrated that vitamin D deficiency is not necessarily a function of long-standing disease by showing 22% of newly diagnosed IBD patients to be vitamin D deficient [144].

Only one prospective human study has been done to examine the effect vitamin D deficiency has on the severity of IBD. Ananthakrishnan et al. studied a large cohort of 3217 IBD patients and found that vitamin D deficiency (<20 ng/mL) was associated with an increased risk of surgery and hospitalization. Impressively, the CD patients who were able to improve their vitamin D levels had a decreased rate of surgery and hospitalization compared to those patients who remained deficient [142]. In a small study, 108 CD patients were supplemented with either 1200 IU of vitamin D or placebo, and the rate of relapse and the improvement in vitamin D levels were measured. Those treated with vitamin D had a significant increase in their vitamin D levels and a trend toward significance in decreased relapse rates (p=0.06) [145]. An open-label trial by Yang et al. examined 18 patients with mild-to-moderate CD treated with 1000 IU daily vitamin D_3 with increasing doses (max dose 5000 IU daily) as needed to achieve a serum vitamin D level of 40 ng/mL. Of the 18 patients, 14 required the

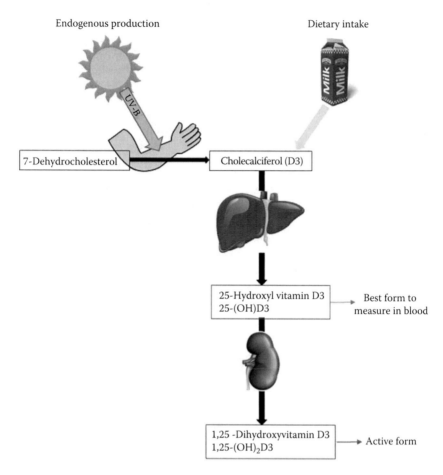

FIGURE 15.1 Vitamin D metabolism. The primary source of vitamin D is via UV-B from sunlight, which moderates the conversion of 7-dehydrocholestrol to cholecalciferol (vitamin D3). Secondary sources of vitamin D3 are from the diet and include fortified milk, fatty fish, and egg yolks. Vitamin D3 is then metabolized in the liver to 25-hydroxyl vitamin D3. 25(OH)D3 is the best form of vitamin D to measure in the blood as it is the major circulating form, although this is a biologically inactive form. The proximal tubules of the kidneys convert 25(OH)D3 into the active form—1,25 dihydroxyvitamin D3. This final conversion step is regulated by multiple factors, including serum calcium, phosphorus, parathyroid hormone, and various growth factors.

highest dose (5000 IU daily) of vitamin D. The authors concluded that vitamin D supplementation significantly reduced CD activity index scores by an average of over 100 points, and quality-of-life scores also improved significantly [146].

It is recommended for all IBD patients to have vitamin D levels assessed on an annual basis and repletion given to those below 30 ng/mL. There are multiple formulations of vitamin D, and there have been inadequate trials to determine which formulation is superior. All of the studies to date using several different formulations of vitamin D have found them to all be safe and well tolerated.

VITAMIN B$_{12}$

Cobalamin, or vitamin B$_{12}$, deficiency is uncommon in the general population but frequently seen in the elderly as well as Crohn's patients. This results in megaloblastic anemia. B$_{12}$ absorption occurs in the terminal ileum, which is frequently inflamed, strictured, or resected in CD. Ileal resection in CD was associated with a sevenfold increased risk of B$_{12}$ deficiency [147]. Repletion of cobalamin in CD patients may be best via subcutaneous injections monthly due to difficult absorption when the ileum is affected, although there are no studies comparing oral to parenteral.

FOLATE

Folate is important for DNA synthesis and red blood cell development. The daily recommended intake is between 400 and 1000 µg of folic acid as this vitamin cannot be stored in large quantities within the body and stores can be quickly depleted [148]. Folate deficiency in the general population is much less common now that cereals and other grain products are enriched with folate, although this deficiency is still common in CD [149]. The cause of folate deficiency in CD has been shown to be multifactorial including inadequate dietary intake, intestinal inflammation causing poor absorption, and medication-induced mechanisms. Both sulfasalazine and methotrexate inhibit the uptake of folate and lead to deficiency; therefore, patients on these two medications must be on daily supplementation of 1 mg of folic acid daily [150].

Folate deficiency has been associated with hyperhomocysteinemia and venous thromboembolisms. IBD patients are already prothrombotic, and folate deficiency can further increase the risk of blood clots [151]. There have been several trials that found an association between low folate levels and sporadic colorectal cancer in the general population [152–155]. IBD studies have also demonstrated an increased risk of colonic dysplasia or cancer in patients with low folate levels [156–158].

VITAMIN A

Vitamin A is a fat-soluble vitamin that has been shown to be important for wound healing. As a fat-soluble vitamin, it requires an intact enterohepatic biliary circulation, which is disrupted in patients with large ileal resection. Adequate pancreatic enzyme secretion is also required for fat-soluble vitamin absorption. It has been suggested that retinol form of vitamin A may help in IBD patients with fistula or postoperatively for wound healing. Vitamin A is stored in the liver, and toxicity is possible when taking high doses.

VITAMIN C

Vitamin C is also important for wound healing. It is an antioxidant and acts as a cofactor for collagen synthesis. Vitamin C also regulates angiogenesis and neutrophil activity [159]. Deficiencies are common in both CD and UC patients [160,161]. Supplementation is suggested for patients postoperatively and those with fistulas [159].

ZINC

Zinc is a mineral that is important as well for wound healing. It also is important in the body's immune function. Zinc deficiency can be hard to measure as serum levels do not correlate with overall zinc deficiency. Chronic diarrhea, small bowel inflammation, and sepsis commonly lead to deficiencies in zinc. Symptoms of severe zinc deficiency include diarrhea, hair loss, dermatitis, and a poor immune status leading to frequent infections. Subclinical deficiencies can be recognized by an impaired sense of taste and smell, difficulty seeing at night, and depressed immune system. Patients with significant diarrhea may benefit from increased supplementation of zinc with 20–40 mg/day [162]. To assist with wound healing, doses of 40 mg of elemental zinc can be given for a maximum length of 2–3 weeks. Over repletion of zinc can affect iron and copper absorption and lead to deficiencies in these minerals [159].

IRON

Iron-deficiency anemia is quite common in the IBD population; reported estimates vary from 36% to 90% [163,164]. This could stem from a decreased intake of iron, a decreased absorption of iron, chronic blood loss, or a combination of these. Iron is absorbed in the duodenum and proximal jejunum. Iron-deficiency anemia can lead to symptoms including fatigue, weakness, decreased exercise tolerance, glossitis, and restless leg syndrome. It has been shown to decrease quality of life in IBD patients [165]. Iron supplementation can be difficult as the ferric and ferrous pills are harsh on the stomach with less than 30% actually absorbed [166]. It is recommended to take iron concomitantly with ascorbic acid (vitamin C) and to stop any antacid therapy, which would inhibit absorption [167]. Oral iron can also cause significant constipation.

Interestingly, oral iron supplementation has been associated with inflammation in the intestines in animal models due to the production of reactive oxygen species [168]. Intravenous iron may be the preferred method of repletion for IBD patients, especially in those with severe deficiency [169]. However, intravenous iron does carry the risk of infusion reactions and anaphylaxis. A newer intravenous iron has been developed, called ferric carboxymaltose, which can be safely administered at higher doses and therefore decrease the number of infusions needed. A multicenter trial found it superior to traditional iron sucrose in regard to efficacy in increasing hemoglobin levels and patient compliance [170]. Iron therapy is relatively contraindicated during active infections such as abscesses. Table 15.3 summarizes the most common vitamin and mineral deficiencies in IBD patients, the daily recommended dose, and foods that contain these vitamins.

BONE HEALTH IN IBD

Bone health is of particular concern in the IBD population. Osteoporosis and osteopenia are more common among IBD patients and occur at an earlier age compared to the general population [171–173]. This unfortunately translates into a higher rate of bone fractures in IBD patients [174]. Important risk factors for osteoporosis in

TABLE 15.3

Food Sources of Commonly Deficient Vitamins and Minerals in IBD Patients

	Natural Sources	Recommended Daily Intake
Vitamin D	UV-B from sun, fatty fishes (tuna, mackerel, salmon), cod-liver oil, beef liver, egg yolks, fortified milk, or orange juice	600 IU
Calcium	Dairy products (milk, yogurt, cheese), sardines, spinach, kale	1000 mg
Magnesium	Dark green vegetables, legumes, beets, peas, nuts	320–420 mg
Folate	Beef liver, spinach, fortified cereals and grains, asparagus, Brussels sprouts, avocado, spinach, broccoli	400 µg
Cobalamin (B_{12})	Clams, beef liver, mackerel, salmon, tuna, red meat, eggs	2.5 mcg
Iron	Red meat, liver, pork, beans, apricots, spinach	8–18 mg
Vitamin A	Dairy products, fish, berries, green leafy vegetables, liver	700–900 µg
Vitamin C	Citrus fruits, tomatoes, potatoes, strawberries, cauliflower, broccoli, cabbage, spinach	75–90 mg
Zinc	Oysters, liver, red meat, sunflower seeds, fortified milk and grain products, pecans	8–11 mg

the general population include advancing age, female gender, postmenopausal status, and low body weight. In addition to these, IBD patients frequently have further increased risks due to the presence of inflammation and corticosteroid use, which are both known to accelerate osteoporosis [171–173]. Furthermore, poor oral intake of calcium and vitamin D and poor absorption contribute to the risk of poor bone health in IBD patients [175].

Calcium is one of the most important minerals for bone health. Calcium intake is frequently poor in the IBD population due to concomitant lactose intolerance. Calcium is absorbed in the proximal small intestines and is regulated by parathyroid hormone and active vitamin D levels. It is theorized that calcium can be lost in the stool during episodes of diarrhea [176]. Low magnesium and low vitamin D levels can lead to the malabsorption of calcium in the gut. Steroids can decrease absorption of calcium from the kidneys as well as the gut. IBD patients may benefit from 1000 mg daily of calcium supplementation in addition to vitamin D supplementation [177].

Vitamin D as mentioned previously is essential for adequate bone health. It is required for the absorption of calcium from the GI tract. Steroids seem to decrease the absorption of vitamin D as shown by several studies [160]. Cholecalciferol (D_3) may be better absorbed and more effective than ergocalciferol (D_2) [178], although current guidelines to not differentiate between the two and suggest at minimum 600–800 IU daily of vitamin D. Higher doses of 1500–2000 IU may be more efficacious in raising serum vitamin D to adequate levels. Obese patients and patients on steroids require at least double the dose of vitamin D.

REFERENCES

1. Kappelman, M.D. et al., The prevalence and geographic distribution of Crohn's disease and ulcerative colitis in the United States. *Clin Gastroenterol Hepatol*, 2007. **5**(12): 1424–1429.
2. Ekbom, A. et al., The epidemiology of inflammatory bowel disease: A large, population-based study in Sweden. *Gastroenterology*, 1991. **100**(2): 350–358.
3. Munkholm, P. et al., Incidence and prevalence of Crohn's disease in the county of Copenhagen, 1962–87: A sixfold increase in incidence. *Scand J Gastroenterol*, 1992. **27**(7): 609–614.
4. Loftus, E.V., Jr. et al., Ulcerative colitis in Olmsted County, Minnesota, 1940–1993: Incidence, prevalence, and survival. *Gut*, 2000. **46**(3): 336–343.
5. Tragnone, A. et al., Dietary habits as risk factors for inflammatory bowel disease. *Eur J Gastroenterol Hepatol*, 1995. **7**(1): 47–51.
6. Persson, P.G., A. Ahlbom, and G. Hellers, Diet and inflammatory bowel disease: A case-control study. *Epidemiology*, 1992. **3**(1): 47–52.
7. Sakamoto, N. et al., Dietary risk factors for inflammatory bowel disease: A multicenter case-control study in Japan. *Inflamm Bowel Dis*, 2005. **11**(2): 154–163.
8. Amre, D.K. et al., Imbalances in dietary consumption of fatty acids, vegetables, and fruits are associated with risk for Crohn's disease in children. *Am J Gastroenterol*, 2007. **102**(9): 2016–2025.
9. Ananthakrishnan, A.N. et al., A prospective study of long-term intake of dietary fiber and risk of Crohn's disease and ulcerative colitis. *Gastroenterology*, 2013. **145**(5): 970–977.
10. Porter, C.K. et al., Infectious gastroenteritis and risk of developing inflammatory bowel disease. *Gastroenterology*, 2008. **135**(3): 781–786.
11. Gradel, K.O. et al., Increased short- and long-term risk of inflammatory bowel disease after salmonella or campylobacter gastroenteritis. *Gastroenterology*, 2009. **137**(2): 495–501.
12. Shaw, S.Y., J.F. Blanchard, and C.N. Bernstein, Association between the use of antibiotics and new diagnoses of Crohn's disease and ulcerative colitis. *Am J Gastroenterol*, 2011. **106**(12): 2133–2142.
13. Hollander, D., Crohn's disease—A permeability disorder of the tight junction? *Gut*, 1988. **29**(12): 1621–1624.
14. Chapman-Kiddell, C.A. et al., Role of diet in the development of inflammatory bowel disease. *Inflamm Bowel Dis*, 2010. **16**(1): 137–151.
15. O'Sullivan, M. and C. O'Morain, Nutrition in inflammatory bowel disease. *Best Pract Res Clin Gastroenterol*, 2006. **20**(3): 561–573.
16. Magee, E.A. et al., Associations between diet and disease activity in ulcerative colitis patients using a novel method of data analysis. *Nutr J*, 2005. **4**: 7.
17. Jowett, S.L. et al., Influence of dietary factors on the clinical course of ulcerative colitis: A prospective cohort study. *Gut*, 2004. **53**(10): 1479–1484.
18. Borrelli, O. et al., Polymeric diet alone versus corticosteroids in the treatment of active pediatric Crohn's disease: A randomized controlled open-label trial. *Clin Gastroenterol Hepatol*, 2006. **4**(6): 744–753.
19. Fell, J.M. et al., Mucosal healing and a fall in mucosal pro-inflammatory cytokine mRNA induced by a specific oral polymeric diet in paediatric Crohn's disease. *Aliment Pharmacol Ther*, 2000. **14**(3): 281–289.
20. Beattie, R.M. et al., Responsiveness of IGF-I and IGFBP-3 to therapeutic intervention in children and adolescents with Crohn's disease. *Clin Endocrinol (Oxf)*, 1998. **49**(4): 483–489.
21. Yamamoto, T. et al., Impact of elemental diet on mucosal inflammation in patients with active Crohn's disease: Cytokine production and endoscopic and histological findings. *Inflamm Bowel Dis*, 2005. **11**(6): 580–588.

22. Breese, E.J. et al., The effect of treatment on lymphokine-secreting cells in the intestinal mucosa of children with Crohn's disease. *Aliment Pharmacol Ther*, 1995. **9**(5): 547–552.

23. Bannerjee, K. et al., Anti-inflammatory and growth-stimulating effects precede nutritional restitution during enteral feeding in Crohn disease. *J Pediatr Gastroenterol Nutr*, 2004. **38**(3): 270–275.

24. Takagi, S. et al., Effectiveness of an "half elemental diet" as maintenance therapy for Crohn's disease: A randomized-controlled trial. *Aliment Pharmacol Ther*, 2006. **24**(9): 1333–1340.

25. Rigaud, D. et al., Controlled trial comparing two types of enteral nutrition in treatment of active Crohn's disease: Elemental versus polymeric diet. *Gut*, 1991. **32**(12): 1492–1497.

26. Ruuska, T. et al., Exclusive whole protein enteral diet versus prednisolone in the treatment of acute Crohn's disease in children. *J Pediatr Gastroenterol Nutr*, 1994. **19**(2): 175–180.

27. Lochs, H. et al., ESPEN guidelines on enteral nutrition: Gastroenterology. *Clin Nutr*, 2006. **25**(2): 260–274.

28. Heuschkel, R., Enteral nutrition in Crohn disease: More than just calories. *J Pediatr Gastroenterol Nutr*, 2004. **38**(3): 239–241.

29. Brown, A.C. and M. Roy, Does evidence exist to include dietary therapy in the treatment of Crohn's disease? *Expert Rev Gastroenterol Hepatol*, 2010. **4**(2): 191–215.

30. Jones, V.A. et al., Crohn's disease: Maintenance of remission by diet. *Lancet*, 1985. **2**(8448): 177–180.

31. Giaffer, M.H., P. Cann, and C.D. Holdsworth, Long-term effects of elemental and exclusion diets for Crohn's disease. *Aliment Pharmacol Ther*, 1991. **5**(2): 115–125.

32. Workman, E.M. et al., Diet in the management of Crohn's disease. *Hum Nutr Appl Nutr*, 1984. **38**(6): 469–473.

33. Jones, V.A., Comparison of total parenteral nutrition and elemental diet in induction of remission of Crohn's disease. Long-term maintenance of remission by personalized food exclusion diets. *Dig Dis Sci*, 1987. **32**(12 Suppl.): 100S–107S.

34. Stange, E.F. et al., Exclusion diet in Crohn disease: A controlled, randomized study. *Z Gastroenterol*, 1990. **28**(10): 561–564.

35. Rajendran, N. and D. Kumar, Food-specific IgG4-guided exclusion diets improve symptoms in Crohn's disease: A pilot study. *Colorectal Dis*, 2011. **13**(9): 1009–1013.

36. Chiba, M. et al., Lifestyle-related disease in Crohn's disease: Relapse prevention by a semi-vegetarian diet. *World J Gastroenterol*, 2010. **16**(20): 2484–2495.

37. Suskind, D.L. et al., Nutritional therapy in pediatric Crohn disease: The specific carbohydrate diet. *J Pediatr Gastroenterol Nutr*, 2014. **58**(1): 87–91.

38. Cohen, S.A. et al., Clinical and mucosal improvement with specific carbohydrate diet in pediatric Crohn disease. *J Pediatr Gastroenterol Nutr*, 2014. **59**(4): 516–521.

39. Nieves, R. and R.T. Jackson, Specific carbohydrate diet in treatment of inflammatory bowel disease. *Tenn Med*, 2004. **97**(9): 407.

40. Teshima, C.W., L.A. Dieleman, and J.B. Meddings, Abnormal intestinal permeability in Crohn's disease pathogenesis. *Ann N Y Acad Sci*, 2012. **1258**: 159–165.

41. Halmos, E.P. et al., A diet low in FODMAPs reduces symptoms of irritable bowel syndrome. *Gastroenterology*, 2014. **146**(1): 67–75 e5.

42. Gearry, R.B. et al., Reduction of dietary poorly absorbed short-chain carbohydrates (FODMAPs) improves abdominal symptoms in patients with inflammatory bowel disease—A pilot study. *J Crohns Colitis*, 2009. **3**(1): 8–14.

43. Croagh, C. et al., Pilot study on the effect of reducing dietary FODMAP intake on bowel function in patients without a colon. *Inflamm Bowel Dis*, 2007. **13**(12): 1522–1528.

44. Hou, J.K., D. Lee, and J. Lewis, Diet and inflammatory bowel disease: Review of patient-targeted recommendations. *Clin Gastroenterol Hepatol*, 2014. **12**(10): 1592–1600.
45. Roberfroid, M., Prebiotics: The concept revisited. *J Nutr*, 2007. **137**(3 Suppl. 2): 830S–837S.
46. Fernandez-Banares, F. et al., Randomized clinical trial of *Plantago ovata* seeds (dietary fiber) as compared with mesalamine in maintaining remission in ulcerative colitis. Spanish Group for the Study of Crohn's Disease and Ulcerative Colitis (GETECCU). *Am J Gastroenterol*, 1999. **94**(2): 427–433.
47. Hallert, C., M. Kaldma, and B.G. Petersson, Ispaghula husk may relieve gastrointestinal symptoms in ulcerative colitis in remission. *Scand J Gastroenterol*, 1991. **26**(7): 747–750.
48. Casellas, F. et al., Oral oligofructose-enriched inulin supplementation in acute ulcerative colitis is well tolerated and associated with lowered faecal calprotectin. *Aliment Pharmacol Ther*, 2007. **25**(9): 1061–1067.
49. Lindsay, J.O. et al., Clinical, microbiological, and immunological effects of fructo-oligosaccharide in patients with Crohn's disease. *Gut*, 2006. **55**(3): 348–355.
50. Benjamin, J.L. et al., Randomised, double-blind, placebo-controlled trial of fructo-oligosaccharides in active Crohn's disease. *Gut*, 2011. **60**(7): 923–929.
51. Kanauchi, O. et al., Treatment of ulcerative colitis patients by long-term administration of germinated barley foodstuff: Multi-center open trial. *Int J Mol Med*, 2003. **12**(5): 701–704.
52. Hanai, H. et al., Germinated barley foodstuff prolongs remission in patients with ulcerative colitis. *Int J Mol Med*, 2004. **13**(5): 643–647.
53. Hill, C. et al., Expert consensus document. The International Scientific Association for Probiotics and Prebiotics consensus statement on the scope and appropriate use of the term probiotic. *Nat Rev Gastroenterol Hepatol*, 2014. **11**(8): 506–514.
54. Garcia Vilela, E. et al., Influence of *Saccharomyces boulardii* on the intestinal permeability of patients with Crohn's disease in remission. *Scand J Gastroenterol*, 2008. **43**(7): 842–848.
55. Jonkers, D. et al., Probiotics in the management of inflammatory bowel disease: A systematic review of intervention studies in adult patients. *Drugs*, 2012. **72**(6): 803–823.
56. Tsuda, Y. et al., Clinical effectiveness of probiotics therapy (BIO-THREE) in patients with ulcerative colitis refractory to conventional therapy. *Scand J Gastroenterol*, 2007. **42**(11): 1306–1311.
57. Rembacken, B.J. et al., Non-pathogenic *Escherichia coli* versus mesalazine for the treatment of ulcerative colitis: A randomised trial. *Lancet*, 1999. **354**(9179): 635–639.
58. Kruis, W. et al., Double-blind comparison of an oral *Escherichia coli* preparation and mesalazine in maintaining remission of ulcerative colitis. *Aliment Pharmacol Ther*, 1997. **11**(5): 853–858.
59. Kruis, W. et al., Maintaining remission of ulcerative colitis with the probiotic *Escherichia coli* Nissle 1917 is as effective as with standard mesalazine. *Gut*, 2004. **53**(11): 1617–1623.
60. Matthes, H. et al., Clinical trial: Probiotic treatment of acute distal ulcerative colitis with rectally administered *Escherichia coli* Nissle 1917 (EcN). *BMC Complement Altern Med*, 2010. **10**: 13.
61. Kato, K. et al., Randomized placebo-controlled trial assessing the effect of bifidobacteria-fermented milk on active ulcerative colitis. *Aliment Pharmacol Ther*, 2004. **20**(10): 1133–1141.
62. Ishikawa, H. et al., Randomized controlled trial of the effect of bifidobacteria-fermented milk on ulcerative colitis. *J Am Coll Nutr*, 2003. **22**(1): 56–63.

63. Oliva, S. et al., Randomised clinical trial: The effectiveness of *Lactobacillus reuteri* ATCC 55730 rectal enema in children with active distal ulcerative colitis. *Aliment Pharmacol Ther*, 2012. **35**(3): 327–334.

64. Guslandi, M., P. Giollo, and P.A. Testoni, A pilot trial of *Saccharomyces boulardii* in ulcerative colitis. *Eur J Gastroenterol Hepatol*, 2003. **15**(6): 697–698.

65. Furrie, E. et al., Synbiotic therapy (*Bifidobacterium longum*/Synergy 1) initiates resolution of inflammation in patients with active ulcerative colitis: A randomised controlled pilot trial. *Gut*, 2005. **54**(2): 242–249.

66. Ishikawa, H. et al., Beneficial effects of probiotic bifidobacterium and galacto-oligosaccharide in patients with ulcerative colitis: A randomized controlled study. *Digestion*, 2011. **84**(2): 128–133.

67. Zocco, M.A. et al., Efficacy of Lactobacillus GG in maintaining remission of ulcerative colitis. *Aliment Pharmacol Ther*, 2006. **23**(11): 1567–1574.

68. Sang, L.X. et al., Remission induction and maintenance effect of probiotics on ulcerative colitis: A meta-analysis. *World J Gastroenterol*, 2010. **16**(15): 1908–1915.

69. Mack, D.R. et al., Extracellular MUC3 mucin secretion follows adherence of Lactobacillus strains to intestinal epithelial cells in vitro. *Gut*, 2003. **52**(6): 827–833.

70. Kuisma, J. et al., Effect of Lactobacillus rhamnosus GG on ileal pouch inflammation and microbial flora. *Aliment Pharmacol Ther*, 2003. **17**(4): 509–515.

71. Gionchetti, P. et al., Oral bacteriotherapy as maintenance treatment in patients with chronic pouchitis: A double-blind, placebo-controlled trial. *Gastroenterology*, 2000. **119**(2): 305–309.

72. Gionchetti, P. et al., Prophylaxis of pouchitis onset with probiotic therapy: A double-blind, placebo-controlled trial. *Gastroenterology*, 2003. **124**(5): 1202–1209.

73. Pardi, D.S. et al., Clinical guidelines for the management of pouchitis. *Inflamm Bowel Dis*, 2009. **15**(9): 1424–1431.

74. Gupta, P. et al., Is lactobacillus GG helpful in children with Crohn's disease? Results of a preliminary, open-label study. *J Pediatr Gastroenterol Nutr*, 2000. **31**(4): 453–457.

75. Schultz, M. et al., Lactobacillus GG in inducing and maintaining remission of Crohn's disease. *BMC Gastroenterol*, 2004. **4**: 5.

76. Fujimori, S. et al., High dose probiotic and prebiotic cotherapy for remission induction of active Crohn's disease. *J Gastroenterol Hepatol*, 2007. **22**(8): 1199–1204.

77. Steed, H. et al., Clinical trial: The microbiological and immunological effects of synbiotic consumption—A randomized double-blind placebo-controlled study in active Crohn's disease. *Aliment Pharmacol Ther*, 2010. **32**(7): 872–883.

78. Guslandi, M. et al., *Saccharomyces boulardii* in maintenance treatment of Crohn's disease. *Dig Dis Sci*, 2000. **45**(7): 1462–1464.

79. Rolfe, V.E. et al., Probiotics for maintenance of remission in Crohn's disease. *Cochrane Database Syst Rev*, 2006. (4): CD004826.

80. Doherty, G. et al., Interventions for prevention of post-operative recurrence of Crohn's disease. *Cochrane Database Syst Rev*, 2009. (4): CD006873.

81. Rahimi, R. et al., A meta-analysis on the efficacy of probiotics for maintenance of remission and prevention of clinical and endoscopic relapse in Crohn's disease. *Dig Dis Sci*, 2008. **53**(9): 2524–2531.

82. Shen, J. et al., Meta-analysis: The effect and adverse events of Lactobacilli versus placebo in maintenance therapy for Crohn disease. *Intern Med J*, 2009. **39**(2): 103–109.

83. Gallai, V. et al., Cytokine secretion and eicosanoid production in the peripheral blood mononuclear cells of MS patients undergoing dietary supplementation with n-3 polyunsaturated fatty acids. *J Neuroimmunol*, 1995. **56**(2): 143–153.

84. Fisher, M. et al., Dietary n-3 fatty acid supplementation reduces superoxide production and chemiluminescence in a monocyte-enriched preparation of leukocytes. *Am J Clin Nutr*, 1990. **51**(5): 804–808.

85. Whiting, C.V., P.W. Bland, and J.F. Tarlton, Dietary n-3 polyunsaturated fatty acids reduce disease and colonic proinflammatory cytokines in a mouse model of colitis. *Inflamm Bowel Dis*, 2005. **11**(4): 340–349.

86. Calder, P.C., Polyunsaturated fatty acids, inflammation, and immunity. *Lipids*, 2001. **36**(9): 1007–1024.

87. Roediger, W.E., The colonic epithelium in ulcerative colitis: An energy-deficiency disease? *Lancet*, 1980. **2**(8197): 712–715.

88. Meijer, K., P. de Vos, and M.G. Priebe, Butyrate and other short-chain fatty acids as modulators of immunity: What relevance for health? *Curr Opin Clin Nutr Metab Care*, 2010. **13**(6): 715–721.

89. Wong, J.M. et al., Colonic health: Fermentation and short chain fatty acids. *J Clin Gastroenterol*, 2006. **40**(3): 235–243.

90. Cummings, J.H., Short-chain fatty acid enemas in the treatment of distal ulcerative colitis. *Eur J Gastroenterol Hepatol*, 1997. **9**(2): 149–153.

91. Breuer, R.I. et al., Rectal irrigation with short-chain fatty acids for distal ulcerative colitis. Preliminary report. *Dig Dis Sci*, 1991. **36**(2): 185–187.

92. Scheppach, W. et al., Effect of butyrate enemas on the colonic mucosa in distal ulcerative colitis. *Gastroenterology*, 1992. **103**(1): 51–56.

93. Breuer, R.I. et al., Short chain fatty acid rectal irrigation for left-sided ulcerative colitis: A randomised, placebo controlled trial. *Gut*, 1997. **40**(4): 485–491.

94. Steinhart, A.H. et al., Treatment of left-sided ulcerative colitis with butyrate enemas: A controlled trial. *Aliment Pharmacol Ther*, 1996. **10**(5): 729–736.

95. Jobin, C. et al., Curcumin blocks cytokine-mediated NF-kappa B activation and proinflammatory gene expression by inhibiting inhibitory factor I-kappa B kinase activity. *J Immunol*, 1999. **163**(6): 3474–3483.

96. Duvoix, A. et al., Chemopreventive and therapeutic effects of curcumin. *Cancer Lett*, 2005. **223**(2): 181–190.

97. Perkins, S. et al., Chemopreventive efficacy and pharmacokinetics of curcumin in the min/+ mouse, a model of familial adenomatous polyposis. *Cancer Epidemiol Biomarkers Prev*, 2002. **11**(6): 535–540.

98. Bengmark, S., Curcumin, an atoxic antioxidant and natural NFkappaB, cyclooxygenase-2, lipooxygenase, and inducible nitric oxide synthase inhibitor: A shield against acute and chronic diseases. *J Parenter Enteral Nutr*, 2006. **30**(1): 45–51.

99. Cheng, A.L. et al., Phase I clinical trial of curcumin, a chemopreventive agent, in patients with high-risk or pre-malignant lesions. *Anticancer Res*, 2001. **21**(4B): 2895–2900.

100. Jian, Y.T. et al., Preventive and therapeutic effects of NF-kappaB inhibitor curcumin in rats colitis induced by trinitrobenzene sulfonic acid. *World J Gastroenterol*, 2005. **11**(12): 1747–1752.

101. Deguchi, Y. et al., Curcumin prevents the development of dextran sulfate Sodium (DSS)-induced experimental colitis. *Dig Dis Sci*, 2007. **52**(11): 2993–2998.

102. Sugimoto, K. et al., Curcumin prevents and ameliorates trinitrobenzene sulfonic acid-induced colitis in mice. *Gastroenterology*, 2002. **123**(6): 1912–1922.

103. Holt, P.R., S. Katz, and R. Kirshoff, Curcumin therapy in inflammatory bowel disease: A pilot study. *Dig Dis Sci*, 2005. **50**(11): 2191–2193.

104. Hanai, H. et al., Curcumin maintenance therapy for ulcerative colitis: Randomized, multicenter, double-blind, placebo-controlled trial. *Clin Gastroenterol Hepatol*, 2006. **4**(12): 1502–1506.

105. Singla, V. et al., Induction with NCB-02 (curcumin) enema for mild-to-moderate distal ulcerative colitis—A randomized, placebo-controlled, pilot study. *J Crohns Colitis*, 2014. **8**(3): 208–214.

106. Gayathri, B. et al., Pure compound from *Boswellia serrata* extract exhibits anti-inflammatory property in human PBMCs and mouse macrophages through inhibition of TNFalpha, IL-1beta, NO and MAP kinases. *Int Immunopharmacol*, 2007. **7**(4): 473–482.

107. Gupta, I. et al., Effects of gum resin of *Boswellia serrata* in patients with chronic colitis. *Planta Med*, 2001. **67**(5): 391–395.

108. Gerhardt, H. et al., Therapy of active Crohn disease with *Boswellia serrata* extract H 15. *Z Gastroenterol*, 2001. **39**(1): 11–17.

109. Holtmeier, W. et al., Randomized, placebo-controlled, double-blind trial of *Boswellia serrata* in maintaining remission of Crohn's disease: Good safety profile but lack of efficacy. *Inflamm Bowel Dis*, 2011. **17**(2): 573–582.

110. Langmead, L., R.J. Makins, and D.S. Rampton, Anti-inflammatory effects of aloe vera gel in human colorectal mucosa in vitro. *Aliment Pharmacol Ther*, 2004. **19**(5): 521–527.

111. Langmead, L. et al., Randomized, double-blind, placebo-controlled trial of oral aloe vera gel for active ulcerative colitis. *Aliment Pharmacol Ther*, 2004. **19**(7): 739–747.

112. Kulkarni, S.D. et al., Evaluation of the antioxidant activity of wheatgrass (Triticum aestivum L.) as a function of growth under different conditions. *Phytother Res*, 2006. **20**(3): 218–227.

113. Nicholas, C. et al., Apigenin blocks lipopolysaccharide-induced lethality in vivo and proinflammatory cytokines expression by inactivating NF-kappaB through the suppression of p65 phosphorylation. *J Immunol*, 2007. **179**(10): 7121–7127.

114. Ben-Arye, E. et al., Wheat grass juice in the treatment of active distal ulcerative colitis: A randomized double-blind placebo-controlled trial. *Scand J Gastroenterol*, 2002. **37**(4): 444–449.

115. Cantorna, M.T. et al., Vitamin D status, 1,25-dihydroxyvitamin D3, and the immune system. *Am J Clin Nutr*, 2004. **80**(6 Suppl.): 1717S–1720S.

116. Cantorna, M.T. and B.D. Mahon, D-hormone and the immune system. *J Rheumatol Suppl*, 2005. **76**: 11–20.

117. Adams, J.S. et al., Vitamin D-directed rheostatic regulation of monocyte antibacterial responses. *J Immunol*, 2009. **182**(7): 4289–4295.

118. Lemire, J.M. et al., 1,25-Dihydroxyvitamin D3 suppresses human T helper/inducer lymphocyte activity in vitro. *J Immunol*, 1985. **134**(5): 3032–3035.

119. Yuk, J.M. et al., Vitamin D3 induces autophagy in human monocytes/macrophages via cathelicidin. *Cell Host Microbe*, 2009. **6**(3): 231–243.

120. Wu, S. and J. Sun, Vitamin D, vitamin D receptor, and macroautophagy in inflammation and infection. *Discov Med*, 2011. **11**(59): 325–335.

121. Toss, G. and T. Symreng, Delayed hypersensitivity response and vitamin D deficiency. *Int J Vitam Nutr Res*, 1983. **53**(1): 27–31.

122. Liu, P.T. et al., Toll-like receptor triggering of a vitamin D-mediated human antimicrobial response. *Science*, 2006. **311**(5768): 1770–1773.

123. Liu, P.T. and R.L. Modlin, Human macrophage host defense against Mycobacterium tuberculosis. *Curr Opin Immunol*, 2008. **20**(4): 371–376.

124. Liu, P.T. et al., Cutting edge: Vitamin D-mediated human antimicrobial activity against Mycobacterium tuberculosis is dependent on the induction of cathelicidin. *J Immunol*, 2007. **179**(4): 2060–2063.

125. Arnedo-Pena, A. et al., Latent tuberculosis infection, tuberculin skin test and vitamin D status in contacts of tuberculosis patients: A cross-sectional and case-control study. *BMC Infect Dis*, 2011. **11**: 349.

126. Ganmaa, D. et al., Vitamin D, tuberculin skin test conversion, and latent tuberculosis in Mongolian school-age children: A randomized, double-blind, placebo-controlled feasibility trial. *Am J Clin Nutr*, 2012. **96**(2): 391–396.
127. Zhang, Y. et al., Vitamin D inhibits monocyte/macrophage proinflammatory cytokine production by targeting MAPK phosphatase-1. *J Immunol*, 2012. **188**(5): 2127–2135.
128. Holick, M.F., Vitamin D deficiency. *N Engl J Med*, 2007. **357**(3): 266–281.
129. Rosen, C.J., Clinical practice. Vitamin D insufficiency. *N Engl J Med*, 2011. **364**(3): 248–254.
130. Sentongo, T.A. et al., Vitamin D status in children, adolescents, and young adults with Crohn disease. *Am J Clin Nutr*, 2002. **76**(5): 1077–1081.
131. Tajika, M. et al., Risk factors for vitamin D deficiency in patients with Crohn's disease. *J Gastroenterol*, 2004. **39**(6): 527–533.
132. Leichtmann, G.A. et al., Intestinal absorption of cholecalciferol and 25-hydroxycholecalciferol in patients with both Crohn's disease and intestinal resection. *Am J Clin Nutr*, 1991. **54**(3): 548–552.
133. Lim, W.C., S.B. Hanauer, and Y.C. Li, Mechanisms of disease: Vitamin D and inflammatory bowel disease. *Nat Clin Pract Gastroenterol Hepatol*, 2005. **2**(7): 308–315.
134. Harries, A.D. et al., Vitamin D status in Crohn's disease: Association with nutrition and disease activity. *Gut*, 1985. **26**(11): 1197–1203.
135. Vogelsang, H. et al., Bone disease in vitamin D-deficient patients with Crohn's disease. *Dig Dis Sci*, 1989. **34**(7): 1094–1099.
136. Joseph, A.J. et al., 25 (OH) vitamin D level in Crohn's disease: Association with sun exposure & disease activity. *Indian J Med Res*, 2009. **130**(2): 133–137.
137. Pappa, H.M. et al., Prevalence and risk factors for hypovitaminosis D in young patients with inflammatory bowel disease. *J Pediatr Gastroenterol Nutr*, 2011. **53**(4): 361–364.
138. Atia, A. et al., Vitamin D status in veterans with inflammatory bowel disease: Relationship to health care costs and services. *Mil Med*, 2011. **176**(6): 711–714.
139. Suibhne, T.N. et al., Vitamin D deficiency in Crohn's disease: Prevalence, risk factors and supplement use in an outpatient setting. *J Crohns Colitis*, 2012. **6**(2): 182–188.
140. Fu, Y.T. et al., Hypovitaminosis D in adults with inflammatory bowel disease: Potential role of ethnicity. *Dig Dis Sci*, 2012. **57**(8): 2144–2148.
141. Hassan, V. et al., Association between serum 25 (OH) vitamin D concentrations and inflammatory bowel diseases (IBDs) activity. *Med J Malaysia*, 2013. **68**(1): 34–38.
142. Ananthakrishnan, A.N. et al., Normalization of plasma 25-hydroxy vitamin D is associated with reduced risk of surgery in Crohn's disease. *Inflamm Bowel Dis*, 2013. **19**(9): 1921–1927.
143. Alkhouri, R.H. et al., Vitamin and mineral status in patients with inflammatory bowel disease. *J Pediatr Gastroenterol Nutr*, 2013. **56**(1): 89–92.
144. Leslie, W.D. et al., Vitamin D status and bone density in recently diagnosed inflammatory bowel disease: The Manitoba IBD Cohort Study. *Am J Gastroenterol*, 2008. **103**(6): 1451–1459.
145. Jorgensen, S.P. et al., Clinical trial: Vitamin D3 treatment in Crohn's disease—A randomized double-blind placebo-controlled study. *Aliment Pharmacol Ther*, 2010. **32**(3): 377–383.
146. Yang, L. et al., Therapeutic effect of vitamin D supplementation in a pilot study of Crohn's patients. *Clin Transl Gastroenterol*, 2013. **4**: e33.
147. Headstrom, P.D., S.J. Rulyak, and S.D. Lee, Prevalence of and risk factors for vitamin B(12) deficiency in patients with Crohn's disease. *Inflamm Bowel Dis*, 2008. **14**(2): 217–223.
148. Yakut, M. et al., Serum vitamin B12 and folate status in patients with inflammatory bowel diseases. *Eur J Intern Med*, 2010. **21**(4): 320–323.

149. Hoffbrand, A.V. et al., Folate deficiency in Crohn's disease: Incidence, pathogenesis, and treatment. *Br Med J*, 1968. **2**(5597): 71–75.

150. Lindenbaum, J., Drugs and vitamin B12 and folate metabolism. *Curr Concepts Nutr*, 1983. **12**: 73–87.

151. Erzin, Y. et al., Hyperhomocysteinemia in inflammatory bowel disease patients without past intestinal resections: Correlations with cobalamin, pyridoxine, folate concentrations, acute phase reactants, disease activity, and prior thromboembolic complications. *J Clin Gastroenterol*, 2008. **42**(5): 481–486.

152. Giovannucci, E. et al., Alcohol, low-methionine—Low-folate diets, and risk of colon cancer in men. *J Natl Cancer Inst*, 1995. **87**(4): 265–273.

153. Konings, E.J. et al., Intake of dietary folate vitamers and risk of colorectal carcinoma: Results from The Netherlands Cohort Study. *Cancer*, 2002. **95**(7): 1421–1433.

154. Meyer, F. and E. White, Alcohol and nutrients in relation to colon cancer in middle-aged adults. *Am J Epidemiol*, 1993. **138**(4): 225–236.

155. Su, L.J. and L. Arab, Nutritional status of folate and colon cancer risk: Evidence from NHANES I epidemiologic follow-up study. *Ann Epidemiol*, 2001. **11**(1): 65–72.

156. Lashner, B.A., Red blood cell folate is associated with the development of dysplasia and cancer in ulcerative colitis. *J Cancer Res Clin Oncol*, 1993. **119**(9): 549–554.

157. Lashner, B.A. et al., Effect of folate supplementation on the incidence of dysplasia and cancer in chronic ulcerative colitis. A case-control study. *Gastroenterology*, 1989. **97**(2): 255–259.

158. Lashner, B.A. et al., The effect of folic acid supplementation on the risk for cancer or dysplasia in ulcerative colitis. *Gastroenterology*, 1997. **112**(1): 29–32.

159. Sinno, S., D.S. Lee, and A. Khachemoune, Vitamins and cutaneous wound healing. *J Wound Care*, 2011. **20**(6): 287–293.

160. Filippi, J. et al., Nutritional deficiencies in patients with Crohn's disease in remission. *Inflamm Bowel Dis*, 2006. **12**(3): 185–191.

161. Hengstermann, S. et al., Altered status of antioxidant vitamins and fatty acids in patients with inactive inflammatory bowel disease. *Clin Nutr*, 2008. **27**(4): 571–578.

162. Lansdown, A.B. et al., Zinc in wound healing: Theoretical, experimental, and clinical aspects. *Wound Repair Regen*, 2007. **15**(1): 2–16.

163. Gasche, C. et al., Iron, anaemia, and inflammatory bowel diseases. *Gut*, 2004. **53**(8): 1190–1197.

164. Kulnigg, S. and C. Gasche, Systematic review: Managing anaemia in Crohn's disease. *Aliment Pharmacol Ther*, 2006. **24**(11–12): 1507–1523.

165. Wells, C.W. et al., Effects of changes in hemoglobin level on quality of life and cognitive function in inflammatory bowel disease patients. *Inflamm Bowel Dis*, 2006. **12**(2): 123–130.

166. Andrews, N.C., Disorders of iron metabolism. *N Engl J Med*, 1999. **341**(26): 1986–1995.

167. Frazer, D.M. and G.J. Anderson, Iron imports. I. Intestinal iron absorption and its regulation. *Am J Physiol Gastrointest Liver Physiol*, 2005. **289**(4): G631–G635.

168. Werner, T. et al., Depletion of luminal iron alters the gut microbiota and prevents Crohn's disease-like ileitis. *Gut*, 2011. **60**(3): 325–333.

169. Gasche, C. et al., Guidelines on the diagnosis and management of iron deficiency and anemia in inflammatory bowel diseases. *Inflamm Bowel Dis*, 2007. **13**(12): 1545–1553.

170. Evstatiev, R. et al., FERGIcor, a randomized controlled trial on ferric carboxymaltose for iron deficiency anemia in inflammatory bowel disease. *Gastroenterology*, 2011. **141**(3): 846–853 e1–e2.

171. Lichtenstein, G.R., B.E. Sands, and M. Pazianas, Prevention and treatment of osteoporosis in inflammatory bowel disease. *Inflamm Bowel Dis*, 2006. **12**(8): 797–813.

172. Bernstein, C.N., Inflammatory bowel diseases as secondary causes of osteoporosis. *Curr Osteoporos Rep*, 2006. **4**(3): 116–123.

173. Bernstein, C.N., Osteoporosis in patients with inflammatory bowel disease. *Clin Gastroenterol Hepatol*, 2006. **4**(2): 152–156.
174. Bernstein, C.N. et al., The incidence of fracture among patients with inflammatory bowel disease. A population-based cohort study. *Ann Intern Med*, 2000. **133**(10): 795–799.
175. Pappa, H.M., R.J. Grand, and C.M. Gordon, Report on the vitamin D status of adult and pediatric patients with inflammatory bowel disease and its significance for bone health and disease. *Inflamm Bowel Dis*, 2006. **12**(12): 1162–1174.
176. Bronner, F., Mechanisms of intestinal calcium absorption. *J Cell Biochem*, 2003. **88**(2): 387–393.
177. Jackson, R.D. et al., Calcium plus vitamin D supplementation and the risk of fractures. *N Engl J Med*, 2006. **354**(7): 669–683.
178. Heaney, R.P. et al., Vitamin D(3) is more potent than vitamin D(2) in humans. *J Clin Endocrinol Metab*, 2011. **96**(3): E447–E452.

16 Use of Complementary and Alternative Therapies in Hepatic Disorders

Alia S. Dadabhai, MD

CONTENTS

It is estimated that half the U.S. adult population consumes herbals and dietary supplements (HDS), with recent reports showing their use to be increasing.[1,2] The heightened interest in alternative therapies has led motivated patients to try HDS for indolent to serious hepatic diseases. The therapies remain controversial as there are little to no federal or internal oversight of their use or production, nor are there consistently reproducible studies to gauge their efficacy. The dose, concentration, and forms of these therapies vary not only between manufacturers, but also from "bottle-to-bottle" and the subsequent absorption in the body can therefore be vastly irregular. The intended use of these supplements has ranged from treating viral hepatitis (i.e., hepatitis C virus [HCV], hepatitis B virus [HBV], or hepatitis A virus), to fatty liver, NASH (nonalcoholic steatohepatitis), hepatic encephalopathy (HE), primary

375

biliary cirrhosis (PBC), Wilson's disease, hemachromatosis, alcoholic liver disease, among others. Most concerning is a recent report by the Drug-Induced Livery Injury Network that quoted 20% of drug-induced liver injury is from HDS.[1] What follows is an examination of popularized HDS that are being used for the treatment of liver diseases (Table 16.1).

HERBAL THERAPIES

MILK THISTLE

Milk thistle, also known as silybin, silybum, silymarin, or Marian thistle, has been used for ages as a food and herbal treatment of liver conditions. Milk thistle has not been implicated in causing liver injury and is still used widely as a liver tonic in patients with acute and chronic liver diseases. Specifically, the impact of milk thistle has been studied for drug toxicity treatment from acetaminophen, carbon tetrachloride, mushroom poisoning (phalloidin), radiation, iron overload, phenyl hydrazine, alcohol, cold ischemia, and thiocetamide.[3]

Extracts of milk thistle seeds contain multiple flavanolignans, known collectively as silymarin, consisting largely of silybinin, silychristin, and silydianin. Silymarin and its active constituent, silybin, have been reported to work as antioxidants scavenging free radicals and inhibiting lipid peroxidation. Studies also suggest that they protect against genomic injury, increase hepatocyte protein synthesis, decrease the activity of tumor promoters, stabilize mast cells, chelate iron, and slow down calcium metabolism.[4]

Milk thistle is marketed as capsules or tablets containing ethanol-extracted silymarin in amounts of 250–750 mg and is purported to be beneficial for liver disease, including alcoholic and viral liver disease. The daily dosage varies, but it is typically taken two to three times daily. Intravenous preparations of purified silibinin are approved in Europe for therapy of *Amanita phalloides* mushroom poisoning. The IV form of silibinin is not currently available in the United States, but is used in Europe; however, an oral form (silymarin) may be obtained. Silibinin is thought to interfere with hepatic uptake of alpha-amanitin, a deadly cyclic peptide. Trials using the impact of milk thistle on liver diseases such as hepatitis C have not been conducted with any validity. The differing virology of hepatitis C based on genotype, IL28B, Q80K, and the rise of ever-evolving therapy in hepatitis C would make the effect of milk thistle difficult to assess.

Despite its widespread use in patients with and without liver disease, milk thistle has not been implicated in causing serum enzyme elevations or clinically apparent acute liver injury. While silymarin has effects on cytochrome P450 enzymes and hepatic transporters in vitro, there is little evidence that it causes clinically significant herb–drug interactions.

GREEN TEA (POLYPHENOLS)

Green tea extract and concentrated infusions of green tea have been implicated in many cases of clinically apparent acute liver injury, including instances of acute

TABLE 16.1
Herbs and Liver Toxicity

Herb	Plant	Active Compound	Uses	Toxicity	Mechanism of Action
Asian herbs	*Dictamnus dasycarpus*, *Rehmannia glutimosa*, *Paeonia* species, *Glycyrrhiza* species, *Lophatherum* species	Combination	Eczema and psoriasis; Traditional Chinese Medicine for fever, flu, bronchitis, lung infections, TB, malaria, jaundice, and hepatitis	Acute liver failure, hepatitis	Unknown
Black Cohosh	*Actaea racemosa*, syn *Cimicifuga racemosa*	Triterpenes glycosides and polyphenols	Menopause symptoms and weight loss	Symptomatic elevations in serum enzymes without jaundice, acute self-limited hepatitis, prolonged hepatitis with cholestasis, autoimmune hepatitis, and acute liver failure requiring liver transplantation	Does not appear to be inherently hepatotoxic, possible liver injury is an idiosyncratic reaction, which may be immunologically mediated; specific component of injury unknown
Kava	*Piper methysticum*	Kava lactones (kava pyrones)	Its sedative, analgesic, and psychotropic properties are used for nervousness and insomnia. Cultural beverage in parts of Polynesia	2 cases of acute hepatitis, 11 cases of necrotizing hepatitis, 6 cases of cholestatic hepatitis, 1 case of lobular hepatitis, 6 cases of fulminant hepatic failure, 2 deaths	Direct hepatotoxin; inhibits oxidative phosphorylation; several kava lactones may act as inhibitors of CYP 450 system (CYP1A2, 2C9, 2C19, 2D6, 3A4 and 4A9/11). Therefore, potential drug interactions with kava are likely. Interactions between kava and CNS depressant, alcohol, levodopa, caffeine, anticonvulsants and MAO inhibitors *(Continued)*

TABLE 16.1 (Continued)
Herbs and Liver Toxicity

Herb	Plant	Active Compound	Uses	Toxicity	Mechanism of Action
Chaparral	*Larrea tridentata*	Nordihydroguaiaretic acid (NDGA)	Cancer (melanoma), bronchitis, colds, rheumatic pain, stomach pain, and chicken pox	Hepatitis, liver toxicity, liver failure. 13 cases of hepatitis reported to FDA between 1992 and 1994. Removed from the GRAS list in 1970.	Unknown mechanism; cholestasis, hepatocyte necrosis
Germander	*Teucrium chamaedrys*	Diterpenes	Weight loss, gout, digestive aid, fever	Liver toxicity, fatal hepatitis. France banned it in 1992 after 26 hepatitis cases	Components including glycosides, flavonoids, saponins, volatile oils and furan containing neoclerodane diterpenoids, the last of which (Teucrin A and Teuchmaedryn A) are considered the hepatotoxins responsible for its liver injury
Greater celandine	*Chelidonium majus*	Isoquinoline alkaloids	Externally for skin conditions (warts, eczema); internally for liver and gallstones	10 cases of hepatitis	Unknown, possibly idiosyncratic

(Continued)

TABLE 16.1 (Continued)
Herbs and Liver Toxicity

Herb	Plant	Active Compound	Uses	Toxicity	Mechanism of Action
Green tea	C. sinensis	Epigallocatechin-3-gallate (EGCG)	Antioxidant properties; prevent cancer and heart disease, decrease serum lipid levels, promote weight loss, decrease periodontal disease, acne, and treat clostridial diarrhea	Liver injury typically arises within 3 months, with latency to onset of symptoms ranging from 10 days to 7 months; acute hepatitis-like syndrome and a markedly hepatocellular pattern of serum enzyme elevations. Most recover rapidly upon stopping the extract or HDS; fatal instances of acute liver failure, rare	EGCG has been shown to induce mitochondrial toxicity and generation of reactive oxygen species. Higher doses of green tea (as in extracts) suggest a component of direct hepatotoxicity. Noted host susceptibility exacerbated by obesity, fasting or glutathionine depletion
Jin bu huan	Lycopodium serratum, Stephania species, Corydalis species	Levo-tetrohydropalamatine; pyrrolizidine alkaloids	Used in Traditional Chinese Medicine as a sedative, analgesic, and for indigestion	Life threatening bradycardia, respiratory distress, liver damage. Acute hepatitis	Unknown
Ma huang Mistletoe	Ephedra species Viscum album	Toxic proteins—phoratoxins and viscotoxins	Calms nerves, high blood pressure, antispasmodic; liver cancer	Hepatitis	Unknown Cytotoxic viscotoxins and mistletoe lectins

(Continued)

TABLE 16.1 (Continued)
Herbs and Liver Toxicity

Herb	Plant	Active Compound	Uses	Toxicity	Mechanism of Action
Pennyroyal	*Mentha puleguim, Hedeoma pulegoides*	Pulegone	Used in Hispanic cultures to treat colic, stimulate menses, and induces abortion	Liver toxicity, death	Reactive oxidative metabolite causes hepatocyte necrosis
Coltsfoot	*Tussilago farfara*	Pyrrolizidine alkaloids	Traditional Austrian medicine internally (as tea or syrup—confections) or externally (directly applied) for treatment of disorders of the respiratory tract, skin, locomotor system, viral infections, flu, colds, fever, rheumatism, gout	Liver toxicity, hepatitis, heavy drug interactions	Direct hepatotoxin; veno-occlusive disease; portal hypertension; centrilobular necrosis; and hepatocellular carcinoma
Comfrey	*Symphytum officinale, Symphytum asperum,* or *Symphytum uplandicum*	Pyrrolizidine alkaloids	Internally for blunt injuries (bruises, sprains, and broken bones), digestive tract (ulcers, diarrhea, inflammation), rheumatism pleuritis. Externally as a gargle for gum disease, pharyngitis, and strep throat	Vino-occlusive disease, liver toxicity and failure, and liver cancer	Direct hepatotoxin; veno-occlusive disease; portal hypertension; centrilobular necrosis; and hepatocellular carcinoma

(Continued)

TABLE 16.1 (Continued)
Herbs and Liver Toxicity

Herb	Plant	Active Compound	Uses	Toxicity	Mechanism of Action
Bush tea	*Crotalaria*	Pyrrolizidine Alkaloids with n-oxide base	Primarily South Africa: treating HIV infection, preventing cancer, anti-aging	Portal HTN, ascites, hepatomegaly	Direct hepatotoxin; veno-occlusive disease; portal hypertension; centrilobular necrosis; and hepatocellular carcinoma
Senecio	*Senecio longilobus*	Pyrrolizidine alkaloids	Folk remedy among the Mexican-American population: Atony of the reproductive organs, with impairment of function; uterine enlargement, with uterine or cervical leucorrhoea; difficult tenesmic micturition; dragging sensations in the testicles; perineal weight and fullness	Acute hepatocellular disease and portal hypertension and hepatic fibrosis	Direct hepatotoxin; veno-occlusive disease; portal hypertension; centrilobular necrosis; and hepatocellular carcinoma
Senna	*Cassia angustifolia*	Menthofuran	Laxative	Hepatitis, potassium loss, finger clubbing, and cathartic colon.	May be direct hepatotoxin; centrilobular necrosis is predominant pattern of injury
Skullcap-valerian combination	*Scutelleria lateriflora* and *Valeriana officinalis*	Cytotoxic flavonoids	Nervousness, insomnia	Hepatitis, liver failure and death	Possible hypersensitivity reaction

liver failure and death, but is generally well tolerated in standard over-the-counter tea preparations.

Both green tea and black tea are produced from the leaves of the Chinese tea tree *Camellia sinensis*. Green tea, as opposed to black tea, is unfermented, preserving its antioxidant polyphenolic catechols. It has been advertised to improve health, prevent cancer and heart disease, decrease serum lipid levels, promote weight loss, decrease periodontal disease, and treat clostridia diarrhea. The multiple polyphenols in green tea are believed to be the active components responsible for its purported chemoprotective, antiproliferative, and antioxidant properties.[5] Bose et al. studied the major effects of green tea polyphenol, (–)-epigallocatechin-3-gallate (EGCG), on high-fat-induced obesity, symptoms of the metabolic syndrome, and fatty liver in mice.[6] In mice fed a high-fat diet (HFD) (60% energy as fat), supplementation with dietary EGCG treatment (3.2 g/kg diet) for 16 weeks reduced body weight (BW) gain, percent body fat, and visceral fat weight ($P < 0.05$) compared with mice without EGCG treatment. The BW decrease was associated with increased fecal lipids in the high-fat-fed groups, attenuated insulin resistance, plasma cholesterol, and also decreased liver weight, liver triglycerides, and plasma alanine aminotransferase concentrations. Histological analyses of liver samples revealed decreased lipid accumulation in hepatocytes in mice treated with EGCG compared with HFD-fed mice without EGCG treatment.

Human clinical studies demonstrate that single doses of up to 1.6 g of green tea extract are well tolerated. The maximum tolerated dose in humans is reported to be 9.9 g/day; a dose equivalent to 24 cups of green tea. Side effects of high doses of green tea extract are usually mild and include headache, dizziness, and nausea.

Liver injury in unregulated forms of green tea such as "mega green tea" or green tea infusions typically arises within 3 months, with latency to onset of symptoms ranging from 10 days to 7 months. The majority of cases present with an acute hepatitis-like syndrome and a markedly hepatocellular pattern of serum enzyme elevations. Most patients recover rapidly upon stopping the extract or HDS, although fatal instances of acute liver failure have been described. Biopsy findings show necrosis, inflammation, and eosinophils in a pattern resembling acute hepatitis. Immunoallergic and autoimmune features are usually absent.

Preclinical and human data implicate the catechin and their gallic-acid esthers as the possible source of hepatotoxicity via effects on mitochondrial membranes.[7] Approximately 10% of the green tea extract is composed of catechins; of these, EGCG is present in highest concentration. There is great variability in the concentration of green tea extract, EGCG, and other components among marketed products, which may explain why some products have been implicated in hepatotoxicity. Exposure of rat hepatocytes to EGCG at high doses has been shown to induce mitochondrial toxicity and generation of reactive oxygen species. The association of liver injury with higher doses of green tea (as in extracts) suggests a component of direct hepatotoxicity, perhaps in the context of some degree of host susceptibility exacerbated by environmental features such as obesity, fasting, or glutathione depletion.

Given the widespread consumption of green tea and its extract in various HDS, liver injury from green tea is rare. Patients who present with acute liver injury particularly with a hepatocellular pattern without an obvious cause should be asked about the use of HDS and green tea extract, and should be advised to stop all herbal medications. In typical cases, recovery is expected in 1–2 months.

WEIGHT LOSS SUPPLEMENTS

Weight loss aids can be separated into several categories: *Prescription*: appetite suppressants (such as diethylpropion and phentermine) and those that block absorption of calories (Orlistat) and *Nonprescription*: Hydroxycut™, SlimQuick™, etc.

PRESCRIPTION WEIGHT LOSS MEDICATIONS

Several medications are directly aimed at sympathomimetic properties to cause anorexia such as amphetamine, diethylpropion, and phentermine. Side effects of other medication can also produce weight loss such as antidepressant serotonin and norepinephrine reuptake inhibitors (bupropion, fenfluramine, fluoxetine), serotonin agonists (lorcaserin), GABAnergic agents (topiramate, zonisamide) and cannabinoid antagonists (rimonabant). In 2012, two new weight loss agents were approved for use in the United States: a combination of phentermine and topiramate (Qsymia) and a serotonin agonist (Lorcaserin: Belviq). Due to heavy regulation by the FDA, liver injury is rare with all of the currently approved medications for weight loss. In contrast, serious hepatotoxicity has been linked to several over the counter and herbal preparations.

OVER-THE-COUNTER

Hydroxycut: The primary active component in the original formulation of Hydroxycut was ephedra prior to the FDA ban of this compound in 2004.[8] The liver injury attributed to ephedrine was possibly in conjunction with other constituents in the formulation leading to an idiosyncratic liver injury pattern. The company went into bankruptcy in 2006, and in 2009 a reformulation led to a revival of Hydroxycut's popularity. As of 2013, Hydroxycut's active ingredients are lady's mantle extract (*Alchemilla vulgaris*), wild olive extract (*Olea europaea*), komijn extract (*Cuminum cyminum*), wild mint extract (*Mentha longifolia*), and, in some products, green coffee bean extract (*Coffear canephora* robusta). The newest formulation has not been reported with liver toxicity.

Herbalife™: Similar to Hydroxycut, Herbalife's original formulation was based on ephedra. Later compositions contain a list of ingredients that varied with their multiple product lines. Several conflicting reports have been published regarding the direct causality of Herbalife and hepatitis. In July 2013, the *World Journal of Hepatology* evaluated the hepatotoxic link to Herbalife products. Their conclusion was using "the liver specific Council for International Organizations of Medical Sciences scale, causality was probable in 1 case, unlikely and excluded in the other cases. Thus, causality levels were much lower than hitherto proposed."[9] Also a recent report published by Navarro et al. speculates that often hepatotoxicity presents unique challenges given multiple ingredients, variable common names, which makes identifying the specific toxic agent difficult. Inclusion of vitamins can make the ingredient list exhausting to evaluate. Lastly, as in the case of Herbalife, foreign and unregulated manufacturing and distribution plants can be subject to less rigorous attention to contamination of herbals with microbials, pharmaceuticals mycotoxins, and heavy metals.[1]

SlimQuick: SlimQuick, a weight loss supplement, has reported rare cases of acute liver failure. The most recent was in a healthy patient that was also fasting for 3 weeks prior to ingestion and another case report was in a patient with heterozygous Alpha-one Antitrypsin disease who was also fasting at the time. The major ingredient in SlimQuick caplets is green tea extract (*C. sinensis* leaf) containing 135 mg of EGCG. EGCG has pro-oxidant effects that can cause hepatotoxicity when administered at high doses. Underlying fasting and aggressive other dieting practices may have contributed to the toxicity of this product in both cases and the reporters were inconclusive regarding direct toxicity.

NUTRITIONALS

CHOCOLATE

The believed impact of chocolate on liver disease is from the cocoa flavonoids, which have antioxidant properties. Increase in portal blood flow has also been implicated in the benefits of chocolate. At the Annual Meeting of the European Association for the Study of Liver (EASL, 2010) and later published in 2012, a study of 21 cirrhotic patients with end-stage liver disease (child score 6.9 ± 1.8; MELD 11 ± 4; hepatic venous pressure gradient (HPVG*) 16.6 ± 3.8 mmHg) were randomized to receive a standard liquid meal containing dark chocolate (containing 85% cocoa) while 11 patients received the liquid meal containing white chocolate that is devoid of cocoa flavonoids (antioxidant properties) according to BW. Both meals caused a highly significant but similar increase in portal blood flow; 24% increase with dark chocolate and a 34% increase with white chocolate. This counteracted the intrinsically decreased portal blood flow in cirrhosis, which leads to ongoing hepatic damage. The most interesting finding from this study was also a postprandial reduction in HPVG in the dark chocolate group. This was perhaps due to improved intrahepatic endothelial dysfunction from diminished oxidative stress. The decrease in gradient implied less resistance of blood supply to the liver, decreasing low-level ischemic damage.[10,11]

CAFFEINE

Coffee was initially believed, via its caffeine component, to have hepatoprotective effects. In a recently published article in *Hepatology*, August 2014, higher coffee consumption was inversely associated with elevated levels of liver enzymatic markers.[12] A total of 27,793 participants, age 20 or older, in the U.S. National Health and

Nutrition Examination Survey (1999–2010) was found to show that coffee at least three cups/day consumption was inversely associated with abnormal levels of all four liver enzymes (AST, ALT, ALP, GGT) and continuous levels of AST, ALP, and GGT.[13] However, the similarly inverse associations for total and decaffeinated coffee with liver enzyme suggested that coffee constituents other than caffeine may be beneficial toward the liver.

Several mechanistic studies have explored possible hepatoprotective effects of candidate coffee compounds. It has been reported that coffee diterpenes, cafestol and kahweol, may offer protective effects against aflatoxin B1-induced damage in rat and in hepatocyte cultures.[14] Cafestol and kahweol may also induce the synthesis of glutathione, which has been suggested to have a role in detoxification and prevention of liver damage. However, filtered coffee, the common type consumed in the United States, is thought to have lower levels of cafestol and kahweol when compared with boiled coffee. Other studies have suggested that polyphenols, which are found in coffee and shown to have potent antioxidant activity, may also be partially responsible for the effects on liver enzymes.[14] Adenosine, a purine nucleoside, is released in response to toxin exposure that can lead to hepatic fibrosis. Chan et al. and Peng et al. demonstrated that caffeine blocks adenosine and therefore can reduce possible fibrosis.[15,16] A review article by Cadden et al. on the further speculated on the beneficial effects of coffee beyond on improving abnormal liver biochemistry, and actually delaying cirrhosis development and hepatocellular carcinoma prevention.[17] The latter was also suggested in 2007 by Bravi et al. among other investigators.[18]

RED WINE

The component of red wine that is thought to be effective in mitigating liver disease is resveratrol, a red wine polyphenol that has shown to attenuate ethanol-induced oxidative stress in rat liver. The involvement of oxidative stress in the pathogenesis of alcoholic diseases in the liver has been repeatedly validated. Resveratrol, which is present in grape skins, is a natural phytoalexin (an antimicrobial and antioxidant substance within plants).[19] Resveratrol has a preventive effect on the main indicators of hepatic oxidative status as an expression of the cellular damage caused by free radicals, and on antioxidant defense mechanism during chronic ethanol treatment. A study by Kasdallah-Grissa et al. determined the mitigating influence of resveratrol on laboratory animals. Wistar rats were treated daily with 35% ethanol solution (3 g/kg/day i.p.) during 6 weeks and fed a standard diet with or without 5 g/kg resveratrol.[19] Experimentally, chronic ethanol administration leads to hepatotoxicity as monitored by the increase in the level of hepatic marker enzymes and the appearance of fatty change, necrosis, fibrosis, and inflammation in liver sections. Ethanol also enhances the lipid peroxidation, a major end point of oxidative damage, and caused drastic alterations in antioxidant defense systems. In this study, the activities of the hepatoprotective enzymes involved in antioxidant defense hepatic superoxide dismutase (SOD), glutathione peroxidase (GPx), and catalase (CAT) were found to be reduced by ethanol treatment while glutathione reductase (GR) activity was unchanged. Dietary supplementation with resveratrol during ethanol treatment inhibited hepatic lipid peroxidation and preserved SOD, GPx, and CAT activities in the liver and prevented hepatic oxidative damage[19] study.

Resveratrol has also shown in vitro antitumor properties in hepatocellular carcinoma. It is thought to inhibit hepatic cell proliferation, induce apoptosis, and impede angiogenesis.[20–22] These studies have not been validated in human subjects.

Notably, the consumption of red wine in patients with liver disease, however, is generally discouraged. According to the *Dietary Guidelines for Americans*,[23] moderate alcohol consumption is defined as having up to one drink per day for women and up to two drinks per day for men. This definition is referring to the amount consumed on any single day and is not intended as an average over several days. Alcohol is a proven hepatotoxin as elucidated earlier. A standard drink is equal to 14.0 g (0.6 oz) of pure alcohol. Generally, this amount of pure alcohol is found in 5 oz of wine (12% alcohol content). Red wine contains on the order of 0.1–14.3 mg/L of resveratrol.[24] Vitaglione et al. and Goldger et al. further studied the bioavailability of resveratrol and concluded the trace amounts of resveratrol reached in the blood are insufficient to explain its suspected ameliorating effects of alcohol. The metabolism and amount of resveratrol can be varying in wines and therefore, may benefit in healthy patients while patients with advanced liver disease may be harmed by red wine. Further studies are speculating that the cardiovascular benefits of wine appear to correlate with the content of procyanidins (flavanols).[25]

Probiotics

A number of studies have evaluated the potential mitigating influence of probiotics on liver disease. Probiotics are live microorganisms supplied from outside the human body, usually in the form of spores that aim to restore the natural balance. The speculated role of probiotic supplements is based on the established "gut–liver axis," which is an interaction between bacterial components like lipopolysaccharide (LPS) and hepatic receptors (Toll-like receptors [TLR]). Dysbiosis and altered intestinal permeability are speculated to alter this interaction and therefore result in hepatic disorders or worsening of hepatic diseases. Cirrhosis patients have colonic microbiota that are different from that of healthy control subjects.[26,27] Microbiota are commensal microbial organisms that coexist with humans in an enormous quantity. Normal gut integrity prevents the movement of these bacteria from the gut outside of the intestinal space that can trigger inflammatory responses.[28] The human gastrointestinal tract is the most heavily colonized site, and the colon contains more than two-thirds of the microbial load. On the whole, our gut has approximately 100 trillion (10^{14}) microbes of 1800 species, which make up approximately 1–2 kg of our weight.[29] Changes in microbiota have also been reported in nonalcoholic fatty liver disease (NAFLD), HE, alcohol-related liver disease, and hepatocellular carcinoma.

The abundance of the major gut microbiota, including Firmicutes and Bacteroidetes, has been considered a potential underlying mechanism of obesity and NAFLD. Gut microbiota may cause NAFLD by luminal ethanol production, causing a leaky gut and metabolic endotoxemia, or by metabolizing choline, a B-complex vitamin. Gut microbiota are a source of TLR ligands, and their compositional change can also increase the amount of TLR ligands delivered to the liver. TLR ligands can stimulate liver cells to produce proinflammatory cytokines.[30] These inflammatory-mediated, intracytoplasmic protein complexes-microbiota–host interactions may have a role in the transition from NAFLD to NASH.[31] Loguercio et al. first reported benefits of a complex preparation of probiotics, prebiotics, vitamins, and minerals in reducing aminotransferase levels in patients with NASH. The same group reported a reduction in parameters of lipid peroxidation in NAFLD patients with use of VSL#3 (Sigma-tau: VSL Pharmaceuticals, Inc.; Gaithersburg, MD).[32] Notably though, another small report by Solga et al., however, indicated an increase in hepatic fat with probiotic use.[33] Two further human studies later evaluated the role of probiotics in NAFLD, and were able to reproduce the findings of Loguercio et al. with reduced transaminase and LPS levels.[34,35]

Changes in microbiota have also been implicated in causation of HE, but the reports are conflicting.[36–38] In regard to HE, benefits of probiotics are modulated by changes in gut microbiota: an increase in nonurease-producing bacteria like lactobacilli and a concomitant reduction in urease producers like *Escherichia coli* and *Staphylococcus aureus*. However, a multistrain probiotic had no benefit in these patients except for a nonsignificant trend toward reduction in serum ammonia levels in those with elevated ammonia.[39] It should be noted that these changes in gut microbiota may also have a role in the pathogenesis of other complications of cirrhosis (e.g., spontaneous bacterial peritonitis, hepatorenal syndrome), which can induce encephalopathy. The 2014 Practice Guidelines by the American Association for the Study of Liver Disease (AASLD) do not support the role of probiotics in the treatment of HE. The guidelines do recommend though daily energy intakes should be 35–40 kcal/kg ideal BW, daily protein intake should be 1.2–1.5 g/kg/day, small meals or liquid nutritional supplements evenly distributed throughout the day and a late night snack should be offered, and oral BCAA supplementation may allow recommended nitrogen intake to be achieved and maintained in patients intolerant of dietary protein.[40]

It has also been suggested that microbiota are involved in the pathogenesis of cholestatic disorders like primary sclerosing cholangitis and PBC. The amount of circulating bile acid pool size is a function of microbial metabolism of bile acids in the intestines.[41] Increasing levels of the primary bile acid cholic acid (CA) causes an increasing production of the harmful secondary bile acid deoxycholic acid (DCA). During progression of cirrhosis, gut microbiome, both through their metabolism, cell wall components (LPS) and translocation lead to inflammation. Inflammation suppresses synthesis of bile acids in the liver leading to a positive-feedback mechanism. Decrease in bile acids entering the intestines (which is intrinsically present in cholestatic liver diseases) appears to favor overgrowth of pathogenic and pro-inflammatory members of the microbiome.[42] However, the role of multistrain probiotic in patients with primary sclerosing cholangitis for 3 months had no benefit for pruritus or liver functions, although there may be some benefit seen when an inflammatory bowel disease is concomitantly diagnosed.[43]

Bacterial displacement has been well documented in the pathogenesis of alcoholic liver disease via impairment of the function of intestinal tight junction[44–46] in conjunction with bacterial proliferation[47,48] by alcohol and/or its metabolites, such as acetaldehyde. These bacterial-derived metabolites (i.e., acetaldehye) enhance bacterial translocation into the liver, which induces activation of immune cells, including Kupffer cells, to release various pro-inflammatory cytokines and che-mokines.[49,50] Endotoxemia is notably often found in patients with cirrhosis, and the degree of endotoxemia correlates with the degree of liver failure.[28,51–53] Recent animal studies have shown that microbial translocation begins early in the course of alcoholic liver disease, leading to increased inflammation and eventually cirrho-sis.[54] Use of *E. coli* Nissle strain was reported to result in improvement in liver func-tion, as measured by Child-Pugh score, and reduction in endotoxin levels.[55] Use of VSL#3 for 2 months in cirrhosis patients with an elevated hepatic venous pressure gradient (>10 mmHg) did not reduce hepatic venous pressure gradient, although reductions in plasma endotoxemia and cytokines (TNF-α, interleukin 6, and inter-leukin 8) were noted.[56] However, these results have not been replicated or validated as clinically significant.

Preoperative and postoperative use of probiotics in cirrhosis and hepatocel-lular carcinoma patients who underwent tumor resection was associated with a lower serum TNF-α level and quicker recovery of hepatic function.[57] In rat mod-els of hepatic carcinogenesis, induction of gut dysbiosis significantly promoted carcinogenesis.[58] Another report indicates that microbiota may not be involved in the initiation of hepatocellular carcinoma, but in promotion and proliferation of hepatocellular carcinoma (PB22). Another interesting report from China evaluated a multistrain probiotic (*Lactobacillus* and *Propionobacterium* species) in healthy indi-viduals and noted a decrease in urinary excretion of aflatoxin metabolite, suggesting that probiotics may reduce exposure to aflatoxin and may have a chemopreventive role in hepatocellular carcinoma.[59] Also, the use of synbiotics (pre- and probiotic combinations) seems to decrease bacterial infections after liver transplantation.[60] In a recent randomized study, preoperative and postoperative use of a synbiotic prepa-ration significantly reduced infectious complications after elective living-donor liver transplantation.[61]

Overall, the gut–liver axis is continuously being studied and has several promis-ing launch points for treatment of liver disease.

VITAMINS AND MINERALS

NIACIN

Niacin, also known as nicotinic acid and vitamin B3, is a water-soluble, essential B vitamin. It is effective in lowering low-density lipoprotein (LDL) cholesterol and raising high-density lipoprotein (HDL) cholesterol, and is effective at regulating dys-lipidemia at high doses. Niacin can cause mild-to-moderate serum aminotransferase elevations and certain formulations of sustained-release niacin have been linked to clinically apparent, fatal fulminant liver injury.[62]

The recommended dietary allowance (RDA) of this vitamin is 14–16 mg daily in adults, for pregnant women (18 mg), and for children (2–12 mg). Niacin given at or around these doses is not associated with significant side effects or liver injury nor do they affect lipid levels. The doses of niacin for hyperlipidemia are higher than the RDA dose ranging from 1 to 6 g daily. The mechanism of action of niacin in hyperlipidemia is theoretically related to inhibition of cAMP signaling pathways in adipocytes, which results in decreased release of lipids from fat cells.

Niacin is available under intermediate release, sustained release, and extended release form in many concentrations from 50 to 1000 mg each. The recommended dosage for hyperlipidemia is 1–6 g daily, starting at low doses (100 mg three times daily) and increasing at weekly intervals based upon tolerance and effect. Common side effects of niacin include nausea, fatigue, pruritus and flushing; flushing being a major dose-limiting side effect. Flushing is thought to be related to the effect on the nicotinic receptors.

Niacin in doses above 500 mg daily causes transient, asymptomatic elevations in serum aminotransferase levels in up to 20% of people. The elevations are rarely greater than three times the upper limit of the normal range and usually resolve spontaneously even with continuation of the drug. The effect is partially dose related and is more common with doses above 3 g/day. Discontinuation of therapy rapidly resolved clinical symptoms usually within a week, whereas biochemical resolution may take months. Rechallenge with the same form leads to rapid recurrence and should be avoided.

Niacin can uncommonly cause serious hepatotoxicity, and is primarily hepatocellular, when the patients present with jaundice, itching, nausea, vomiting, and fatigue. Early during the injury serum aminotransferase levels are very high and then usually fall rapidly with discontinuation or dose lowering. It is believed to cause a direct toxic effect. Liver imaging may reveal areas of hypodensity ("starry sky liver") interpreted as focal fatty infiltration that resolves after stopping the drug. Liver biopsy typically shows varying degrees of centrolobular necrosis with only mild inflammation.

ZINC

Zinc deficiency/altered metabolism is observed in many types of liver diseases, including alcoholic liver disease (ALD) and viral liver disease.[63] Purported mechanisms speculated for zinc deficiency/altered metabolism include decreased dietary intake, increased urinary excretion, activation of certain zinc transporters, and induction of hepatic metallothionein.[63] Deficiency may manifest as skin lesions, poor wound healing/liver regeneration, altered mental status, or altered immune function.[63,64]

Zinc is an essential trace element required for normal cell growth, development, and differentiation. It is involved in DNA synthesis, RNA transcription, and cell division and activation. Zinc is a critical component in many zinc protein/enzymes, including critical zinc transcription factors.[65] Supplementation has been documented to block/attenuate experimental ALD through multiple processes, including stabilization of gut–barrier function, decreasing endotoxemia, decreasing proinflammatory cytokine production, decreasing oxidative stress, and attenuating apoptotic hepatocyte death.[66] Studies suggest improvement in liver function in both ALD and hepatitis C following zinc supplementation, and one study suggested improved fibrosis markers in hepatitis C patients.[67] Use in muscle cramps related to cirrhosis has also been attempted with mixed results at doses of 220 mg zinc sulfate twice daily.[68] The dose of zinc used for the treatment of liver disease is usually 50 mg of elemental zinc (or 220 mg zinc sulfate) taken with a meal to decrease the potential side effect of nausea.[63]

Zinc has also been used widely for the treatment of HE. In a study published in the *Lancet*, of 22 cirrhotic patients with chronic encephalopathy who were given oral zinc supplementation or placebo in a double-blind randomized trial there was a significant improvement in cognition. In the group that received zinc acetate 600 mg a day for 7 days, serum zinc had been restored to normal by day 8. On day 8 HE, as assessed by a trail making test, was improved in the supplemented group but not in the placebo group. There was also a significant increase in blood urea nitrogen in the supplemented group. Short-term oral zinc supplementation probably improved HE by correcting the zinc deficiency that compromises conversion of ammonia to urea.[69] A systematic review and meta-analysis of the use of oral zinc in the treatment of HE by Chavez-Tapia et al. further validated the improved performance on the number connection test, with the use of zinc.[70]

The critical role of zinc in Wilson's disease is well documented as a treatment.[71] Wilson's disease is an autosomal-recessive disorder of excessive copper accumulation. The defect in Wilson's disease is in the ATP-7B gene that downstream encodes ATPase that functions in the transmembrane transport of the copper within the hepatocytes. Absent ATPase leads to decreased hepatocellular excretion of copper into the bile. Subsequent accumulation of hepatic copper occurs with related injury. By inducing the enterocyte metallothionein protein (which is copper avid), zinc inhibits absorption of copper into the portal circulation. The copper is then excreted through fecal matter.[71] The dose of elemental zinc to use in Wilson's disease is 50 mg three times daily. Long-term supplemental zinc ingestion will cause copper depletion and have potential adverse consequences ranging from anemia to myelopathy and paresis.[72]

Vitamin C and Iron

Vitamin C, or ascorbic acid, is a popular supplement aids in collagen synthesis, and increases the production of neurotransmitters such as norepinephrine and serotonin, as well as supplementing with the nutrients that have been depleted due to the alcohol consumption.[73] Vitamin C enhances the absorption of iron. Notably, many patients with liver disease—up to 50%—have alteration in iron metabolism, but only 10% of all cases have excess hepatic iron deposition.[74,75] In the usual state of health, excess dietary iron is not absorbed and is excreted in the stool. In the setting of many chronic liver diseases, there is a propensity for excess iron to accumulate in the hepatic parenchyma. Patients with chronic hepatitis C and alcoholic liver disease have a tendency toward secondary hemosiderosis. The mechanism for iron overload in chronic liver disease is speculated to be from several mechanisms that include increased iron release from injured hepatocytes with secondary uptake by Kupffer cells, acute-phase reactions associated with chronic inflammatory states, increased gastrointestinal absorption of iron, and ineffective erythropoiesis with redistribution from sites of utilization to sites of storage.[75] Iron induces hepatotoxicity through the increased generation of free radicals and increased peroxidation of lipids, which in turn lead to organelle dysfunction, lysosomal fragility, mitochondrial dysfunction, and ultimately cell death.[76] Iron and vitamin C are therefore not generally recommended in chronic liver disease.

Vitamin D

The liver produces 25-hydroxy (25-OH) vitamin D, also known as calcidiol, the immediate precursor to the metabolically active form of vitamin D, also known as calcitriol. 25-OH vitamin D is the most abundant circulating form of vitamin D, and its measurement is used to assess vitamin D deficiency (VDD).[77] In patients with liver failure, the levels of 25-OH vitamin D can be low due to impaired synthesis. Liver disease could also lead to impaired absorption of vitamin D, which is possibly connected to impaired bile acid production or gut edema associated with portal hypertension. VDD has been proposed as fibrogenic through the vitamin D nuclear receptor.[78]

Low vitamin D levels and bone disease are well-recognized complications of "cholestatic" liver disease, which decreases the production or flow of bile. More recently, studies have confirmed low vitamin D levels in noncholestatic liver disease as well.[77] VDD or insufficiency is recognized for its association with NASH, while the underlying mechanism remains unknown.[79] In animal models, VDD promoted the HFD initiated simple steatosis into typical NASH, characterized by elevated hepatic inflammation and fat degeneration.[80] In alcoholic liver patients, there has been shown to be a direct toxicity of low vitamin D levels to bone cells and impaired calcium metabolism.[81] Alcoholics independently also may be disposed to deficiency due to poor nutrition, cholestasis, and pancreatic insufficiency.[81]

Vitamin D3 (cholecalciferol) has varied preparations with standard being 400 IU of vitamin D and calcium. Vitamin D3 at 50,000 international units are available. Vitamin D2 (ergo calciferol) is also available as 400 and 50,000 units. Calcidiol, which does not require hepatic hydroxylation, is also available in patients with liver disease as 25–50 µg capsules. The active form of vitamin D calcitriol is also available, but is associated with a higher risk of hypercalcemia, if not monitored closely. The goal for all patients with chronic liver disease should be a 25-OH vitamin D level of 30 ng/mL. Anything less than 15–20 ng/mL is considered a deficiency.

Vitamin E

Vitamin E, or tocopherol, has been widely studied for its role in the therapy of nonalcoholic fatty liver disease. In both alcoholic and nonalcoholic fatty liver disease, tumor necrosis factor alpha (TNF-α) and nuclear factor kappa B (NF-κB) are implicated in the pro-inflammatory pathway.[82] Vitamin E treatments in vitro have decreased the activation of both of the cytokines. Additionally, it has been shown to block stellate cell activity that induces fibrosis.

In the pioglitazone (30 mg daily) versus vitamin E (800 IU daily) versus placebo for the treatment of nondiabetic patients with nonalcoholic steatohepatitis (PIVENS) trial, vitamin E therapy demonstrated a significant improvement in steatosis, inflammation, ballooning, and resolution of steatohepatitis in adult patients with aggressive NASH (without cirrhosis).[83]Although vitamin E showed a significant resolution of

NASH in the pediatric population, a sustained reduction of alanine aminotransferase was not attained in the treatment of NAFLD in children (TONIC) trial.[84]

Enthusiasm for vitamin E as a preventative measure for NASH patients to progress to cirrhosis was later curbed, as vitamin E, was also found to demonstrate possible risks. One concern with vitamin E is the controversial issue of whether it increases all-cause mortality. Some meta-analyses have reported an increase in all-cause mortality with high-dose vitamin E, but others failed to confirm such an association.[85–87] In a review by Dietrich et al., vitamin E supplements were associated with an increased incidence of cardiovascular disease and all-cause mortality specifically in patients with underlying heart disease and diabetes in the Framingham Heart Study.[85] Another study described the increased risk of prostate cancer with vitamin E intake.[88]

The prevalence of NAFLD is likely to increase over time due to the epidemics of obesity and diabetes. Presently, there is no definitive treatment for NAFLD. Based on available evidence, vitamin E (RRR-α-tocopherol) at 800 IU/day is only recommended in NASH adults without diabetes or cirrhosis and with aggressive histology.

CONCLUSIONS

The challenges in causality assessment of liver toxicity and HDS are from limitations in complete case ascertainment, complexity, and multiplicity of HDS, possibility of adulterants in manufacturing (such as pharmaceuticals, microbes, chemicals, heavy metals), and HDS–drug interactions. Certainly, given the popularity of these agents among the public, further attention to investigate their pros/cons is warranted. More importantly, the impact of these therapies in conjunction with standard medical therapies as opposed to in lieu of them can be areas of investigation in the future.

REFERENCES

1. Navarro VJ, Barnhart H, Bonkovsky HL et al. Liver injury from herbals and dietary supplements in the U.S. drug-induced liver injury network. *Hepatology.* 2014;60(4):1399–1408.
2. Radimer K, Bindewald B, Hughes J, Ervin B, Swanson C, Picciano MF. Dietary supplement use by US adults: Data from the national health and nutrition examination survey, 1999–2000. *Am J Epidemiol.* 2004;160(4):339–349.
3. Abenavoli L, Capasso R, Milic N, Capasso F. Milk thistle in liver diseases: Past, present, future. *Phytother Res.* 2010;24(10):1423–1432.
4. Flora K, Hahn M, Rosen H, Benner K. Milk thistle (*Silybum marianum*) for the therapy of liver disease. *Am J Gastroenterol.* 1998;93(2):139–143.
5. Seeff L, Stickel F, Navarro VJ. Hepatotoxicity of herbals and dietary supplements. In Kaplowitz N, DeLeve LD, eds. *Drug-Induced Liver Disease*, 3rd edn. Amsterdam, the Netherlands: Elsevier, 2013, pp. 631–658. (Review of hepatotoxicity of herbal and dietary supplements [HDS] mentions that there have been at least 58 case reports of liver injury attributed to green tea extracts, powdered leaves or infusions including 1 fatal case.)
6. Bose M, Lambert JD, Ju J, Reuhl KR, Shapses SA, Yang CS. The major green tea polyphenol, (–)-epigallocatechin-3-gallate, inhibits obesity, metabolic syndrome, and fatty liver disease in high-fat-fed mice. *J Nutr.* 2008;138(9):1677–1683.

7. Galati G, Lin A, Sultan AM, O'Brien PJ. Cellular and in vivo hepatotoxicity caused by green tea phenolic acids and catechins. *Free Radic Biol Med.* 2006;40(4):570–580.

8. Fessenden, F. Studies of dietary supplements come under growing scrutiny. *The New York Times, 1-3.* June 23, 2003. http://www.nytimes.com/2003/06/23/us/studies-of-dietary-supplements-come-under-growing-scrutiny.html. Retrieved May 2, 2009.

9. Teschke R, Wolff A, Frenzel C, Schwarzenboeck A, Schulze J, Eickhoff A. Drug and herb induced liver injury: Council for international organizations of medical sciences scale for causality assessment. *World J Hepatol.* 2014;6(1):17–32.

10. De Gottardi A, Berzigotti A, Seijo S et al. 19 dark chocolate attenuates the post-prandial increase in HVPG in patients with cirrhosis and portal hypertension. *J Hepatol.* 2010;52:S9.

11. De Gottardi A, Berzigotti A, Seijo S et al. Postprandial effects of dark chocolate on portal hypertension in patients with cirrhosis: Results of a phase 2, double-blind, randomized controlled trial. *Am J Clin Nutr.* 2012;96(3):584–590.

12. Goh GB, Chow WC, Wang R, Yuan JM, Koh WP. Coffee, alcohol and other beverages in relation to cirrhosis mortality: The Singapore Chinese health study. *Hepatology.* 2014;60(2):661–669.

13. Ruhl CE, Everhart JE. Coffee and caffeine consumption reduce the risk of elevated serum alanine aminotransferase activity in the United States. *Gastroenterology.* 2005;128(1):24–32.

14. Higdon JV, Frei B. Coffee and health: A review of recent human research. *Crit Rev Food Sci Nutr.* 2006;46(2):101–123.

15. Peng Z, Fernandez P, Wilder T et al. Ecto-5′-nucleotidase (CD73)-mediated extracellular adenosine production plays a critical role in hepatic fibrosis. *FASEB J.* 2008;22(7):2263–2272.

16. Chan ES, Montesinos MC, Fernandez P et al. Adenosine A(2A) receptors play a role in the pathogenesis of hepatic cirrhosis. *Br J Pharmacol.* 2006;148(8):1144–1155.

17. Cadden IS, Partovi N, Yoshida EM. Review article: Possible beneficial effects of coffee on liver disease and function. *Aliment Pharmacol Ther.* 2007;26(1):1–8.

18. Bravi F, Bosetti C, Tavani A et al. Coffee drinking and hepatocellular carcinoma risk: A meta-analysis. *Hepatology.* 2007;46(2):430–435.

19. Kasdallah-Grissa A, Mornagui B, Aouani E et al. Resveratrol, a red wine polyphenol, attenuates ethanol-induced oxidative stress in rat liver. *Life Sci.* 2007;80(11):1033–1039.

20. Delmas D, Jannin B, Cherkaoui Malki M, Latruffe N. Inhibitory effect of resveratrol on the proliferation of human and rat hepatic derived cell lines. *Oncol Rep.* 2000;7(4):847–852.

21. Carbo N, Costelli P, Baccino FM, Lopez-Soriano FJ, Argiles JM. Resveratrol, a natural product present in wine, decreases tumour growth in a rat tumour model. *Biochem Biophys Res Commun.* 1999;254(3):739–743.

22. Bishayee A, Politis T, Darvesh AS. Resveratrol in the chemoprevention and treatment of hepatocellular carcinoma. *Cancer Treat Rev.* 2010;36(1):43–53.

23. U.S. Department of Agriculture and U.S. Department of Health and Human Services. *Dietary Guidelines for Americans*, 7th Edn., Washington, DC: U.S. Government Printing Office, December 2010, pp. 30–32.

24. Baur JA, Sinclair DA. Therapeutic potential of resveratrol: The in vivo evidence. *Nat Rev Drug Discov.* 2006;5(6):493–506.

25. Corder R, Mullen W, Khan NQ et al. Oenology: Red wine procyanidins and vascular health. *Nature.* 2006;444(7119):566.

26. Liu J, Wu D, Ahmed A et al. Comparison of the gut microbe profiles and numbers between patients with liver cirrhosis and healthy individuals. *Curr Microbiol.* 2012;65(1):7–13.

27. Chen Y, Yang F, Lu H et al. Characterization of fecal microbial communities in patients with liver cirrhosis. *Hepatology.* 2011;54(2):562–572.

28. Seo YS, Shah VH. The role of gut-liver axis in the pathogenesis of liver cirrhosis and portal hypertension. *Clin Mol Hepatol.* 2012;18(4):337–346.

29. Sharma V, Garg S, Aggarwal S. Probiotics and liver disease. *Perm J.* 2013;17(4):62–67.

30. Miura K, Ohnishi H. Role of gut microbiota and toll-like receptors in nonalcoholic fatty liver disease. *World J Gastroenterol.* 2014;20(23):7381–7391.

31. Henao-Mejia J, Elinav E, Jin C et al. Inflammasome-mediated dysbiosis regulates progression of NAFLD and obesity. *Nature.* 2012;482(7384):179–185.

32. Loguercio C, Federico A, Tuccillo C et al. Beneficial effects of a probiotic VSL#3 on parameters of liver dysfunction in chronic liver diseases. *J Clin Gastroenterol.* 2005;39(6):540–543.

33. Solga SF, Buckley G, Clark JM, Horska A, Diehl AM. The effect of a probiotic on hepatic steatosis. *J Clin Gastroenterol.* 2008;42(10):1117–1119.

34. Aller R, De Luis DA, Izaola O et al. Effect of a probiotic on liver aminotransferases in nonalcoholic fatty liver disease patients: A double blind randomized clinical trial. *Eur Rev Med Pharmacol Sci.* 2011;15(9):1090–1095.

35. Vajro P, Mandato C, Licenziati MR et al. Effects of lactobacillus rhamnosus strain GG in pediatric obesity-related liver disease. *J Pediatr Gastroenterol Nutr.* 2011;52(6):740–743.

36. Bajaj JS, Hylemon PB, Ridlon JM et al. Colonic mucosal microbiome differs from stool microbiome in cirrhosis and hepatic encephalopathy and is linked to cognition and inflammation. *Am J Physiol Gastrointest Liver Physiol.* 2012;303(6):G675–G685.

37. Bajaj JS, Ridlon JM, Hylemon PB et al. Linkage of gut microbiome with cognition in hepatic encephalopathy. *Am J Physiol Gastrointest Liver Physiol.* 2012;302(1):G168–G175.

38. Shawcross DL, Sharifi Y, Canavan JB et al. Infection and systemic inflammation, not ammonia, are associated with grade 3/4 hepatic encephalopathy, but not mortality in cirrhosis. *J Hepatol.* 2011;54(4):640–649.

39. Pereg D, Kotliroff A, Gadoth N, Hadary R, Lishner M, Kitay-Cohen Y. Probiotics for patients with compensated liver cirrhosis: A double-blind placebo-controlled study. *Nutrition.* 2011;27(2):177–181.

40. Vilstrup H, Amodio P, Bajaj J et al. Hepatic encephalopathy in chronic liver disease: 2014 practice guideline by the American Association for the Study of Liver Diseases and the European Association for the Study of the Liver. *Hepatology.* 2014;60(2):715–735.

41. Ridlon JM, Kang DJ, Hylemon PB, Bajaj JS. Bile acids and the gut microbiome. *Curr Opin Gastroenterol.* 2014;30(3):332–338.

42. Ridlon JM, Alves JM, Hylemon PB, Bajaj JS. Cirrhosis, bile acids and gut microbiota: Unraveling a complex relationship. *Gut Microbes.* 2013;4(5):382–387.

43. Vleggaar FP, Monkelbaan JF, van Erpecum KJ. Probiotics in primary sclerosing cholangitis: A randomized placebo-controlled crossover pilot study. *Eur J Gastroenterol Hepatol.* 2008;20(7):688–692.

44. Rao RK, Seth A, Sheth P. Recent advances in alcoholic liver disease I. Role of intestinal permeability and endotoxemia in alcoholic liver disease. *Am J Physiol Gastrointest Liver Physiol.* 2004;286(6):G881–G884.

45. Rao RK. Acetaldehyde-induced increase in paracellular permeability in caco-2 cell monolayer. *Alcohol Clin Exp Res.* 1998;22(8):1724–1730.

46. Keshavarzian A, Farhadi A, Forsyth CB et al. Evidence that chronic alcohol exposure promotes intestinal oxidative stress, intestinal hyperpermeability and endotoxemia prior to development of alcoholic steatohepatitis in rats. *J Hepatol.* 2009;50(3):538–547.

47. Yumuk Z, Ozdemirci S, Erden BF, Dundar V. The effect of long-term ethanol feeding on *Brucella melitensis* infection of rats. *Alcohol Alcohol.* 2001;36(4):314–317.

48. Kavanaugh MJ, Clark C, Goto M et al. Effect of acute alcohol ingestion prior to burn injury on intestinal bacterial growth and barrier function. *Burns.* 2005;31(3):290–296.

49. Wheeler MD, Kono H, Yin M et al. The role of Kupffer cell oxidant production in early ethanol-induced liver disease. *Free Radic Biol Med.* 2001;31(12):1544–1549.

50. Thakur V, McMullen MR, Pritchard MT, Nagy LE. Regulation of macrophage activation in alcoholic liver disease. *J Gastroenterol Hepatol.* 2007;22(Suppl. 1):S53–S56.

51. Bigatello LM, Broitman SA, Fattori L et al. Endotoxemia, encephalopathy, and mortality in cirrhotic patients. *Am J Gastroenterol.* 1987;82(1):11–15.

52. Lin RS, Lee FY, Lee SD et al. Endotoxemia in patients with chronic liver diseases: Relationship to severity of liver diseases, presence of esophageal varices, and hyperdynamic circulation. *J Hepatol.* 1995;22(2):165–172.

53. Michie HR, Manogue KR, Spriggs DR et al. Detection of circulating tumor necrosis factor after endotoxin administration. *N Engl J Med.* 1988;318(23):1481–1486.

54. Schaffert CS, Duryee MJ, Hunter CD et al. Alcohol metabolites and lipopolysaccharide: Roles in the development and/or progression of alcoholic liver disease. *World J Gastroenterol.* 2009;15(10):1209–1218.

55. Lata J, Novotny I, Pribramska V et al. The effect of probiotics on gut flora, level of endotoxin and child-pugh score in cirrhotic patients: Results of a double-blind randomized study. *Eur J Gastroenterol Hepatol.* 2007;19(12):1111–1113.

56. Tandon P, Moncrief K, Madsen K et al. Effects of probiotic therapy on portal pressure in patients with cirrhosis: A pilot study. *Liver Int.* 2009;29(7):1110–1115.

57. Rifatbegovic Z, Mesic D, Ljuca F et al. Effect of probiotics on liver function after surgery resection for malignancy in the liver cirrhotic. *Med Arh.* 2010;64(4):208–211.

58. Zhang HL, Yu LX, Yang W et al. Profound impact of gut homeostasis on chemically-induced pro-tumorigenic inflammation and hepatocarcinogenesis in rats. *J Hepatol.* 2012;57(4):803–812.

59. El-Nezami HS, Polychronaki NN, Ma J et al. Probiotic supplementation reduces a biomarker for increased risk of liver cancer in young men from southern China. *Am J Clin Nutr.* 2006;83(5):1199–1203.

60. Rayes N, Seehofer D, Theruvath T et al. Supply of pre- and probiotics reduces bacterial infection rates after liver transplantation—A randomized, double-blind trial. *Am J Transplant.* 2005;5(1):125–130.

61. Eguchi S, Takatsuki M, Hidaka M, Soyama A, Ichikawa T, Kanematsu T. Perioperative synbiotic treatment to prevent infectious complications in patients after elective living donor liver transplantation: A prospective randomized study. *Am J Surg.* 2011;201(4):498–502.

62. Mullin GE, Greenson JK, Mitchell MC. Fulminant hepatic failure after ingestion of sustained-release nicotinic acid. *Ann Intern Med.* 1989;111(3):253–255.

63. Mohammad MK, Zhou Z, Cave M, Barve A, McClain CJ. Zinc and liver disease. *Nutr Clin Pract.* 2012;27(1):8–20.

64. Prasad AS. Zinc: An overview. *Nutrition.* 1995;11(1 Suppl.):93–99.

65. Chasapis CT, Loutsidou AC, Spiliopoulou CA, Stefanidou ME. Zinc and human health: An update. *Arch Toxicol.* 2012;86(4):521–534.

66. Zhou Z, Wang L, Song Z, Saari JT, McClain CJ, Kang YJ. Zinc supplementation prevents alcoholic liver injury in mice through attenuation of oxidative stress. *Am J Pathol.* 2005;166(6):1681–1690.

67. Kang YJ, Zhou Z. Zinc prevention and treatment of alcoholic liver disease. *Mol Aspects Med.* 2005;26(4–5):391–404.

68. Kugelmas M. Preliminary observation: Oral zinc sulfate replacement is effective in treating muscle cramps in cirrhotic patients. *J Am Coll Nutr.* 2000;19(1):13–15.

69. Reding P, Duchateau J, Bataille C. Oral zinc supplementation improves hepatic encephalopathy. Results of a randomised controlled trial. *Lancet.* 1984;2(8401):493–495.

70. Chavez-Tapia NC, Cesar-Arce A, Barrientos-Gutierrez T, Villegas-Lopez FA, Mendez-Sanchez N, Uribe M. A systematic review and meta-analysis of the use of oral zinc in the treatment of hepatic encephalopathy. *Nutr J.* 2013;12:74.

71. Brewer GJ. Zinc acetate for the treatment of Wilson's disease. *Expert Opin Pharmacother.* 2001;2(9):1473–1477.

72. Ala A, Walker AP, Ashkan K, Dooley JS, Schilsky ML. Wilson's disease. *Lancet.* 2007;369(9559):397–408.

73. Leevy CM, Thompson A, Baker H. Vitamins and liver injury. *Am J Clin Nutr.* 1970;23(4):493–498.

74. Riggio O, Montagnese F, Fiore P et al. Iron overload in patients with chronic viral hepatitis: How common is it? *Am J Gastroenterol.* 1997;92(8):1298–1301.

75. Di Bisceglie AM, Axiotis CA, Hoofnagle JH, Bacon BR. Measurements of iron status in patients with chronic hepatitis. *Gastroenterology.* 1992;102(6):2108–2113.

76. Stal P, Hultcrantz R. Iron increases ethanol toxicity in rat liver. *J Hepatol.* 1993;17(1):108–115.

77. Nair S. Vitamin D deficiency and liver disease. *Gastroenterol Hepatol (N Y).* 2010;6(8):491–493.

78. Timms PM, Mannan N, Hitman GA et al. Circulating MMP9, vitamin D and variation in the TIMP-1 response with VDR genotype: Mechanisms for inflammatory damage in chronic disorders? *QJM.* 2002;95(12):787–796.

79. Kitson MT, Roberts SK. D-livering the message: The importance of vitamin D status in chronic liver disease. *J Hepatol.* 2012;57(4):897–909.

80. Kong M, Zhu L, Bai L et al. Vitamin D deficiency promotes nonalcoholic steato-hepatitis through impaired enterohepatic circulation in animal model. *Am J Physiol Gastrointest Liver Physiol.* 2014;307(9):G883–G893.

81. Malik P, Gasser RW, Kemmler G et al. Low bone mineral density and impaired bone metabolism in young alcoholic patients without liver cirrhosis: A cross-sectional study. *Alcohol Clin Exp Res.* 2009;33(2):375–381.

82. Tilg H, Diehl AM. Cytokines in alcoholic and nonalcoholic steatohepatitis. *N Engl J Med.* 2000;343(20):1467–1476.

83. Chalasani NP, Sanyal AJ, Kowdley KV et al. Pioglitazone versus vitamin E versus placebo for the treatment of non-diabetic patients with non-alcoholic steatohepatitis: PIVENS trial design. *Contemp Clin Trials.* 2009;30(1):88–96.

84. Athinarayanan S, Wei R, Zhang M et al. Genetic polymorphism of cytochrome P450 4F2, vitamin E level and histological response in adults and children with nonalcoholic fatty liver disease who participated in PIVENS and TONIC clinical trials. *PLoS ONE.* 2014;9(4):e95366.

85. Dietrich M, Jacques PF, Pencina MJ et al. Vitamin E supplement use and the incidence of cardiovascular disease and all-cause mortality in the Framingham heart study: Does the underlying health status play a role? *Atherosclerosis.* 2009;205(2):549–553.

86. Gerss J, Kopcke W. The questionable association of vitamin E supplementation and mortality—Inconsistent results of different meta-analytic approaches. *Cell Mol Biol (Noisy-le-grand).* 2009;55(Suppl.):OL1111–OL1120.

87. Berry D, Wathen JK, Newell M. Bayesian model averaging in meta-analysis: Vitamin E supplementation and mortality. *Clin Trials.* 2009;6(1):28–41.

88. Klein EA, Thompson IM, Jr, Tangen CM et al. Vitamin E and the risk of prostate cancer: The selenium and vitamin E cancer prevention trial (SELECT). *JAMA.* 2011;306(14):1549–1556.

17 Nutrition in Acute and Chronic Pancreatitis

Neha Jakhete, MD and Vikesh K. Singh, MD, MSc

CONTENTS

INTRODUCTION

The pancreas plays an important role in digestion—producing and releasing enzymes that help to break down carbohydrates, fats, and proteins. When food enters the stomach and passes into the small intestine, a variety of hormonal signals stimulate the acinar cells of the pancreas to release stored enzymes into the lumen of the small intestine to assist in the digestion of macromolecules. The islet cells of the pancreas also make insulin and glucagon, playing a key role in glucose control. Inflammation and fibrosis of the pancreas can lead to disruptions of its exocrine and endocrine functions that can lead to nutritional complications. Nutrition has a critical role in healing and is especially important in acute and chronic pancreatitis given its central function in the digestive process. The type and route of nutritional support differs depending on duration and severity of pancreatic inflammation and fibrosis.

ACUTE PANCREATITIS

Patients with acute pancreatitis often present with acute onset epigastric abdominal pain, nausea, and vomiting. The diagnosis is made when two of following three features are present: acute epigastric abdominal pain, elevated serum amylase and/or lipase levels ≥3 times the upper limit of normal, and/or characteristic imaging findings of pancreatitis on abdominal imaging studies [1]. Imaging is not required to make the diagnosis of acute pancreatitis but is recommended if an alternative diagnosis is being entertained at the time of patient presentation or to monitor for complications.

Acute pancreatitis is categorized as mild, moderate, or severe. These classifications are based on the presence of local/systemic complications and/or organ failure (renal, pulmonary, and/or cardiovascular). Mild acute pancreatitis (the most common form of acute pancreatitis) usually resolves within a week and does not involve any organ failure. In moderate acute pancreatitis, transient organ failure (<48 h) may be present and local complications may result (peripancreatic fluid collections, pancreatic necrosis). When organ failure is persistent (>48 h), acute pancreatitis is classified as severe [1].

Acute pancreatitis can also be divided into two different morphological subtypes: interstitial edematous pancreatitis and necrotizing pancreatitis, based on the revised Atlanta Classification. In interstitial edematous pancreatitis, the pancreas enlarges due to interstitial edema from inflammation (present in a majority of patients with acute pancreatitis). Necrotizing pancreatitis is present in 5%–10% of patients and results from necrosis of pancreatic parenchyma and surrounding tissues. Pseudocysts and walled-off necrosis can occur >4 weeks after the onset of symptoms in patients with interstitial and necrotizing pancreatitis, respectively [1]. It should be noted that infected necrosis is classified as "moderately" severe acute pancreatitis by the revised Atlanta classification but severe acute pancreatitis by the determinant-based classification [2].

Patients with severe acute pancreatitis should be admitted to the intensive care unit for management. Mortality is based on the presence of persistent organ failure and/or infected necrosis. Various prognostic scoring systems have been developed (APACHE II, Ranson's criteria, BISAP) that can help predict the mortality of acute pancreatitis [1,3]. However, the primary role of these prognostic scoring systems in clinical practice is their high negative predictive value (i.e., patients without positive scores are likely to have mild acute pancreatitis).

Management of Nutrition

The metabolic demands in patients with acute pancreatitis increase due to the systemic inflammatory response syndrome (SIRS); however, the body is unable to absorb nutrients to meet this demand. This results in a catabolic state that can delay healing and lead to poor outcomes. Historically, prolonged fasting was the mainstay of treatment in acute pancreatitis because it was thought that oral intake would release secretin and CCK, resulting in further pancreatic stimulation leading to worsening acute inflammation. However, multiple studies have shown that early oral or enteral feeding can lead to shortened hospitalizations, decreased infectious complications, decreased morbidity, and decreased mortality [3–9]. A 2013 meta-analysis found that initiation of enteral feeding within 48 h showed improved clinical outcomes including decreased incidence of hyperglycemia, organ failure, and infections in both mild and severe acute pancreatitis [10]. Of note, the PYTHON trial did not show superiority of early nasoenteric tube feeding, as compared with an oral diet after 72 h, in reducing the rate of infection or death in patients with acute pancreatitis at high risk for complications; however, there were many limitations to the study including using scoring systems (which have poor positive predictive value) to predict severity of pancreatitis [11]. In general, nutritional support should not be delayed for more than 5–7 days to prevent severe net nitrogen losses [12]. The type and route of nutritional support in acute pancreatitis depends on the severity of the pancreatitis.

Mild Acute Pancreatitis

Patients with mild acute pancreatitis are initially managed with intravenous hydration, nil per os, and analgesics. When analgesic requirements decrease, symptoms improve (decreased abdominal pain, nausea, bloating; increased hunger) and physical examination demonstrates the presence of bowel sounds and decreased abdominal tenderness, an oral diet can be gradually introduced. This usually occurs within 1 week of presentation. Patients will typically be started on a clear liquid diet and then advanced to a solid diet as tolerated. A low fat and low-residue (low-fiber) diet is often recommended on the premise that a low fat diet will decrease stimulation of the pancreas. There are no formal guidelines for what constitutes a "low"-fat diet with studies reporting anywhere from 2–4 g fat/meal to 30–35 g fat/day [13–16]. A few clinical trials have shown mixed results in starting immediately with soft diet, with some studies reporting no difference and others showing shorter length of hospital stay [8,15–18]. Initiation of feeding with a low fat solid diet appears as safe as a clear liquid diet [16].

It is important to note, however, that discharging a patient before he/she is able to tolerate a solid diet is a risk factor for readmission [19].

Moderate/Severe Acute Pancreatitis

Patients suffering from moderate/severe pancreatitis will need to have nutritional support as they will have a delay in resuming oral intake due to gastrointestinal inflammation and/or pancreatic/peripancreatic fluid. Enteral feeding is preferred over total parenteral nutrition (TPN), as long as there is no ileus present [7,20]. Using enteral feeding has been shown to help maintain the intestinal barrier by preventing intestinal mucosal atrophy that, in turn, prevents the translocation of bacteria [21–24]. Enteral feeding also avoids the complications of parenteral nutrition including catheter-related bloodstream infections. Studies have shown a reduction in mortality, organ dysfunction, and infections with enteral nutrition [25,26]. Enteral feedings can be initiated in most cases even in the presence of fluid collections within or surrounding the pancreas. Parental nutrition should only be used if the patient is unable to tolerate enteral feeds (<10% of goal rate), if there is ileus present, or if the patient is not meeting sufficient caloric requirements [3].

Enteral feeding can be introduced via a nasogastric tube as studies have shown no significant difference in outcomes and are comparable in safety when compared to nasojejunal feeding [27,28]. There has been one small study showing increased pulmonary complications (risk of aspiration) with nasogastric tube feedings; however, additional studies are needed to determine whether the nasogastric route is truly inferior to the nasojejunal. For now, positioning patients in an upright position and following aspiration precautions is recommended. One disadvantage of enteral feeding via nasojejunal tube instead of nasogastric is the necessity for endoscopic or radiological tube placement. This can lead to delays in initiating nutrition depending on the ability to have the procedure. Placement of a nasojejunal tube is associated with higher costs and is associated with an increased risk of proximal migration [3,26–31]. Complications of nasogastric or nasojejunal feedings include nasopharyngeal discomfort, mucosal irritation, and sinusitis [12].

Enteral Tube Feedings High-protein, low fat feedings are recommended because of decreased stimulation of the pancreas and a reduction in pancreatic enzyme release. Studies comparing elemental formulas (completely predigested formula composed of amino acids, simple sugars, and essential fatty acids) to polymeric or semi-elemental formulas (nonhydrolyzed proteins, complex carbohydrates, and long chain fatty acids) have shown no difference in risk of infectious complications and death [32]. The rate of tube feeds should be advanced as tolerated to reach calorie goal (about 25–35 kcal/kg and 0.8–1.5 g/kg protein in adults) and patients should be monitored for abdominal pain, vomiting, and diarrhea. Continuous feedings are preferred to bolus feedings although more studies are needed. Typically, feedings can be started at 25 mL/h for 24 h and then advanced by 25 mL/h daily over the next 48 h to reach caloric goal [3,12].

A 2009 review evaluated the use of probiotics in pancreatitis and found that a majority of the studies demonstrated reduced bacterial infection rates [33]. However, probiotic supplementation is not recommended in severe acute pancreatitis as there was a significant increase in mortality in one RCT [34].

CHRONIC PANCREATITIS

Chronic pancreatitis results from progressive fibrosis of the pancreas from chronic inflammation that can lead to permanent and irreversible loss of pancreatic exocrine and endocrine function. The development of chronic pancreatitis depends on a complex interaction between environmental exposures and genetics. Alcohol, tobacco, smoking, hypertriglyceridemia, and gene mutations can all play a role in disease development. The progression of fibrosis depends on the etiology of chronic pancreatitis [35,36].

The most common presenting symptom of chronic pancreatitis is abdominal pain (usually begins as intermittent pain and then becomes constant). While patients with abdominal pain and calcifications are easily diagnosed as having chronic pancreatitis, the diagnosis of noncalcific chronic pancreatitis can be challenging for many reasons. There are many other conditions and diseases that can present with similar symptoms and no tests that accurately differentiate early or mild chronic pancreatitis from these other conditions and diseases. In addition, diagnostic endoscopic and radiological imaging studies are used to detect structural changes of the pancreas that may be correlated fibrosis but it should be emphasized that pancreatic fibrosis can be seen in asymptomatic patients who consume alcohol or smoke, are obese, or who are older. The single strongest risk factor for chronic pancreatitis is a prior history of acute recurrent pancreatitis [35,36].

Management of Nutrition

Exocrine Insufficiency

Fibrosis of the pancreatic parenchyma in chronic pancreatitis results in malabsorption of fat, protein, and carbohydrates due to decreased production of pancreatic enzymes. Fat malabsorption is the primary presentation of severe exocrine insufficiency as enzymes involved in lipid breakdown are affected before enzymes involved in protein breakdown because lipase is more susceptible to acidic and proteolytic degradation [35–37]. Steatorrhea occurs when 90% of the glandular function has been lost due to progressive fibrosis and acinar cell death. Steatorrhea presents as foul smelling and greasy stools. It can be diagnosed with a 72 h fecal fat collection (>7 g/day when on 100 g fat restricted diet for 3 days) or fecal elastase (most commonly <100 mcg/g). Unfortunately, it is much harder to diagnose mild/moderate exocrine insufficiency. Fecal elastase testing has limited sensitivity for mild/moderate exocrine insufficiency. The only available test for the diagnosis of moderate exocrine insufficiency is the 13C mixed triglyceride breath test [38,39], but this test is limited by the fact that it takes 6 h to complete.

The mainstay of treatment is following a fat-restricted diet, usually <20 g/day, with monitoring of stools and bloating. It should be noted that there is no strong evidence for fat restriction in pancreatic insufficiency and this is usually recommended for symptom control. The malabsorption of fat contributes to weight loss in chronic pancreatitis patients and there is controversy regarding fat restriction given the importance of maintaining adequate nutrition [35,36]. In addition, pancreatic enzymes work best when administered with fat.

Amylase and trypsin deficiencies develop after lipase deficiency, resulting in impairment in breakdown and absorption of carbohydrates and proteins, respectively. Fecal protein loss can result in fluid retention and edema when >2.5 g are lost in the stool per day. However, there are other mechanisms for the breakdown and absorption for these molecules that do not involve pancreatic enzymes and therefore, carbohydrate and protein metabolism can still proceed [35,40].

Patients should be treated with lipase supplementation to help control steatorrhea. The healthy pancreas secretes approximately 700,000–1,000,000 units of lipase (USP) per meal. It is recommended that patients receive 10% of this amount to achieve symptom control. The amount of lipase supplementation can be adjusted based on symptoms and nutrition goals, for example, the dose can be increased in patients trying to achieve weight gain [41]. Enzymes should be taken during or after meals for greatest effect as endogenous pancreatic enzymes release peaks at 20–60 min after consumption of meals [35,42].

Treatment with pancreatic enzymes is thought to reduce pancreatic enzyme secretion and therefore reduce pain [43]. The presence of exogenous enzymes suppresses CCK release that prevents stimulation of endogenous pancreatic enzyme release [44]. However, there have been mixed results in clinical trials with some showing enzyme supplements are no better than placebo for the treatment of pain. Many different doses of enzymes supplements have been studied with no one dose showing increased benefit over any other dose [45]. Nonenteric-coated enzymes should be used with H2 blockers to prevent the activation of enzymes by stomach acid. Fecal chymotrypsin can be measured to assess response to pancreatic enzyme supplementation with decreasing quantities of chymotrypsin indicating adequate dosing [46].

Patients with chronic pancreatitis can also be supplemented with medium-chain triglycerides (MCTs). MCTs are absorbed directly by the intestinal mucosa without requiring prior breakdown with lipase or bile salts, both of which are decreased in chronic pancreatitis [35].

In general, 80% of patients can be treated with a normal diet and pancreatic enzyme supplementation as long as they can tolerate a high-calorie diet of at least

35 kcal/kg/day. The increased caloric intake is needed to match the increased resting energy expenditure that is present in chronic pancreatitis [35].

Endocrine Dysfunction

Endocrine dysfunction is due to loss of alpha and beta cells within the pancreas and can lead to derangements in glucose control, known as type 3c diabetes. Type 3c diabetes makes up about 5%–10% of all diabetes, and 80% of these cases are due to chronic pancreatitis, typically chronic calcific pancreatitis [47,48]. Brittle diabetes can result from impairments in both insulin and glucagon production. It is therefore important to screen chronic pancreatitis patients with fasting blood sugar and hemoglobin A1c [35,49]. Metformin is typically the first drug of choice in patients with type 3c diabetes; however, this may not be tolerated due to its gastrointestinal side effects. Insulin secretagogues can also be used, such as sulfonylureas to help boost insulin secretion. Incretin-based therapies also enhance insulin secretion. Of note, the data on GLP1 agonists and DPP4 inhibitors causing acute pancreatitis is weak—they can cause low-grade amylase and lipase elevations, but this is commonly in asymptomatic patients [50–52]. Many patients will eventually end up on insulin therapy and in cases of severe malnutrition, insulin therapy should be initiated immediately [53]. It is important that MCTs be used with caution in diabetics as they can induce ketogenesis [54].

Vitamin Deficiencies

It is also important to monitor for vitamin deficiencies in chronic pancreatitis, especially the fat-soluble vitamins A, D, E, and K. Levels should be checked and supplemented as needed. Periodic screening of bone density should be done in certain patients given malabsorption of calcium and vitamin D as this can lead to increased fracture risk [35,55,56].

CONCLUSION

Nutrition management in pancreatitis plays a key role in the treatment plan as the pancreas recovers. The type and route of nutrition varies based on severity and chronicity of disease. Bowel rest is no longer recommended, and nutrition should be initiated early in acute pancreatitis. In chronic pancreatitis, enzyme supplementation is the main treatment recommendation with close monitoring of abdominal pain, bloating, stool consistency, and weight. More studies are needed to determine the ideal amount of fat consumption in both acute and chronic pancreatitis.

REFERENCES

1. Banks, P., Bollen, T., Dervenis, C. et al. 2013. Classification of acute pancreatitis—2012: Revision of the Atlanta classification and definitions by international consensus. *Gut* 62: 102–111.
2. Dellinger, E.P., Forsmark, C.E., Layer, P. et al. 2012. Determinant-based classification of acute pancreatitis severity. *Ann Surg* 256: 875–880.
3. Tenner, S., Baillie, J., DeWitt, J. et al. 2013. American College of Gastroenterology guideline: Management of acute pancreatitis. http://gi.org/guideline/acute-pancreatitis/. Accessed Novemeber 8, 2014.

4. Louie, B.E., Noseworthy, T., Hailey, D. et al. 2005. 2004 MacLean-Mueller Prize enteral or parenteral nutrition for severe pancreatitis: A randomized controlled trial and health technology assessment. *Can J Surg* 48: 298–306.
5. Casas, M., Mora, J., Fort, E. et al. 2007. Total enteral nutrition vs. total parenteral nutrition in patients with severe acute pancreatitis. *Rev Esp Enferm Dig* 99: 264–269.
6. Gupta, R., Patel, K., Calder, P.C. et al. 2003. A randomised clinical trial to assess the effect of total enteral and total parenteral nutritional support on metabolic, inflammatory and oxidative markers in patients with predicted severe acute pancreatitis II (APACHE ≥ 6). *Pancreatology* 3: 406–413.
7. Yi, F., Ge, L., Zhao, J. et al. 2012. Meta-analysis: Total parenteral nutrition versus total enteral nutrition in predicted severe acute pancreatitis. *Intern Med* 51: 523–530.
8. Li, J., Xue, G.J., Liu, Y.L. et al. 2013. Early oral refeeding wisdom in patients with mild acute pancreatitis. *Pancreas* 42: 88–91.
9. Wereszczynska-Siemiatkowska, U., Swidnicka-Siergiejko, A., Siematkowski, A. et al. 2013. Early enteral nutrition is superior to delayed enteral nutrition for the prevention of infected necrosis and mortality in acute pancreatitis. *Pancreas* 42: 640–646.
10. Li, J.Y., Yu, T., Chen, G.C. et al. 2013. Enteral nutrition within 48 hours improves clinical outcomes of acute pancreatitis by reducing complications: A meta-analysis. *PLoS ONE* 8: 1–12.
11. Bakker, O.J., van Brunschot, S., van Santvoort, H.C. et al. 2014. Early versus on-demand nasoenteric tube feeding in acute pancreatitis. *N Engl J Med* 371: 1983–1993.
12. Vipperla, K. and O'Keefe, S.J. 2015. Nutrition in severe acute pancreatitis. In *Prediction and Management of Severe Acute Pancreatitis*, Forsmark, C.E. and Gardner, T.B. (eds.), pp. 123–132. Springer Science + Business Media, New York.
13. Mirtallo, J.M., Forbes, A., McClave, S.A. et al. 2012. International consensus guidelines for nutrition therapy in pancreatitis. *JPEN J Parenter Enteral Nutr* 36: 284.
14. LaRusch, J., Solomon, S., and Whitcomb, D.C. 1993–2014. Pancreatitis overview. In *GeneReviews®* [Internet], Pagon, R.A., Adam, M.P., Ardinger, H.H., Bird, T.D., Dolan, C.R., Fong, C.T., Smith, R.J.H., and Stephens, K. (eds.). Seattle, WA: University of Washington.
15. Jacobson, B.C., Vander Vliet, M.B., Hughes, M.D. et al. 2007. A prospective, randomized trial of clear liquids versus low-fat solid diet as the initial meal in mild acute pancreatitis. *Clin Gastroenterol Hepatol* 5: 946–951.
16. Moraes, J.M., Felga, G.E., Chebli, L.A. et al. 2010. A full solid diet as the initial meal in mild acute pancreatitis is safe and result in a shorter length of hospitalization: Results from a prospective, randomized, controlled, double-blind clinical trial. *J Clin Gastroenterol* 44: 517e22.
17. Sathiaraj, E., Murthy, S., Mansard, M.J. et al. 2008. Clinical trial: Oral feeding with a soft diet compared with clear liquid diet as initial meal in mild acute pancreatitis. *Aliment Pharmacol Ther* 28: 777–781.
18. Rajkumar, N., Karthikeyan, V.S., Ali, S.M. et al. 2013. Clear liquid diet vs soft diet as the initial meal in patients with mild acute pancreatitis: A randomized interventional trial. *Nutr Clin Pract* 28: 365–370.
19. Whitlock, T.L., Repas, K., Tignor, A. et al. 2010. Early readmission in acute pancreatitis: Incidence and risk factors. *Am J Gastroenterol* 105: 2492–2497.
20. Kalfarentzos, F., Kehagias, J., Mead, N. et al. 1997. Enteral nutrition is superior to parenteral nutrition in severe acute pancreatitis: Results of a randomized prospective trial. *Br J Surg* 84: 1665–1669.
21. Ammori, B.J., Leeder, P.C., King, R. et al. 1999. Early increase in intestinal permeability in patients with severe acute pancreatitis: Correlation with endotoxemia, organ failure, and mortality. *J Gastrointest Surg* 3: 252–262.

22. Qin, H.L., Su, Z.D., Gao, Q. et al. 2002. Early intrajejunal nutrition: Bacterial translocation and gut barrier function of severe acute pancreatitis in dogs. *Hepatobiliary Pancreat Dis Int* 1: 150–154.
23. Qin, H.L., Su, Z.D., Hu, L.G. et al. 2002. Effect of early intrajejunal nutrition on pancreatic pathological features and gut barrier function in dogs with acute pancreatitis. *Clin Nutr* 21: 469–473.
24. Abou-Assi, S., Craig, K., and O'Keefe, S.J. 2002. Hypocaloric jejunal feeding is better than total parenteral nutrition in acute pancreatitis: Results of a randomized comparative study. *Am J Gastroenterol* 97: 2255–2262.
25. Forsmark, C.E., Baillie, J., AGA Institute Clinical Practice and Economics Committee, and AGA Institute Governing Board. 2007. AGA Institute technical review on acute pancreatitis. *Gastroenterology* 132: 2022.
26. Al-Omran, M., Albalawi, Z.H., Tashkandi, M.F. et al. 2010. Enteral versus parenteral nutrition for acute pancreatitis. *Cochrane Database Syst Rev* Issue 1. Art. No.: CD002837.
27. Eatock, F.C., Brombacher, G.D., Steven, A. et al. 2000. Nasogastric feeding in severe acute pancreatitis may be practical and safe. *Int J Pancreatol* 28: 23–29. Taylor & Francis Group, Boca Raton, FL.
28. Eatock, F.C., Chong, P., Menezes, N. et al. 2005. A randomized study of early nasogastric versus nasojejunal feeding in severe acute pancreatitis. *Am J Gastroenterol* 100: 432–439.
29. Singh, N., Sharma, B., Sharma, M. et al. 2012. Evaluation of early enteral feeding through nasogastric and nasojejunal tube in severe acute pancreatitis: A noninferiority randomized controlled trial. *Pancreas* 41(1): 153–159.
30. Kumar, A., Singh, N., Prakash, S. et al. 2006. Early enteral nutrition in severe acute pancreatitis: A prospective randomized controlled trial comparing nasojejunal and nasogastric routes. *J Clin Gastroenterol* 40: 431–434.
31. Olah, A. and Romics, L. Jr. 2010. Evidence-based use of enteral nutrition in acute pancreatitis. *Langenbecks Arch Surg* 395: 309–316.
32. Petrov, M.S., Loveday, B.P., Pylypchuk, R.D. et al. 2009. Systematic review and meta-analysis of enteral nutrition formulations in acute pancreatitis. *Br J Surg* 96: 1243–1252.
33. Rayes, N., Seehofer, D., and Neuhaus, P. 2009. Prebiotics, probiotics, synbiotics in surgery—Are they only trend, truly effective or even dangerous? *Langenbecks Arch Surg* 394: 547–555.
34. Besselink, M.G., van Santvoort, H.C., Buskens, E. et al. 2008. Probiotic prophylaxis in predicted severe acute pancreatitis: A randomised, double-blind, placebo-controlled trial. *Lancet* 371: 651–659.
35. Afghani, E., Sinha, A., and Singh, V.K. 2014. An overview of the diagnosis and management of nutrition in chronic pancreatitis. *Nutr Clin Pract* 29: 295–311.
36. Steer, M.L., Waxman, I., and Freedman, S. 1995. Chronic pancreatitis. *N Engl J Med* 332: 1482.
37. Gosine, D., Kaleel, M.R., and Singh, V.K. 2011. Nutritional considerations in acute and chronic pancreatitis. In *Gastrointestinal and Liver Disease Nutrition Desk Reference*, Mullin, M. Matarese, G., and Palmar, L.E. (eds.), pp. 171–180.
38. Keller, J., Aghdassi, A.A., Lerch, M.M. et al. 2009. Tests of pancreatic exocrine function—Clinical significance in pancreatic and non-pancreatic disorders. *Best Pract Res Clin Gastroenterol* 23: 425–439.
39. Keller, J., Meier, V., Wolfram, K.U. et al. 2014. Sensitivity and specificity of an abbreviated (13)C-mixed triglyceride breath test for measurement of pancreatic exocrine function. *United European Gastroenterol J* 2: 288–294.

40. Airinei, G., Gaudichon, C., Bos, C. et al. 2011. Postprandial protein metabolism but not a fecal test reveals protein malabsorption in patients with pancreatic exocrine insufficiency. *Clin Nutr* 30: 831–837.

41. Keller, J. and Layer, P. 2005. Human pancreatic exocrine response to nutrients in health and disease. *Gut* 54(Suppl. 6): vi1.

42. Dominguez-Munoz, J.E., Iglesias-Garcia, J., Iglesias-Rey, M. et al. 2005. Effect of the administration schedule on the therapeutic efficacy of oral pancreatic enzyme supplements in patients with exocrine pancreatic insufficiency: A randomized, three-way crossover study. *Aliment Pharmacol Ther* 21: 993–1000.

43. Singh, V.V. and Toskes, P.P. 2003. Medical therapy for chronic pancreatitis pain. *Curr Gastroenterol Rep* 5: 110.

44. Owyang, C. 1994. Negative feedback control of exocrine pancreatic secretion: Role of cholecystokinin and cholinergic pathway. *J Nutr* 124: 1321S.

45. Brown, A., Hughes, M., Tenner, S. et al. 1997. Does pancreatic enzyme supplementation reduce pain in patients with chronic pancreatitis: A meta-analysis. *Am J Gastroenterol* 92: 2032.

46. Chowdhury, R.S. and Forsmark, C.E. 2003. Review article: Pancreatic function testing. *Aliment Pharmacol Ther* 17: 733–750.

47. Ewald, N., Kaufmann, C., Raspe, A. et al. 2012. Prevalence of diabetes mellitus secondary to pancreatic diseases (type 3c). *Diabetes Metab Res Rev* 28: 338–342.

48. Cui, Y. and Andersen, D.K. 2011. Pancreatogenic diabetes: Special considerations for management. *Pancreatology* 11:279–294.

49. Rickels, M.R., Bellin, M., Toledo, F.G. et al. 2013. Detection, evaluation and treatment of diabetes mellitus in chronic pancreatitis: Recommendations from Pancreas Fest. *Pancreatology* 13: 336–342.

50. Giorda, C.B., Sacerdote, C., Nada, E. et al. 2014. Incretin-based therapies and acute-pancreatitis risk: A systematic review and meta-analysis of observational studies. *Endocrine* 48: 461–471.

51. Shetty, A.S., Nandith, A., Snehalath, C. et al. 2013. Treatment with DPP-4 inhibitors does not increase the chance of pancreatitis in patients with type 2 diabetes. *J Assoc Physicians India* 61: 543–544.

52. Delfino, M., Motola, D., Benini, A. et al. 2014. Incretin-mimetics associated pancreatitis: Evidence from the spontaneous adverse drug reactions reporting in Italy. *Expert Opin Drug Saf* 13: 151–156.

53. Ewald, N. and Hardt, P.D. 2013. Diagnosis and treatment of diabetes mellitus in chronic pancreatitis. *World J Gastroenterol* 19: 7276–7281.

54. Yeh, Y.Y. and Zee, P. 1976. Relation of ketosis to metabolic changes induced by acute medium-chain triglyceride feeding in rats. *J Nutr* 106: 58–67.

55. Bernstein, C.N., Leslie, W.D., and Leboff, M.S. 2003. AGA technical review on osteoporosis in gastrointestinal diseases. *Gastroenterology* 124: 795–841.

56. Tignor, A.S., Wu, B.U., Whitlock, T.L. et al. 2010. High prevalence of low-trauma fracture in chronic pancreatitis. *Am J Gastroenterol* 105: 2680–2686.

18 Nutrition and Mental Health

Nora Galil, MD, MPH, FAACAP
and Robert Hedaya, MD, DLFAPA

CONTENTS

INTRODUCTION

Psychiatric illnesses and disabilities are on the rise as much as other chronic illnesses. To this end, the burden of mental health and substance abuse disorders has increased 37.6% from 1990 to 2010 (Whiteford et al. 2013, 1575–1586). Despite the progression in disease burden, the solutions remain limited in a conventional medicine model. In contrast, in a functional medicine (Jones and Quinn 2006) model of psychiatry, nutrition is one of the major biopsychosocial factors to explore when a previously successful medication regimen suddenly *stops working*. It is the authors' view that barring high-risk situations requiring immediate relief, medication changes (other than dose adjustments) should not be the primary focus of treatment until other causes of medication failure are explored (nutrition, inflammation, etc.). While psychiatric medications clearly have their place in the medical armamentarium, they also have their limitations. Among these limitations is the fact that some of these medications are known to deplete certain nutrients. For example, valproic acid depletes carnitine in young children (Abd and El-Serogy 2012, 275–281), and metformin and gastric acid inhibitors are associated with vitamin B_{12} deficiencies (Lam et al. 2013, 2435–2442; Reinstatler et al. 2012, 327–333).

Improving nutrition can frequently correct many of the symptoms of mental and emotional disorders and, for some, completely restore health without the use of medication. Others will be able to decrease their use of medication and/or ameliorate side effects.

Furthermore, the stresses of modern life place a burden on bodily systems and increase the need for many nutrients. Nutrient-depleted soils, antibiotic/grain-fed meats, excessive sugar intake, and diets low in anti-inflammatory fats and rich in pro-inflammatory foods (Fallon and Enig 2001) are thought to be harming our health. One of the authors has been routinely successful in treating bipolar type II and obsessive compulsive disorder (OCD) without medication using a functional medicine model (Jones and Quinn 2006). Importantly, nutrition is an important cornerstone of this model.

In this chapter, we describe how nutritional science is applicable to mental health, highlight some of the more common nutrient deficiencies associated with compromised mental health, and review some of the evidence for various nutraceuticals commonly used in psychiatric disorders. Finally, we provide a basic template of useful laboratory tests that are important in the integration of nutrition into an overall plan for improved mental and physical health.

DIET AND MENTAL HEALTH

Most psychiatric patients consume diets heavy in carbohydrates and deficient in protein (Ventura et al. 2014, 252–256), a practice that flies in the face of current core dietary guidelines generally deemed important for mental and physical health. These guidelines include minimal amounts of processed foods, good-quality fats with an emphasis on omega-3 fatty acids, complex carbohydrates, minimal or no sugar, adequate but not excessive protein from clean (no antibiotics or hormones, grass-fed) animal or plant sources, and plenty of clean water. Of course, given the biochemical and genetic diversity of the human race, one diet cannot be the appropriate one for everyone. It is important to note that Weston Price described various cultures that enjoyed good health and longevity on varied diets: some were mostly seafood with no fruit and few vegetables (Alaskan Eskimos), others were primarily rye bread and cheese (Swiss farmers), while the Masai warriors' diet consisted of animal blood and milk (Planck 2006).

Processed foods do not contain the needed micronutrients and often contain trans fats and significant amounts of sugar (often high-fructose corn syrup [HFCS]) and salt. The chronic consumption of these *foods* causes structural change of membrane phospholipids, affecting brain neurotransmission, and has been shown to increase anxiety (Bakhtiyari et al. 2013, 107–112; Jacka et al. 2011, 483–490) and depression (Jacka et al. 2010, 305–311). Trans fats, created by hydrogenation to make them artificially saturated fats (and solid at room temperature), raise LDL (Brouwer et al. 2013, 541–547) and cause heart disease (Brouwer et al. 2013, 541–547). Low cholesterol is associated with increased impulsivity and suicide (Troisi 2011, 83–87; Zhang 2011, 268–287).

Sugar consumption has increased dramatically as well in recent years, in part because of the advent of HFCS, the main caloric sweetener in *junk food*. The body is not equipped to deal with either the high doses of sugar (unbound by fiber and without micronutrients) or the compensatory release of insulin; high serum glucose levels lead to a surge in adrenalin, one of the acute stress hormones (Jones et al. 1995, 171–177). Thus, intraday depression, anxiety, panic, fatigue, difficulty concentrating, etc., can be traced back to diet-based dysglycemia and have numerous downstream consequences.

Essential fatty acids, which make up much of the cell membranes, are enormously important in mental health. However, since the 1960s, *low-fat diets* and the consumption of *polyunsaturated vegetable fats* have been championed. More recently, these assumptions are coming into question as a new debate emerges about fats and health and, by extension, mental health. A 2010 review of 21 studies looking at saturated fats did not find evidence of increased cardiac risk (Siri-Tarino et al. 2010, 535–546). It has been established that the membrane phospholipids mediate the entry of neurotransmitters (NTs) into the cell. Inadequate amounts of these essential fatty acids (omega-3s, primarily) and structural substitution by dietary trans fats are thought to alter normal neurotransmission. Studies in rats indicate that trans fats result in a preference for and augmentation of amphetamine effects. Kuhn et al. (2015) support the idea that trans fats may have a negative influence on mental health. On the other hand, the omega-3 fatty acids (found in certain fish, seaweed, algae, and eggs (hatched from chickens fed only on flaxseeds and fish meal), are clearly effective in mood disorders (Grosso et al. 2014). A wide palette of color in the vegetable category provides much needed antioxidant and nutrient benefit, with a more minor emphasis on fruit.

Patients should be educated to balance every meal and every snack with protein, fat, and complex carbohydrates, barring medical reasons to the contrary. Generally, this approach enhances mental stability and energy within 5–6 days (Hedaya 2000).

Caffeine may be healthy for some people due to its antioxidant content, but in the psychiatric population too, often it causes unstable blood sugar, depression, irritability, adrenal depletion, nutrient depletion, and irritable bowel with concomitant malabsorption, among other difficulties (Bergin and Kendler 2012, 473–482).

GENERAL RECOMMENDATIONS FOR NUTRITIONAL DEFICIENCIES

While individuals differ in their needs for certain nutrients, there are certain nutritional deficiencies that are extremely common and relevant to the psychiatric population. Most commonly, these deficiencies include omega-3 fatty acids, zinc, iron, vitamin D, and methylated B vitamins (Pfeiffer et al. 2013, 938S–947S), hence our discussion later.

Because of individual variation, it is best to conduct appropriate lab tests before recommending many, if not most of these supplements. In cases where deficiencies are identified, it is useful to supplement with the single micronutrient necessary. However, many other micronutrient deficiencies can exist and can affect mental health. Given that (1) individuals vary in their specific needs for certain nutrients and (2) micronutrients work in concert, it is also useful to consider a broad-spectrum micronutrient mixture in patients with mental illness. For an excellent review of the literature on single and broad-spectrum micronutrient supplementation affecting mental health, Popper's review in *Child and Adolescent Clinics of North America* is much recommended (Popper 2014, 591–672).

OMEGA-3 ESSENTIAL FATTY ACIDS

Omega-3 fatty acids, one of the nutrients most commonly deficient in Western diets, have been implicated in attention-deficit hyperactivity disorder (Arnold et al. 2013, 381–402), depression, bipolar disorder (Song 2013, 75–89), alcoholism, and violence (Simopoulos 2011, 203–215). The two omega-3 essential fatty acids of note are EPA and DHA.

While studies examining the relevance of omega-3s in ADHD are somewhat mixed, the generally recommended dose for ADHD is 2–3 g/day, with a preponderance of DHA (Richardson 2006, 155–172). A meta-analysis of the use of omega-3s in bipolar disorder found "strong evidence that bipolar depressive but not manic symptoms may be improved by adjunctive use of omega-3 fatty acids" (Sarris et al. 2012, 81–86). The doses used in various studies for unipolar depression range from 1 to 4 g of EPA daily with 1 g being more efficacious than 4 g (Osher and Belmaker 2009, 128–133).

It is safe to say that the best dose for optimal mental health is yet to be determined. Different forms of fish and krill oil are available; when using high doses, liquid may be better tolerated. When using omega-3 essential fatty acids, some clinicians also recommend balancing them with GLA (from primrose or borage oil), an anti-inflammatory omega-6 and a precursor to prostaglandin E_1 (Vasquez 2009, 561).

When recommending omega-3 fatty acids, be cautious of their use in patients with diabetes or coagulation disorders.

ZINC

The highest concentration of zinc is normally in the brain. It is necessary for efficient serotonergic neurotransmission and immune function, yet it is one of the most commonly deficient minerals. Low zinc is associated with learning difficulties (Yorbik et al. 2008, 662–667) and ADHD (Bloch and Mulqueen 2014). Zinc deficiency is quite common in adolescence (Schenkel et al. 2007, 264–271), leaving young people more vulnerable to mood disorders, irritability, and OCD (Ozuguz et al. 2013). Because requirements for zinc vary, based on copper status, genetic factors, and soil content, testing must be done.

IRON

Many micronutrient deficiencies can be linked to inadequate dietary intake, and certainly vegetarians/vegans are at increased risk for low iron. But so are women of childbearing age. Iron is necessary to ensure oxygenation and for the synthesis of NTs and myelin and affects behavior in a variety of ways (Kim and Wessling-Resnick, 2014). Deficiency is found in children with ADHD (Bourre 2006, 377–385) and is often implicated in fatigue.

VITAMIN D

Vitamin D is necessary for the function of every cell in the body; and so, it is critical to mental health. In psychiatry, deficiency has been associated with seasonal affective disorder and depression, although causality has not been established (Parker and Brotchie 2011, 243–249). Still, given modern lifestyles with often minimal sun exposure and a paucity of vitamin D–rich food sources, supplementation to bring levels into the normal range may be useful. However, there are dangers to oversupplementing, and vitamin D functions in a balance with other nutrients, such as vitamin A. High levels of vitamin A can decrease the benefits/levels of vitamin D (Oh et al. 2007, 1178–1186). Testing and retesting are always recommended.

B COMPLEX VITAMINS

Deficiencies of B vitamins, particularly folate, B_6 and B_{12}, are overwhelmingly linked to mood disorders and depression (Herbison et al. 2012, 634–638; Mischoulon and Raab 2007, 28–33; Penninx et al. 2000, 715–721). Vitamins B_6 and B_{12} also play crucial roles in methylation (see discussion later) and NT metabolism (Midttun et al. 2007, 131–138; Miller 2008, 216–226).

DIGESTION AND MENTAL HEALTH

ABSORPTION

Even the best diet cannot overcome persistent difficulties in the digestion and absorption of food. Digestion requires normal gastric function (including production of appropriate levels of hydrochloric acid [HCl]) and pancreatic digestive enzymes. HCl (whose production is commonly reduced with age and acid blocking agents often used for acid reflux) serves at least three functions. First, it helps break down protein components of the diet, so that amino acids such as tryptophan and tyrosine (essential for the production of NTs) can be available for absorption by facilitating the action of pepsin in the small intestine. Second, it helps maintain normal bacterial flora in the proximal small intestine, which facilitates normal absorption and digestion, and bacterial production of micronutrients such as B_{12} (Dukowicz et al. 2007, 112–122). Finally, when administered as a supplement (betaine HCl), the betaine moiety supplies an alternative pathway in the methylation cycle (Crider et al. 2012, 21–38), which is a critical factor in the regulation of NT availability. The parietal cell, which produces HCl, also assists in the absorption of B_{12}. Thus, all factors that affect parietal cell function (e.g., age and medications used for gastroesophageal reflux) affect the earlier processes, which in turn affect NT availability.

Pancreatic digestive enzymes are needed for the breakdown and absorption of fats, complex carbohydrates, and proteins, and so decreased production of pancreatic enzymes will have broad effects on the availability of multiple micronutrients.

INFLAMMATION

Gastrointestinal (GI) inflammation is relevant to brain function, hence mental illness (Rosenblat et al. 2014, 23–34). A large portion of the immune system is associated with the gut. Inflammatory processes originating in the GI tract affect brain function both through impaired nutrient absorption and through cytokine-mediated vagal endocrine signaling (Mayer et al. 2014, 1500–1512) to the brain. Therefore, all factors affecting the GI inflammation must be a consideration in establishing good mental health.

GLUTEN SENSITIVITY

A growing concern in the mental health field is gluten sensitivity (of which celiac disease is a subcategory) since it is well known to cause absorptive abnormalities. Gluten intolerance has been implicated in the pathophysiology of ADHD, schizophrenia, anxiety, depression, and autism even without any obvious GI manifestations (Genuis and Lobo 2014; Jackson et al. 2012, 91–102; Peters et al. 2014, 1104–1112).

NUTRACEUTICALS FOR PSYCHIATRIC SYMPTOMS AND DISORDERS

L-METHYLFOLATE

Methylation, one of the fundamental processes of the body, is central to numerous physiological processes including NT and hormonal regulation, mitochondrial function, protein manufacture, detoxification, inflammatory regulation, DNA expression, and epigenetic programming (Crider et al. 2012, 21–38). It has been established that normal function of methylation is necessary for normal brain function (Martin 2008, 377–387), and folic acid has been proven to be effective as an augmentation strategy in the treatment of depression (Papakostas et al. 2014, 855–863; Sarris et al. 2011, 454–465). Establishing normal methylation function via the judicious use of folic acid (or, in the case of those with the MTHFR C677T single-nucleotide polymorphism [SNP], 5-methylfolate; Davis and Uthus 2004, 988–995), B_{12}, betaine HCl (Obeid 2013, 3481–3495), and B_6 should be a part of the nutritional evaluation of patients with psychiatric and neurological disorders. Moderation in the use of methylation factors is important as there are emerging data that hypermethylation may be associated with neuronal diseases such as genetically based frontotemporal dementia (Banz-Strathmann 2013, 16). Laboratory testing is important to establish the need for methylation-modulating nutrients in individual patients, as there is insufficient evidence that augmenting methylation in the absence of abnormalities is efficacious in psychiatric patients.

SAM-E (S-Adenosyl Methionine)

SAM-E occurs naturally in the body and is used to treat depression (Bressa 1994, 7–14), fibromyalgia (Dibenedetto et al. 1993, 222–229), and ADHD (Shekim et al. 1990, 249–253). SAM-E works to balance NT levels, by both increasing the ability of COMT (catechol-*o*-methyltransferase) to degrade synaptic molecules (NTs and hormones) and increasing the production of NTs. Doses may be as low as 200 mg twice a day to as high as 1600 mg twice a day and require folate and B_{12} for proper utilization (Goldberg 1999, 4).

Inositol

Inositol has been shown in several studies to be helpful for depression, OCD, panic disorder, and anxiety (Benjamin et al. 1995, 167–175; Mukai et al. 2014, 55–63). The dose must be gradually increased to minimize the laxative effect (it is often used in infants for constipation). The target is a total of 9 g twice daily. Full response can take as long as 12 weeks. However, because of the large amounts needed, some patients are reluctant to try this.

N-Acetylcysteine

N-acetylcysteine (NAC) is an antioxidant derived from the amino acid L-cysteine. In psychiatry, it has shown promise as a treatment for adult trichotillomania and self-grooming behaviors, OCD, addiction (cannabis cocaine, heroin, alcohol, nicotine) via an effect on *N*-methyl-D-aspartate receptors in the nucleus accumbens, augmentation in refractory bipolar and unipolar depression, and negative symptoms in schizophrenia (Dean et al. 2011, 78–86). It is useful as a liver support for those taking valproic acid. The starting dose is 600 mg twice a day and is raised as tolerated to 1200 mg twice a day in 2 weeks, with a maximum daily dose of 2400 mg/day (Dean et al., 2011) when used for stereotypy and irritability in autism.

Specific Amino Acids

Tyrosine and tryptophan are necessary for NT production and are therefore essential to normal mental health and medication response. Normal levels are conditional on adequate diet, digestion, and absorption. Tryptophan and tyrosine depletion studies (Altman et al. 2010, 171–176; McLean et al. 2004, 286–297) consistently demonstrate that 60% of responders to serotonin-, dopamine-, or norepinephrine-acting antidepressants relapse into depression within 5–6 days when fed a diet deficient in these amino acids. This loss of response is specific to the medication being used, for example, tryptophan affecting response to selective serotonin reuptake inhibitors (SSRIs) and tyrosine affecting response to bupropion. One can use tryptophan when attempting to augment production of serotonin; however, this can cause anxiety and agitation when inflammation is part of the picture. Using 5-hydroxytryptophan (5-HTP), a metabolic intermediate in the biosynthesis of serotonin from tryptophan, avoids this risk. Dosages of 5-HTP can range between 12.5 and 100 mg given at bedtime. Care must be taken to avoid serotonin syndrome with those taking SSRIs, whether using tryptophan or 5-HTP. Tyrosine, a precursor to dopamine as well as epinephrine and norepinephrine, can be used in doses of 250–1000 mg BID, with attention to blood pressure in the elderly.

TESTING

This list is by no means definitive, but is meant to be a basic template.

CONVENTIONAL LABS

1. CBC: r/o anemia (microcytic iron deficiency, macrocytic B_{12} deficiency), infections, respiratory allergies (eosinophilia).
2. Fe: ++, TIBC, Ferritin: r/o anemia, iron malabsorption common in hypothyroidism.
3. Fasting insulin, fasting glucose, 2 h glucose tolerance test, hemoglobin A1C.
4. RBC magnesium, selenium, copper, zinc.
5. Celiac panel with antigliadin antibodies (IgG, secretory IgA), HLA DQ2 and DQ8 (only a positive response is helpful; too many false negatives); anti-IgA tissue transglutaminase antibodies, endomysium antibodies. None of these tests, however, is definitive, so the entire clinical picture must be considered.
6. Lipid profile (NMR preferable): cholesterol is a precursor to adrenal hormones.
7. Homocysteine: Used as a functional marker of methylation processes, it should be kept at a level of approximately 7. Levels are affected by B_{12}, folate, and B_6.
8. hsCRP, ESR: As general inflammatory status markers.

SPECIALTY LABS

1. IgG and IgA food sensitivity testing useful when restoring gut health.
2. Comprehensive stool tests in cases where GI symptoms are present.
3. NT testing: There is little use in this testing procedure since urinary output of NTs is mostly reflective of NT function in body compartments other than the brain.
4. Genotype testing: to identify SNPs affecting the CYP 450 enzyme systems, which can influence medication dosing and side effects.
5. Genotype testing to identify MTHFR status.
6. Pyroluria: evaluate for kryptopyrolluria (genetically based increased need for B_6 and zinc).

SUMMARY

The best medicine is personalized, and most mental health patients would benefit from an individually tailored nutritional program that is ideally based on a thorough history, physical exam, and laboratory testing. For those patients who do not respond fully to such an approach, we recommend a full functional medicine assessment. However, we feel strongly that a sound nutritional program is a necessary basis for successful mental health treatment.

REFERENCES

Abd and H. El-Serogy. 2012. Plasma carnitine levels in children with idiopathic epilepsy treated with old and new antiepileptic drugs. *Journal of Pediatric Neurology* 10 (4): 275–281.

Altman, S. E., S. A. Shankman, and B. Spring. 2010. Effect of acute tryptophan depletion on emotions in individuals with personal and family history of depression following a mood induction. *Neuropsychobiology* 62 (3): 171–176.

Arnold, L. E., E. Hurt, and N. Lofthouse. 2013. Attention-deficit/hyperactivity disorder: Dietary and nutritional treatments. *Child and Adolescent Psychiatric Clinics of North America* 22 (3): 381–402.

Bakhtiyari, M., E. Ehrampoush, N. Enayati, G. Joodi, S. Sadr, A. Delpisheh, J. Alihaydari, and R. Homayounfar. 2013. Anxiety as a consequence of modern dietary pattern in adults in tehran-iran. *Eating Behaviors* 14 (2): 107–112.

Banz-Strathmann, J. 2013. Promoter DNA methylation regulates progranulin expression and is altered in FTLD. *Acta Neuropathologica Communications* 1: 16.

Benjamin, J., G. Agam, J. Levine, Y. Bersudsky, O. Kofman, and R. H. Belmaker. 1995. Inositol treatment in psychiatry. *Psychopharmacology Bulletin* 31 (1): 167–175.

Bergin, J. E. and K. S. Kendler. 2012. Common psychiatric disorders and caffeine use, tolerance, and withdrawal: An examination of shared genetic and environmental effects. *Twin Research and Human Genetics: The Official Journal of the International Society for Twin Studies* 15 (4): 473–482.

Bloch, M. H. and J. Mulqueen. 2014. Nutritional supplements for the treatment of attention-deficit hyperactivity disorder. *Child and Adolescent Psychiatric Clinics of North America* 22 (3): 381–402.

Bourre, J. M. 2006. Effects of nutrients (in food) on the structure and function of the nervous system: Update on dietary requirements for brain. Part 1: Micronutrients. *Journal of Nutrition, Health and Aging* 10 (5): 377–385.

Bressa, G. M. 1994. S-adenosyl-L-methionine (same) as antidepressant—Metaanalysis of clinical-studies. *Acta Neurologica Scandinavica* 89 (154): 7–14.

Brouwer, I. A., A. J. Wanders, and M. B. Katan. 2013. Trans fatty acids and cardiovascular health: Research completed? *European Journal of Clinical Nutrition* 67 (5): 541–547.

Crider, K. S., T. P. Yang, R. J. Berry, and L. B. Bailey. 2012. Folate and DNA methylation: A review of molecular mechanisms and the evidence for folate's role. *Advances in Nutrition* 3 (1): 21–38.

Davis, C. D. and E. O. Uthus. 2004. DNA methylation, cancer susceptibility, and nutrient interactions. *Experimental Biology and Medicine* 229 (10): 988–995.

Dean, O., F. Giorlando, and M. Berk. 2011. N-acetylcysteine in psychiatry: Current therapeutic evidence and potential mechanisms of action. *Journal of Psychiatry and Neuroscience: JPN* 36 (2): 78–86.

Dibenedetto, P., L. G. Iona, and V. Zidarich. 1993. Clinical-evaluation of S-adenosyl-L-methionine versus transcutaneous electrical nerve-stimulation in primary fibromyalgia. *Current Therapeutic Research* 53 (2): 222–229.

Dukowicz, A. C., B. E. Lacy, and G. M. Levine. 2007. Small intestinal bacterial overgrowth: A comprehensive review. *Gastroenterology and Hepatology* 3 (2): 112–122.

Fallon, S. and M. Enig. 2001. *Nourishing Traditions*. pp. 1–3. Washington, DC: New Trends Publishing.

Genuis, S. J. and R. A. Lobo. 2014. Gluten sensitivity presenting as a neuropsychiatric disorder. *Gastroenterology Research and Practice* 2014 (5): 1–6.

Goldberg, I. K. 1999. What should I tell my patients regarding the new over-the-counter antidepressant compound SAM-e? *Brown University Psychopharmacology Update* 10 (12): 4.

Grosso, G., A. Pajak, S. Marventano, S. Castellano, F. Galvano, C. Bucolo, F. Drago, and F. Caraci. 2014. Role of omega-3 fatty acids in the treatment of depressive disorders: A comprehensive meta-analysis of randomized clinical trials. *PLoS ONE* 9 (5): e96905.

Hedaya, R. 2000. *The Antidepressant Survival Guide*. p. 75. New York: Three Rivers Press.

Herbison, C. E., S. Hickling, K. L. Allen, T. A. O'Sullivan, M. Robinson, A. P. Bremner, R.-C. Huang, L. J. Beilin, T. A. Mori, and W. H. Oddy. 2012. Low intake of B-vitamins is associated with poor adolescent mental health and behaviour. *Preventive Medicine* 55 (6): 634–638.

Jacka, F. N., A. Mykletun, M. Berk, I. Bjelland, and G. S. Tell. 2011. The association between habitual diet quality and the common mental disorders in community-dwelling adults: The Hordaland health study. *Psychosomatic Medicine* 73 (6): 483–490.

Jacka, F. N., J. A. Pasco, A. Mykletun, L. J. Williams, A. M. Hodge, S. L. O'Reilly, G. C. Nicholson, M. A. Kotowicz, and M. Berk. 2010. Association of western and traditional diets with depression and anxiety in women. *American Journal of Psychiatry* 167 (3): 305–311.

Jackson, J. R., W. W. Eaton, N. G. Cascella, A. Fasano, and D. L. Kelly. 2012. Neurologic and psychiatric manifestations of celiac disease and gluten sensitivity. *Psychiatric Quarterly* 83 (1): 91–102.

Jones, D. and S. Quinn. 2006. *Textbook of Functional Medicine*. p. 5. Gig Harbor, WA: Institute for Functional Medicine.

Jones, T. W., W. P. Borg, S. D. Boulware, G. McCarthy, R. S. Sherwin, and W. V. Tamborlane. 1995. Enhanced adrenomedullary response and increased susceptibility to neuroglycopenia: Mechanisms underlying the adverse effects of sugar ingestion in healthy children. *Journal of Pediatrics* 126 (2): 171–177.

Kim, J. and M. Wessling-Resnick. 2014. Iron and mechanisms of emotional behavior. *Journal of Nutrition Biochemistry* 25 (11): 1101–1107.

Kuhn, F. T., F. Trevizol, V. T. Dias, R. C. Barcelos, C. S. Pase, K. Roversi, C. T. Antoniazzi et al. 2015. Toxicological aspects of trans fat consumption over two sequential generations of rats: Oxidative damage and preference for amphetamine. *Toxicology Letters* 232 (1): 58–67 (October 5, 2015).

Lam, J. R., J. L. Schneider, W. Zhao, and D. A. Corley. 2013. Proton pump inhibitor and histamine 2 receptor antagonist use and vitamin B12 deficiency. *JAMA: Journal of the American Medical Association* 310 (22): 2435–2442.

Martin, L. J. 2008. DNA damage and repair: Relevance to mechanisms of neurodegeneration. *Journal of Neuropathology and Experimental Neurology* 67 (5): 377–387.

Mayer, E. A., T. Savidge, and R. J. Shulman. 2014. Brain-gut microbiome interactions and functional bowel disorders. *Gastroenterology* 146 (6): 1500–1512.

McLean, A., J. S. Rubinsztein, T. W. Robbins, and B. J. Sahakian. 2004. The effects of tyrosine depletion in normal healthy volunteers: Implications for unipolar depression. *Psychopharmacology* 171 (3): 286–297.

Midttun, O., S. Hustad, J. Schneede, S. E. Vollset, and P. M. Ueland. 2007. Plasma vitamin B-6 forms and their relation to transsulfuration metabolites in a large, population-based study. *American Journal of Clinical Nutrition* 86: 131–138.

Miller, A. L. 2008. The methylation, neurotransmitter, and antioxidant connections between folate and depression. *Alternative Medicine Review* 13 (3): 216–226.

Mischoulon, D. and M. F. Raab. 2007. The role of folate in depression and dementia. *Journal of Clinical Psychiatry* 68 (Suppl. 10): 28–33.

Mukai, T., T. Kishi, Y. Matsuda, and N. Iwata. 2014. A meta-analysis of inositol for depression and anxiety disorders. *Human Psychopharmacology* 29 (1): 55–63.

Obeid, R. 2013. The metabolic burden of methyl donor deficiency with focus on the betaine homocysteine methyltransferase pathway. *Nutrients* 5 (9): 3481–3495.

Oh, K., W. C. Willett, K. Wu, C. S. Fuchs, and E. L. Giovannucci. 2007. Calcium and vitamin D intakes in relation to risk of distal colorectal adenoma in women. *American Journal of Epidemiology* 165 (10): 1178–1186.

Osher, Y. and R. H. Belmaker. 2009. Omega-3 fatty acids in depression: A review of three studies. *CNS Neuroscience and Therapeutics* 15 (2): 128–133.

Ozuguz, P., S. Dogruk Kacar, O. Ekiz, Z. Takci, I. Balta, and G. Kalkan. 2013. Evaluation of serum vitamins A and E and zinc levels according to the severity of acne vulgaris. *Cutaneous and Ocular Toxicology* 33 (2): 99–102 (July 5, 2013).

Papakostas, G. I., R. C. Shelton, J. M. Zajecka, T. Bottiglieri, J. Roffman, C. Cassiello, S. M. Stahl, and M. Fava. 2014. Effect of adjunctive L-methylfolate 15 mg among inadequate responders to SSRIs in depressed patients who were stratified by biomarker levels and genotype: Results from a randomized clinical trial. *The Journal of Clinical Psychiatry* 75 (8): 855–863.

Parker, G. and H. Brotchie. 2011. 'D' for depression: Any role for vitamin D?: 'Food for thought' II parker and brotchie vitamin D and depression. *Acta Psychiatrica Scandinavica* 124 (4): 243–249.

Penninx, B. W. J. H., J. M. Guralnik, L. Ferrucci, L. P. Fried, R. H. Allen, and S. P. Stabler. 2000. Vitamin B12 deficiency and depression in physically disabled older women: Epidemiologic evidence from the women's health and aging study. *American Journal of Psychiatry* 157 (5): 715–721.

Peters, S. L., J. R. Biesiekierski, G. W. Yelland, J. G. Muir, and P. R. Gibson. 2014. Randomised clinical trial: Gluten may cause depression in subjects with non-coeliac gluten sensitivity—An exploratory clinical study. *Alimentary Pharmacology and Therapeutics* 39 (10): 1104–1112.

Pfeiffer, C. M., M. R. Sternberg, R. L. Schleicher, B. M. H. Haynes, M. E. Rybak, and J. L. Pirkle. 2013. The CDC's second national report on biochemical indicators of diet and nutrition in the U.S. population is a valuable tool for researchers and policy makers. *Journal of Nutrition* 143 (6): 938S–947S.

Planck, N. 2006. *Real Food: What To Eat and Why.* p. 26. New York: Bloomsbury.

Popper, C. W. 2014. Single-micronutrient and broad-spectrum micronutrient approaches for treating mood disorders in youth and adults. *Child and Adolescent Psychiatric Clinics of North America* 23 (3): 591–672.

Reinstatler, L., Y. P. Qi, R. S. Williamson, J. V. Garn, and G. P. Oakley, Jr. 2012. Association of biochemical B_{12} deficiency with metformin therapy and vitamin B_{12} supplements: The national health and nutrition examination survey, 1999–2006. *Diabetes Care* 35 (2): 327–333.

Richardson, A. J. 2006. Omega-3 fatty acids in ADHD and related neurodevelopmental disorders. *International Review of Psychiatry (Abingdon, England)* 18 (2): 155–172.

Rosenblat, J. D., D. S. Cha, R. B. Mansur, and R. S. McIntyre. 2014. Inflamed moods: A review of the interactions between inflammation and mood disorders. *Progress in Neuro-Psychopharmacology and Biological Psychiatry* 53: 23–34.

Sarris, J., D. Mischoulon, and I. Schweitzer. 2011. Adjunctive nutraceuticals with standard pharmacotherapies in bipolar disorder: A systematic review of clinical trials. *Bipolar Disorders* 13 (5–6): 454–465.

Sarris, J., D. Mischoulon, and I. Schweitzer. 2012. Omega-3 for bipolar disorder: Meta-analyses of use in mania and bipolar depression. *The Journal of Clinical Psychiatry* 73 (1): 81–86.

Schenkel, T. C., N. K. A. Stockman, J. N. Brown, and A. M. Duncan. 2007. Evaluation of energy, nutrient and dietary fiber intakes of adolescent males. *Journal of the American College of Nutrition* 26 (3): 264–271.

Shekim, W. O., F. Antun, G. L. Hanna, J. T. McCracken, and E. B. Hess. 1990. *S*-adenosyl-L-methionine (SAM) in adults with ADHD, RS: Preliminary results from an open trial. *Psychopharmacology Bulletin* 26 (2): 249–253.

Simopoulos, A. P. 2011. Evolutionary aspects of diet: The omega-6/omega-3 ratio and the brain. *Molecular Neurobiology* 44 (3): 203–215.

Siri-Tarino, P., Q. Sun, F. B. Hu, and R. M. Krauss. 2010. Meta-analysis of prospective cohort studies evaluating the association of saturated fat with cardiovascular disease. *The American Journal of Clinical Nutrition* 91 (3): 535–546.

Song, C. 2013. Essential fatty acids as potential anti-inflammatory agents in the treatment of affective disorders. *Modern Trends in Pharmacopsychiatry* 28: 75–89.

Troisi, A. 2011. Low cholesterol is a risk factor for attentional impulsivity in patients with mood symptoms. *Psychiatry Research* 188 (1): 83–87.

Vasquez, A. 2009. *Chiropractic and Naturopathic Mastery of Common Clinical Disorders: The Art of Co-Creating Wellness while Effectively Managing Acute and Chronic Health Disorders.* p. 561. Fort Worth, TX: Integrative and Biological Medicine Research and Consulting, LLC.

Ventura, T., J. Santander, R. Torres, and A. M. Contreras. 2014. Neurobiologic basis of craving for carbohydrates. *Nutrition* 30 (3): 252–256.

Whiteford, H. A., L. Degenhardt, J. Rehm, A. J. Baxter, A. J. Ferrari, H. E. Erskine, F. J. Charlson et al. 2013. Global burden of disease attributable to mental and substance use disorders: Findings from the global burden of disease study 2010. *The Lancet* 382 (9904): 1575–1586.

Yorbik, O., M. F. Ozdag, A. Olgun, M. G. Senol, S. Bek, and S. Akman. 2008. Potential effects of zinc on information processing in boys with attention deficit hyperactivity disorder. *Progress in Neuro-Psychopharmacology and Biological Psychiatry* 32 (3): 662–667.

Zhang, J. 2011. Epidemiological link between low cholesterol and suicidality: A puzzle never finished. *Nutritional Neuroscience* 14 (6): 268–287.

19 Neurology and Nutrition

Maya Shetreat-Klein, MD

CONTENTS

INTRODUCTION

Food plays a significant role in the treatment of neurological conditions in many ways. Eating nutrient-dense food provides nutritional resources for all components of the nervous system, and indeed, the entire body, to function optimally. Beyond the obvious macro- and micronutrients necessary for cellular function, phytochemicals in fruits and vegetables directly interact with our genes and influence the function of our nervous system. Eating cruciferous vegetables rich in isothiocyanates, for example, directly upregulates nuclear factor-like 2, or NRF-2, a gene transcription factor that controls learning and memory, detoxification, and other physiological functions necessary for optimal brain function.[1]

Conversely, food toxicants can act as significant stressors to the nervous systems of vulnerable people. For instance, pesticides have been shown to contribute to the development of Parkinson's disease in people with certain genetic polymorphisms such as aldehyde dehydrogenase,[2] or cytochrome p450 2D6,[3,4] but not in those without.[5]

Similarly, children who have high pesticide metabolites in the urine are more likely to have attention deficit-hyperactivity disorder (ADHD) symptoms, such as hyperactivity. In another study, children who consumed a combination of food dyes and preservatives were more likely to display hyperactive behavior than their nonexposed counterparts, but those with a polymorphism in their histamine degradation gene polymorphisms HNMT T939C and HNMT Thr105Ile carried a much higher risk of such a reaction than those without.[6]

Beyond direct components of food such as vitamins and minerals, the diversity of the gut microflora we consume and subsequently feed through diet cause the nervous system to behave differently. Mice with sterile guts displayed greater anxiety behaviors and had lower levels of markers related to learning and memory than those with well-established gut flora.[7,8] When their guts were repopulated with lactobacillus alone, many of the neurological markers improved. Anxiety, however, only improved with the introduction of additional bifidobacterium strains. Probiotics can provide commensal gut microflora, as can cultured or fermented foods like yogurt and others rich in diverse probiotic bacteria.

Most importantly, the relationship between gut and brain, now well established in the scientific literature, both directly and indirectly influences neuroinflammation among other aspects of neuronal function. From mood to cognition to function, the nervous system is deeply impacted by food and nutrition.

While nature's unique ratios of macronutrients, micronutrients, and antioxidants in food are superior in theory to any company's manufactured supplements, many people now eat vast amounts of processed food and suffer the consequences. Soil itself has become more depleted in the industrial agriculture system,[9] which may lead to those who eat whole-food-based diets consuming lower levels of some or even several nutrients.[10] Further, some people have a higher biological demand for a particular nutrient due to increased environmental challenges such as detoxification or stress, or due to genetic polymorphisms. For instance, children with the methylenetetrahydrofolate reductase gene polymorphism may have a greater demand for vitamins such as folate, B_6, and B_{12}.[11]

Though there is controversy over whether people benefit from taking a high-quality multivitamin or derive all they need from their diet, people with neurological disorders require closer examination of their nutritional status.[12] Nutritional requirements, however, differ depending on genetic polymorphisms and biological demands. Although studies on supplements are useful for safety as well as for efficacy, every study can only tell a piece of the puzzle, and can only act as a guide to an individual patient.

MIGRAINES

DIET

Nearly a quarter of children with migraine are considered to be refractory to pharmaceutical approaches.[13] Migraines are a clinical manifestation of a body and nervous system in distress. As such, successful therapy requires a multipronged approach. A regimen of normal sleep, regular eating schedules, and preferably, exercise, is imperative.[14]

However, migraine has well-known connections to food and drink. Food additives of all types may trigger migraine, including artificial sweeteners, monosodium glutamate, and preservatives, which disrupt normal neurochemistry by triggering aberrant metabolic processes in the neuron such as excitotoxicity.[15] In addition, food and environmental allergies play a significant role. Increased Th2 immune response and associated abnormal inflammatory cytokine levels in migraineurs supports the role of immune dysfunction in the etiology of migraine.[16,17] Further, high prevalence of red-ear syndrome in children with migraine as well as in food allergy further supports the allergic-migraine connection.[18,19]

In one large-scale double-blind trial of an elimination diet involving 88 patients treated with an oligoantigenic diet, eliminating all but a few sensitizing food antigens, 93% with severe frequent migraine were free of headaches.[20] The diet consisted of lamb or chicken, rice or potato, banana or apple, Brassicas, water, and vitamin supplements. Of the 82 patients who improved on the diet, all but eight patients relapsed upon the reintroduction of one or more foods. A remarkable fondness for migraine-provoking foods was a common finding, with some patients craving them and eating them in large amounts. These cravings for foods that provoke neurological or other problematic symptoms are an often observed hallmark of food sensitivities or allergies. Cow's milk and cheese caused headaches in most of the patients in the study, but none of the patients complained of headaches after substituting goat's milk with cheese. Another double-blind, placebo-controlled provocation study by the same group found that 89% of children ($n = 36$) who had comorbid migraines and refractory epilepsy experienced statistically significant reduction in migraine and seizure symptoms on the oligoantigenic diet.[21] Gluten sensitivity or celiac, too, can be a significant trigger for migraine. Migraine sufferers have been shown to have a slightly higher risk of celiac disease than controls as measured by tissue transglutaminase antibodies.[22] Conversely, those with celiac are more likely to have neurological symptoms, including migraines, than the general population.[23]

Despite the evidence supporting the role of food in migraine, the concept of food removal remains controversial. In part due to the lack of education in nutrition, many neurologists and allergists are skeptical of the use of elimination diets in treatment. However, by recording events in a headache diary, patients are able to compare headache frequency and intensity before and after diet to objectively assess improvement. Foods can then be reintroduced one at a time in order to assess for exacerbation of headaches. This option should be one that is offered to patients with appropriate support from a physician or nutritionist.

By any standard, the elimination diet is the gold-standard approach to elucidating which foods, if any, impact health. A headache diary, including daily meals, may be helpful in the process of identifying triggers. While it is worthwhile to measure IgE and in some cases, IgG panels, of common food allergens, these panels represent an inexact science—a negative result should never take priority over the observations of food reactivity from patients themselves. Skin testing identifies food allergies less effectively than blood testing, as noted in studies on eosinophilic esophagitis.[24] Conversely, even low or equivocal positivity should trigger investigation due to the limitations of testing for food allergens in skin or blood.

The practitioner must monitor for and address specific nutrient deficiencies when applicable. Before considering the elimination of a broad array of foods, careful logging of diet and symptoms can often identify specific triggers. Often, one or two triggers can be identified without the induction of the oligoantigenic diet. Common food allergens to investigate include dairy, egg, soy, wheat, corn, citrus, peanut, tree nuts, and shellfish.

SUPPLEMENTS

Those prone to migraine have been shown to have increased vulnerability to oxidative stress,[25] lipid peroxidation,[26] as well as mitochondrial dysfunction.[27] In addition, those with migraine are more likely to have polymorphisms of their 5,10-methylenetetrahydrofolate reductase gene (MTHFR),[28,29] as well as increased hypercoagulability markers associated with stroke such as homocysteine and lipoprotein A.[30] The use of supplements and botanicals target these areas of vulnerability.

Riboflavin: High-dose riboflavin (200 or 400 mg) alone may contribute to decreased frequency of headaches, with better response to abortive therapy than placebo.[31,32] Though riboflavin has not been shown to effectively prevent pediatric migraine in some studies at doses of 50–200 mg,[33,34] these studies were complicated by unprecedented response to placebo treatments. In general, riboflavin may improve the cumulative effect of combination therapy in migraine, as seen further in studies outlined below.

Magnesium: Intracellular magnesium levels have been found to be reduced in population with migraines.[35,36] Ongoing oral repletion of magnesium reduces frequency and intensity of events.[37] In a randomized, double-blind, placebo-controlled trial, magnesium oxide supplements led to significant reduction in headache days in people who suffered from migraine.[38] Average doses may range from 400 to 600 mg.

CoQ10: Patients with migraine commonly have deficiency in CoQ10 levels and show improvement in headache frequency and intensity with repletion.[39] In a randomized, double-blind, placebo-controlled, crossover trial of pediatric and adolescent migraine, CoQ10 at 1–3 mg/kg/day was shown to improve frequency significantly in the first 4 weeks of treatment, though both groups showed benefit by the last 4 weeks.[40] Other studies support this finding.[41] Seventy-five percent of children with refractory cyclic vomiting syndrome, also thought to stem in part from mitochondrial dysfunction, improved or resolved with a combination of CoQ10 (10 mg/kg/day, max 200 mg/day), L-carnitine (100 mg/kg/day divided bid, max 2 g/day), and amitryptiline.[42]

Feverfew: Botanical approaches, such as feverfew, have been shown to have efficacy in migraineurs. In one study, a sublingual feverfew-ginger product was found to be effective as an abortive therapy in the early stages of a migraine.[43]

Large-scale review of the data on feverfew suggest that while it is not uniformly effective, it is safe and some subsets of patients suffering from migraine may benefit.[44]

ADHD

DIET

Diet has been a controversial topic of interest for treating ADHD. For years, parents claimed improvement with low sugar diets, diets without additives and salicylates, even gluten-free/casein free diets in ADHD. Most doctors were skeptical of these claims and awaited evidence. The past 30 years have seen more research that suggests a link between food and ADHD, though more well-designed studies are needed.[45,46] Meanwhile, our understanding of mechanism is beginning to take shape. As seen in the area of pathophysiology, basic science research offers growing understanding of underlying connections between gut and brain. Clinical studies support the presence of certain nutritional deficiencies, increased immune reactivity, and neurological vulnerability to food and environmental toxins in particular groups of children.

Even in the face of this growing evidence, however, the medical community overall has remained dismissive of parents' claims that diet changes seem to improve neurological symptoms. A 2010 paper published in the *Journal of Family Practice* concluded that dietary interventions "probably [do] not" improve ADHD symptoms in children and cited studies from three categories to support this conclusion: sugar, artificial food coloring, and EFAs.[47]

In 1989, *Pediatrics*, the respected journal for the American Academy of Pediatrics, published a small study ($n = 23$) that documented improvement in hyperactive preschool-aged boys diagnosed with ADHD by changing diet.[48] After replacing food over 10 weeks with similar foods free of MSG, Aspartame, food dyes, caffeine, and other substances that could be bothersome (including milk in those who were thought to be reactive to milk), over 40% of parents observed 50% or greater improvement in their children. Further, other symptoms improved, such as halitosis, night awakenings, and latency to sleep onset. Over the years, other groups have replicated the findings that diets high in processed foods contribute to deficits in learning and behavior.[49,50] A recent large-scale study from the United Kingdom examined the link between "junk food" intake at age 4 years (as defined by approximately 57 foods with particular ingredients) and behavior issues in 4000 children from birth cohort in the Avon Longitudinal Study of Parents and Children. Children who ate a diet with a one standard deviation increase in "junk food" at age 4½ years were likely to be in the top 33% on the Strengths and Difficulties (SDQ) hyperactivity subscale at age 7 years.[51]

It is tempting to hope for a simple answer to explain childhood neurological diseases. However, most convincing studies point toward a combination of risk factors and exposures together. Many children are incredibly adaptable and can compensate for smaller, potentially toxic challenges; others, however, cannot compensate. Once the threshold of toxic load is reached, clinical symptoms may find expression in the form of one or any combination of disorders, including neurological.

Fish Oil

Omega-3 fatty acids have anti-inflammatory properties and can alter central nervous system cell membrane fluidity and phospholipid composition. Cell membrane fluidity can alter serotonin and dopamine neurotransmission.[52] The omega-3 fatty acids derived from marine animals primarily consist of EPA and DHA, and, therefore, serve as good dietary sources of DHA. The only rich sources of omega-3 fatty acids are cold water fish, including anchovies, krill, herring, tuna, mackerel, salmon, and sardines; cod liver oil; and other fish oils. At present, the recommended daily dietary intakes of ALA and of EPA and DHA in combination are 1200 and 500 mg, respectively.[53] These recommended dietary levels are achieved by less than one-third of the North American population, mainly because the North American diet has low levels of omega-3 fatty acids and high levels of omega-6 fatty acids.[54,55] Within this population, those with neurological, cognitive, or psychiatric disorders have been shown to have lower levels of omega-3 fatty acids than controls.[50,56–60]

Epidemiologic and clinical evidence suggests that omega-3 fatty acid–enriched diets and supplements may be beneficial treatment for a variety of cognitive and psychiatric disorders.[61] Many studies have found a beneficial effect of omega-3 PUFA supplementation in ADHD.[62] In particular, some studies have shown that children with ADHD may have lower concentrations of polyunsaturated fatty acids (PUFAs), particularly omega-3, in their red blood cells and plasma, and that supplementation with omega-3 fatty acids may alleviate behavioral symptoms in this population.[63] Richardson et al. measured fatty acid levels in a mainstream school population to determine if levels relate to learning and behavior. Though measures of reading, spelling, and intelligence did not show any association, they noted associations between level of omega-3 fatty acids and problematic behavior, with some evidence that higher omega-3 levels were associated with decreased inattention, hyperactivity, emotional and conduct difficulties, and better social behavior.[64]

Despite the fact that low levels of DHA were found in children with ADHD, supplementing with DHA alone or in high amounts relative to other essential fatty acids (EFAs) have not been shown to be effective in improving behavior.[65,66] Researchers have begun to look at other fatty acids and found that a combination of EFAs and in particular EPA may be more effective in the modulation of behavior disorders. Forty-one children with learning difficulties were randomly assigned to supplementation with EPA 186 mg, DHA 480 mg, gamma linolenic acid (GLA) 96 mg, linoleic acid 864 mg, and AA 42 mg or placebo (olive oil) for 12 weeks. The group receiving the fish oil supplement had significant improvements in learning and behavioral scores and other ADHD-related symptoms compared to the group given olive oil.[67] In a later study, 117 children with developmental coordination disorder were given either 558 mg EPA, 174 mg DHA, and 60 mg GLA or placebo.[68] The children receiving the fish oil supplement demonstrated significant improvements in reading, spelling, and behavior after 3 months of treatment compared to placebo. In an open-label pilot study, Sorgi et al.[69] gave a high-dose EPA/DHA supplement containing 10.8 g of EPA and 5.4 g of DHA per day to nine children for 8 weeks. They found significant improvements in behavior including inattention, hyperactivity, oppositional behavior, and conduct disorder. Sinn and Bryan administered 558 mg EPA, 174 mg DHA, and 60 mg GLA/day to 36 children for 15 weeks and improvements were found for inattention and hyperactivity and impulsivity compared with the control group.[70] Recently both Johnson et al.[71] and Belanger et al.[72] found improvement in inattention in a subgroup of children with ADHD when supplemented with a mixture of these essential fatty acids. The literature supporting omega-3s for ADHD, however, supports the benefit of a combination of PUFAs. Despite the very low concentration in the brain of EPA, more evidence points to EPA as having particular benefit for neuropsychiatric disorders including schizophrenia and depression.[73]

Phosphatidylserine

Phosphatidylserine (PS) is one of several types of phospholipids that play critical roles in the nervous system, as a building block of neuron cell membrane structure as well as neurotransmitter production. Vaisman et al.[74] conducted a double-blind trial investigating omega-3 with phosphatidylserine for ADHD. They recruited 60 children (3:1 ratio of boys:girls; average age 9 years) with ADHD symptoms who were subsequently randomized to three groups (1) canola oil (controls), (2) fish oil (providing 250 mg DHA/EPA daily), and (3) an omega-3/PS combination (providing 300 mg PS and 250 mg DHA/EPA daily). No stimulant medications or other dietary supplements were administered during the trial period (80–100 days; average 91 days). The group receiving PS and omega-3 had the highest proportion of children whose symptoms improved. The children's sustained visual attention and discrimination were assessed using the Test of Variables of Attention (TOVA). This score improved for subjects over controls for both the omega-3 PS and the fish oil groups, but significantly more in the PS group ($p < 0.001$). This indicates that omega-3 PS improved attention performance (and more dramatically than fish oil) compared to the control group. Omega-3 PS ameliorated the inattention symptoms of ADHD to a greater degree than equivalent amounts of DHA/EPA from other dietary sources.[74] Further, these results suggest that a lower dose of omega-3 fatty acids may achieve better outcome when bound to phospholipids, which also addresses such issues as overfishing and ocean conservation as well as patient cost for supplements. Another study investigated phosphatidylserine (200 mg/day vs. placebo) in 36 children ages 4–14 and found improvements in ADHD, inattention, and short-term auditory memory.[75]

Iron

Supplementation of iron is complicated in that the range of benefit is very narrow. Low iron is obviously problematic for many reasons, but so too can iron contribute to oxidative stress. Free radicals generated by iron damages membrane lipids and DNA within the cell. Several studies have shown that as many as 84% of children with ADHD have low ferritin levels.[76] Moreover, ferritin levels are proportional to worse behavior in children with ADHD.[77,78] Of note, most studies do not find anemia, but simply low ferritin levels. Other studies examining ferritin and ADHD found that low ferritin (<45) was linked not only with more severe scores on Connors' scale but also increased restless leg or abnormal movements in sleep.[79]

Zinc

The ADHD population has been found to be at particular risk of zinc deficiency.[80,81] One randomized, double-blind, placebo-controlled trial investigated zinc as adjunct treatment to methylphenidate. Children who received a combination of zinc and methylphenidate showed improvement significantly better than methylphenidate alone.[82] Further, there was a significant correlation between serum zinc and serum-free fatty acid (FFA) levels in patients with ADHD, who had significantly lower FFA and zinc than those of healthy controls.[83] One randomized, double-blind, placebo-controlled study evaluated the effects of zinc supplementation in 400 children with documented ADHD. Supplementing these children significantly reduced hyperactivity, impulsivity, and impaired socialization scores, especially in children with low levels of EFAs.[82,84]

Magnesium

Both magnesium and zinc are needed to help convert the 18-carbon, plant-derived essential fatty acids (EFAs) to long chain fatty acids, notably DHA and EPA.[85] Many children with ADHD are deficient in these nutrients and may therefore have difficulty elongating the 18-carbon fatty acids.[86] In a sample of 116 children with ADHD, researchers found that 95% had a magnesium deficiency.[87] In 1997, researchers found that a combination of magnesium aspartate and magnesium lactate supplemented at a dose of 200 mg daily for 6 months significantly reduced disruptive behavior in children with ADHD compared to a control group.[88]

SEIZURES

DIET

Patients with epilepsy have a greater incidence of celiac and gluten sensitivity than those in the general population.[89,90] Several studies describe improvement in patients who have intractable epilepsy and are then found to have celiac.[91,92] These patients then improve following removal of gluten from their diets.[93,94] Though molecular mimicry likely plays a role in the neurological symptoms of celiac disease, intestinal malabsorption with subsequent vitamin and mineral deficiencies may also contribute. Gluten sensitivity has been implicated in hippocampal sclerosis, a common pathological finding in people with seizures.[95] Further, gluten sensitivity has been found at a much higher rate in people with epilepsy.

Dairy consumption also may play a role in seizure activity for those who are sensitive or allergic to dairy. Cow's milk allergy, eczema, and asthma are more common in children with epilepsy[96] and can be considered red flags for food allergy even in a child presenting primarily with a neurological syndrome. A case study and a small study suggest that removal of dairy led to improvement of seizure activity, EEG abnormalities, and other behavioral and cognitive symptoms. First, a child with skin positivity to dairy showed sustained improvement in seizures and EEG following removal of dairy from his diet.[97] In a follow-up study, a series of three unmedicated children with partial cryptogenic epilepsy were skin test positive to dairy. These children had comorbid problems with sleep, handwriting, or behavior. Dairy was removed from their diets, with subsequent improvement of seizures, EEG abnormalities, and comorbid issues. All of these problems subsequently returned shortly after dairy was reintroduced, and then improved again upon removal of dairy.[98] More recent studies have shown that removing dairy in a group of dairy-allergic children with rolandic epilepsy reduced seizure activity significantly.[99]

Modified Atkins diet (MAD) is a low-carbohydrate, high-protein diet used in people with seizures refractory to medications. Unlike the traditionally used ketogenic diet, MAD does not require an initial fast, allows unlimited fat and protein, and does not restrict calories or fluids.[100] Kossoff et al.[101] published their experience with the modified Atkins diet in 20 children with intractable epilepsy in 2006. Eighty percent of the patients stayed on the diet for 6 months. At 6 months on the diet, 65% had a >50% response, and 35% had a >90% response. Kang et al. evaluated the efficacy, safety, and tolerability of the modified Atkins diet in 14 Korean children with refractory epilepsy. Six months after diet initiation, seven (50%) remained on the diet, five (36%) had >50% seizure reduction, and three (21%) were seizure free.[102] Side effects were limited to some cases of constipation and occasional weight loss. To date, the few open-label studies in adults with epilepsy have had less impressive results. Well-designed studies are necessary to assess efficacy in seizures, though there are reports of improvement in adults with Parkinson's, Alzheimer's, mitochondrial disorders, and bipolar disorder.[103,104]

SUPPLEMENTS

Omega-3

Omega-3 fatty acids have been found to be a basic component of normal neural development and maintenance of neural plasticity.[105] In part, DHA protects neurons and glia from death by maintaining brain-derived neurotrophic factor (BDNF), a small protein produced in the brain that is pivotal to learning and memory.[106,107] Wu et al.[108] found that dietary omega-3 fatty acids in the form of DHA not only normalize BDNF but also reduce oxidative damage and counteract learning disability after traumatic brain injury in rats. Moreover, both DHA and EPA have been shown to modify hippocampal excitability during excitotoxicity with glutamate, which plays an important role in damage from seizures.[109]

Several animal and human studies support that DHA increases seizure threshold.[110,111] In one randomized, double-blind study, patients with intractable epilepsy were given daily 1 g EPA and 0.7 g of DHA or mineral oil (placebo). Fifty-six patients with epilepsy (29 PUFAs/27 placebos) completed the 12-week trial. Seizure frequency was slightly reduced over a 6-week period of treatment in the supplemented group (5 of 29 supplemented vs. 0 of 27 control), but the effect was of only short duration.[112] Two following studies, however, found no improvement in a 12-week or shorter trial. This may be explained by the fact that these studies were of relatively short duration and low dose. Another possibility is that the benefits of omega-3s in vivo are part of a synergistic response with other as yet-undefined components.

People with epilepsy are well known to be at increased risk of sudden death. Sudden unexpected death in epilepsy (SUDEP) is defined as the sudden, unexpected, witnessed or unwitnessed, nontraumatic, and nondrowning death of patients with epilepsy with or without evidence of a seizure, excluding documented status epilepticus, and in whom postmortem examination does not reveal a structural or toxicological cause for death.[113] People with epilepsy have a two- to threefold increased risk of dying prematurely than those without epilepsy, and the most common epilepsy-related category of death is SUDEP. Though the exact causes of SUDEP remain unclear, it is likely that cardiac arrhythmia during and between seizures plays a potential role.[114] Omega-3 fatty acid deficiency has an interesting role in this scenario. Animal and clinical studies have demonstrated that omega-3 fatty acids may be useful in the prevention and treatment of epilepsy.[115] As omega-3 fatty acids per se have been shown to reduce cardiac arrhythmias[116-118] and sudden cardiac deaths,[119-122] omega-3 fatty acid supplementation has been shown to act as a means of reducing refractory seizures, seizure-associated arrhythmias, and SUDEP in patients with refractory seizures may reduce seizures and seizure-associated cardiac arrhythmias.

Magnesium

Magnesium (Mg^{2+}) plays an essential role in mitigating excitotoxicity related to seizures. Magnesium deficiency has been shown to be damaging. In vitro, reduction of extracellular Mg^{2+} lowers the threshold level of excitatory amino acids necessary to activate *N*-methyl-D-aspartate (NMDA) receptor and induces spontaneous epileptiform activity in cortical neurons.[123] Depletion increases oxidative cell death,[124] while elevation of magnesium levels was shown to confer protection.[125] Similarly, dietary Mg^{2+} deficiency was documented to enhance oxidative stress.[126,127] Severe magnesium depletion can cause seizures[128,129] or increase susceptibility to seizure-inducing stimuli.[130] Magnesium concentrations in serum and cerebrospinal fluid (CSF) were significantly lower in 40 patients with grand mal epilepsy than in controls.[131] Serum and CSF magnesium levels fell with increasing duration and frequency of seizures. Pronounced hypomagnesemia is documented in epileptic patients and those on certain AEDs[132]; lower CSF magnesium levels correlate with increased frequency of seizures, poor control, and prolonged events.[133]

Growing literature supports that magnesium can counteract antioxidant damage from toxins.[134] Indeed, magnesium's antioxidant potential is widely reported,[135,136] and it is thought to protect against free radicals surge linked with epileptic convulsions. Magnesium supplementation improved efficacy of a common seizure medication.[137] IV magnesium is used as an effective treatment for the seizures of neonatal tetany[138] and eclampsia and possibly for those associated with ethanol withdrawal and acute intermittent porphyria.[139] Oral administration of magnesium has been associated in some cases with an improvement in EEG findings and a reduction in seizure frequency.[140]

Zinc

About 25% of the human population worldwide is at risk of zinc deficiency, and zinc supplementation can be beneficial for neurological issues.[141] The hippocampus and cerebral cortex are particularly rich in zinc.[142,143] Zinc supplementation is postulated as an adjuvant in the therapy of mood disorders in adults and children.[144] In pre-clinical studies, oral zinc supplementation has been shown to have an antidepressant effect.[145] Zinc also protects against oxidative damage induced by chronic alcohol ingestion,[146] organophosphates,[147] or by lithium.[148]

Zinc is also pivotal in brain function and can be neuroprotective.[149] Zinc plays an important role in glutamate transmission and excitotoxicity. Stored in synaptic vesicles, it is released simultaneously with glutamate, acting as a neuromodulator.[143] Further, zinc has protective effects against excitotoxic insults,[150] partly by antagonism of NMDA receptors.[151,152] Zinc modulates inhibitory GABA neurotransmission by blocking GABA transporters in the hippocampus. Zinc may bridge excitatory and inhibitory neurotransmission, especially during epileptic seizures.[153] Zinc also modulates neurogenesis, neuronal migration, and synaptogenesis.[150]

The temporal lobes have the highest zinc content in the brain and that zinc plays a major role in reducing NMDA excitability.[154] Lower zinc concentration in the brains of epileptic mice as compared to that of control mice suggests that decreased hippocampal zinc may play a role as a trigger of convulsive seizures.[155] Zinc loading reduces seizure susceptibility, while susceptibility is increased by dietary zinc deficiency.[156] Furthermore, low intracellular zinc has consistently been found to enhance seizure susceptibility.[150,157] Though more is not necessarily better, sufficient levels of zinc appear to reduce excitotoxicity and convulsant potential.

B6 (Pyridoxine)

Vitamin B6 is necessary for the proper function of more than 100 different enzymes that participate in amino acid, carbohydrate, and fat metabolism, among its other roles.[158] Pyridoxine is involved in the synthesis of the neurotransmitters serotonin, dopamine, norepinephrine, and gamma-aminobutyric acid (GABA) in the brain and nerve cells, and may support mental function (mood) and nerve conduction. Any deficiency of pyridoxine can quickly lead to insomnia and a profound malfunctioning of the central nervous system.

Pyridoxine helps maintain normal brain functions; therefore, vitamin B6 deficiency leads to a range of neurological dysfunctions, such as anxiety, depression, seizures, and neuropathy.[159] It has been shown that vitamin B6 improves glutamate-induced neurotoxicity,[160] which can result from prolonged or frequent seizures, and protects against neuronal death in experimentally induced seizures.[161–164] Furthermore, vitamin B6 has been reported to promote neuronal survival and improve cognitive functions such as memory in patients with epilepsy.[161,165] These findings suggest that vitamin B6 is not only required for normal brain function, but also plays a protective role against excitotoxicity to the brain.

Take-home points for prevention:

1. Eat whole foods: Minimize processed foods that are nutritionally depleted.
2. Read labels: Eat a diet free of food chemicals.
3. Look for USDA organic labels to minimize toxins.
4. Consider a trial off of dairy and/or gluten.

5. If other dietary interventions do not help, consider a trial of high-fat, high-protein, minimal carbohydrate diet with the help of an experienced health-care provider.
6. An array of nutritional supplements can be preventive for an array of neurological disorders, including but not limited to: omega-3s, zinc, magnesium, B complex vitamins (B2 and B6, among others), CoQ10, and phosphatidylserine.

REFERENCES

1. Santana-Martínez RA et al. Sulforaphane reduces the alterations induced by quinolinic acid: Modulation of glutathione levels. *Neuroscience.* July 11, 2014;272:188–198.
2. Fitzmaurice AGI, Rhodes SL, Cockburn M, Ritz B, Bronstein JM. Aldehyde dehydrogenase variation enhances effect of pesticides associated with Parkinson disease. *Neurology.* February 4, 2014;82(5):419–426.
3. Singh NK, Banerjee BD, Bala K, Chhillar M, Chhillar N. Gene-gene and gene-environment interaction on the risk of Parkinson's disease. *Curr Aging Sci.* 2014;7(2):101–109.
4. Ryan SD et al. Isogenic human iPSC Parkinson's model shows nitrosative stress-induced dysfunction in MEF2-PGC1a transcription. *Cell.* December 5, 2013;155(6):1351–1364.
5. Barnhill LM, Bronstein JM. Pesticides and Parkinson's disease: Is it in your genes? *Neurodegener Dis Manag.* June 2014;4(3):197–200.
6. Stevenson J et al. The role of histamine degradation gene polymorphisms in moderating the effects of food additives on children's ADHD symptoms. *Am J Psychiatry.* September 2010;167(9):1108–1115.
7. Bercik P et al. The anxiolytic effect of *Bifidobacterium longum* NCC3001 involves vagal pathways for gut-brain communication. *Neurogastroenterol Motil.* December 2011;23(12):1132–1139.
8. Neufeld KM, Kang N, Bienenstock J, Foster JA. Reduced anxiety-like behavior and central neurochemical change in germ-free mice. *Neurogastroenterol Motil.* March 2011;23(3):255–264, e119.
9. Horrigan L, Lawrence RS, Walker P. How sustainable agriculture can address the environmental and human health harms of industrial agriculture. *Environ Health Perspect.* May 2002;110(5):445–456.
10. Gopalan C. The changing nutrition scenario. *Indian J Med Res.* September 2013;138(3):392–397.
11. Mitchell ES, Conus N, Kaput J. B vitamin polymorphisms and behavior: Evidence of associations with neurodevelopment, depression, schizophrenia, bipolar disorder and cognitive decline. *Neurosci Biobehav Rev.* August 27, 2014;47C:307–320.
12. Ward E. Addressing nutritional gaps with multivitamin and mineral supplements. *Nutr J.* July 15, 2014;13:72.
13. Kung TA, Totonchi A, Eshraghi Y, Scher MS, Gosain AK. Review of pediatric migraine headaches refractory to medical management. *J Craniofac Surg.* January 2009;20(1):125–128.
14. Powers SW, Mitchell MJ, Byars KC, Bentti A-L, LeCates SL, Hershey AD. A pilot study of one-session biofeedback training in pediatric headache. *Neurology.* 2000;56:133.
15. Millichap JG, Yee MM. The diet factor in pediatric and adolescent migraine. *Pediatr Neurol.* January 2003;28(1):9–15.
16. Boćkowski L, Smigielska-Kuzia J, Sobaniec W, Zelazowska-Rutkowska B, Kułak W, Sendrowski K. Anti-inflammatory plasma cytokines in children and adolescents with migraine headaches. *Pharmacol Rep.* March–April 2010;62(2):287–291.

17. Boćkowski L, Sobaniec W, Zelazowska-Rutkowska B. Proinflammatory plasma cytokines in children with migraine. *Pediatr Neurol.* July 2009;41(1):17–21.

18. Raieli V, Compagno A, Brighina F, La Franca G, Puma D, Ragusa D, Savettieri G, D'Amelio M. Prevalence of red ear syndrome in juvenile primary headaches. *Cephalalgia.* April 2011;31(5):597–602.

19. Raieli V, Monastero R, Santangelo G, Eliseo GL, Eliseo M, Camarda R. Red ear syndrome and migraine: Report of eight cases. *Headache.* February 2002;42(2): 147–151.

20. Egger J, Carter CM, Wilson J, Turner MW, Soothill JF. Is migraine food allergy? A double-blind controlled trial of oligoantigenic diet treatment. *Lancet.* 1983;2: 865–869.

21. Egger J, Carter CM, Soothill JF, Wilson J. Oligoantigenic diet treatment of children with epilepsy and migraine. *J Pediatr.* 1989;114:51–58.

22. Alehan F, Ozçay F, Erol I, Canan O, Cemil T. Increased risk for coeliac disease in paediatric patients with migraine. *Cephalalgia.* September 2008;28(9):945–949.

23. Zelnik N, Pacht A, Obeid R, Lerner A. Range of neurologic disorders in patients with celiac disease. *Pediatrics.* June 2004;113(6):1672–1676.

24. Erwin EA et al. Serum IgE measurement and detection of food allergy in pediatric patients with eosinophilic esophagitis. *Ann Allergy Asthma Immunol.* June 2010;104(6):496–502.

25. Erol I, Alehan F, Aldemir D, Ogus E. Increased vulnerability to oxidative stress in pediatric migraine patients. *Pediatr Neurol.* July 2010;43(1):21–24.

26. Boćkowski L, Sobaniec W, Kułak W, Smigielska-Kuzia Serum and intraerythrocyte antioxidant enzymes and lipid peroxides in children with migraine. *J Pharmacol Rep.* July–August 2008;60(4):542–548.

27. Zaki EA, Freilinger T, Klopstock T, Baldwin EE, Heisner KR, Adams K, Dichgans M, Wagler S, Boles RG. Two common mitochondrial DNA polymorphisms are highly associated with migraine headache and cyclic vomiting syndrome. *Cephalalgia.* July 2009;29(7):719–728.

28. Alsayouf H, Zamel KM, Heyer GL, Khuhro AL, Kahwash SB, de los Reyes EC. Role of methylenetetrahydrofolate reductase gene (MTHFR) 677C>T polymorphism in pediatric cerebrovascular disorders. *J Child Neurol.* March 2011;26(3):318–321.

29. Bottini F et al. Metabolic and genetic risk factors for migraine in children. *Cephalalgia.* 2006;26:731–737.

30. Teber S, Bektas Ö, Yılmaz A, Aksoy E, Akar N, Deda G. Lipoprotein a levels in pediatric migraine. *Pediatr Neurol.* October 2011;45(4):225–228.

31. Condò M, Posar A, Arbizzani A, Parmeggiani A. Riboflavin prophylaxis in pediatric and adolescent migraine. *Headache Pain.* October 2009;10(5):361–365.

32. Schiapparelli P, Allais G, Castagnoli Gabellari I, Rolando S, Terzi MG, Benedetto C. Non-pharmacological approach to migraine prophylaxis: Part II. *Neurol Sci.* June 2010;31 Suppl. 1:S137–S139.

33. MacLennan SC, Wade FM, Forrest KM, Ratanayake PD, Fagan E, Antony J. High-dose riboflavin for migraine prophylaxis in children: A double-blind, randomized, placebo-controlled trial. *J Child Neurol.* November 2008;23(11):1300–1304.

34. Bruijn J, Duivenvoorden H, Passchier J, Locher H, Dijkstra N, Arts WF. Medium-dose riboflavin as a prophylactic agent in children with migraine: A preliminary placebo-controlled, randomised, double-blind, cross-over trial. *Cephalalgia.* December 2010;30(12):1426–1434.

35. Smeets MC, Vernooy CB, Souverijn JH, Ferrari MD. Intracellular and plasma magnesium in familial hemiplegic migraine and migraine with and without aura. *Cephalalgia.* February 1994;14(1):29–32.

36. Talebi M, Savadi-Oskouei D, Farhoudi M, Mohammadzade S, Ghaemmaghamihezaveh S, Hasani A, Hamdi A. Relation between serum magnesium level and migraine attacks. *Neurosciences (Riyadh)*. October 2011;16(4):320–323.

37. Sun-Edelstein C, Mauskop A. Foods and supplements in the management of migraine headaches. *Clin J Pain*. June 2009;25(5):446–452.

38. Wang F, Van Den Eeden SK, Ackerson LM, Salk SE, Reince RH, Elin RJ. Oral magnesium oxide prophylaxis of frequent migrainous headache in children: A randomized, double-blind, placebo-controlled trial. *Headache*. June 2003;43(6):601–610.

39. Hershey AD, Powers SW, Vockell AL, Lecates SL, Ellinor PL, Segers A, Burdine D, Manning P, Kabbouche MA. Coenzyme Q10 deficiency and response to supplementation in pediatric and adolescent migraine. *Headache*. January 2007;47(1):73–80.

40. Slater SK, Nelson TD, Kabbouche MA, LeCates SL, Horn P, Segers A, Manning P, Powers SW, Hershey AD. A randomized, double-blinded, placebo-controlled, crossover, add-on study of CoEnzyme Q10 in the prevention of pediatric and adolescent migraine. *Cephalalgia*. June 2011;31(8):897–905.

41. Hershey AD et al. Coenzyme Q10 deficiency and response to supplementation in pediatric and adolescent migraine. *Headache*. January 2007;47(1):73–80.

42. Boles RG. High degree of efficacy in the treatment of cyclic vomiting syndrome with combined co-enzyme Q10, L-carnitine and amitriptyline, a case series. *BMC Neurol*. August 16, 2011;11:102.

43 Cady RK, Goldstein J, Nett R, Mitchell R, Beach ME, Browning R. A double-blind placebo-controlled pilot study of sublingual feverfew and ginger (LipiGesic™ M) in the treatment of migraine. *Headache*. July–August 2011;51(7):1078–1086.

44. Saranitzky E. Feverfew for migraine prophylaxis: A systematic review. *J Diet Suppl*. 2009;6(2):91–103.

45. Nigg JT, Holton K. Restriction and elimination diets in ADHD treatment. *Child Adolesc Psychiatr Clin N Am*. October 2014;23(4):937–953.

46. Millichap JG, Yee MM. The diet factor in attention-deficit/hyperactivity disorder. *Pediatrics*. February 2012;129(2):330–337.

47. Ballard W, Hall MN, Kaufmann L. Clinical inquiries. Do dietary interventions improve ADHD symptoms in children? *J Fam Pract*. April 2010;59(4):234–235.

48. Kaplan BJ, McNicol J, Conte RA, Moghadam HK. Dietary replacement in preschool-aged hyperactive boys. *Pediatrics*. January 1989;83(1):7–17.

49. Molteni R, Barnard R, Ying Z, Roberts K, Gomez-Pinilla F. A high-fat, refined sugar diet reduces hippocampal brain-derived neurotrophic factor, neuronal plasticity, and learning. *Neuroscience*. 2002;112(4):803–814.

50. Ottoboni F, Ottoboni A. Can attention deficit-hyperactivity disorder result from nutritional deficiency? *J Am Phys Surg*. 2003;8(2):58–60.

51. Wiles NJ, Northstone K, Emmett P, Lewis G. 'Junk food' diet and childhood behavioural problems: Results from the ALSPAC cohort. *Eur J Clin Nutr*. April 2009;63(4): 491–498.

52. Bloch MH, Qawasmi A. Omega-3 fatty acid supplementation for the treatment of children with attention-deficit/hyperactivity disorder symptomatology: Systematic review and meta-analysis. *J Am Acad Child Adolesc Psychiatry*. October 2011;50(10):991–1000.

53. Harris WS, Mozaffarian D, Lefevre M, Toner CD, Colombo J, Cunnane SC, Holden JM, Klurfeld DM, Morris MC, Whelan J. Towards establishing dietary reference intakes for eicosapentaenoic and docosahexaenoic acids. *J Nutr*. 2009;139:804S–819S.

54. Denomme J, Stark KD, Holub BJ. Directly quantitated dietary (n-3) fatty acid intakes of pregnant Canadian women are lower than current dietary recommendations. *J Nutr*. 2005;135:206–211.

55. Lucas M, Asselin G, Plourde M, Cunnane SC, Dewailly E, Dodin S. n-3 Fatty acid intake from marine food products among Quebecers: Comparison to worldwide recommendations. *Public Health Nutr.* 2010;13:63–70.
56. Hallahan B, Garland MR. Essential fatty acids and their role in the treatment of impulsivity disorders. *Prostaglandins Leuko Essent Fatty Acids.* October 2004;71(4):211–216.
57. Stevens LJ et al. Essential fatty acid metabolism in boys with attention-deficit hyperactivity disorder. *J Clin Nutr.* 1995;62(4):761–768.
58. Mitchell EA, Aman MG, Turbott SH, Manku M. Clinical characteristics and serum essential fatty acid levels in hyperactive children. *Clin Pediatr (Phila).* 1987;26(8):406–411.
59. Colter AL, Cutler C, Meckling KA. Fatty acid status and behavioural symptoms of attention deficit hyperactivity disorder in adolescents: A case control study. *Nutr J.* 2008;14(7):8.
60. Dufault R et al. Mercury exposure, nutritional deficiencies and metabolic disruptions may affect learning in children. *Behav Brain Funct.* 2009;5:44.
61. Crawford MA, Bazinet RP, Sinclair AJ. Fat intake and CNS functioning: Ageing and disease. *Ann Nutr Metab.* 2009;55:202–228.
62. Antalis CJ, Stevens LJ, Campbell M, Pazdro R, Ericson K, Burgess JR. Omega-3 fatty acid status in attention-deficit/hyperactivity disorder. *Prostaglandins Leukot Essent Fatty Acids.* 2006;75:299–308.
63. Richardson A. The importance of omega 3 fatty acids for behaviour, cognition and mood. *Scand J Food Nutr.* 2003;47(2):92–98.
64. Kirby A, Woodward A, Jackson S, Wang Y, Crawford MA. Childrens' learning and behaviour and the association with cheek cell polyunsaturated fatty acid levels. *Res Dev Disabil.* May–June 2010;31(3):731–742.
65. Voigt RG et al. A randomized double-blind, placebo-controlled trial of docosahexaenoic acid supplementation in children with attention deficit/hyperactivity disorder. *J Pediatr.* 2001;139(2):189–196.
66. Hirayama S, Hamazaki T, Terasawa K. Effect of docosahexaenoic acid-containing food administration on symptoms of attention-deficit/hyperactivity disorder—A placebo-controlled double blind study. *Eur J Clin Nutr.* 2003;58:467–473.
67. Richardson AJ, Puri BK. A randomized double-blind, placebo-controlled study of the effects of supplementation with highly unsaturated fatty acids on ADHD-related symptoms in children with specific learning difficulties. *Prog Neuropsychopharmacol Biol Psychiatry.* February 2002;26(2):233–239.
68. Richardson AJ, Montgomery P. The Oxford-Durham study: A randomized, controlled trial of dietary supplementation with fatty acids in children with developmental coordination disorder. *Pediatrics.* 2005;115(5):1360–1366.
69. Sorgi PJ, Hallowell EM, Hutchins HL, Sears B. Effects of an open-label pilot study with high-dose EPA/DHA concentrates on plasma phospholipids and behavior in children with attention deficit hyperactivity disorder. *Nutr J.* 2007;13(6):16.
70. Sinn N, Bryan J. Effect of supplementation with polyunsaturated fatty acids and micronutrients on learning and behavior problems associated with child ADHD. *J Dev Behav Pediatr.* 2007;28(2):82–91.
71. Johnson M, Ostlund S, Fransson G, Kadesjo B, Gillberg C. Omega-3/omega-6 fatty acids for attention deficit hyperactivity disorder: A randomized placebo-controlled trial in children and adolescents. *J Atten Disord.* 2009;12(5):394–401.
72. Belanger SA et al. Omega-3 fatty acid treatment of children with attention-deficit hyperactivity disorder: A randomized, double-blind, placebo-controlled study. *Paediatr Child Health.* 2009;14(2):89–98.

73. Peet M. Eicosapentaenoic acid in the treatment of schizophrenia and depression: Rationale and preliminary double-blind clinical trial results. *Prostaglandins Leukot Essent Fatty Acids*. December 2003;69(6):477–485.

74. Vaisman N et al. Correlation between changes in blood fatty acid composition and visual sustained attention performance in children with inattention: Effect of dietary n-3 fatty acids containing phospholipids. *Am J Clin Nutr*. May 2008;87(5):1170–1180.

75. Hirayama S et al. The effect of phosphatidylserine administration on memory and symptoms of attention-deficit hyperactivity disorder: A randomised, double-blind, placebo-controlled clinical trial. *J Hum Nutr Diet*. April 2014;27 Suppl. 2:284–291.

76. Konofal E, Lecendreux M, Arnulf I, Mouren MC. Iron deficiency in children with attention-deficit/hyperactivity disorder. *Arch Pediatr Adolesc Med*. December 2004;158(12):1113–1115.

77. Oner O, Alkar OY, Oner P. Relation of ferritin levels with symptom ratings and cognitive performance in children with attention deficit-hyperactivity disorder. *Pediatr Int*. February 2008;50(1):40–44.

78. Oner P, Oner O. Relationship of ferritin to symptom ratings children with attention deficit hyperactivity disorder: Effect of comorbidity. *Child Psychiatry Hum Dev*. September 2008;39(3):323–330.

79. Konofal E et al. Impact of restless legs syndrome and iron deficiency on attention-deficit/hyperactivity disorder in children. *Sleep Med*. November 2007;8(7–8):711–715.

80. Toren, P et al. Zinc deficiency in ADHD. *Biol Psychiatry*. 1996;40:1308–1310.

81. Kozielec T, Starobrat-Hermelin B, Kotkowiak L. Deficiency of certain trace elements in children with hyperactivity. *Psychiatry Pol*. 1994;28:345–353.

82. Bilici M et al. Double-blind, placebo-controlled study of zinc sulfate in the treatment of attention deficit hyperactivity disorder. *Prog Neuropsychopharmacol Biol Psychiatry*. January 2004;28(1):181–190.

83. Bekaroglu M et al. Relationships between serum free fatty acids and zinc, and attention deficit hyperactivity disorder: A research note. *J Child Psychol Psychiatry*. February 1996;37(2):225–227.

84. Arnold LE, DiSilvestro RA. Zinc in attention-deficit/hyperactivity disorder. *J Child Adolesc Psychopharmacol*. 2005;15(4):619–627.

85. Arnold LE. Treatment alternatives for attention-deficit/hyperactivity disorder (ADHD). *J Atten Disord*. 1999;3(1):30–48.

86. Burgess JR, Stevens L, Zhang W, Peck L. Long-chain polyunsaturated fatty acids in children with attention-deficit hyperactivity disorder. *Am J Clin Nutr*. 2000;71:327S–330S.

87. Kozielec T, Starobrat-Hermelin B. Assessment of magnesium levels in children with attention deficit hyperactivity disorder (ADHD). *Magnes Res*. 1997;10(2):143–148.

88. Starobrat-Hermelin B, Kozielec T. The effects of magnesium physiological supplementation on hyperactivity in children with attention deficit hyperactivity disorder (ADHD): Positive response to magnesium oral loading test. *Magnes Res*. 1997;10(2):149–156.

89. Vieira C, Jatobá I, Matos M, Diniz-Santos D, Silva LR. Prevalence of celiac disease in children with epilepsy. *Arq Gastroenterol*. October–December 2013;50(4):290–296.

90. Diaconu G et al. Celiac disease with neurologic manifestations in children. *Rev Med Chir Soc Med Nat Iasi*. January–March 2013;117(1):88–94.

91. Canales P, Mery VP, Larrondo FJ, Bravo FL, Godoy J. Epilepsy and celiac disease: Favorable outcome with a gluten-free diet in a patient refractory to antiepileptic drugs. *Neurologist*. November 2006;12(6):318–321.

92. Gobbi G. Coeliac disease, epilepsy and cerebral calcifications. *Brain Dev*. April 2005;27(3):189–200.

93. Pratesi R, Modelli IC, Martins RC, Almeida PL, Gandolfi L. Celiac disease and epilepsy: Favorable outcome in a child with difficult to control seizures. *Acta Neurol Scand*. October 2003;108(4):290–293.

94. Hernández MA, Colina G, Ortigosa L. Epilepsy, cerebral calcifications and clinical or subclinical coeliac disease. Course and follow up with gluten-free diet. *Seizure.* February 1998;7(1):49–54.

95. Peltola M, Kaukinen K, Dastidar P, Haimila K, Partanen J, Haapala AM, Mäki M, Keränen T, Peltola J. Hippocampal sclerosis in refractory temporal lobe epilepsy is associated with gluten sensitivity. *J Neurol Neurosurg Psychiatry.* June 2009;80(6):626–630.

96. Frediani T et al. Allergy and childhood epilepsy: A close relationship? *Acta Neurol Scand.* December 2001;104(6):349–352.

97. Frediani T, Pelliccia A, Aprile A, Ferri E, Lucarelli S. Partial idiopathic epilepsy: Recovery after allergen-free diet. *Pediatr Med Chir.* May–June 2004;26(3):196–197.

98. Pelliccia A et al. Partial cryptogenetic epilepsy and food allergy/intolerance. A causal or a chance relationship? Reflections on three clinical cases. *Minerva Pediatr.* May 1999;51(5):153–157.

99. Lucarelli S, Spalice A, D'Alfonso Y, Lastrucci G, Sodano S, Topazio L, Frediani T. Cow's milk allergy and rolandic epilepsy: A close relationship? *Arch Dis Child.* May 2012;97(5):481.

100. Sharma S, Jain P. The modified Atkins diet in refractory epilepsy. *Epilepsy Res Treat.* 2014;2014:404202.

101. Kossoff EH, McGrogan JR, Bluml RM, Pillas DJ, Rubenstein JE, Vining EP. A modified Atkins diet is effective for the treatment of intractable pediatric epilepsy. *Epilepsia.* 2006;47(2):421–424.

102. Kang HC, Lee HS, You SJ, Kang du C, Ko TS, Kim HD. Use of a modified Atkins diet in intractable childhood epilepsy. *Epilepsia.* January 2007;48(1):182–186.

103. Paoli A, Bianco A, Damiani E, Bosco G. Ketogenic diet in neuromuscular and neurodegenerative diseases. *Biomed Res Int.* 2014;2014:474296.

104. Phelps JR, Siemers SV, El-Mallakh RS. The ketogenic diet for type II bipolar disorder. *Neurocase.* 2013;19(5):423–426.

105. Wainwright PE. Dietary essential fatty acids and brain function: A developmental perspective on mechanisms. *Proc Nutr Soc.* 2002;61(1):61–69.

106. Lukiw WJ, Bazan NG. Docosahexaenoic acid and the aging brain. *J Nutr.* 2008;138(12):2510–2514.

107. Lukiw WJ. Docosahexaenoic acid and amyloid-beta peptide signaling in Alzheimer's disease. *World Rev Nutr Diet.* 2009;99:55–70.

108. Wu A, Ying Z, Gomez-Pinilla F. Dietary omega-3 fatty acids normalize BDNF levels, reduce oxidative damage, and counteract learning disability after traumatic brain injury in rats. *J Neurotrauma.* 2004;21(10):1457–1467.

109. Xiao Y, Li X. Polyunsaturated fatty acids modify mouse hippocampal neuronal excitability during excitotoxic or convulsant stimulation. *Brain Res.* October 30, 1999;846(1):112–21.

110. Gilby KL, Jans J, McIntyre DC. Chronic omega-3 supplementation in seizure-prone versus seizure-resistant rat strains: A cautionary tale. *Neuroscience.* 2009;163:750–758.

111. Taha AY, Burnham WM, Auvin S. Polyunsaturated fatty acids and epilepsy. *Epilepsia.* 2010;51:1348–1358.

112. Yuen AW, Sander JW, Fluegel D, Patsalos PN, Bell GS, Johnson T, Koepp MJ. Omega-3 fatty acid supplementation in patients with chronic epilepsy: A randomized trial. *Epilepsy Behav.* 2005;7:253–258.

113. Nashef L. Sudden unexpected death in epilepsy: Terminology and definitions. *Epilepsia.* 1997;38 (Suppl. 11):S6–S8.

114. Stollberger C, Finsterer J. Cardiorespiratory findings in sudden unexplained/unexpected death in epilepsy (SUDEP). *Epilepsy Res.* 2004;59:51–60.

115. Voskuyl RA, Vreugdenhil M, Kang JX, Leaf A. Anticonvulsant effect of polyunsaturated fatty acids in rats, using the cortical stimulation model. *Eur J Pharmacol.* 1998;341:145–152.

116. Gudbjarnason S, Hallgrimsson J. Prostaglandins and polyunsaturated fatty acids in heart muscle. *Acta Biol Med Geriatr.* 1976;35:1069–1080.

117. McLennan PL, Bridle TM, Abeywardena MY, Charnock JS. Dietary lipid modulation of ventricular fibrillation threshold in the marmoset monkey. *Am Heart J.* 1992;123:1555–1561.

118. McLennan PL. Relative effects of dietary saturated, monounsaturated, and polyunsaturated fatty acids on cardiac arrhythmias in rats. *Am J Clin Nutr.* 1993;57:207–212.

119. Billman GE, Kang JX, Leaf A. Prevention of ischemia-induced cardiac sudden death by n -3 polyunsaturated fatty acids in dogs. *Lipids.* 1997;32:1161–1168.

120. Albert CM et al. Fish consumption and risk of sudden cardiac death. *JAMA.* 1998;279:23–28.

121. Siscovick DS, Lemaitre RN, Mozaffarian D. The fish story: A diet–heart hypothesis with clinical implications: n-3 polyunsaturated fatty acids, myocardial vulnerability, and sudden death. *Circulation.* 2003;107:2632–2634.

122. Marchioli R et al. and for the GISSI-Prevenzione Investigators, Early protection against sudden death by n-3 polyunsaturated fatty acids after myocardial infarction: Time-course analysis of the results of the Gruppo Italiano per lo Studio della Sopravvivenza nell'Infarto Miocardico (GISSI)-Prevenzione. *Circulation.* 2002;105:1897–1903.

123. Cao H, Jiang Y, He Q, Chen Y, Yuan L, Wu X. Effect of intracellular-free Ca^{2+} concentration on transient magnesium-free treatment induced epileptic injury in developing cortical neurons of rats. *Beijing Da Xue Xue Bao.* October 2003;35(5):466–470.

124. Altura BM, Gebrewold A, Zhang A, Altura BT. Low extracellular magnesium ions induce lipid peroxidation and activation of nuclear factor-kappa B in canine cerebral vascular smooth muscle: Possible relation to traumatic brain injury and strokes. *Neurosci Lett.* May 8, 2003;341(3):189–192.

125. Regan RF, Jasper E, Guo Y, Panter SS. The effect of magnesium on oxidative neuronal injury in vitro. *J Neurochem.* January 1998;70(1):77–85.

126. Bussière FI, Gueux E, Rock E, Mazur A, Rayssiguier Y. Protective effect of calcium deficiency on the inflammatory response in magnesium-deficient rats. *Eur J Nutr.* October 2002;41(5):197–202.

127. Shafiee H et al. Prevention of malathion-induced depletion of cardiac cells mitochondrial energy and free radical damage by a magnetic magnesium-carrying nanoparticle. *Toxicol Mech Methods.* November 2010;20(9):538–543.

128. Arnold JD, Oldfield RK. Pollard AC, Silink M. Primary hypomagnesaemia: Case report. *Aust Paediatr J.* 1983;19:45–46.

129. Nuytten D, Van Hees J, Meulemans A, Carton H. Magnesium deliciency as a cause of acute intractable seizures. *J Neurol.* 1991;238:262–264.

130. Borges LF, Gucer G. Effect of magnesium on epileptic foci. *Epilepsia.* 1978;19:81–91.

131. Govil MK et al. Serum and cerebrospinal fluid calcium and magnesium levels in cases of idiopathic grand mal epilepsy and induced convulsions. *J Assoc Phys India.* 1981;29:695–697.

132. Dharnidharka VR, Carney PR. Isolated idiopathic hypomagnesemia presenting as aphasia and seizures. *Pediatr Neurol.* July 2005;33(1):61–65.

133. Sood AK, Handa R, Malhotra RC, Gupta BS. Serum, CSF, RBC & urinary levels of magnesium & calcium in idiopathic generalised tonic clonic seizures. *Indian J Med Res.* June 1993;98:152–154.

134. Srivastava D, Subramanian RB, Madamwar D, Flora SJ. Protective effects of selenium, calcium, and magnesium against arsenic-induced oxidative stress in male rats. *Arh Hig Rada Toksikol.* June 1, 2010;61(2):153–159.

135. Ariza AC et al. Effects of magnesium sulfate on lipid peroxidation and blood pressure regulators in preeclampsia. *Clin Biochem.* February 2005;38(2):128–133.

136. Turkoglu OF et al. A comparative study of treatment for brain edema: Magnesium sulphate versus dexamethasone sodium phosphate. *J Clin Neurosci.* January 2008;15(1):60–65.

137. Safar MM, Abdallah DM, Arafa NM, Abdel-Aziz MT. Magnesium supplementation enhances the anticonvulsant potential of valproate in pentylenetetrazol-treated rats. *Brain Res.* June 2, 2010;1334:58–64.

138. Turner TL, Cockburn F, Forfar JO. Magnesium therapy in neonatal tetany. *Lancet.* 1977;1:283–284.

139. Sadch M et al. Treatment of porphyric convulsions with magnesium sulfate. *Epilepsia.* 1991;32:712–715.

140. Steidl L, Tolde I, Svomova V. Metabolism of magnesium and zinc in patients treated with antiepileptic drugs and with magnesium lactate. *Magnesium.* 1987;6:284–295.

141. Maret W, Sandstead HH. Zinc requirements and the risks and benefits of zinc supplementation. *J Trace Elem Med Biol.* 2006;20(1):3–18.

142. Vallee BL, Falchuk KH. The biochemical basis of zinc physiology. *Phys Rev.* January 1993 ;73(1):79–118.

143. Frederickson CJ, Koh JY, Bush AI. The neurobiology of zinc in health and disease. *Nat Rev Neurosci.* June 2005;6(6):449–462.

144. Digirolamo AM et al. Randomized trial of the effect of zinc supplementation on the mental health of school-age children in Guatemala. *Am J Clin Nutr.* September 29, 2010.

145. Cope EC, Levenson CW. Role of zinc in the development and treatment of mood disorders. Role of zinc in the development and treatment of mood disorders. *Curr Opin Clin Nutr Metab Care.* November 2010;13(6):685–689.

146. Zhou Z et al. Zinc supplementation prevents alcoholic liver injury in mice through attenuation of oxidative stress. *Am J Pathol.* June 2005;166(6):1681–1690.

147. Goel A, Dani V, Dhawan DK. Chlorpyrifos-induced alterations in the activities of carbohydrate metabolizing enzymes in rat liver: The role of zinc. *Toxicol Lett.* June 1, 2006;163(3):235–241.

148. Bhalla P, Chadha VD, Dhar R, Dhawan DK. Neuroprotective effects of zinc on antioxidant defense system in lithium treated rat brain. *Indian J Exp Biol.* November 2007;45(11):954–958.

149. Cuajungco MP, Lees GJ. Zinc metabolism in the brain: Relevance to human neurodegenerative disorders. *Neurobiol Dis.* 1997;4:137–169.

150. Cole TB, Robbins CA, Wenzel HJ, Schwartzkroin PA, Palmiter RD. Seizures and neuronal damage in mice lacking vesicular zinc. *Epilepsy Res.* April 2000;39(2):153–169.

151. Chen N, Moshaver A, Raymond LA. Differential sensitivity of recombinant N-methyl-D-aspartate receptor subtypes to zinc inhibition. *Mol Pharmacol.* June 1997;51(6):1015–1023.

152. Paoletti P, Ascher P, Neyton J. High-affinity zinc inhibition of NMDA NR1-NR2A receptors. *J Neurosci.* August 1, 1997;17(15):5711–5725.

153. Cohen-Kfir E, Lee W, Eskandari S, Nelson N. Zinc inhibition of gamma-aminobutyric acid transporter 4 (GAT4) reveals a link between excitatory and inhibitory neurotransmission. *Proc Natl Acad Sci USA.* April 26, 2005;102(17):6154–6159.

154. Williamson A, Spencer D. Zinc reduces dentate granule cell hyperexcitability in epileptic humans. *Neuroreport.* July 31, 1995;6(11):1562–1564.

155. Fukahori M, Itoh M, Oomagari K, Kawasaki H. Zinc content in discrete hippocampal and amygdaloid areas of the epilepsy (El) mouse and normal mice. *Brain Res.* 1988;455:381–384.

156. Fukahori M, Itoh M. Effects of dietary zinc status on seizure susceptibility and hippocampal zinc content in the El (epilepsy) mouse. *Brain Res.* 1990;529:16–22.

157. Blasco-Ibáñez JM et al. Chelation of synaptic zinc induces overexcitation in the hilar mossy cells of the rat hippocampus. *Neurosci Lett.* 2004;355:101–104.

158. Tong Y. Seizures caused by pyridoxine (vitamin B6) deficiency in adults: A case report and literature review. *Intractable Rare Dis Res.* May 2014;3(2):52–56.

159. Baxter P. Pyridoxine-dependent seizures: A clinical and biochemical conundrum. *Biochim Biophys Acta.* 2003;1647:36–41.

160. Yang TT, Wang SJ. Pyridoxine inhibits depolarization-evoked glutamate release in nerve terminals from rat cerebral cortex: A possible neuroprotective mechanism? *J Pharmacol Exp Ther.* October 2009;331(1):244–254.

161. Geng MY, Saito H, Nishiyama N. Protective effects of pyridoxal phosphate against glucose deprivation-induced damage in cultured hippocampal neurons. *J Neurochem.* 1997;68:2500–2506.

162. YamashimaT, Zhao L, Wang XD, Tsukada T, Tonchev AB. Neuroprotective effects of pyridoxal phosphate and pyridoxal against ischemia in monkeys. *Nutr Neurosci.* 2001;4:389–397.

163. Wang XD, Kashii S, Zhao L, Tonchev AB, Katsuki H, Akaike A, Honda Y, Yamashita J, Yamashima T. Vitamin B6 protects primate retinal neurons from ischemic injury. *Brain Res.* 2002;940:36–43.

164. Dakshinamurti K, Sharma SK, Geiger JD. Neuroprotective actions of pyridoxine. *Biochim Biophys Acta.* 2003;1647:225–229.

165. Araujo JA, Landsberg GM, Milgram NW, Miolo A. Improvement of short-term memory performance in aged beagles by a nutraceutical supplement containing phosphatidylserine, *Ginkgo biloba*, vitamin E, and pyridoxine. *Can Vet.* 2008; J49:379–385.

20 Physical Activity

Karen M. Gibson, RDN, CD, CSSD

CONTENTS

BENEFITS OF PHYSICAL ACTIVITY

The health benefits of regular exercise and physical activity are hard to ignore and are one of the most important things that can be done to maintain or improve health. Regardless of age, sex, or physical ability, the benefits of exercise have been shown to prevent or help manage a wide number of health-related conditions.

Although the terms "physical activity" and "exercise" are often used interchangeably, these terms represent different behaviors. Physical activity and exercise are two separate, but related, activities. Physical activity is any bodily movement resulting in energy expenditure and often is unstructured and can include activities of daily living and active transportation.[1] Alternatively, exercise has been defined as a subset of physical activity, one that is planned, structured, and repetitive and is of a sufficient intensity to lead to improved physical fitness or changes in body composition. In this context, and in accordance with the Department of Health and Human Services *2008 Physical Activity Guidelines for Americans*, physical activity generally refers to movement that enhances health.[2,3] Examples of physical activity are swimming, yoga, walking, and running, while examples of exercise might include taking an aerobics class or playing on a sports team. This chapter details the effects of physical activity, which for some individuals might mean exercise, and its relationship to various disease processes.

TYPES OF PHYSICAL ACTIVITY

Before this relationship is explored, it is important to understand the four main types of physical activity; aerobic, muscle-strengthening, bone-strengthening, and stretching. Aerobic activity benefits your heart and lungs the most, whereas the other types benefit the body in other ways. Aerobic activity is any activity that moves the large muscles of the body such as the arms and legs. This type of activity makes the heart beat faster than usual and the individual to breathe harder than normal. With time, regular aerobic activity makes the heart and lungs stronger and able to work better. Three other types of physical activity that may be less well known than aerobic activity include muscle-strengthening, bone strengthening, and stretching. These types of physical activity are important and contribute to overall health and well-being. Muscle-strengthening activities improve the strength, power, and endurance of muscles. Doing pushups and sit-ups, lifting weights, climbing stairs, and digging in the garden are examples of muscle-strengthening activities. With bone-strengthening activities, feet, legs, or arms support the body's weight, and the muscles push against the bones. This helps make bones strong. Running, walking, jumping rope, and lifting weights are examples of bone-strengthening activities. Muscle-strengthening and bone-strengthening activities also can be aerobic. Whether they are considered both types of activities depends on if they make the heart and lungs work harder than normal. For example, running is an aerobic activity and a bone-strengthening activity. Stretching helps improve flexibility and joint mobility. Touching toes, doing side stretches, and yoga exercises are examples of stretching.

CURRENT PHYSICAL ACTIVITY RECOMMENDATIONS

The 2008 Physical Activity Guidelines for Adults recommends that adults need to do two types of physical activity each week to improve health—aerobic and muscle-strengthening. Guidelines for aerobic activities, for substantial health benefits, are included in Table 20.1.

The amount of physical activity recommended for older adults depends on their level of fitness and the presence of any condition that might limit activity. Engaging in regular physical activity is one of the most important things older adults can do for their health by helping to prevent many health problems that may come with age.

If adults aged 65 years of age or older are generally fit, they can follow the guidelines listed in Table 20.2.

If older adults have a chronic disease or other health condition that might limit activity and prevent them from meeting the guidelines, they should talk with their healthcare provider about setting physical activity goals. They should avoid an inactive lifestyle. Inactive older adults should increase their amount of physical

TABLE 20.1
Guidelines for Adults

Type of Activity	Recommendation	Frequency	For Additional Health Benefits
Aerobic	150 min each week of moderate-intensity aerobic activity, or 75 min of vigorous-intensity aerobic activity, or an equivalent mix of moderate- and vigorous-intensity aerobic activity.	This type of activity should be spread throughout the week and performed for at least 10 min at a time.	5 h (300 min) each week of moderate-intensity aerobic activity, or 2 h and 30 min (150 min) a week of vigorous-intensity aerobic activity, or an equivalent mix of moderate- and vigorous-intensity aerobic activity.
Muscle strengthening	All major muscle groups including the arms, legs, hips, back, abdomen, chest, and shoulders should be worked.	These activities should be done two or more days a week. Exercises for each muscle groups should be repeated 8–12 times per set. As each exercise becomes easier, the weight should be increased or another set should be added.	

activity gradually. Older adults should also do exercises that maintain or improve balance if they are at risk of falling.

The physical activity guidelines for children and adolescents aged 6–17 focuses on three types of activity: aerobic, muscle-strengthening, and bone-strengthening. Each type has important health benefits. Current recommendations call for youth to engage in moderate to vigorous physical activity 5 or more days per week for at least 1 h/day (Table 20.3).[4]

Youth should be encouraged to engage in physical activities that are appropriate for their age, enjoyable, and offer variety. No period of activity is too short to count toward meeting these guidelines. Whether a child or adolescent, the evidence is conclusive that physical activity is conducive to a healthy lifestyle and prevention of disease. Habitual physical activity established during the early years may provide the greatest likelihood of impact on mortality and longevity. It is evident that environmental factors need to change if physical activity strategies are to have a significant impact on increasing habitual physical activity levels in children and adolescents.

Physical activity guidelines not only provide the number of recommended minutes, but also indicate level of intensity. Aerobic activity can be accomplished with light, moderate, or vigorous intensity. Although these guidelines may seem fairly clear, it is not uncommon for terms "moderate" and "vigorous" to be misinterpreted. For example, an unfit individual may consider a slow-paced walk vigorous because they feel out of breath and an increase in their heart rate. Relative to their fitness level,

TABLE 20.2
Guidelines for Adults >65

Type of Activity	Recommendation	Frequency	For Additional Health Benefits
Aerobic	2 h and 30 min (150 min) each week of relatively moderate-intensity aerobic activity, or 1 h 15 min (75 min) of relatively vigorous intensity aerobic activity, or a mix of moderate- and vigorous-intensity aerobic activity.	This type of activity should be spread throughout the week and performed for at least 10 min at a time.	5 h (300 min) each week of relatively moderate-intensity aerobic activity, or 2 h and 30 min (150 min) a week of relatively vigorous-intensity aerobic activity or a mix of moderate- and vigorous-intensity aerobic activity.
Muscle strengthening	All major muscle groups including the arms, legs, hips, back, abdomen, chest, and shoulders should be worked.	These activities should be done two or more days a week. Exercises for each muscle groups should be repeated 8–12 times per set. As each exercise becomes easier, the weight should be increased or another set should be added.	

TABLE 20.3
Guidelines for Children

Aerobic activities—1 h/day at least 5 days per week	Most of the 1 h a day should be either moderate- or vigorous-intensity aerobic physical activity, and include vigorous-intensity physical activity at least 3 days a week.
Muscle strengthening—as part of the 1 h/day of physical activity—at least 3 days a week	These activities make muscles do more work than usual during daily life. They should involve a moderate to high level of effort and work the major muscle groups of the body: legs, hips, back, abdomen, chest, shoulders, and arms.
Bone-strengthening on at least 3 days of the week	These activities produce a force on the bones that promotes bone growth and strength through impact with the ground.

they may truthfully feel that the activity is vigorous. The level of intensity depends on how hard the individual has to work to do the activity. People who are less fit usually have to work harder to do an activity than people who are more fit. Thus, what is light-intensity activity for one person may be moderate intensity for another. In general, moderate- and vigorous-intensity aerobic activity is better for the heart than light-intensity activity. Either moderate- or vigorous-intensity exercise, or both, can be undertaken to meet current exercise recommendations, provided the criterion for total volume of energy expended is satisfied. However, even light-intensity activity is better than no activity at all. Light-intensity activities are common daily tasks that do not require much effort. Aerobic intensity is often viewed or determined using a scale system. On a scale of 0–10, moderate-intensity activity is a 5 or 6. It causes noticeable increases in breathing and heart rate. A person doing moderate-intensity activity can talk but not sing. Using that same scale, vigorous-intensity activity is a 7 or 8. A person doing vigorous-intensity activity cannot say more than a few words without stopping for a breath. Another common measurement scale is the RPE, or Rate of Perceived Exertion scale. The RPE scale measures feelings of effort, strain, discomfort, and/or fatigue experienced during both aerobic and resistance training. Although this is a subjective measure, a person's exertion rating may provide a fairly good estimate of the actual heart rate during physical activity.[5] The level of perceived exertion is often measured with a 15 category scale that was developed by the Swedish psychologist Gunnar Borg.[5] This scale is shown here:

Rating	Perceived Exertion/Examples
6	No exertion at all. No effort—sitting and doing nothing.
7	Extremely light. Your effort is just noticeable.
8	
9	Very light; walking slowly at his/her own pace for some minutes.
10	
11	Light.
12	
13	Somewhat hard, but still feels okay to continue.
14	
15	Hard (heavy).
16	
17	Very hard, a healthy person can still go on, but he or she really has to push themselves. If feels very heavy, and the person is very tired.
18	
19	Extremely strenuous or hard, for most people this is the most strenuous exercise they have ever experienced.
20	Maximal exertion.

Practitioners generally agree that perceived exertion ratings between 12 and 14 on the Borg Scale suggests that physical activity is being performed at a moderate level of intensity.[6]

CURRENT RATES OF PHYSICAL ACTIVITY

Although a substantial amount of evidence exists regarding the myriad benefits of physical activity, most Americans fail to meet current recommendations. The Behavioral Risk Factor Surveillance System (BRFSS) included new questions in 2011 to assess participation in aerobic, physical, and muscle-strengthening activities among adults in the United States.[7] This data, analyzed by the Center for Disease Control and Prevention (CDC), revealed that less than half (48%) of all adults met the 2008 Physical Activity Guidelines.[8] During the past decade, there has been no overall improvement in the percentage of adults reporting any physical activity in the BRFSS: for men, the rate was 22.5% in 2001 and 22.4% in 2011; for women, the rate was 28.1% in 2001 and 25.9% in 2011.[9] Less than 30% of high school students get a least 60 min of physical activity.[8] Physical activity rates also vary across ethnicities and regions. Americans living in the South are less active than are individuals living in other parts of the United States.[8] In addition, some groups tend to be more physically active than other groups. Men are more likely than women (52.1% vs. 42.6%, respectively) to meet the 2008 guidelines and younger adults are more likely to meet the guidelines for aerobic activity than older adults.[8] Non-Hispanic white adults (22.8%) are more likely to meet aerobic and muscle-strengthening activity than either non-Hispanic black adults (17.3%) or Hispanic adults (14.4%).[8] In addition, families with an income above the poverty level are more likely to meet the 2008 guidelines for aerobic activity than adults with a family income at or near the poverty level. In addition, adults with a higher education level are more likely to meet the aerobic activity guidelines than adults with less education are.[8] Few older adults achieve the minimum recommended 30 or more minutes of moderate physical activity on 5 or more days per week. Data from the CDC indicate that about 28%–34% of adults aged 65–74 and 35%–44% of adults ages 75 or older are inactive, meaning they engage in no leisure-time physical activity. Inactivity is more common in older people than in middle-aged men and women. Women were more likely than men to report no leisure-time activity.[10]

The physical activity guidelines focus on preventive effects of physical activity, which include lowering the risk of developing chronic diseases such as heart

---

TABLE 20.4
Benefits of Physical Activity

Type of Activity	Benefits
Any exercise	Improved glycemic control
	Reduced risk of diabetes, cancer, and heart disease
	Reduced stress, reduced risk of depression
Aerobic	Improves overall glycemic control
	Improves mood; reduced risk of depression
	Improves lipid levels and cardiovascular risk profile
	Intense aerobic activity—effective for weight loss
	Improved cognitive function
Resistance/strength training	Improved insulin sensitivity
	Increased lean muscle tissue
	Reduced blood pressure
	Improved bone density
	Helpful for weight loss
Balance/flexibility training	Reduced risk of falling
	Improved core strength and stability
	Improved mobility

disease and type 2 diabetes. In addition, physical activity has beneficial therapeutic effects and is commonly recommended as part of the treatment plan for a variety of medical conditions. Table 20.4 lists benefits associated with various types of physical activity.

BARRIERS TO PHYSICAL ACTIVITY

Physical activity is a complex phenomenon influenced by a host of varied psychosocial factors or determinants, such as personal perceptions related to the behavior. Physical activity, like many other health behaviors, such as weight loss, is often cyclical or episodic. People begin an exercise program; participate for a time, and then stop, only to resume again later. Among adults in the United States who begin an exercise program, approximately 50% drop out during the first 3–6 months.[11] Individuals may be motivated to change exercise habits but fall short when confronted with barriers presented by everyday life, ultimately discontinuing the activity completely. Research supports this pattern, finding that an individual's perceived barriers to physical activity are an important determinant of activity level.[12] Research suggests that lowering perceived barriers to exercise is an effective strategy for encouraging physical activity. For health-related behavior change, two important dimensions play an important role: a behavioral dimension and a motivational dimension. Understanding the interaction of these dimensions within the process of changing particular behaviors is a key issue. In order to establish positive behavioral patterns of moderate to vigorous physical activity, health professionals need to understand the factors that may motivate or interfere with participation in physical activity. Several investigations have reported that helping people overcome their perceived barriers has more influence on encouraging people to be physically active than does enhancing perceived benefits of exercise.[13] In fact, knowledge of health benefits is not correlated with activity levels.[11]

The health promotion model, which is derived from social cognitive theory, provides an important framework to guide behavior change interventions for reducing high-risk health behaviors, such as physical inactivity.[14] Behavior-specific cognitions identified in the health promotion model, such as the perceived benefits of the action, the perceived barriers to the action, self-efficacy, and interpersonal influences (social support, norms, and models), as well as affect (enjoyment), represent critical areas to assess and target as means to motivate individuals to engage in health-promoting behaviors.[15] Among the psychological correlates of exercise that have been examined, exercise self-efficacy is the strongest and most consistent predictor of exercise behavior. Exercise self-efficacy is the degree of confidence an individual has in his/her ability to be physically active under a number of specific/different circumstances, or in other words, efficacy to overcome barriers to exercise.[16] Self-efficacy is thought to be particularly important in the early stages of exercise.[16] In the early stage of an exercise program, exercise frequency is related to one's general beliefs regarding physical abilities and one's confidence that continuing to exercise in the face of barriers will pay off. Individuals with greater self-efficacy are more likely to adhere to exercise programs with sufficient regularity to reach a point where the behavior has become, to a certain extent, habitual.

In addition to assessing an individual's degree of self-efficacy, it is also important to explore and be cognizant of barriers to physical activity. Age- and gender-related perceived benefits of and barriers to physical activity have been identified as important mediators of physical activity participation.

Qualitative research involving adolescents has elicited some of this information. For adolescents, the predominant perceived barriers to moderate to vigorous physical activity include lack of time, preferred involvement in technology-related activities, having no one to be active with, safety issues, injury or appearance concerns, fear of failure or not doing well, and laziness.[17] The reported perceived benefits of moderate to vigorous physical activity include staying in shape and having a healthy and attractive body, running around and being active, playing sports and developing athletic skills, gaining energy and recognition, working toward a challenging goal, having fun and socializing, and decreasing stress or anger.[17]

A 2011 systematic review by Siddiqi et al. reported that individual barriers to physical activity among African-American women included a lack of time, a lack of motivation, and a lack of knowledge; lack of childcare, family responsibilities, and costs.[18]

In a review of physical activity determinants in rural women, Olson concluded: "determinants considered as barriers included the physical characteristics of poor health, fear of injury and lack of energy; the social force of family and childcare demands; and physical environment factors such as lack of access, safety concerns, and structural inadequacies."[19]

A variety of barriers may make it harder for older persons to increase and maintain their physical activity. Some neighborhoods and communities are poorly designed or unsafe, a particular obstacle for elderly persons who may feel especially vulnerable to crime or traffic. Many have chronic medical conditions that require more care and planning in how they exercise. Older adults may have trouble getting to facilities and programs, and those facilities may not provide adequate training and monitoring for older adults beginning a program.[9] Additional barriers identified in the older adult population include lack of time (due to multiple regular volunteer and other activities), potential for injury, self-discipline, motivation, boredom, and intimidation.[20] Motivators for this group of individuals included health concerns, socialization, and staff/programming.[20]

Barriers exist not only with the patient/client side, but also with healthcare providers. Lack of time and reimbursement are the preeminent obstacles providers may face in participating in health promotion interventions which limits the scientific data available on physical activity counseling as a pragmatic tool to contain healthcare costs. Other deterrents identified that may limit healthcare providers' routinely counseling patients on physical activity include cost, practice capacity and availability of resources; inadequate knowledge of specific physical activity recommendations to make and resources to refer patients to; low self-efficacy for their ability to change patients' participation in physical activity; and the hesitation prompted by the providers' own failure to meet physical activity recommendations.[21]

ASSESSING LEVEL OF PHYSICAL ACTIVITY

Physical activities are often classified into domains that reflect the purpose of the activity. A common four-category classification is as follows:

- Occupational (work-related)
- Domestic (housework, yard work, physically active child care, and chores)
- Transportation (walking or bicycling for the purposes of going somewhere)
- Leisure time (discretionary or recreational time for hobbies, sports, and exercise)

Existing physical activity (PA) assessment questionnaires differ as to which domains are measured and few assess multiple domains. Historically, strategies to promote physical activity have emphasized increases in leisure-time physical activity and consequently, many questionnaires focus on only this domain. More recently, strategies to promote physical activity have emphasized the health benefits of all kinds of physical activity. Consequently, more physical activity assessment questionnaires are being designed to measure more than one, if not all four, domains of activity. Physical activity can be assessed in three general ways: questionnaire, observation and direct measurement, or diary. Survey measures of PA continue to be the most practical mode of measurement of PA due to cost and ease of administration, and despite the issues related to validity among surveys of PA. Knowing what an individual believes he/she is doing in terms of PA is critical to establishing appropriate PA goals. There are several tools available to measure an individual's level of physical activity. One is the Physical Activity Rating (PA-R), a tool for categorizing a person's level of physical activity. The individual selects the number that best describes their overall level of physical activity for the previous 6 months according to the following[22]:

	Does not participate regularly in programmed recreation, sport, or physical activity
0 points	Avoids walking or exercise (e.g., always uses elevators, drives whenever possible instead of walking)
1 points	Walks for pleasure, routinely uses stairs, occasionally exercises sufficiently to cause heavy breathing or perspiration
	Participates regularly in recreation or work requiring modest physical activity (such as golf, horseback riding, calisthenics, gymnastics, table tennis, bowling, weight lifting, or yard work)
2 points	10–60 min/week
3 points	Over 1 h/week
	Participates regularly in heavy physical exercise (such as running or jogging, swimming, cycling, rowing, skipping rope, and running in place) or engages in vigorous aerobic type activity (such as tennis, basketball, or handball)
4 points	Runs less than 1 mile/week or spends less than 30 min/week in comparable physical activity
5 points	Runs 1–5 miles/week or spends 30–60 min/week in comparable physical activity
6 points	Runs 5–10 miles/week or spends 1–3 h/week in comparable physical activity
7 points	Runs more than 10 miles/week or spends more than 3 h/week in comparable physical activity

In response to the global demand for comparable and valid measures of physical activity within and between countries, the International Physical Activity Questionnaire (IPAQ) was developed for surveillance activities and to guide policy development related to health-enhancing physical activity across various life domains.[23]

The purpose of the IPAQ is to provide a set of well-developed instruments that can be used internationally to obtain comparable estimates of physical activity. There are two versions of the questionnaire. The short version is suitable for use in national and regional surveillance systems. The long version provides more detailed information often required in research work or for evaluation purposes. The IPAQ is available in 15 languages.[24] The long, self-administered IPAQ questionnaire has acceptable validity when assessing levels and patterns of physical activity in healthy adults.[25]

The Physical Activity Readiness Questionnaire can be used by individuals looking to start an exercise program, to increase their current activity level, or partake in a fitness testing assessment.

Physical Activity Readiness Questionnaire[26]

Yes	No	
☐	☐	Has your doctor ever said that you have a heart condition and that you should only do physical activity recommended by a doctor?
☐	☐	Do you feel pain in your chest when you do physical activity?
☐	☐	In the past month, have you had chest pain when you were not doing physical activity?
☐	☐	Do you lose your balance because of dizziness or do you ever lose consciousness?
☐	☐	Do you have a bone or joint problem that could be made worse by a change in your physical activity?
☐	☐	Is your doctor currently prescribing drugs (e.g., water pills) for your blood pressure or heart condition?
☐	☐	Do you know of any other reason why you should not do physical activity?

Source: Hagstromer, M. et al., *Public Health Nutr.*, 9(6), 755, 2006.

If "yes" is marked for any question, a more thorough assessment is completed prior to beginning or increasing activity level. If "no" is marked for all questions, you can be reasonably sure that becoming active or increasing activity level is safe.

The Rapid Assessment of Physical Activity (RAPA) was developed to provide an easily administered and interpreted means of assessing levels of physical activity among adults older than 50 years.[27] The RAPA, developed by the Health Promotion Research Center, a CDC Prevention Research Center, can be accessed at http://depts.washington.edu/hprc/rapa. The Community Health Activities Model Program for Seniors (Champs) PA Questionnaire, developed by the Institute for Health & Aging at the University of California, San Francisco is another instrument that can be used to assess physical activity level in seniors and is available at http://dne2.ucsf.edu/public/champs/resources/qxn/.

PRESCRIPTIONS FOR PHYSICAL ACTIVITY

While the importance of promoting PA is widely acknowledged, the most effective way of supporting a patient's behavior is still unclear and thus presents a challenge to those charged with this task. Providing patients with individually tailored advice, supported by written materials, which include details of local facilities, may be as effective as referral to supervised exercise classes as well as being a more cost-effective option.[28]

Healthcare providers are uniquely positioned to influence participation rates by prescribing physical activity more frequently and precisely. The most utilized method of prescribing cardiovascular exercise intensity is the target heart rate method, typically 60%–90% of age-predicted maximal heart rate [206.9 − (0.67 × age)].[29] Although this method is effective at prescribing relative exercise intensity, it does not truly quantify the actual amount of physical work being performed during exercise for reasons including the variability of predicting maximal heart rate as well as the influence of environmental factors on heart rate.

Ratings of perceived exertion can also be used to prescribe and monitor exercise intensity during a workout. A common approach is to periodically ask a person to rate his/her perceived exertion for a given exercise intensity during a stress test and then match it to an appropriate exercise intensity prescription. Attempting to keep the RPE within a training range similar to heart rate training ranges can be effective. Using this procedure, the target RPE ratings are based upon prior test results, and the person is requested to produce intensity perceived to be similar to the target rating during a workout. The key is close approximation to heart rate in aerobic exercise, where the RPE scale is most often used. A high correlation exists between a person's perceived exertion rating times 10 and the actual heart rate during physical activity; so a person's exertion rating may provide a fairly good estimate of the actual heart rate during activity.[5] For example, if a person's rating of perceived exertion (RPE) is 12, then $12 \times 10 = 120$; so the heart rate should be approximately 120 beats/min.[6] It should be noted that this calculation is only an approximation of heart rate, and the actual heart rate can vary quite a bit depending on age and physical condition.

Specific written exercise prescriptions can increase patient compliance substantially.[30] The FITT principle—frequency, intensity, timing, and type of exercise—can be used to tailor physical activity recommendations to the needs and the goals of the individual patient. Exercise intensity is usually measured by a percent of maximal capacity. For individual exercise prescription, a relative measure of intensity (i.e., the energy cost of the activity relative to the individual's maximal capacity) is more appropriate, especially for older and deconditioned persons.[31] There are several commonly used methods of estimating relative exercise intensity during cardiorespiratory exercise but two common measures are percent of the maximum HR (%HRmax) and percent of maximal oxygen uptake (%VO$_2$max). Each of these methods for prescribing exercise intensity has been shown to result in improvements in cardiorespiratory fitness when used for exercise prescription; thus can be recommended when prescribing exercise for an individual.[31] The American College of Sports Medicine classifies exercise intensity as[31]:

Intensity	% HRmax	%VO$_2$max	RPE
Very light	<57	<37	<Very light (RPE <9)
Light	57–63	37–45	Very light-fairly light (RPE 9–11)
Moderate	64–76	46–63	Fairly light to somewhat hard (RPE 12–13)
Vigorous	77–95	64–90	Somewhat hard to very hard (RPE 14–17)
Near-maximal to maximal	≥96	≥91	≥Very hard (RPE ≥ 18)

Direct measurements of HR and oxygen uptake are recommended for individualized exercise prescription for greater accuracy, but when not feasible, estimation of exercise intensity is acceptable.

Frequency is prescribed in sessions per day and in days per week while timing is the duration, such as 10 or 30 min. The "type" of exercise would include the classifications described previously, that is, aerobic, balance, flexibility, and bone or muscle strengthening. Simply providing individuals with an exercise prescription outlining the recommended frequency, intensity, and duration is insufficient. Individuals need to develop an understanding of how to use behavior change strategies to successfully adhere to a regular physical activity program. Thus, a one-time prescription is not useful, if conversation with the client does not include a discussion of behavior change strategies. The health professional addresses periodic progression in order to maintain the exercise stimulus needed to promote continued health improvements. Just as attention is paid to medication dosage, delivery forms, and frequency, similar precision should be applied to prescriptions for physical activity. Frequency can be prioritized when health goals relate to preventing chronic diseases.[30] Intensity has maximum impact on weight loss and athletic conditioning, whereas timing is particularly relevant for people with diabetes and blood sugar dysregulation.[30] All types (aerobic, balance, flexibility, and resistance) help achieve different health goals. Two types of physical activity prescription programs have been examined to determine if they differed in perceived barriers, benefits, or motives for physical activity. The prescription programs were either a pedometer-based or a time-based Green Prescription. A Green Prescription, a term used by health practitioners in New Zealand, is a referral given by a doctor or nurse to a patient, with exercise and lifestyle goals written on them. This prescription is written after discussing the issues and goals in consultation with the patient. A number of studies have demonstrated the efficacy of the Green Prescription in increasing physical activity and health-related benefits in a number of studies. A pedometer can also be used to monitor habitual step-count physical activity. Using a pedometer to monitor one's accumulation of daily physical activity may be a better motivator and adherence tool than standard time-based goal setting. Patel et al. concluded that the addition of a pedometer to the standard Green Prescription does not appear to increase perceived motives or benefits or decrease perceived barriers for physical activity in low-active adults.[32] It therefore appeared that weekly goal setting helped participants increase their walking with or without the aid of pedometer step-count information.[32]

Whether the healthcare provider includes physical activity counseling or guidelines may depend on their self-efficacy or confidence in their own abilities to counsel on physical activity and exercise. Schields et al. reported that may diabetes educators indicated they are ill trained and lack the skills, experience, and knowledge to counsel their patients in the areas of physical activity and exercise.[33] This low confidence may reduce the likelihood that they will counsel individuals with diabetes regarding lifestyle behaviors. This low level of self-confidence may similarly be found in other healthcare providers. A study involving internal medicine residents reported the following: "few demonstrated adequate knowledge useful for patient counseling (e.g., listing three ways to integrate physical activity into daily life [27%], calculating target heart rate [29%], and identifying personal exercise stages of change [25%]).[34] Personal use of behavior modification techniques was reported infrequently. Although 88% reported confidence in the knowledge of exercise benefits, less than half reported confidence in the knowledge of local facilities, American College of Sports Medicine (ACSM) guidelines, and behavior modification techniques.[34]

Multiple linear regression demonstrated that a higher level of training ($p = 0.02$) and a greater confidence in the knowledge of ACSM guidelines ($p = 0.048$, total R2 = 0.21) independently predicted more frequent self-reported counseling."[34] Additional training, or the use of an "exercise toolkit," may be necessary to increase providers' confidence and ease in counseling for physical activity.

The ACSM's Exercise is Medicine's website, http://exerciseismedicine. org, is a useful site that provides information for a variety of audiences, including healthcare providers. This site has exercise prescription available to download http://exerciseismedicine.org/assets/page_documents/Appendix%20G%20-%20 Prescription%20Form%20(2).pdf.

PHYSICAL ACTIVITY AND CHRONIC DISEASE PREVENTION

PHYSICAL ACTIVITY AND CANCER

According to the World Cancer Research Fund/American Institute for Cancer Research, nearly one-third of the more than 572,000 cancer deaths that occur in the United States each year can be attributed to diet and physical activity habits.[35] Behaviors, such as staying physically active throughout life, can substantially reduce one's lifetime risk of developing, or dying from, cancer.[36] Due to the complexity of factors involved in cancer development and the difficulty in conducting randomized controlled trials to answer questions about how diet, physical activity, and obesity relate to cancer, guidelines have been developed by the American Cancer Society (ACS) based on the synthesis of the current scientific evidence. The recommendation from ACS regarding physical activity and cancer prevention are consistent with the *2008 Physical Activity Guidelines for Americans* detailed earlier in this chapter and restated here.

Adults should engage in at least 150 min of moderately intensity or 75 min of vigorous-intensity activity each week, or an equivalent combination, preferably spread throughout the week

- Children and adolescents should engage in at least 1 h of moderate- or vigorous-intensity activity each day, with vigorous-intensity activity occurring at least 3 days each week.
- Limit sedentary behavior such as sitting, lying down, watching television, or other forms of screen-based entertainment
- Doing some physical activity above usual activities, no matter what one's level of activity, can have many health benefits.

These guidelines indicate that, when individuals with chronic conditions such as cancer are unable to meet the stated recommendations based on their health status, they "should be as physically active as their abilities and conditions allow."[4] An explicit recommendation was made to "avoid inactivity" and it is clearly stated, "some physical activity is better than none."

In addition to encouraging individual physical activity, the ACS encourages community involvement and recommends that organizations should work collaboratively to implement policy and environmental changes that provide safe, enjoyable, and accessible environments for physical activity in schools and worksites, and for transportation and recreation in communities.[36]

Not only does physical activity play a role in the prevention of cancer, but is also an important aspect for the cancer survivor. A cancer survivor is defined as anyone who has been diagnosed with cancer, from the time of diagnosis through the rest of their life.[37] Due to advances in the detection and treatment of cancer, the number of cancer survivors in the United States is approximately 13.7 million and is expected to rise by 31% to 18 million by 2022.[38] Many cancer survivors are highly motivated to seek information and make informed lifestyle choices to improve response to treatment, speed recovery, reduce their risk of recurrence, and improve their quality of life.[39] In discussing cancer survivorship, it is important to recognize the four phases of the continuum of cancer: treatment and recovery; long-term disease-free living or living with stable disease; and, for some, living with advanced cancer. As each of these phases has different needs and challenges with respect to physical activity, it is vital to recognize, and discuss, each phase separately.

The value of exercise during primary cancer treatment has been examined in an increasing number of studies. Existing evidence strongly suggests that exercise is not only safe and feasible during cancer treatment, but that it can also improve physical functioning, fatigue, and multiple aspects of quality of life.[40] Some studies have suggested that physical activity may even increase the rate of completion of chemotherapy.[41] Although physical activity certainly appears beneficial, the decision regarding when to initiate, and how to maintain, physical activity should be individualized to the patient's condition and personal preferences. Those individuals that were active and now receiving chemotherapy and/or radiation therapy may need to exercise at a lower intensity and/or a shorter duration, but the goal is to maintain activity as much as possible. For those individuals who were sedentary prior to cancer treatment, low-intensity exercises, such as slow walks and stretching, should be adopted and slowly increased. If bone metastases or osteoporosis are a concern, careful attention should be given to balance and safety to reduce risk of falls and injuries. If periods of bed rest are mandated, physical therapy is advised to maintain strength and range of motion and can help counteract fatigue and depression.

The next stage in cancer survivorship, after cancer therapy has been completed, is recovery. Many symptoms and side effects that occurred during the treatment phase are subsiding, although some may continue. In addition, latent effects of treatment may appear long after treatment ceases. Survivors may require ongoing nutritional assessment and intervention during the phase of survival based on lingering or latent side effects, but a program of regular physical activity is an essential aid in the process of recovery and improved fitness.

The third phase, long-term disease-free living or stable disease, involves many lifestyle components, physical activity is one. An increasing number of studies have examined the impact of physical activity on cancer recurrence and long-term survival. Because individuals who have been diagnosed with cancer are at a significantly higher risk of developing second primary cancers and may also be at an increased risk of other chronic diseases such as diabetes, cardiovascular disease, and osteoporosis, both nutrition and physical activity guidelines established to prevent those diseases are particularly important for cancer survivors. Exercise has been shown to improve not only cardiovascular fitness, muscle strength, and body composition, but also fatigue, anxiety, depression, self-esteem, and several components of quality of life in cancer survivors. In addition, exercise may have beneficial effects that are cancer specific, such as lymphedema in breast cancer survivors. In the past, there were concerns that cancer survivors with upper extremity lymphedema should not engage in upper extremity resistance training or vigorous aerobic physical activity. Several trials have demonstrated that physical activity is not only safe, but also actually reduces the incidence and severity of lymphedema.[41–43] Although additional studies are needed, over 20 prospective observational studies have shown that physically active cancer survivors have a lower risk of cancer recurrences and improved survival compared with those who are sedentary.[40] Among breast cancer survivors, physical activity after diagnosis has consistently been associated with reduced risk of breast cancer recurrence and breast-cancer-specific mortality. A meta-analysis demonstrated that postdiagnosis exercise was associated with a 34% lower risk of death from breast cancer, a 41% lower risk of all-cause mortality, and a 24% lower risk of breast cancer recurrence.[44] Among survivors of colorectal cancer, at least four large cohort studies have found an inverse association between being physically active after diagnosis and recurrence, colorectal cancer-specific mortality, and/or overall mortality.[45–48] A 2011 meta-analysis of 78 exercise intervention trials showed that exercise interventions resulted in clinically meaningful improvements in quality of life that persisted after the completion of the intervention.[49] In another meta-analysis of 44 studies that included over 3000 participants with varying cancer types, cancer survivors randomized to an exercise intervention had significantly reduced cancer-related fatigue levels, with evidence of a linear relationship to the intensity of resistance exercise.[50]

Despite the many benefits of exercise for cancer survivors, particular issues may affect the ability of survivors to exercise. Effects of treatment may also increase the risk of exercise-related injuries and adverse effects, and therefore specific precautions may be advisable. According to the Nutrition and Physical Activity Guidelines for Cancer Survivors, these include the following [40]:

Survivors with severe anemia should delay exercise, other than activities of daily living, until the anemia is improved.

Survivors with compromised immune function should avoid public gyms and public pools until their white blood cell counts return to safe levels. Survivors who have completed a bone marrow transplant are usually advised to avoid such exposures for 1 year after transplantation.

Survivors experiencing severe fatigue from their therapy may not feel up to an exercise program, and therefore they may be encouraged to do 10 min of light exercises daily.

Survivors undergoing radiation should avoid chlorine exposure to irradiated skin (e.g., from swimming pools).

Survivors with indwelling catheters or feeding tubes should be cautious or avoid pool, lake, or ocean water or other microbial exposures that may result in infections, as well as resistance training of muscles in the area of the catheter to avoid dislodgment.

Survivors with multiple or uncontrolled comorbidities need to consider modifications to their exercise program in consultation with their physicians.

Survivors with significant peripheral neuropathies or ataxia may have a reduced ability to use the affected limbs because of weakness or loss of balance. They may do better with a stationary reclining bicycle, for example, than walking on a treadmill.

After consideration of these and other specific precautions, it is recommended that cancer survivors follow the survivor-specific guidelines written by an expert panel convened by the American College of Sports Medicine.[51] The ACSM panel recommended that individuals avoid inactivity and return to normal activity as soon as possible after diagnosis or treatment.

For individuals living with advanced cancer, both physical activity and a healthy diet may be important factors in establishing and maintaining a sense of well-being and enhancing quality of life. Several systematic reviews have suggested that some level of physical activity is feasible and may improve quality of life and physical function in persons with advanced cancer although this may be specific to certain cancer types.[52,53] At present, there is insufficient evidence to make general recommendations for physical activity for those living with advanced cancer and are best based on individual physical abilities.

PHYSICAL ACTIVITY AND BODY WEIGHT

Overweight and obesity are major public health problems as they pose a major risk factor for serious chronic diseases, including type 2 diabetes, cardiovascular disease, hypertension and stroke, and certain forms of cancer.[54] According to data from the 2009 to 2010 National Health and Nutrition Examination Survey, more than 2 in adults are considered to be overweight or obese.[54] In addition, more than 1 in 3 adults are considered to be obese, and 1 in 20 are considered to have extreme obesity.[55] This is not just a problem faced in adulthood. About 1/3rd of children and adolescents ages 6–19 are considered to be overweight or obese and more than 1 in 6 children are considered to be obese.[56] As the prevalence of childhood obesity increases, so do its related health problems. The rise in overweight/obesity is a global phenomenon as similar changes are seen in all Western countries and many non-Western countries as well.[57] The rising prevalence of obesity has been attributed in part to population-level changes in physical activity. Physical inactivity is leading to a global epidemic of childhood obesity. Physical inactivity is one of the leading causes of major chronic illness tracking from childhood into adulthood. Overweight and obese children are four times more likely to become overweight adults, thus leading to major chronic illnesses such as type 2 diabetes, heart disease, and cancer. In 2010, The World Health Organization (WHO) stated that physical inactivity is the fourth leading risk factor for global mortality.[58]

Clearly, body weight and physical activity are inextricably linked. The extent to which weight status is a barrier to physical activity, a consequence of physical inactivity, or a motivating factor for initiating activity is unclear. Most studies report on longitudinal associations between physical activity and BMI or body weight; with most reporting a negative association (lower physical activity predicts higher subsequent weight gain). Interestingly, one study reported a reverse association, suggesting that higher baseline levels of BMI predict future low levels of physical activity.[59] Results from a large population-based prospective cohort study in Europe involving 25,639 men and women aged 39–79 followed over a 10-year period supported this idea. The study concluded that weight gain is a significant determinant of future physical inactivity independent of baseline weight and activity.[60] Compared with maintaining weight, moderate (1.0–4 lb) and large (>4 lb/year) weight gains significantly predict future inactivity which may lead to a potentially vicious cycle including further weight gain, obesity, and complications associated with a sedentary lifestyle.[60] Due to this relationship, it is vital that routine weights are taken by the medical profession during visits so that early intervention can be initiated to break this cycle. Results published in a separate trial using the EPIC cohort of 84,511 men and 203,987 women followed for 5.1 years suggested that a higher level of physical activity reduces abdominal adiposity independent of baseline and changes in body weight and is thus a useful strategy for preventing chronic disease and premature deaths.[61]

Effective weight management for individuals and groups with overweight and obesity involves a range of strategies including reducing energy intake through dietary change and increasing energy expenditure by increasing physical activity. Clinical trials have shown that exercise in adults with overweight or obesity can reduce body weight; and a systematic review published in The Cochrane Library has supported this view.[62] The results of this systematic review, which included 43 studies with 3476 participants, support the use of exercise as a weight loss intervention, particularly when combined with dietary changes. For successful long-term weight loss, physical activity alone is insufficient and must be combined with low-energy intake. Exercise is also associated with improved cardiovascular disease risk factors even if no weight loss occurs.[62]

Individuals may resist an increase in physical activity under the mistaken assumption that physical activity can increase hunger and that people may reward themselves by eating foods with high energy density after physical activity. A 2009 study that investigated the effect of physical activity on appetite found that levels of peptide YY, an appetite-suppressing hormone, were increased immediately after vigorous physical activity while levels of ghrelin, an appetite-stimulating hormone, were suppressed.[63] Appetite did return after approximately 1 h, but at no point were people hungrier after physical activity than the control group who had not exercised.[63] It was concluded that for most people, over a short-term period of 1–2 days, there was an incomplete compensation for the energy expended by physical activity of more energy from food and drink. In the longer term, there is a partial compensation for the energy expended, but it is typically insufficient to account for the energy cost of the physical activity and so will result in weight loss over time.[64] Another study published in 2013 examined the acute effects of high-intensity intermittent exercise on energy intake, perception of appetite, and appetite-related hormones in a small group of overweight, sedentary men.[65] The results showed that ad lib energy intake was lower after both the high- and very high-intensity activity compared to the control group ($p = 0.038$ and $p = 0.004$ respectively) and the very high intensity was also lower than the continuous moderate-intensity exercise ($p = 0.028$).[65] Energy intake in the subsequent 38 h remained less than control or moderate-intensity groups. These observations were associated with a lower active ghrelin ($p = 0.05$). No differences were found in perceived appetite between the groups and the ratings of physical activity enjoyment were similar between all exercise trials indicating the high-intensity format was well tolerated in an overweight, sedentary population.[65] The physical activity does not need to be "structured" in order to achieve an energy deficient.

Levine et al. measured nonexercise activity in two groups of individuals. The results of the study suggested that less-structured physical activity (i.e., simply moving around more) can make a significant contribution to energy expenditure and therefore to help prevent weight gain.[66]

PHYSICAL ACTIVITY AND DIABETES

Type 1 Diabetes Mellitus

Diet and physical activity form a solid foundation for both the prevention and treatment of diabetes mellitus. Regular physical activity increases insulin sensitivity, improves pharmacotherapy, lowers blood sugar concentrations, reduces body fat content, builds muscle, and improves cardiovascular fitness and function.[67] A number of studies have demonstrated the effectiveness of regular exercise in improving metabolic control and overall health in persons with diabetes, although the clinical management of physically active patients with type 1 diabetes (T1DM) remains a challenge. Most activities that include varying intensity can be performed by most people with T1DM who have optimum metabolic control of diabetes and have no complications. The most important issue for these individuals is an understanding of how exercise affects blood glucose control and developing the knowledge and skills to avoid hypo- and hyperglycemia. This can be achieved by knowing how to adjust insulin administration and carbohydrate intake prior to, during, and after exercise. The American Diabetes Association Position Statement asserts that: "All levels of exercise, including leisure activities, recreational sports, and competitive professional performance, can be performed by people with T1DM who do not have complications and are in good blood glucose control." The vast majorities of sports are open to individuals with T1DM and impose no restrictions.[68] The ABCD position statement on physical activity and exercise provides excellent tables to use as guidelines and/or educational tools for the physically active diabetic.

For the majority of children diagnosed with T1DM, physical activity can provide benefits of improved cardiovascular fitness, increased lean mass, improved blood lipid profile, and decreased body adiposity.[69] Exercise benefits are particularly important for this population because exercise may lower the risk of cardiovascular disease, a primary cause of morbidity, and mortality among those diagnosed with T1DM.[70] Studies have shown that there is a positive relationship between regular physical activity and glycemic control as well as glucose metabolism in children and adolescents with T1DM, and experts have concluded that physical activity is an important lifestyle component of T1DM management in children.[69–72]

Type 2 Diabetes Mellitus

The prevalence type of type 2 diabetes mellitus (T2DM) is projected to increase to 300 million worldwide by 2025.[73] Diabetes affects 25.8 million people (or 8.3% of the U.S. population) of all ages, with estimated total costs, both direct and indirect, of $174 billion.[74] Although there are multiple genetic and environmental factors that increase the risk for diabetes, recent epidemiologic research suggests that the global epidemic rise in the incidence of diabetes over the past two decades is largely due to changes in lifestyle factors such as diet and physical activity.[75] A review of studies investigating the role of physical activity and risk of type 2 diabetes found that it is protective in the general population, with a reduction in risk of 10%–40%. This has been observed in men and women, across the BMI range and across ethnic groups.[76] For the individual with type 2 diabetes (T2DM), regular moderate-intensity physical activity improves both short- and long-term glycemic control as a result of increased hepatic and peripheral insulin sensitivity. Increased physical activity in diabetes may enable reductions, or even discontinuation, of pharmacological treatment in a substantial proportion of patients.[68] A meta-analysis of the effects of exercise on glycemic control and body weight concluded that exercise reduces HbA1c by approximately 0.66%, an amount that may be clinically significant in the long run.[77] Interventions comprising diet alone, exercise alone, or diet and exercise combined, all produce similar reductions in diabetes risk.[78] Each intervention can produce the weight loss critical for risk reduction. The relative contribution of diet, physical activity, and weight change on the risk of developing diabetes was analyzed by Hamman et al.[79] In a population of 1079 middle-aged, obese Americans, weight loss was the dominant predictor of reduced diabetes incidence (HR per 5 kg weight loss 0.42; 95% CI 0.35–0.51; $p < 0.0001$).[79] Increased physical activity was found to be of particular importance in the absence of weight loss. Among the 495 participants who failed to meet the weight loss goal after the first year, those who achieved the physical activity goal had a 44% lower diabetes incidence than those who did not, whereas the Da Qing IGT and Diabetes Study showed that exercise alone reduced risk of disease progression by 46%.[79,80] When weight loss proves difficult, exercise alone can reduce diabetes risk by increasing insulin-mediated glucose disposal to muscle.

Although physical activity has been documented to improve patient outcomes, research has noted that healthcare professionals inadequately address this issue, resulting in physical activity being an underutilized therapy.[81] In a meta-analysis conducted by Avery et al., 10 behavior change techniques were associated with potential clinically significant improvements in HbA1c: prompting generalization of a target behavior (e.g., once PA is performed in one situation, the individual is encouraged to try it in another); use of follow-up prompts (e.g., telephone calls to support maintenance); prompt review of behavioral goals (e.g., review whether PA goals were achieved followed by revisions or adjustments); providing information on where and when to be active (e.g., tips on places and times to access local PA and exercise clubs); plan social support and social change (e.g., encourage individuals to elicit social support from others to help achieve a PA related goal); goal setting (e.g., supporting individuals to formulate specific, measurable, achievable, relevant, and timely PA-related goals); time management (e.g., making time to be active); prompting focus on past success (e.g., identifying previous successful attempts at PA); barrier identification/problem solving (e.g., identifying potential barriers to PA and ways to overcome them); and providing information on the consequences of PA specific to the individual (e.g., information about the benefits and costs of PA to individuals).[82] This list of behavior change techniques is not definitive but serves as a starting point to begin the discussion of physical activity with the individual with T2D.

There is strong and consistent evidence that promotion of physical activity plays a critical role in *primary prevention* of type 2 diabetes, and efforts to increase physical activity behavior needs to be targeted to individuals within the clinical setting and the social and physical environments within communities.[83] In 2005–2008, based on fasting glucose or A1c levels, 35% of adults in the United States ages 20 years or older had prediabetes, which correlates to an estimated 79 million Americans using current population numbers.[74] Studies have shown that people with prediabetes who lose weight and increase their physical activity can prevent or delay type 2 diabetes and, in some cases, return their blood glucose levels to normal.[74] The Diabetes Prevention Program (DPP), a large prevention study of people at high risk for diabetes, showed that lifestyle intervention to lose weight and increase physical activity reduced the development of type 2 diabetes by 58% during a 3-year period. The reduction was even greater, 71%, among adults age 60 years or older.[84] The drug metformin also reduced disease risk, although less dramatically. The 10-year follow-up study reported the effects of the DPP persisted for years, with a 43% reduced incidence of diabetes in the lifestyle groups and 18% in those taking metformin compared to the placebo group. Again, the results were even more dramatic for participates age 60 and older, a 49% reduced incidence of diabetes.[84]

Studies performed in children and adolescents demonstrate a positive association between physical activity and insulin dynamics, with increased activity significantly related to lower fasting insulin and greater insulin sensitivity.[85] Resistance training may provide additional benefits. Compared to endurance training, resistance training may substantially increase skeletal muscle mass and strength and, thus, whole-body glucose disposal capacity. Results from the Nurses' Health Study (NHS) showed that resistance exercise and lower-intensity muscular conditioning exercises were each independently associated with lower risk of T2DM in pooled analysis.[86] Thus, resistance or strength training should be considered a safe and effective modality of exercise in individuals at risk for developing type 2 diabetes. This coincides with the Physical Activity Guidelines for American Children and Adolescents, which include bone- and muscle-strengthening activities for inclusion into each day's minimum of 60 min of physical activity.

PHYSICAL ACTIVITY AND BLOOD PRESSURE

The *2008 Physical Activity Guidelines for Americans* included an extensive review of the literature and concluded that individuals engaged in physical activity have a 25%–30% lower risk of stroke than inactive individuals.[87] Publications since that 2008 review further support the recommendations. In a meta-analysis of 25 studies looking at the effects of physical activity on blood pressure, there was an average reduction of 11 and 8 mmHg respectively, in systolic and diastolic blood pressures.[87] This magnitude of blood pressure reduction may be particularly useful in those with mild hypertension and in early stages of the disease.[88] Considerable evidence supports the inclusion of physical activity as an integral component of ischemic stroke prevention. Many observational studies have confirmed that people who are physically active have lower rates of ischemic stroke than those who are sedentary.[89]

However, observational studies offer little insight into the mechanisms of stroke prevention. One possibility is that physical activity improves vascular function and reduces the likelihood of vascular risk factors that contribute to ischemic stroke risk.[90,91] Another role could be that exercise improves the response to an ischemic event and so reduces infarct size after stroke and thereby minimizes the frequency or severity of overt symptoms. In a meta-analysis that included studies using a variety of populations, ages, study designs, and definitions of physical activity, men and women who were most physically active had 25% lower risk of incident ischemic stroke than those who were least physically active (odds ratio [OR], 95% confidence interval [95% CI]: 0.75, 0.67–0.84).[89] This reduction of ischemic stroke risk associated with physical activity appears to be approximately the same in men and in women.[89,92] A 2010 meta-analysis of studies was performed to quantify the association between physical activity level and risk of stroke outcomes.[93] The outcome measures were stroke incidence, stroke mortality, or both. A total of 992 studies were identified, of which, 13 satisfied all eligibility criteria. Compared with low physical activity, moderate physical activity was associated with an 11% reduction in risk of stroke outcome, and a high physical activity level a 19% reduction. When women were singled out, high physical activity resulted in a 24% reduction in risk, but no significant risk reduction was associated with moderate physical activity in women.[93] Therefore, higher levels of physical activity may be required in women to achieve the same risk reduction seen in men. In contrast, a large-scale prospective epidemiological data testing the association between physical activity and cerebrovascular disease (CVD) risk showed that recreational activity was inversely associated with risk of CVD in women but not in men.[94]

PHYSICAL ACTIVITY AND OTHER HEALTH CONCERNS

GALLSTONE DISEASE

Gallstone disease affects approximately 20 million people in the United States.[95] Risk factors for gallstone disease include advancing age, obesity, parity, race and ethnicity, gender, as well as genetic predisposition.[96] Physical inactivity has also been suggested as a risk factor for gallstone disease.[97–101] Although the exact mechanism by which physical activity may reduce gallstone risk is unclear, physical activity may reduce hypomobility of the gallbladder. Hypomobility is a key factor in the pathogenesis of gallstone disease. The relationship between physical activity and gallstone disease was examined as a secondary analysis in a cohort of postmenopausal women who participated in the Study of Osteoporotic Fractures (SOF).[102] Multivariate logistic regression indicated women in the lowest two quartiles of physical activity, according to questionnaire, had a 59% (OR = 1.59 (1.11–2.29), $p = 0.02$) and a 57% higher risk (OR = 1.57 (1.11–2.23), $p = 0.01$) of developing gallstone disease compared to women in the highest quartile of activity (PTrend ≤ 0.0001).[102] Additionally, this relationship was examined in a cohort of 182 postmenopausal women (mean age 74.2 years, SD = 4.1) who participated in a randomized controlled trial of a walking intervention. Women in the randomized clinical trial in the lowest tertile of physical activity determined by a physical activity monitor had a higher risk of developing gallstone disease than women in the highest tertile of physical activity, 13% (OR = 1.13 [1.01–1.28], $p = 0.05$, PTrend ≤ 0.04).[102]

PSYCHOLOGICAL HEALTH

The benefits of physical activity extend beyond their contributions to physical well-being and also include mental well-being.[103] The twentieth century witnessed an exponential growth in the literature regarding the positive effects of physical activity on psychological health.[104] Psychological health is defined as "a state characterized by psychological integrity; ability to perform valued family, work, and community roles; ability to deal with psychological stress; a feeling of well-being; and freedom from the risk of disease and untimely death."[105] Psychological health concerns itself with how you cope, how you are doing in response, and whether you find life to be interesting and enjoyable. Although life is better when we are feeling good, there is no avoiding the fact that there will be ups and downs. In the end, psychological health and well-being is basically about "how are you doing?" Anxiety and depression disorders constitute one of the major health issues of our time and their impact is increasing.[106] Depression is a widespread health issue with a lifetime prevalence of 17% currently affecting 121 million people with the World Health Organization (WHO) predicting that depression will become the most prevalent cause of disability in the world by 2020.[104,107] The evidence is consistent across meta-analytic or narrative reviews and large-scale epidemiological surveys, and points to a convincing relationship between physical activity and improved positive mood.[104,108,109] Despite the convincing evidence base regarding the relationship between physical activity and depression, the mechanisms explaining the association remain inconclusive and likely result from a combination of effects. According to a review by Lotan et al., many researchers have established a relationship between physical activity and self-esteem, self-efficacy, and psychological functioning.[110] Additionally, physical activity can improve physical self-esteem.[111] The positive effects are likely to be greater for those with initially low self-esteem and can be experienced by all age groups, but there is strongest evidence for change in children and middle-aged adults.[112] Several reviews have concluded that there is good evidence that physical activity and can reduce the risk of clinical depression.[111,113,114] Taliaferro et al. explored associations among types physical activity and hopelessness, depression, and suicidal behavior among college students based on the 2005 National College Health Assessment data.[115] The study established an association between physical activity, especially aerobic activity, and reduced risk of hopelessness, depression, and suicidal behavior among college students.[115] Biddle et al. state that the evidence is strong enough to conclude that there is support for a causal link between physical activity and reduced clinically defined depression along with evidence that physical activity has an important effect on anxiety.[109] The beneficial effects of PA on anxiety appear equal to those achieved via meditation or relaxation.[111] Although studies of older adults and children/adolescents are more limited, the benefits of physical activity are seen across the lifespan. Furthermore, lower levels of physical activity in childhood may be a risk factor for adult depression.[103,113] Physical activity also plays a role in management of depression. There are a variety of medications that can be used in the treatment of depression, but it can take several weeks to months before any effect is seen, and it may be several months before the full effect is apparent. Individuals may vary widely in the susceptibility to both the benefits and side effects of antidepressant drugs. None of the available guidelines suggest that drugs alone are sufficient treatment for depression of any severity.[116] Suggested general measures include, in part, a physical activity program as increasing exercise is of proven benefit in all severities of depression and works more quickly than medication.[116,117] A variety of physical exercise interventions have been used in studies and positive findings of both aerobic and strength activities have been shown, although aerobic conditions have been studied more frequently. The results of Dunn et al. and Singh et al. focus on the importance of the intensity of physical exercise rather than the type of physical exercise.[118,119] Positive results have been shown concerning intensity in progressive resistance training as well as aerobic exercise. A focus on intensity of physical activity is more important than a focus on frequency of physical activity according to Dunn et al.[118]

In addition to the multiple reasons for engaging in physical activity, preserving brain health could be a strong and convincing argument to promote activity in the population and one that could have a major impact on medical practice and public health education. In 2012, an estimated 5.4 million Americans of all ages have Alzheimer's disease.[120] As the number of older Americans grows rapidly, so too will the numbers of new and existing cases of Alzheimer's disease. As this number increases, aggregate payments for their care will increase dramatically from an estimated $200 billion in 2012 to $1.1 trillion in 2050.[120] Results from intervention studies are inconclusive, but findings from meta-analyses indicate a small but significant improvement in cognitive functioning of older adults who experience an increase in aerobic fitness.[109] Furthermore, there is some evidence from clinical trials that shows exercise can help reduce the risk of dementia and Alzheimer's disease.[110,111]

OSTEOARTHRITIS

Approximately 27 million adults 65 and older are affected by osteoarthritis (OA) and it is the second most common health condition in community-dwelling older Americans.[121] OA is a progressive and debilitating disease that commonly affects the hand, knee, hip, and spine joints.[122] Although not fatal, OA is associated with pain, stiffness, decreased physical functioning, incontinence, depression, and overall poorer quality of life for affected older adults.[123] Physical function is an important predictor of health outcomes and the capacity to perform basic physical aspects is a central aspect of health-related quality of life. Maintaining independent functioning is a critical factor in preserving health and well-being. Examples of physical function are things such as climbing stairs or carrying groceries. To date, physical exercise is the only intervention that has been consistently demonstrated to attenuate functional decline, but the change is quite variable.[124] Brach et al. examined whether older adults who exercise demonstrate higher levels of physical function than those who do not exercise but are physically active throughout the day.[125] After examining baseline data from 3075 participants in the Health, Aging and Body Composition study, they concluded that older adults who participate in 20–30 min of moderate-intensity exercise on most days of the week have better physical function than older persons who are active throughout the day or who are inactive.[125] Any type of physical activity is better than no activity for protection against functional limitations, but exercise confers greater benefit for physical capacity.

In relation to OA, major risk factors include: older age, overweight and obesity, physical inactivity, previous joint injury, repeated overuse of certain joints, and heredity.[126] The health benefits of physical activity are well established, including prevention of obesity, delay of onset of physical limitation, and importance to normal joint health.[127] Vigorous activity has been associated with better joint health in people age 50–79, and Ding et al. reported that women who were regular walkers were less likely to have early signs of joint abnormalities, such as cartilage degeneration.[126,128] Older adults with a higher muscle mass, presumably from regular exercise, have decreased cartilage loss, suggesting that increased muscle mass and strength protect joints from degenerative changes.[126] Aerobic and resistance exercise have been shown to reduce pain and disability among those with OA, while increasing physical performance; however, individuals with arthritis are often wary of exercise because activity can initially increase pain or because they inaccurately believe physical activity will worsen their arthritis. A summary of a Cochrane review examining exercise for OA of the knee discovered small, statistically significant benefit for exercise effects on pain and self-reported physical function.[121,129] Adults with arthritis should follow either the Active Adult or the Active Older Adult Guidelines, whichever meets their personal health goals and matches their abilities. Many people with arthritis have joint stiffness that makes daily tasks such as bathing and fixing meals difficult. Doing daily flexibility exercises for all upper (e.g., neck, shoulder, elbow, wrist, and finger) and lower (e.g., low back, hip, knee, ankle, and toes) joints of the body helps maintain essential range of motion. Many older adults and some adults with arthritis and other chronic diseases may be prone to falling. If this a concern, activities that improve balance such as Tai Chi, backward walking, side stepping, heel and toe walking, and/or standing on one foot should be included at least 3 days/week as part of the activity plan.

ALL-CAUSE MORTALITY

Regular exercise increases cardiorespiratory endurance, tolerance to physical exertion, high density lipoprotein cholesterol, and insulin sensitivity while decreasing adiposity, blood pressure, blood triglycerides, and inflammatory markers. Thus, those who are physically active on a regular basis are more fit and generally have a better risk factor profile for a variety of common chronic disorders. They also, on average, have a lower risk of premature death. Samitz et al. conducted a system review and meta-analysis to determine the association of all-cause mortality of different domains of physical activity and of defined increases in physical activity and energy expenditure.[130] Data from 80 studies that included ~1,340,000 participants revealed that higher levels of total and domain-specific physical activity were associated with reduced all-cause mortality.[130] The risk reduction per unit of time increase was largest for vigorous exercise. Moderate-intensity activities of daily living were to a lesser extent beneficial in reducing mortality.

PHYSICALLY ACTIVE LIFESTYLE

Physical activity has repeatedly been shown to be associated with reductions in the onset/major causes of death, such as cardiovascular disease, cancer, and all-cause mortality. Physical activity is increasingly recognized as a key component of a healthy lifestyle; humankind was designed to be active and has become more sedentary in recent decades. Changes in work environment, entertainment, transport, and domestic life mean that very little physical activity is required in our day-to-day life. In recent times, there has been a general reluctance to give children the freedom to be active. If children do not develop the habit of being physically active at a young age, it is unlikely that they will be active as adults. Levine et al. measured nonexercise activity thermogenesis in a group of self-reported "inactive" lean and obese individuals.[66] The lean group performed a significant amount of "nonexercise" physical activity, whereas the obese individuals spent more time sitting and being still. The difference in energy expenditure between the obese and lean individuals was 350 kcal/day on average. This study suggests that less-structured physical activity, that is, simply moving around more, can make a significant contribution to energy expenditure and therefore help to prevent weight gain, which may translate to reduced risk of the chronic conditions associated with overweight and obesity. Physical activity can be an important lifestyle factor at all stages of cancer progression, from prediagnosis, to treatment, to end-of-life care or rehabilitation in survival.

Physical activity and other health-promoting behaviors are complex and are associated with different factors, but are also associated with one another. Common barriers to changing physical activity and other health-promoting behaviors such as time, resources, access/opportunity, and support need to be identified and discussed in order for behavior change to occur. Those with a responsibility for the health and well-being of the population must work together to consider ways to encourage people to be active and to educate people on the implications of an inactive lifestyle.

REFERENCES

1. National Heart, Lung, and Blood Institute. What is physical activity? September 26, 2011. Available at: http://www.nhlbi.nih.gov/health/health-topics/topics/phys/. Accessed July 20, 2013.
2. U.S. Department of Health & Human Services, 2008. Physical activity guidelines for Americans 2008. Available at: http://www.health.gov/paguidelines/guidelines/default. aspx. Accessed April 20, 2015.
3. U.S. Department of Health & Human Services, 2008. *Physical Activity Guidelines Advisory Committee Report 2008. Nutr Rev.* 2009;67(2):114–120.
4. Department of Health & Human Services. HHS announces physical activity guidelines for Americans. 2008. Available at: http://www.health.gov/paguidelines/guidelines/. Accessed April 19, 2015.
5. Borg GA. Psychophysical bases of perceived exertion. *Med Sci Sports Exerc.* 1982;14:377–381.

6. Centers for Disease Control and Prevention (CDC) website. 2011. Physical activity page. Perceived exertion. Available at http://www.cdc.gov/physicalactivity/everyone/measuring/exertion.html. Accessed April 20, 2015.

7. Behavioral Risk Factor Surveillance System. 2014. BRFSS today: Facts and highlights. Available at: http://www.cdc.gov/brfss/about/brfss_today.htm. Accessed March 19, 2013.

8. Patel N, Keglar S. Adult participation in aerobic and muscle-strengthening physical activities—United States, 2011. *Morb Mortal Wkly Rep.* May 3, 2013;62(17):326–330.

9. Dwyer-Lindgren L, Freedman G, Engell RE et al. Prevalence of physical activity and obesity in US countries, 2001–2011: A roadmap for action. *Popul Health Metr.* 2013;11:7.

10. Agency for Healthcare Research and Quality and the Centers for Disease Control. Physical activity and older Americans: Benefits and strategies, June 2002. Available at: http://www.ahrq.gov/ppip/activity.htm. Accessed January 20, 2014.

11. Toscos T, Consolvo S, McDonald DW. Barriers to physical activity: A study of self-revelation in an online community. *J Med Syst.* 2011;35:1225–1242.

12. Trost SG, Owen N, Bauman AE et al. Correlates of adults' participation in physical activity: Review and update. *Med Sci Sports Exerc.* 2002;34(12):1996–2001.

13. Ransdell LG, Detling N, Hildebrand K et al. Can physical activity interventions change perceived exercise benefits and barriers. *Am J Health Stud.* 2004;19(4):195–204.

14. Bandura A. Health promotion by social cognitive means. *Health Educ Behav.* 2004;31(2):143–164.

15. White SM, Mailey EL, McAuley E. Leading a physically active lifestyle: Effective behavior characteristics. *ACSM's Health Fitness J.* 2010;14(1):8–15.

16. Sherwood NE, Jeffery RW. The behavioral determinants of exercise: Implications for physical activity interventions. *Annu Rev Nutr.* 2000;20:21–44.

17. Robbins LB, Wu T, Sikorskii A, Morley B. Psychometric assessment of the adolescent physical activity perceived benefits and barriers scales. *J Nurs Meas.* 2008;16(2):98–112.

18. Siddiqi Z, Tiro J, Shuval K. Understanding Impediments and enablers to physical activity among African American adults: A systematic review of qualitative studies. *Health Educ Res.* 2011;26(6):1010–1024.

19. Olson JM. An integrative review of literature on the determinants of physical activity among rural women. *Public Health Nurs.* 2013;30(4):288–311.

20. Costello E, Kafchinski M, Vrazel J, Sullivan P. Motivators, barriers, and beliefs regarding physical activity in an older population. *J Geriatr Phys Ther.* 2011;34:138–147.

21. Josyula LK, Lyle RM. Barriers in the implementation of a physical activity intervention in primary care settings: Lessons learned. *Health Promot Pract.* 2013;14(1):81–87.

22. Jackson AS, Blair SN, Mahar MT et al. Prediction of functional aerobic capacity without exercise testing. *Med Sci Sports Exerc.* 1990;22(6):863–870.

23. Hagstromer, M. International physical activity questionnaire 2002. Available at https://sites.google.com/site/theipaq/home. Accessed April 20, 2015.

24. Agency for Healthcare Research & Quality. 2002. U.S. Department of Health & Human Services. Available at: https://innovations.ahrq.gov/qualitytools/international-physical-activity-questionnaires-ipaq. Accessed April 29, 2015.

25. Hagstromer M, Oja P, Sjostrom M. The international physical activity questionnaire (IPAQ): A study of concurrent and construct validity. *Public Health Nutr.* 2006;9(6):755–762.

26. British Columbia Ministry of Health. Physical activity readiness questionnaire, Department of National Health and Welfare, Canada, revised 1992.

27. Topolski TD, LoGerfo J, Patrick DL et al. The rapid assessment of physical activity (RAPA) among older adults. *Prev Chronic Dis.* 2006;3(4):A118.

28. Barrett EM, Darker CD, Hussey J. Promotion of physical activity in primary care: Knowledge and practice of general practitioners and physiotherapists. *J Public Health.* 2013;21:63–69.

29. American College of Sports Medicine. *ACSM's Guidelines for Exercise Testing and Prescription*, 8th edn. Baltimore, MD: Lippincott Williams & Wilkins, 2010.

30. Oberg E. Physical activity prescription: Our best medicine. *Integrative Med.* 2007; 6(5):18–22.

31. ASCM Position Stand. Quantity and quality of exercise for developing and maintaining cardiorespiratory, musculoskeletal, and neuromotor fitness in apparently healthy adults: Guidance for prescribing exercise. *Med Sci Sports Exerc.* 2011; 43(7):1334–1359.

32. Patel A, Schofield GM, Kolt GS, Keogh JW. Perceived barriers, benefits, and motives for physical activity: Two primary-care physical activity prescription programs. *J Aging Phys Activity.* 2013;21:85–99.

33. Schields CA, Fowles JR, Dunbar P et al. Increasing diabetes educators' confidence in physical activity and exercise counseling: The effectiveness of the "physical activity and exercise toolkit" training intervention. *Can J Diabetes.* 2013;37:381–387.

34. Rogers LQ, Gutin B, Humphries MC et al. Evaluation of internal medicine residents as exercise role models and associations with self-reported counseling behavior, confidence, and perceived success. *Teach Learn Med.* 2006;18(3):215–221.

35. World Cancer Research Fund/American Institute for Cancer Research. *Food, Nutrition, Physical Activity, and the Prevention of Cancer: A Global Perspective.* Washington, DC: World Cancer Research Fund/American Institute for Cancer Research, 2007.

36. Kushi LH, Doyle C, McCullough M et al. American Cancer Society guidelines on nutrition and physical activity for cancer prevention: Reducing the risk of cancer with healthy food choices and physical activity. *CA Cancer J Clin.* 2102;62:30–67.

37. Centers for Disease Control and Prevention (CDC). Cancer survivors—United States 2007. *Morb Mortal Wkly Rep.* 2011;60:269–272.

38. American Cancer Society. *Cancer Treatment and Survivorship Facts and Figures 2012–2013.* Atlanta, GA: American Cancer Society, 2012. Available at: http://www.cancer.org/acs/groups/content/@epidemiologysurveilance/documents/document/acspc-033876.pdf. Accessed July 8, 2013.

39. Jones LW, Demark-Wahnefried W. Diet, exercise, and complementary therapies after primary treatment for cancer. *Lancet Oncol.* 2006;7:1017–1026.

40. Rock CL, Doyle C, Denmark-Wahnfried W et al. Nutrition and physical activity guidelines for cancer survivors. *CA Cancer J Clin.* 2012;62:242–274.

41. Courneya KS, Segal RJ, Mackey JR et al. Effects of aerobic and resistance exercise in breast cancer patients receiving adjuvant chemotherapy: A multicenter randomized controlled trial. *J Clin Oncol.* 2007;25:4396–4404.

42. Schmitz KH, Ahmed RL, Troxel A et al. Weight lifting in women with breast cancer-related lymphedema. *N Engl J Med.* 2009;361:664–673.

43. Schmitz KH, Ahmed RL, Troxel AB et al. Weight lifting for women at risk for breast cancer-related lymphedema: A randomized trial. *JAMA.* 2010;304:2699–2705.

44. Ibrahim EM, Al-Homaidh A. Physical activity and survival after breast cancer diagnosis: Meta-analysis of published studies. *Med Oncol.* 2011;28:753–765.

45. Meyerhardt JA, Giovannucci EL, Holmes MD et al. Physical activity and survival after colorectal cancer diagnosis. *J Clin Oncol.* 2006;24:3527–3534.

46. Meyerhardt JA, Giovannucci EL, Ogino S et al. Physical activity and male colorectal cancer survival. *Arch Intern Med.* 2009;169:2102–2108.

47. Meyerhardt JA, Heseltine D, Niedzwiecki D et al. Impact of physical activity on cancer recurrence and survival in patients with stage III colon cancer: Findings from CALGB 89803. *J Clin Oncol.* 2006;24:3535–3541.

48. Haydon AM, Macinnis RJ, English D, Giles GG. Effect of physical activity and body size on survival after diagnosis with colorectal cancer. *Gut.* 2006;55:62–67.

49. Ferrer RA, Huedo-Medina TB, Johnson BT et al. Exercise interventions for cancer survivors: A meta-analysis of quality of life outcomes. *Ann Behav Med.* 2011;41:32–47.

50. Brown JC, Huedo-Medina TB, Pescatello LS et al. Efficacy of exercise interventions in modulating cancer-related fatigue among adult cancer survivors: A meta-analysis. *Cancer Epidemiol Biomarkers Prev.* 2011;20:123–133.

51. Schmitz KH, Courneya KS, Matthews C et al. American College of Sports Medicine roundtable on exercise guidelines for cancer survivors. *Med Sci Sports Exerc.* 2010; 42:1409–1426.

52. Beaton R, Pagdin-Friesen W, Robertson A et al. Effects of exercise intervention on persons with metastatic cancer: A systematic review. *Physiother Can.* 2009;61:141–153.

53. Lowe SS, Watanabe S, Courneya KS. Physical activity as a supportive care intervention in palliative cancer patients: A systematic review. *J Support Oncol.* 2009;7:27–34.

54. Centers for Disease Control and Prevention (CDC) website. Adult obesity facts. Available at: http://www.cdc.gov/obesity/data/adult.html. Accessed April 20, 2015.

55. Ogden CL, Carroll MD, Kit BK, Flegal KM. Prevalence of obesity and trends in body mass index among US children and adolescents, 1999–2010. *JAMA.* 2012;307(5):483–490. Available online: http://jama.ama-assn.org/content/307/5/483.

56. Centers for Disease Control and Prevention (CDC) website. 2011–2012. Data and Statistics page. Available at: http://www.cdc.gov/obesity/data/childhood.html. Accessed April 20, 2015.

57. Wareham NJ, van Sluijs EM, Ekelund U. Physical activity and obesity prevention: A review of the current evidence. *Proc Nutr Soc.* 2005;64:229–247.

58. World Health Organization website. 2014 Physical activity page. Available at: http://www.who.int/topics/physical_activity/en/. Accessed April 20, 2015.

59. Petersen L, Schnohr P, Sorensen TI. Longitudinal study of the long-term relation between physical activity and obesity in adults. *Int J Obes Relat Metab Disord.* 2004;28:105–112.

60. Golubic R, Ekelund U, Wijndaele K et al. Rate of weight gain predicts change in physical activity levels: A longitudinal analysis of the EPIC-Norfolk cohort. *Int J Obes.* 2013;37:404–409.

61. Ekelund U, Besson H, Luan J et al. Physical activity and gain in abdominal adiposity and body weight: Prospective cohort study in 288,498 men and women. *Am J Clin Nutr.* 2011;93:826–835.

62. Shaw KA, Gennat HC, O'Rourke P et al. Exercise for overweight or obesity. *Cochrane Database Syst Rev.* 2006;(4):Art No. CD003817.

63. Watson R, Benelam B. Physical activity: The latest on its contribution to energy balance and health. *Nutr Bull.* 2012;37:78–85.

64. Broom DR, Batterham RL, King JA et al. Influence of resistance and aerobic exercise on hunger, circulating levels of acylated ghrelin and peptide YY in healthy males. *Am J Physiol.* 2009;296:R29–R35.

65. Sim AY, Wallman KE, Fairchild TJ et al. High intensity intermittent exercise attenuates ad-libitum energy intake. *Int J Obes.* 2014;38:417–422.

66. Levine J, Lanningham-Foster LM, McCrady SK et al. Interindividual variation in posture allocation: Possible role in human obesity. *Science.* 2005;307:584–586.

67. Zisser H, Sueyoshi M, Krigstein K et al. Advances in exercise, physical activity and diabetes mellitus. *Int J Clin Pract.* 2012;66(Suppl. 175):62–71.

68. Nagi D. Gallen I. ABCD position statement on physical activity and exercise in diabetes. *Pract Diab.* 2010;27(4):158–163.

69. Giannini C, de Giorgis T, Mohn A et al. Role of physical exercise in children and adolescents with diabetes mellitus. *J Pediatr Endocrinol Metab.* 2007;20:173–184.

70. Lipman TH, Hayman LL, Fabian CV et al. Risk factors for cardiovascular disease in children with type I diabetes. *Nurs Res.* 2000;49:160–166.

71. Ruzic L, Sporis G, Matkovic BR. High volume-low intensity exercise camp and glycemic control in diabetic children. *J Pediatr Child Health.* 2008;44(3):122–128.

72. Sackey AH, Jefferson IG. Physical activity and glycemic control in children with diabetes mellitus. *J Brit Diab Assoc.* 1996;13(9):789–793.

73. Senemmari B. Combating the diabetes epidemic. *Caring.* 2005;24(6):6–12.

74. National Diabetes Information Clearinghouse (NDIC). National diabetes statistics, National Institute of Diabetes and Digestive and Kidney Disease, National Institute of Health, 2011. Available at: http://www.diabetes.niddk.nih.gov/dm/pubs/statistics/#fast. Accessed January 20, 2014.

75. van Dam RM. The epidemiology of lifestyle and risk for type 2 diabetes. *Eur J Epidemiol.* 2003;18:1115–1125.

76. Boule NG, Haddad E, Kenny GP et al. Effects of exercise on glycemic control and body mass in type 2 diabetes mellitus. A meta-analysis of controlled clinical trials. *JAMA.* 2001;286:1218–1227.

77. Gillies CL, Abrams KR, Lambert PC et al. Pharmacological and lifestyle interventions to prevent or delay type 2 diabetes in people with impaired glucose tolerance: Systematic review and meta-analysis. *BMJ.* 2007;334:299–313.

78. Gill JM, Cooper A. Physical activity and prevention of type 2 diabetes mellitus. *Sports Med.* 2008;38:807–824.

79. Hamman RF, Wing RR, Edelstein SL et al. Effect of weight loss with lifestyle intervention on risk of diabetes. *Diabetes Care.* 2006;29:2102–2107.

80. Pan XR, Li GW, Hu YH et al. Effects of diet and exercise in preventing NIDDM in people with impaired glucose tolerance: The Da Qing IGT and Diabetes Study. *Diabetes Care.* 2002;20:537–544.

81. Waryasz GR, McDermott AY. Exercise prescription and the patient with type 2 diabetes: A clinical approach to optimizing patient outcomes. *J Am Acad Nurse Pract.* 2010;22:217–227.

82. Avery L, Flynn D, van Wersch A et al. Changing physical activity behavior in type 2 diabetes. *Diabetes Care.* 2012;35:2681–2689.

83. Deshpande AD, Dodson EA, Gorman I et al. Physical activity and diabetes: Opportunities for prevention through policy. *Phys Ther.* 88(11):1425–1435.

84. Knowler WC, Fowler SE, Hamman RF et al. Diabetes Prevention Research Group. 10-year follow-up of diabetes incidence and weight loss in the Diabetes Prevention Program Outcomes Study. *Lancet.* 2009;374(9702):1677–1686.

85. Tompkins C, Soros A, Sothern MS et al. Effects of physical activity on diabetes management and lowering risk for type 2 diabetes. *J Health Educ.* 2009;40(5):86–290.

86. Grontved A, Pan A, Mekary RA et al. Muscle-strengthening and conditioning activities and risk of type 2 diabetes: A prospective study in two cohorts of US women. *PLoS Med.* 2014;11(1):1–15.

87. Carlson SA, Fulton JE, Schoenborn CA et al. Trend and prevalence estimates based on the 2008 Physical Activity Guidelines for Americans. *Am J Prev Med.* 2010;39:305–313.

88. Hagberg JM. Exercise, fitness and hypertension. In *Exercise, Fitness and Health: A Consensus of Current Knowledge.* Bouchard C, Shephard RJ, Thomas Stephens T et al. (eds.). Champaign, IL: Human Kinetics Books, 1990.

89. Reimers, CD, Knapp G, Reimers AK. Exercise as stroke prophylaxis. *Deutsches Ärzteblatt Int.* 2009;106:715–721.

90. Leung FP, Yun LM, Laher I, Yao X, Chen ZY, Huang Y. Exercise, vascular wall and cardiovascular diseases: An update (part 1). *Sports Med.* 2012;38:1009–1024.

91. Yung LM, Laher I, Yao X, Chen ZY, Huang Y, Leung FP. Exercise, vascular wall and cardiovascular diseases: An update (part 2). *Sports Med.* 2009;39:45–63.

92. Wendel-Vos GC, Schuit AJ, Feskens EJ et al. Physical activity and stroke. A meta-analysis of observational data. *Int J Epidemiol.* 2004;33:787–798.

93. Diep L, Kwagyan J, Kurantsin-Mills J et al. Association of physical activity level and stroke outcomes in men and women: A meta-analysis. *J Women's Health.* 2010;19(10):1815–1822.

94. Huerta JM, Chirlaque MD, Tormo MJ et al. Physical activity and risk of cerebrovascular disease in the European Prospective Investigation into Cancer and Nutrition—Spain Study. *Stroke.* 2013;44:111–118.

95. Shaffer EA. Epidemiology of gallbladder stone disease. *Best Pract Res Clin Gastroenterol.* 2006;20(6):981–196.

96. National Digestive Diseases Information Clearinghouse (NDDIC). Gallstone fact sheet. NIH Publication No. 07-2897, 2010. Available at: http://digestive.niddk.nih.gov/ddiseases/pubs/gallstones/index.aspx#3. Accessed July 2, 2013.

97. Utter AC, Goss FL. Exercise and gallbladder function. *Sports Med.* 1997;23:218–227.

98. Utter AC, Goss FL, Whitcomb DC et al. The effects of acute exercise on gallbladder function in an adult female population. *Med Sci Sports Exerc.* 1996;28:280–284.

99. Kato I, Nomura A, Stemmerman GN et al. Prospective study of clinical gallbladder disease and its association with obesity, physical activity, and other factors. *Dig Dis Sci.* 1992;37:784–790.

100. Leitzmann MF, Giovannucci E, Rimm EB et al. The relation of physical activity to risk of symptomatic gallstone disease in men. *Ann Int Med.* 1998;128:417–425.

101. Leitzmann MF, Rimm EB, Willett WC et al. Recreational physical activity and the risk of cholecystectomy in women. *N Engl J Med.* 1999;341:777–784.

102. Storti KL, Brach JS, FitzGerald SJ et al. Physical activity and decreased risk of clinical gallstone disease among post-menopausal women. *Prev Med.* 2005;41:772–777.

103. Pasco JA, Jacka FN, Williams LJ et al. Don't worry, be active: Positive affect and habitual physical activity. *Aust N Z J Psychiatr.* 2011;45:1047–1052.

104. Cripps F. Exercise your mind: Physical activity as a therapeutic technique for depression. *Int J Ther Rehabil.* 2008;15(10):460–465.

105. Stedmen TL. *Stedman's Medical Dictionary for the Health Professions and Nursing*, 7th edn. Philadelphia, PA: Wolters Kluwer Health/LWW, 2012.

106. Eriksson S, Gard G. Physical exercise and depression. *Phys Ther Rev.* 2011;16(4):261–268.

107. World Health Organization. October 2012. Depression fact sheet. Available from: http://www.who.int/mediacentre/factsheets/fs369/en/. Accessed April 20, 2015.

108. Stathopoulou G, Powers MB, Berry AC et al. Exercise interventions for mental health: A quantitative and qualitative review. *Clin Psychol Sci Pract.* 2006;13:179–193.

109. Biddle SH, Fox KR, Boutcher SH (eds.). *Physical Activity and Psychological Well-Being.* New York: Routledge 2010.

110. Lotan M, Merrick J, Carmeli E. A review of physical activity and well-being. *Int J Adolesc Med Health.* 2005;17:23–31.

111. Miles L. Physical activity and health. *Nutr Bull.* 2007;32:31–363.

112. Biddle SH, Gorely T, Stensel DJ. Health-enhancing physical activity and sedentary behaviour in children and adolescents. *J Sports Sci.* 2004;22:679–701.

113. Korniloff K, Vanhala M, Kautiainen H et al. Lifetime leisure-time physical activity and the risk of depressive symptoms at the ages of 65–74 years: The FIN-D2D survey. *Prevent Med.* 2012;54:313–315.

114. Teychenne M, Ball K, Salmon J. Sedentary behavior and depression among adults: A review. *Int J Behav Med.* 2010;17:246–254.

115. Taliaferro LA, Rienzo BA, Pigg M et al. Associations between physical activity and reduced rates of hopelessness, depression, and suicidal behavior among college students. *J Am College Health.* 2008;57(4):427–435.
116. Warren E. Prescribing in depression. *Practice Nurse.* 2011;41(20):26–30.
117. Smeaton J. Physical exercise and mental health. *Psychiatr Practice.* 1995;14(3):16–18.
118. Dunn DL, Madhukar H, Trivedi MD et al. Exercise treatment for depression—Efficacy and dose response. *Am J Prev Med.* 2005;28:1–8.
119. Singh NA, Stavrinos TM, Scarbek Y et al. A randomized controlled trial of high versus low intensity weight training versus general practitioner care for clinical depression in older adults. *J Gerontol A Biol Sci Med Sci.* 2005;60:768–776.
120. Alzheimer's Association. 2012. Alzheimer's disease facts and figures. *Alzheimers Dement.* 2012;8(2):4. Available at: http://www.alz.org/downloads/facts_figures_2012.pdf. Accessed April 20, 2015.
121. Egan BA, Mentes JC. Benefits of physical activity for knee osteoarthritis. *J Gerontol Nurs.* 2010;36(9):9–14.
122. Goldring SR, Goldring MB. Clinical aspects, pathology and pathophysiology of osteoarthritis. *J Musculoskel Neuronal Interact.* 2006;6:376–378.
123. Arthritis Foundation. Osteoarthritis fact sheet. Retrieved from http://www.arthritis.org/files/images/newsroom/media-kits/Osteoarthritis_fact_sheet.pdf. Accessed July 24, 2013.
124. Buford TW, Anton SD, Clark DJ, Higgins TJ, Cooke MB. Optimizing the benefits of exercise on physical functioning in older adults. *PM&R.* 2014(6);528–543.
125. Brach JS, Simonsick EM, Kritchevsky S, Yaffe K, Newman AM. The association between physical function and lifestyle activity and exercise in the Health, Aging and Body Composition study. *J Am Geriatr Soc.* 2004;54(4):502–509.
126. Ding C, Jones G, Wluka A et al. What can we learn about osteoarthritis by studying people from the healthy to those with early disease? *Curr Opin Rheumatol.* 2010;22(5):520–527.
127. Hootman JM, Macera CA, Ham SA et al. Physical activity levels among the general US adult population and in adults with and without arthritis. *Arthritis Rheum.* 2003;49:129–135.
128. Racunica TL, Teichtahl AJ, Wang Y et al. Effect of physical activity on articular knee joint structures in community based adults. *Arthritis Rheum.* 2007;57:1261–1268.
129. Lin CW, Taylor D, Bierma-Zeinstra SM, Maher CG. Exercise for osteoarthritis of the knee. *Phys Ther.* 2010;90:839–842.
130. Samitz G, Egger M, Zwahlen M. Domains of physical activity and all-cause mortality: Systematic review and dose–response meta-analysis of cohort studies. *Int J Epidemiol.* 2011;40:1382–1400.

Index

A

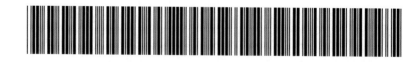